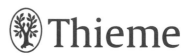

PET and PET/CT

A Clinical Guide

Third Edition

Eugene C. Lin, MD
Diagnostic and Nuclear Radiologist
Virginia Mason Medical Center
Seattle, Washington

Abass Alavi, MD, PhD
Professor and Director of Research Education
Department of Radiology
Perelman School of Medicine
University of Pennsylvania
Philadelphia, Pennsylvania

335 illustrations

Thieme
New York • Stuttgart • Delhi • Rio de Janeiro

Executive Editor: William Lamsback
Managing Editor: Nikole Y. Connors
Director, Editorial Services: Mary Jo Casey
Production Editor: Naamah Schwartz
International Production Director: Andreas Schabert
Editorial Director: Sue Hodgson
International Marketing Director: Fiona Henderson
International Sales Director: Louisa Turrell
Director of Institutional Sales: Adam Bernacki
Senior Vice President and Chief Operating Officer:
  Sarah Vanderbilt
President: Brian D. Scanlan

Library of Congress Cataloging-in-Publication Data
Names: Lin, Eugene, editor. | Alavi, Abass, editor.
Title: PET and PET/CT : a clinical guide / [edited by]
  Eugene C. Lin, MD, Clinical Assistant Professor of Radiology,
  Department of Radiology, Virginia Mason Medical Center, Uni-
  versity of Washington, Seattle, Washington, USA, Abass Alavi,
  MD, MD(Hon), PhD(Hon), DSc(Hon), Professor of Radiology and
  Neurology, Director of Research Education, Department of Radi-
  ology, Hospital of the University of Pennsylvania, Philadelphia,
  Pennsylvania, USA.
Description: Third edition. | New York : Thieme, [2019] |
  Revision of: PET and PET/CT / Eugene Lin, Abass Alavi. c2005. |
  Includes bibliographical references and index. |
Identifiers: LCCN 2018046986 (print) | LCCN 2018047117
  (ebook) | ISBN 9781626231351 (e-book) | ISBN
  9781626231344 (print : alk. paper)
Subjects: LCSH: Tomography, Emission.
Classification: LCC RC78.7.T62 (ebook) | LCC RC78.7.T62 L56
  2019 (print) | DDC 616.07/575--dc23
LC record available at https://lccn.loc.gov/2018046986

© 2019 Thieme Medical Publishers, Inc.

Thieme Publishers New York
333 Seventh Avenue, New York, NY 10001 USA
+1 800 782 3488, customerservice@thieme.com

Thieme Publishers Stuttgart
Rüdigerstrasse 14, 70469 Stuttgart, Germany
+49 [0]711 8931 421, customerservice@thieme.de

Thieme Publishers Delhi
A-12, Second Floor, Sector-2, Noida-201301
Uttar Pradesh, India
+91 120 45 566 00, customerservice@thieme.in

Thieme Publishers Rio de Janeiro, Thieme Publicações Ltda.
Edifício Rodolpho de Paoli, 25º andar
Av. Nilo Peçanha, 50 – Sala 2508
Rio de Janeiro 20020-906 Brasil
+55 21 3172-2297 / +55 21 3172-1896
www.thiemerevinter.com.br

Cover design: Thieme Publishing Group
Typesetting by Thomson Digital, India

Printed in Germany
by Beltz Grafische Betriebe   5 4

ISBN 978-1-62623-134-4

Also available as an e-book:
eISBN 978-1-62623-135-1

Important note: Medicine is an ever-changing science undergoing continual development. Research and clinical experience are continually expanding our knowledge, in particular our knowledge of proper treatment and drug therapy. Insofar as this book mentions any dosage or application, readers may rest assured that the authors, editors, and publishers have made every effort to ensure that such references are in accordance with **the state of knowledge at the time of production of the book.**

Nevertheless, this does not involve, imply, or express any guarantee or responsibility on the part of the publishers in respect to any dosage instructions and forms of applications stated in the book. **Every user is requested to examine carefully** the manufacturers' leaflets accompanying each drug and to check, if necessary in consultation with a physician or specialist, whether the dosage schedules mentioned therein or the contraindications stated by the manufacturers differ from the statements made in the present book. Such examination is particularly important with drugs that are either rarely used or have been newly released on the market. Every dosage schedule or every form of application used is entirely at the user's own risk and responsibility. The authors and publishers request every user to report to the publishers any discrepancies or inaccuracies noticed. If errors in this work are found after publication, errata will be posted at www.thieme. com on the product description page.

Some of the product names, patents, and registered designs referred to in this book are in fact registered trademarks or proprietary names even though specific reference to this fact is not always made in the text. Therefore, the appearance of a name without designation as proprietary is not to be construed as a representation by the publisher that it is in the public domain.

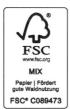

FSC
www.fsc.org
MIX
Papier | Fördert
gute Waldnutzung
FSC® C089473

I would like to thank my colleagues at Virginia Mason Medical Center for providing
an environment which allowed me to write this book and Drs. Marie Lee and Paul Sicuro
for help in obtaining many of the images in this book. My parents instilled in me a love of
learning and working with residents and fellows throughout my career has
inspired me to continually seek out new knowledge.

Eugene C. Lin

I wish to dedicate this book to my mother Fatemeh and my wife Jane for sacrifices
they have made to make my life most rewarding; I cannot thank them enough
for their enormous encouragements all along.

Abass Alavi

Contents

Preface.. xi

Contributors xiii

Part I Basic Science

1 The Physics of PET/CT Scanners 2
Ruth E. Schmitz, Adam M. Alessio, and Paul E. Kinahan

2 The Basics of 2-[F-18]Fluoro-2-deoxy-D-glucose Radiochemistry and Biology 12
N. Scott Mason and Eugene C. Lin

3 The Role of Glucose and FDG Metabolism in the Interpretation of PET Studies.. 18
Ronald L. Korn, Melissa Singer Pressman, and John Millstine

Part II Clinical Basics

4 Patient Preparation 28
Eugene C. Lin

5 Standardized Uptake Value.. 36
Eugene C. Lin and Paul E. Kinahan

6 Quantitative Whole-Body PET/CT Imaging............................. 42
Sina Houshmand, Ali Salavati, Abass Alavi, and Habib Zaidi

7 Normal Variants and Benign Findings 51
Eugene C. Lin

8 Interpretation of FDG PET Studies 89
Eugene C. Lin

9 PET/CT 98
Eugene C. Lin and Paul E. Kinahan

10 PET/MRI: Introduction to Clinical Applications 109
Ali Salavati, Sina Houshmand, Cory Daignault, Abass Alavi, and Drew Torigian

Part III Oncologic Applications

11 Oncological PET by Anatomic Region................................. 128
Eugene C. Lin

12 Therapy Response.. 142
Sandip Basu and Eugene C. Lin

13 Brain Neoplasms 150
Eugene C. Lin

14 Head and Neck Cancer.. 157
Eugene C. Lin

15 Thyroid Cancer 169
Eugene C. Lin

16 Thoracic Neoplasms.. 177
Eugene C. Lin

17 Breast Cancer 195
Eugene C. Lin

18 Gastric, Esophageal, and Gastrointestinal Stromal Tumors 208
Eugene C. Lin

19 Lymphoma.. 220
Eugene C. Lin

20 Melanoma 232
Eugene C. Lin

21 Hepatobiliary Tumors.. 238
Eugene C. Lin

22 Pancreatic Cancer 245
Eugene C. Lin

23 Gynecological Tumors 253
Eugene C. Lin

24 Urological Tumors... 264
Eugene C. Lin and Evan Sirc

25 Colorectal Cancer 280
Eugene C. Lin

26 Musculoskeletal Tumors.. 291
Eugene C. Lin

27 ^{18}F Sodium Fluoride PET/CT in Bone................................... 303
Alireza Rezaee, Poul Høilund-Carlsen, Søren Hess, Werner Langsteger, and Mohsen Beheshti

28   **^{68}Ga-Based Imaging Techniques**   311
Paolo Castellucci, Cristina Nanni, and Valentina Ambrosini

Part IV Nononcologic Applications

29   **Pediatric PET/CT**   324
M. Beth McCarville

30   **PET/CT in Radiation Therapy Planning**   331
Sandip Basu and Guobin Song

31   **FDG-PET/CT in the Evaluation of Infection and Inflammation**   338
Sandip Basu, Abass Alavi, and Eugene C. Lin

32   **Neurological Applications of Fluorodeoxyglucose PET**   352
Eugene C. Lin

33   **Neurological Applications of Nonfluorodeoxyglucose Tracers**   360
Mohsen Khosravi, Andrew B. Newberg, and Abass Alavi

34   **Cardiac PET and PET/CT**   372
Amol Takalkar, Umesh Sharma, and Eugene C. Lin

        Index   387

Preface

The discovery of X-rays by Roentgen in 1895 began a true revolution in medicine which accelerated its pace over the past 5 decades. The invention of the scintillation camera by Anger in the 1960s led to the establishment of the field of nuclear medicine as a specialty in medical imaging. Planar images generated by this approach suffered from suboptimal contrast between the abnormal sites and the background activity. The concept of radiotracer-based tomography became a reality when David Kuhl at the University of Pennsylvania (Penn) designed and built several instruments in the '60s and '70s. In 1971, Hounsfield performed the first x-ray-based tomographic images (XCT) of the brain, which revolutionized the field. The CT technology has been improved substantially over the years and modern tomographic instruments can scan the entire body with high resolution and great speed to improve the sensitivity and specificity of XCT.

Initial radiotracer-based tomographic scans were acquired by designing specialized instruments that focused on imaging brain disorders. The concept of tomographic imaging by Anger camera was introduced by investigators at the University of Michigan and Berkeley, which led to initiation of emission tomography as a powerful modality in medicine. Over the past 3 decades, single photon emission computed tomography (SPECT) has been the main modality in the specialty worldwide. Unfortunately, this technology has suffered due to the lack of progress in synthesizing novel tracers for research and clinical purposes. This has impeded its application in various metabolic disorders.

This frustration led investigators at Penn to explore the possibility of labeling positron emitting radionuclides to novel compounds to assess disease activity in different organs at the molecular level. This major effort eventually resulted in synthesizing 18F-fluorodeoxyglucose (FDG) and administering this preparation to two human beings in 1976. In parallel with these developments, over the years, instrumentation for imaging positron emitters has been improved by investigators at Washington University led by Ter-Pogossian and other scientists in the field.

Research and clinical applications of FDG and other PET tracers along with advances in PET instrumentation have enormously strengthened the field of molecular imaging in medicine.

Development of PET/CT by investigators at the University of Pittsburgh in the late 1990s resulted in a paradigm shift in medical imaging. This novel technology allows co-registration of structural images provided by CT and molecular images by PET for both research and clinical purposes. These advances have rejuvenated the field of molecular imaging with PET. Since 2001 when the first commercial PET/CT instruments were introduced to medicine, PET/CT has become the workhorse of modern nuclear medicine laboratories. Currently, the main compound used for PET/CT imaging is FDG and it is used primarily for managing patients with cancer. During the past decade, PET/MRI has opened up a new domain for molecular imaging and its role as a powerful imaging modality is being explored at this time. It is expected that this technique will play a major role in three fields: disorders of the brain, cardiovascular system and musculoskeletal (MSK) structures. The main challenge for PET/MRI is suboptimal attenuation correction of gamma rays emitted from deep structures in the body and therefore optimal quantification of tracer concentrations in normal and disease sites.

By employing these imaging modalities during the past century, we have realized that structural imaging is quite insensitive in detecting most diseases in their early stages and also in assessing response following therapeutic interventions. To overcome these shortcomings, attempts have been made to measure certain physiologic parameters through the available imaging techniques. Specifically, measurement of blood flow to the brain and the heart has been extensively explored over the past 5 decades. Cerebral blood flow measurement was primarily used for research purposes, and therefore, its clinical significance has been somewhat uncertain. In contrast, imaging of coronary artery perfusion as a means to detect atherosclerosis has become a powerful functional imaging approach in cardiology since the 1980s. Currently, perfusion imaging with technetium labeled preparations is the most common imaging methodology employed for detection of coronary artery disease. This methodology is based on imaging with SPECT, which is widely available. Recently, perfusion imaging with PET has gained some acceptance because of the availability of the rubidium generators, and this provides high resolution images of cardiac blood flow within a short period of time. Furthermore, radiation exposure from this approach is substantially lower than that of SPECT.

Based on experience gained with various imaging techniques, it has become quite evident that changes that occur in the molecular level precede those of either physiological or structural alterations due to normal aging or pathologic states. In particular, since the introduction of FDG-PET in the late 1970s, we have realized the critical role that molecular imaging can play in assessing almost every disease and disorder due to its extraordinary sensitivity. Since molecular changes occur far in advance of structural alterations, early interventions can be employed before advanced stages of the disease, and therefore lead to successful outcome. In other words, the sensitivity of molecular imaging with PET far exceeds that of conventional as well as advanced structural imaging techniques.

PET imaging allows accurate quantification of disease activity in various stages and levels. Not only can PET provide quantitative assessment at the regional level, but it also can provide global disease measurement throughout the body by recently introduced methodologies. This is unique to this modality compared to other imaging techniques, which are primarily used as qualitative modalities. This further enhances PET-based imaging as the modality of choice for following the course of the disease.

Based on experience gained, we believe that PET/CT and PET/MRI will become the modalities of choice for examining many human maladies and will rapidly expand to the daily practice of medicine worldwide. The role of pure structural imaging such as CT and MRI may become limited to interventions that require precise structural definition of the disease sites for radiotherapy or surgical interventions. Otherwise, combination of PET with these structural modalities will increasingly become the main instruments for diagnosis and monitoring both benign and malignant disorders.

Eugene C. Lin
Abass Alavi

Contributors

Abass Alavi, MD, PhD
Professor and Director of Research Education
Department of Radiology
Perelman School of Medicine
University of Pennsylvania
Philadelphia, Pennsylvania

Adam M. Alessio, PhD
Research Assistant
Department of Radiology
University of Washington
Seattle, Washington

Valentina Ambrosini, MD
Associate Professor
Department of Specialized, Diagnostic and
    Experimental Medicine
University of Bologna
Bologna, Italy

Sandip Basu, MBBS(Hons), DRM, DNB, MNAMS
Head, Nuclear Medicine Academic Programme
Department of Radiation Medicine Centre
Bombay, India

Mohsen Beheshti, MD, FASNC, FEBNM
Head, PET-CT Center LINZ
Professor in Nuclear Medicine
Ordensklinikum Linz
Department of Nuclear Medicine and Endocrinology
St. Vincent's Hospital
Linz, Austria

Paolo Castellucci, MD
Service of Nuclear Medicine
S. Orsola-Malpighi University Hospital
University of Bologna
Bologna, Italy

Cory Daignault, MD
Minneapolis VA Medical Center
Nuclear Radiologist
St. Paul, Minneapolis

Søren Hess, MD
Senior Consultant, Clinical Associate Professor
Department of Radiology
Head of Section (Nuclear Medicine)
Hospital Southwest Jutland
Esbjerg, Denmark

Poul Høilund-Carlsen, MD, DMSci, Prof (Hon)
Professor, Head of Research & International
    Relations
Department of Nuclear Medicine
Odense University Hospital
Department of Clinical Research
University of Southern Denmark
Odense, Denmark

Sina Houshmand, MD
Resident
Department of Radiology
University of Pittsburgh
Pittsburgh, Pennsylvania

Mohsen Khosravi, MD
Postdoctoral Research Fellow
Marcus Institute of Integrative Health
Thomas Jefferson University
Philadelphia, Pennsylvania

Paul E. Kinahan, PhD
Associate Professor of Radiology, Bioengineering,
    and Electrical Engineering
Director of PET/CT Physics
Department of Radiology
University of Washington
Seattle, Washington

Ronald L. Korn, MD, PhD
Chairman, CMO and Founder
Imaging Endpoints Core Lab
Scottsdale, Arizona

Werner Langsteger, MD
PET-CT Center Linz
Department of Nuclear Medicine and Endocrinology
Ordensklinikum, St. Vincent's Hospital
Linz, Austria

Eugene C. Lin, MD
Diagnostic and Nuclear Radiologist
Virginia Mason Medical Center
Seattle, Washington

N. Scott Mason, PhD
Research Assistant, Professor of Radiology
Department of Radiology
University of Pittsburgh
Pittsburgh, Pennsylvania

M. Beth McCarville, MD
Associate Member
Division of Diagnostic Imaging
Department of Radiological Sciences
St. Jude Children's Research Hospital
Memphis, Tennessee

John Millstine, MD
Director of Clinical Nuclear Medicine
Department of Radiology and Nuclear Medicine
Scottsdale Medical Imaging Ltd.
Scottsdale, Arizona

Cristina Nanni, MD
Adjunct Professor
Institute of Nuclear Medicine
University of Bologna
Bologna, Italy

Andrew B. Newberg, MD
Professor and Director of Research
Marcus Institute of Integrative Health
Thomas Jefferson University and Hospital
Philadelphia, Pennsylvania

Alireza Rezaee, MD
PET-CT Center LINZ
St. Vincent's Hospital
Linz, Austria

Ali Salavati, MD, MPH
Postdoctoral Research Fellow
Quantitative Medical Imaging Lab
University of Pennsylvania
Philadelphia, Pennsylvania

Ruth E. Schmitz, PhD
Senior Fellow
Department of Radiology
University of Washington
Seattle, Washington

Umesh Sharma, MD, PhD
Division of Cardiovascular Medicine
Department of Medicine
Clinical and Translational Research Center
University at Buffalo
Buffalo, New York

Melissa Singer Pressman, PhD
Chief Clinical Research Officer
Scottsdale Medical Imaging Research Institute
Master Methodologist
Grand Canyon University
Associate Professor of Research
University of Arizona, College of Medicine
Scottsdale, Arizona

Evan Sirc, MD
Radiologist
Bay Imaging Consultants
Walnut Creek, California

Guobin Song, MD, PhD
Department of Radiation Oncology
Virginia Mason Medical Center
Seattle, Washington

Amol Takalkar, MD
Assistant Professor of Clinical Radiology
Department of Radiology
Louisiana State University
Associate Medical Director
PET Imaging Center
Biomedical Research Foundation of Northwest
    Louisiana
Shreveport, Louisiana

Drew Torigian, MD, MA, FSAR, FACR
Clinical Director, Medical Image Processing
    Group (MIPG)
Professor of Radiology
University of Pennsylvania School of Medicine
Philadelphia, Pennsylvania

Habib Zaidi, MD
Head of PET Instrumentation and Neuroimaging
    Laboratory
Geneva University Hospital
Geneva, Switzerland

Part I

Basic Science

1 The Physics of PET/CT
   Scanners   *2*

2 The Basics of 2-[F-18]Fluoro-2-
   deoxy-D-glucose
   Radiochemistry and Biology   *12*

3 The Role of Glucose and FDG
   Metabolism in the
   Interpretation of PET Studies   *18*

I

1 The Physics of PET/CT Scanners

Ruth E. Schmitz, Adam M. Alessio, and Paul E. Kinahan

1.1 What Makes PET Useful?

Positron emission tomography (PET) offers several unique advantages compared with other imaging modalities. PET measures the two annihilation photons that are produced back-to-back after positron emission from a radionuclide-tagged tracer molecule, which is chosen to mark a specific function in the body on a biochemical level (▶ Fig. 1.1). Hence, PET provides molecular imaging of biological function instead of anatomy. The detection of both annihilation photons in coincidence, providing inherent collimation, yields increased sensitivity over single-photon imaging. Furthermore, PET allows for accurate attenuation correction (AC) either from a dedicated transmission scan or from computed tomography (CT) images with combined PET/CT scanners. Accurate correction for attenuation (and scatter, etc.) allows extraction of accurate quantitative as well as qualitative information from PET images. Only minute amounts of radiolabeled tracer need to be injected because of the high sensitivity of PET. In addition, positron emitters (^{11}C, ^{13}N, ^{15}O, ^{18}F, etc.) are relatively short-lived, which enables optimal use of imaging photons while keeping patient radiation dose low. Furthermore, many of these isotopes can be incorporated into biological substrates (glucose, H_2O, NH_3, CO_2, O_2, etc.) and pharmaceuticals, without altering their biological activity.

Compared with CT scans and magnetic resonance imaging (MRI), PET images generally appear much blurrier or noisier, due to the relatively limited number of photons that can be collected during an imaging study. In addition, detector spatial resolution is poorer due to the detector physics. X-ray CT scanners can easily resolve points less than 1 mm in size, whereas PET scanners cannot reliably resolve the size of point sources less than 4 to 5 mm at best, and closer to 10 mm in practice. However, this does not impair their high sensitivity to focal tracer concentrations or their usefulness in accurate quantitative functional imaging.

In this chapter, we introduce the physics of PET imaging. Several textbooks provide a more in-depth treatment and are included in the References section.[1,2,3]

1.2 Radioactive Decay

1.2.1 General Principles

Radioactive isotopes are atoms whose inner core, their nucleus, is unstable, in a state with too much energy. Nuclei consist of a densely packed arrangement of protons and neutrons. By undergoing decay, the nuclei change their composition and properties to arrive in a less energetic and more stable state.

The decay process follows an exponential law: the number of decays per second is always proportional to the number of undecayed nuclei present. The rate of decay is level of radioactivity, also called activity, which is determined by the half-life of the particular nuclide—the time it takes for half of the original nuclei to decay. The most common isotope in PET is fluorine 18 (^{18}F), which has a half-life of 109 minutes. After some time, t, the activity left, $A(t)$, is proportional to the initial number, $A(0)$, and an exponential term involving the half-life, τ, of the nuclide:

$$A(t) = A(0)e^{-t(\ln 2/\tau)}$$

Radioactive rates (or activity) are measured in units of becquerel (1 Bq = 1 decay/s) in the International System of Units (SI) or the traditional curie (1 Ci = 3.7×10^{10} decay/s). A common scale factor used in the clinic is 1 mCi = 37 MBq.

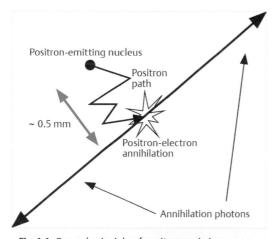

Fig. 1.1 General principle of positron emission tomography imaging: decay of radionuclide, positron (β⁺) emission, multiple scatter in tissue, annihilation with electron, and production of two back-to-back 511-keV annihilation photons. (Not to scale.)

Positron-emitting nucleus

Positron path

~ 0.5 mm

Positron-electron annihilation

Annihilation photons

1.2.2 Positron Emission and Annihilation

In β^+ (positron) decay (▶ Fig. 1.1), a nuclide transforms one of its core protons (p) into a neutron (n) and emits a positron (β^+), essentially a positively charged electron, and a neutrino (v): $p \rightarrow n + \beta^+ + v$. The average positron range in matter depends on the positron's energy and material characteristics, such as the density and the atomic number. For [fluorine 18]fluorodeoxyglucose ([^{18}F]FDG), positron ranges are rather short, typically less than 1 mm.

At the end of its path, the positron, being antimatter to electrons, will annihilate (recombine) with an atomic electron. In the annihilation, electron and positron convert their mass into energy and produce a pair of 511-keV annihilation photons traveling in opposite directions. The 511-keV photon energy (E) comes from Einstein's famous equation $E = mc^2$, where m is the mass of the electron or positron (a very small number) and c is the speed of light (a very large number, which is then squared). This annihilation radiation is what is detected in PET and what is used to form images of tracer concentration in the body.

1.2.3 Interaction of Photons with Matter

The dominant annihilation photon interaction in human tissue is *Compton scatter.* The photon interacts with an electron, ejecting it from its atomic shell. The photon experiences a loss of energy and an associated change of direction, typically out of the active detector range, and so is unavailable for image formation.

Compton scatter and other interactions lead to an attenuation of the annihilation photons along a straight line. In other words, the number of photons that are observed in a straight line from where they were produced decreases exponentially with increasing length of the material traversed. The thickness of soft tissue required to reduce the intensity of a 511-keV photon beam by one-half is approximately 7 cm, as opposed to 3 to 4 cm for lower energy X-rays. Thus, for approximately 14 cm of soft tissue, the 511-keV annihilation photon flux would be reduced to one-fourth of its original intensity; through the abdomen, the photon flux can be reduced to 1/50 of its original intensity. Thus, attenuation is often the dominant factor in PET image quality, especially for thicker patients.

1.3 Data Acquisition

1.3.1 Photon Detection and Scintillation Detectors

The general goal of photon detection is to measure the total energy deposited by the photon when it traverses the detector. For highest sensitivity and accuracy, all of the photon's energy should be deposited, but in practice this is not always possible.

In most PET scanners today, scintillation detectors are used as detection elements. They couple inorganic scintillation crystals that emit visible or near-ultraviolet light after interaction with an incident high-energy (511 keV) photon to photo detectors that detect and measure the scintillation photons.

In scintillation crystals, the incident annihilation photon (nominally 511,000-eV energy) interacts and creates tens of thousands of visible wavelength photons (~1-eV energy each) in a very short flash, or "scintillation." The number of scintillation photons produced in the crystal is proportional to the energy deposited by the annihilation photon.

Scintillators for PET photon detection can be rated on four of their characteristic properties:

1. The *stopping power* is the inverse of the mean distance traveled by photons before they deposit energy in the crystal. This length depends on density and effective atomic number (Z) of the material. A short travel distance is favorable because it will yield more interactions with the 511-keV photons and a better efficiency for detecting them in crystal of fixed size.

2. The *decay constant* describes how long the scintillation flash lasts in the crystal. Shorter decay constants are desirable because they allow for counting higher photon rates and lower background rates.

3. Good *energy resolution*—a small ratio of energy variance over energy—means that there are only small fluctuations in the energy measurement. This gives a means to distinguish against PET photons that have Compton scattered (and lost energy) before being measured. The energy resolution depends on the light output and the intrinsic energy resolution of the crystal.

4. The *light output*, as the name indicates, is the number of scintillation photons produced by each incident photon. Again, this should be as high as possible, allowing the best spatial and energy resolution.

Table 1.1 Scintillators used in PET scanners

Material	Cost	Light output[a]	Effective density[b]	Decay time[c]
NaI(TI)	Inexpensive	Highest	Lowest	Long
BGO	Expensive	Lowest	Highest	Long
LSO (or LYSO, or LFS)	Most expensive	High	High	Very short

Abbreviations: BGO, bismuth germinate; LFS, lutetium fine silicate; LSO, lutetium oxyorthosilicate; LYSO, lutetium yttrium orthosilicate; NaI(TI), thallium-doped sodium iodide.
[a]Determines energy and spatial resolution.
[b]Determines scanner sensitivity.
[c]Determines dead time, random coincidences rate, and time-of-flight resolution.

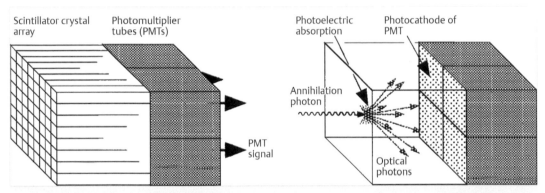

Fig. 1.2 Schematic of a block detector with finely segmented scintillator crystals read out by four photomultiplier tubes.

The most commonly used PET scintillators are listed in ▶ Table 1.1. Other materials are being evaluated (e.g., lanthanum bromide [LaBr]). Historically, manufacturers have adopted different materials for their systems. Current time-of-flight PET scanners (TOF-PET) use the LSO (lutetium orthosilicate)-type scintillators because of their favorable decay constant, providing very short decay time.

The most commonly used photodetectors for PET are photomultiplier tubes (PMTs). PMTs are vacuum tubes with a photocathode, which produce electrons from incoming light photons that are accelerated and amplified. The resulting electrical current is proportional to the number of initial scintillation photons and therefore to the energy deposited in the scintillation crystal by the PET photon. Recently, a new class of photodetectors is being offered in newer PET scanners called silicon photomultipliers (SiPMs). These are silicon-based solid-state detectors that are smaller that PMTs and offer advantages in size, price, and performance.

By segmenting the scintillator blocks, using many small PMTs or SiPMs, the location of the photon detection can be determined. The most commonly used setup today is the *block detector*

(▶ Fig. 1.2). Here, small individual scintillation crystals, a few millimeters in size where they face the patient, are tightly packed into blocks, which are typically coupled to four or more small PMTs or SiPMs. To determine the interaction position of the annihilation photon from the spread-out scintillation photon signals, the relative outputs from the PMT or SiPM signals are compared. The calculated location then determines the crystal element to which the photon is assigned.

Spatial resolution (in the detector) of a few millimeters is possible with this scheme, as it is mainly determined by the size of the crystal cross section.

A conventional clinical PET scanner is constructed as a cylindrical assembly of block detectors, stacked together as multiple rings. The sensitive volume inside the detector cylinder that a patient can occupy is called the imaging field of view (FOV), which in human scanners is typically 70 cm in diameter and 16 to 25 cm in axial length (▶ Fig. 1.3).

1.3.2 Coincident Photon Events

Because of the positron annihilation, we expect to observe two photons at roughly the same time (in coincidence) in the detector ring. The annihilation event, occurring very close to the radioactive tracer of interest, will be located somewhere on the line connecting the two photon-detection points. This knowledge of the photon direction is a huge advantage over single-photon emission computed tomography (SPECT), where collimators have to be used to restrict possible photon directions at the detectors at the cost of a large reduction in sensitivity.

Several factors lead to the photon detections not occurring at the exact same time: the annihilation may occur closer to one detector surface than the other, which will result in a slight but measurable delay of one photon, where the photons travel at the speed of light, or 1 m in 3.3 nanoseconds. Most important for temporal mismatches is the finite timing resolution of the detector, its timing uncertainty, which arises from the decay time of the scintillation in the crystal and the processing time of the PMT signals. These effects lead to the use of a coincidence time window of the order of 6 to 10 nanoseconds. If two photons are detected within a coincidence window, they are assumed to be arising from the same annihilation, and an event is attributed to the line of response (LOR) that connects the two detection points in the sensitive imaging volume.

The detected coincidence events (called *coincidences*) can be classified into true coincidences and background events (▶ Fig. 1.4). The latter are distinguished as either accidental (or random) coincidences, where the two photons did not originate from the same annihilation event, or scattered coincidences that did originate from the same annihilation. Scattered coincidences occur when one or both of the annihilation photons from a single annihilation experience Compton scatter within the patient and therefore have a change of direction leading to a paired detection where the

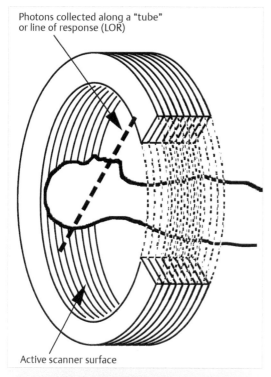

Fig. 1.3 Schematic of positron emission tomography scanner, constructed from multiple cylindrical detector rings, with an example line of response of two annihilation photons exiting the head in opposite directions.

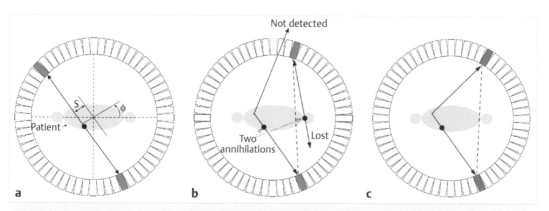

Fig. 1.4 Types of coincident events. From left to right: (a) true coincidence, (b) random (accidental) coincidence, and (c) scattered coincidence. In the last two types, the annihilation event (*black circle*) does not lie on the apparent line of response between the two photon detections.

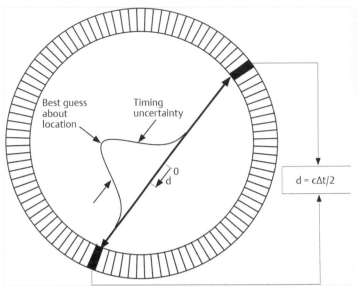

Fig. 1.5 Schematic showing basics of time-of-flight PET imaging. The difference in arrival times of the photons provides information about the origin of the annihilation along the line of response.

true annihilation position does not lie on the line connecting the two photon positions.

1.3.3 Time-of-Flight

With TOF-PET imaging, the relative time difference (Δt) between the detection of the two annihilation photons is used to help determine the most likely location (d) of the annihilation event along the LOR (▶ Fig. 1.5), where c is the speed of light. In the early development of PET technology, TOF-PET imaging was investigated, but not fully adopted due to limitations in hardware. The recent development of scintillators suitable for TOF-PET (i.e., LSO, LYSO [lutetium yttrium orthosilicate], LFS [lutetium fine silicate]) combined with advances in timing resolution and timing stability of detector electronics has led to a resurgence of interest in TOF-PET scanners, with most vendors offering TOF-enabled models. In general, TOF-PET provides advantageous noise properties, particularly for larger patients, and helps mitigate artifacts from erroneous correction factors.

1.3.4 Two-Dimensional versus Three-Dimensional Acquisitions

Axially, PET scanners consist of several rings of detector elements that may or may not be separated by thin annular rings or septa of photon-absorptive material, typically tungsten, that provide collimation. With collimation, all data are acquired in two-dimensional (2D) slices between the septa. This type of acquisition is therefore called 2D, even though the reconstructed stack of images gives three-dimensional (3D) information about the tracer uptake throughout the patient. When a scanner is operated without collimation (i.e., no septa), coincidences from all axial angles in the FOV will be accepted, making this a fully 3D acquisition protocol. Data storage, correction, and image reconstruction are considerably more complex in the fully 3D case.

▶ Fig. 1.6 shows the effect that collimation has on the acquisition of coincidence counts: the septa block a large number of true coincidences from ever reaching the detector surface, decreasing sensitivity. However, they also reduce scattered and random coincidences, thus improving contrast, and may be beneficial for high count rate applications such as dynamic imaging. In dynamic imaging, the radiotracer is often imaged during the first circulatory pass of the injected activity, leading to very high count levels that might exceed the count rate of highly sensitive 3D geometries. That said, most commercial systems are now 3D-only because this approach has been shown to be advantageous for the most common imaging applications (oncology, neuro) and 2D- and 3D-enabled systems require expensive mechanical components to switch modes.

1.3.5 Sinograms

In the scanner, coincidence events are observed and identified along their LORs between pairs of detector elements (▶ Fig. 1.5). To organize these

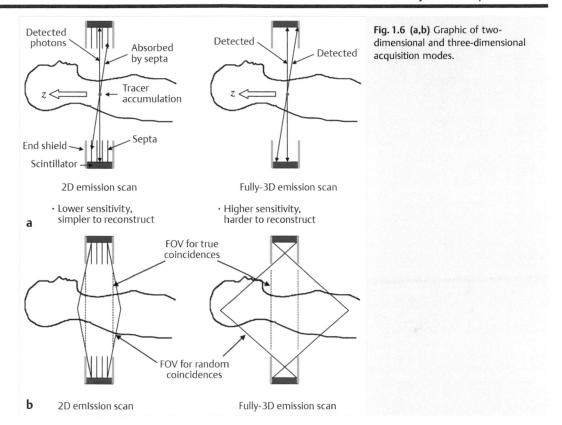

Fig. 1.6 (a,b) Graphic of two-dimensional and three-dimensional acquisition modes.

raw data as they are acquired, each coincident event is catalogued in a histogram matrix based on the angle and distance from the center of the LOR. This is the common data organization used in tomography and leads to matrices in which a single point in the patient traces a sinusoid curve in the raw data histogram, hence the term *sinogram* for the raw data format.

1.3.6 Corrections

The PET data acquisition process is not perfect. Interactions in the patient attenuate the emitted photons, detector elements vary in their detection efficiency, and random and scattered coincidences are recorded along with the true coincidence events. These effects need to be corrected to obtain clinically useful images and accurate quantitative information from PET studies.

The most important of the corrections is AC: photons that encounter more or denser material on their path from the annihilation site to the detectors are more likely to be absorbed or scattered (i.e., attenuated) than photons that travel through sparser parts of the body. If images are

reconstructed from sinograms without AC, this can lead to less dense areas, such as the lungs, appearing darker (emitting more photons) than surrounding denser tissue, such as the mediastinum (► Fig. 1.7). This is clearly an artifact that arises from the fact that lung tissue exhibits lower attenuation, not higher uptake. It not only impairs the visual appearance of the image, but also leads to wildly inaccurate quantitation of tracer uptake. To apply AC, it is necessary to determine the attenuation through the patient for all LORs. On earlier stand-alone PET scanners, this was done with a *transmission scan*, where an external positron source is rotated around the patient, and the attenuation of the transmitted photons is determined. In the now-standard PET/CT scanners, the acquired CT image is used for PET AC. AC from MR images in the new class of PET/MR scanners is a work in progress at this point.

1.4 Image Reconstruction

After the acquisition of PET data in sinograms and their corrections for attenuation and other effects, as described above, the next stage in the PET

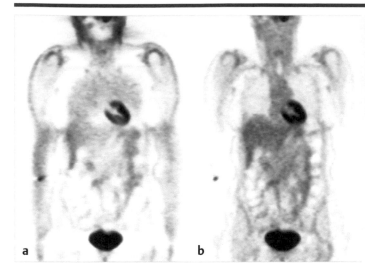

Fig. 1.7 Whole-body positron emission tomography coronal image **(a)** without and **(b)** with attenuation correction. Artifacts from not performing attenuation correction include the lungs and skin showing higher tracer uptake than muscle. In these images, darker regions represent higher tracer uptake using the common inverse-gray color table.

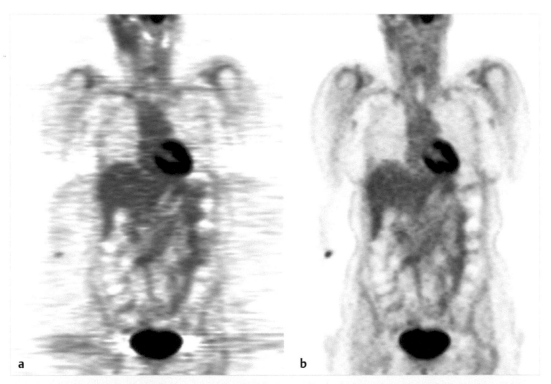

Fig. 1.8 Comparison of coronal sections of positron emission tomography images reconstructed with **(a)** filtered back-projection (FBP) and **(b)** ordered-subsets expectation maximization (OSEM). The FBP image shows characteristic streak artifacts, while the noise texture in OSEM image has a blob nature.

processing chain is to reconstruct an estimate of the in vivo tracer distribution. This process of *image reconstruction* is the most mathematically complex step and is well described elsewhere.[1,2,3] Here, we point out the differences between the two most common methods: filtered back-projection (FBP) and ordered-subsets expectation maximization (OSEM). ▸ Fig. 1.8 shows a visual comparison of FBP and OSEM images, reconstructed from the same patient sinogram.

FBP is an analytic approach known to provide an exact image reconstruction of tomographic data for the conditions of noiseless, fully sampled data. It remains the core of most methods used in CT. In PET, the data contain a lot of noise and have limited spatial resolution, making FBP suboptimal for most PET applications. Furthermore, additional system modeling, such as the TOF information and resolution loss at the detector surface, requires more advanced methods. Methods incorporating models of the photon noise and system generally require iterative solutions, such as the expectation maximization (EM) algorithm. Initially, EM was too slow for clinical needs, but with the advent of the ordered-subsets acceleration of the EM algorithm (OSEM) and faster processors, iterative methods are now the industry standard. It should be stressed that iterative methods have varied substantially over the years and between vendors. These methods have varying levels of sophistication in how (1) corrections are incorporated in the process, (2) the noise is modeled, and (3) the system is modeled.

1.4.1 Noise/Resolution Trade-offs and Image Quality

If images appear very noisy after reconstruction, they may be *smoothed* in a further step to give the eye an easier task, especially for localizing disease. However, because smoothing averages together neighboring image pixels, it is connected to a loss of spatial resolution and small structures may not be distinguishable anymore. ▶ Fig. 1.9 illustrates that changing the reconstruction parameters in OSEM results in images with different noise/resolution trade-offs with increasing iterations and subsets leading to higher spatial resolution at the detriment of increased noise. It is task-dependent and observer-dependent to define an optimal region in the noise/resolution space.

1.5 PET/CT Scanner Components and Function

The primary purpose of combining CT and PET systems in a single scanner is the precise anatomical localization of regions identified on the PET tracer uptake images. Although it is possible to use nonrigid image registration to align separately acquired whole-body PET and CT images, challenges remain in the practical implementation and validation of software-based methods. The advent of combined PET/CT systems has pushed dedicated pure PET scanners almost completely off the market due to the convenience and ease of creating coregistered PET and CT images for oncology, radiation oncology, and cardiology applications.

1.5.1 Basic Components

PET/CT systems are a combination of stand-alone CT and PET scanners in one gantry with a shared patient bed.[4] The patient bed is an important and nontrivial component because there should be no differential bending in the bed between the PET and CT scans. ▶ Fig. 1.10 shows a schematic of a PET/CT scanner. The typical PET/CT protocol begins with an X-ray localization scan (performed by the CT scanner) to define the subsequent scan areas, followed by a CT scan, and finally the PET scan.

The data flow in the combined PET/CT acquisition is outlined in the schematic in ▶ Fig. 1.11. The X-ray CT scan provides anatomical images that after some processing can also be used for AC in PET, and the PET/CT software can display both images side-by-side or overlaid (fused) (▶ Fig. 1.12). It is to be noted that there are no "fused" images in PET/CT—the PET and CT images always remain separate entities. Displaying them together is an overlay process rather than creating a new type of image.

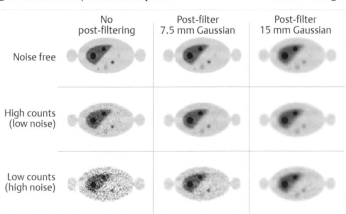

	No post-filtering	Post-filter 7.5 mm Gaussian	Post-filter 15 mm Gaussian
Noise free			
High counts (low noise)			
Low counts (high noise)			

Fig. 1.9 Ordered-subsets expectation maximization images of a digital phantom demonstrating some of the trade-offs between noise and smoothing with different reconstruction settings.

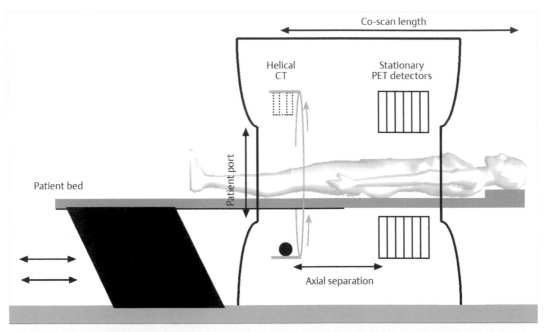

Fig. 1.10 Illustration of the main components of a positron emission tomography/computed tomography (PET/CT) scanner.

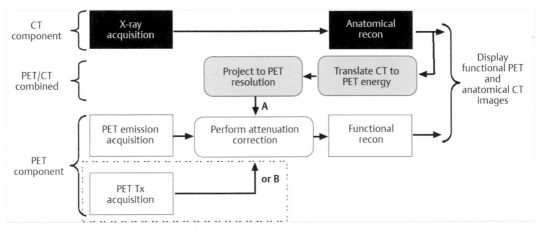

Fig. 1.11 Data flow in a positron emission tomography/computed tomography (PET/CT) scanner.

1.5.2 CT-Based Attenuation Correction

An important synergy of PET/CT scanners is the use of the CT images for AC of the PET emission data. All manufacturers of PET/CT scanners incorporate X-ray CT-based attenuation correction (CTAC) algorithms in their systems. CTAC offers the significant advantage over the original PET transmission scans for AC in that the CT data have much lower statistical noise and can be acquired in a shorter time than a standard PET transmission scan. CT transmission scans can also be acquired after the PET tracer is injected, giving the ability to collect unbiased postinjection transmission scans. This shortens the time spent by a patient on the scanner bed and provides more efficient use of scanner time.

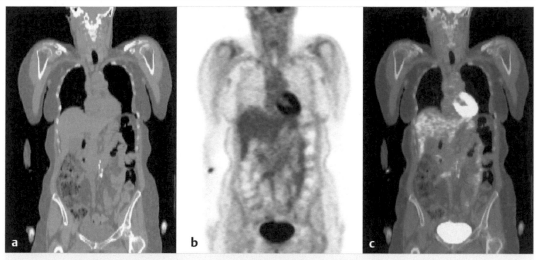

Fig. 1.12 Images from a positron emission tomography/computed tomography (PET/CT) scanner: **(a)** anatomical CT image, **(b)** functional PET image, and **(c)** overlaid image of a whole-body scan.

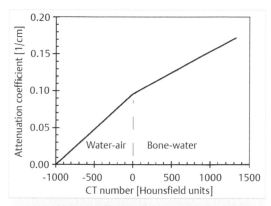

Fig. 1.13 Bilinear scaling transform used to convert computed tomography (CT) image values to positron emission tomography attenuation coefficients.

To be used for AC, the CT data must be transformed to an estimate of the attenuation coefficients at 511 keV. In the bilinear scaling method,[4] the attenuation map at 511 keV is estimated by using separate scaling factors for bone and non-bone components based on the CT image values (▶ Fig. 1.13).

There is, however, no unique transformation from CT energies (~30–140 keV) to 511 keV due to the possibility of independent variations in density and atomic number Z, which can allow two

materials with different atomic numbers to have similar CT values and different attenuation coefficients at 511 keV. Conversely, it is possible for two distinct materials with the same value of attenuation coefficient at 511 keV to yield different CT numbers, and errors in the CTAC image will propagate to errors in the PET image in the same location. This case arises if contrast agent or metallic or high-density implants are present in the CT image. Also, if there are positional mismatches between the PET and CT images due to, for example, respiratory motion, there will also be errors introduced into the PET image. Thus, although CTAC can lead to significant improvements in PET image quality, artifacts can arise from the presence of contrast agent, metallic or high-density implants, and patient motion.

References

[1] Cherry SR, Sorensen JA, Phelps ME. Physics in Nuclear Medicine. Orlando, FL: Grune & Stratton; 2003
[2] Valk PE, Bailey DE, Townsend DW, Maisey MN. Positron Emission Tomography: Basic Science and Clinical Practice. London: Springer-Verlag; 2003
[3] Wernick MN, Aarsvold JN. Emission Tomography. San Diego, CA: Elsevier Academic Press; 2004
[4] Alessio AM, Kinahan PE, Cheng PM, Vesselle H, Karp JS. PET/CT scanner instrumentation, challenges, and solutions. Radiol Clin North Am. 2004; 42(6):1017–1032, vii

2 The Basics of 2-[F-18]Fluoro-2-deoxy-D-glucose Radiochemistry and Biology

N. Scott Mason and Eugene C. Lin

2.1 Introduction

This chapter will present an introduction to the basics of 2-[F-18]fluoro-2-deoxy-D-glucose ([F-18]FDG) radiochemistry and biology. Without question, [F-18]FDG is the most commonly utilized positron emission tomography (PET) radiotracer and has demonstrated utility in a variety of applications including neuroscience, cardiology, and oncology.[1,2,3,4] A brief discussion regarding the historical development of [F-18]FDG will be presented, but more detailed discussions can be found in several other publications.[5,6] In general, there are several chemistry concerns inherent in the production of PET radiotracers. A primary concern is the impact of the relatively short half-lives of the radionuclides on the synthetic process. As a matter of practical necessity, PET radiosyntheses are designed so that the radionuclide is introduced as close to the end of the synthesis as possible. While it is clearly advantageous to have the incorporation of the radionuclide occur as the final step in the synthetic method, this is sometimes not feasible (as is the case in the production of [F-18] FDG). In most circumstances, the radiopharmaceutical for injection must be isolated from the crude reaction mixture using a variety of methods including solid-phase extraction methods, high-performance liquid chromatography methods, or some combination of the two methods.

The design of [F-18]FDG was predicated upon the utility of [C-14]-2-DG, a derivative of glucose where a hydrogen atom replaces the C-2 hydroxyl group (▶ Fig. 2.1).

In many ways, 2-DG (and by extension FDG) and glucose are very similar. Both compounds are transported from the plasma via facilitated transport and both compounds serve as substrates for phosphorylation by the enzyme hexokinase. However, the next enzyme in the metabolic route for these sugars, phosphohexose isomerase, requires the presence of a hydroxyl group on C-2. Consequently, 2-DG and, in a similar fashion, FDG are trapped in the cell as their respective 6-phosphate derivatives that are not substrates for either phosphohexose isomerase or glucose-6-phosphate dehydrogenase. It is this metabolic trapping that leads to the utility of [F-18]FDG in imaging and will be discussed further in the brief section concerning rate constants and pharmacokinetics. The demonstration that 2-FDG, in its unlabeled form, was a reasonable substrate for hexokinase and that the potential alternative substitution positions (i.e., 3-F and 4-F-deoxy-D-glucose, respectively) possessed significantly lower affinities for hexokinase[7,8] further supported the choice of FDG as a reasonable model compound for the development of an in vivo imaging agent.

2.2 First Synthesis

The first radiosynthesis of [F-18]FDG took place in 1976 as the result of a long collaboration between investigators at the National Institutes of Health, the University of Pennsylvania, and Brookhaven National Laboratory.[5] The first radiosynthesis of [F-18]FDG was based on the availability of [F-18]F$_2$ via the deuterium bombardment of a nickel target loaded with neon-20 (^{20}Ne(d,α)^{18}F, indicating the collision of an accelerated deuteron [d] with the stable nuclide neon-20 to produce an alpha

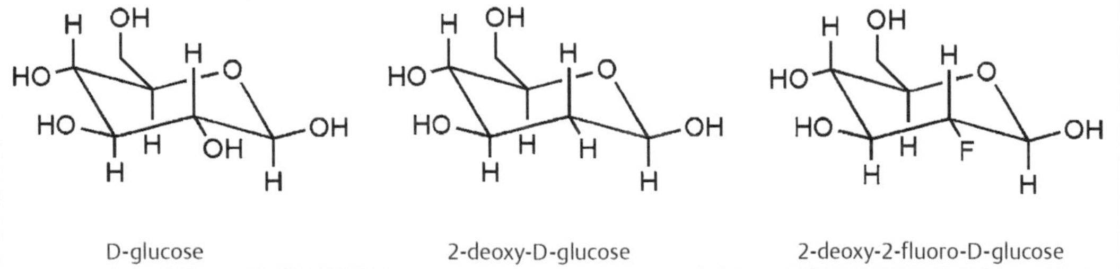

Fig. 2.1 Chemical structures of glucose analogs.

D-glucose

2-deoxy-D-glucose

2-deoxy-2-fluoro-D-glucose

particle [α] and the fluorine-18 radionuclide). The reaction of [F-18]F$_2$ with a protected D-glucal (3,4,6-tri-O-acetyl-D-glucal) yielded a mixture of mannose and glucose isomers that were separable by preparative gas chromatographic methods. Acidic hydrolysis of the glucose derivative yielded [F-18]FDG in yields sufficient for human studies (▶ Fig. 2.2).[9]

2.3 Further Development

A variety of different approaches for the optimization of an electrophilic route to [F-18]FDG were investigated.[10,11,12] The use of [F-18]acetyl hypofluorite ([F-18]CH$_3$CO$_2$F) became one of the methods of choice. However, it was eventually demonstrated that the use of [F-18]acetyl hypofluorite yielded varying amounts of the undesired isomer (2-deoxy-2[F-18]fluoro-D-mannose) depending on the reaction conditions (▶ Fig. 2.2).[13]

One drawback of the electrophilic method (either [F-18]F$_2$ or [F-18]CH$_3$CO$_2$F) is that only half of the label is available for incorporation into the target molecule. Another drawback is the use of carrier fluorine gas in the production that leads to

reductions in specific activity. A third drawback, especially in light of the increasing utilization of [F-18]FDG, was the yield limitation of the production of fluorine-18 from the ^{20}Ne(d,α)^{18}F reaction. The cross-sectional energies for particles in the 10- to 18-MeV range for this reaction are approximately 60 to 90 mCi/uA. This is significantly lower than the corresponding cross section for the ^{18}O(p,n)^{18}F reaction (150–260 mCi/uA).[14] Interest in a nucleophilic radiolabeling route to [F-18]FDG increased with the development of [O-18]water targets capable of producing [F-18]fluoride in high-yield and high-specific activity. The most common method to produce nucleophilic [^{18}F]fluoride is the ^{18}O(p,n)^{18}F reaction (indicating the collision of an accelerated proton [p] with the stable nuclide oxygen-18 to produce a neutron [n] and the fluorine-18 radionuclide). The oxygen-18 target material most commonly consists of enriched [^{18}O]water.[15,16] Irradiation of enriched [^{18}O]water is capable of producing multiCurie (>70 GBq) quantities of [^{18}F]fluoride with high-specific activity in relatively short irradiation times depending on target load volumes and beam geometry. In addition, there are now methods for the

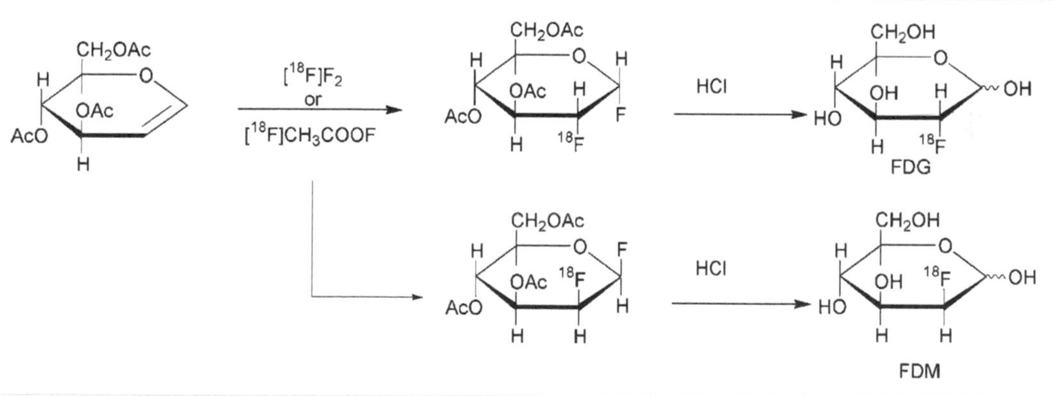

Fig. 2.2 Electrophilic radiosynthetic scheme for [F-18]FDG.

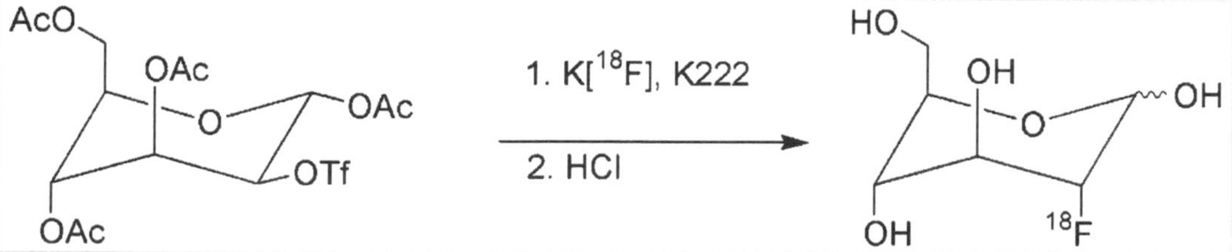

Fig. 2.3 Nucleophilic radiosynthetic scheme for [F-18]FDG.

separation and recovery of the enriched target material from the [^{18}F]fluoride.[17,18,19]

The potential for higher [F-18]fluoride yields prompted significant efforts aimed at the development of a reliable, high-yielding nucleophilic route to [F-18]FDG. In most instances, [F-18]FDG is synthesized using an adaptation of the Julich method (▸ Fig. 2.3).[20] In the original application of this method, aqueous [F-18]fluoride is added to a solution consisting of Kryptofix [2.2.2] and potassium carbonate dissolved in aqueous acetonitrile. The residual water is removed by azeotropic distillation using anhydrous acetonitrile and a stream of inert gas such as nitrogen or argon. A relatively small amount of precursor (~10–20 mg of 1,3,4,6-tetra-O-acetyl-2-O-trifluoromethanesulfonyl-β-D-mannopyranose) dissolved in anhydrous acetonitrile is added to the dried [F-18]fluoride. The reaction mixture is heated to reflux for several minutes. Ethyl ether is used to transfer the reaction solution after cooling across a Sep-Pak silica cartridge (Waters) into a second reaction vessel. This preliminary purification removes the unreacted [F-18]fluoride and the Kryptofix [2.2.2]. The solvents are removed and aqueous hydrochloric acid is added to the intermediate product, 2-deoxy-2-[F-18]fluoro-1,3,4,6-tetra-O-acetyl-β-D-glucopyrranose. The aqueous acid solution is heated to reflux for a short period of time and then purified by passage across an ion-retardation resin followed by an alumina-N Sep-Pak (Waters) and a C-18 Sep-Pak (Waters). Several aliquots of water are subsequently used to transfer all the product material from the hydrolysis vessel across the purification columns. This methodology leads to the presence of D-mannose, D-glucose, and 2-chloro-2-deoxy-D-glucose as chemical impurities in the radiosynthesis of FDG.[21]

This reaction scheme has been utilized as the basis of a computer-controlled automated synthesizer[22] for the routine production of [F-18]FDG (CTI, Knoxville, TN; now part of Siemens—as of September 2016, Siemens has discontinued its cyclotron and biomarker radiochemistry production systems). Further modifications of this methodology have led to the development of "one-pot" syntheses for the production of [F-18]FDG. These modifications include the substitution of tetramethylammonium carbonate for Kryptofix [2.2.2]/potassium carbonate as the phase-transfer reagent and subsequent elimination of the silica Sep-Pak purification step. As a result of these modifications, the acidic hydrolysis was performed in the same reaction vessel.[23] A similar "one-pot" modifi-

cation was reported that retained Kryptofix [2.2.2] as the phase-transfer reagent. This method also eliminated the intermediate silica Sep-Pak purification step, as well as adding an additional cation exchange resin to the purification column (to remove the unwanted Kryptofix [2.2.2]) and an additional alumina N Sep-Pak (Waters) to prevent fluoride ion breakthrough.[24]

The toxicity concerns associated with Kryptofix [2.2.2] (LD$_{50}$ in rats of 35 mg/kg) have prompted the use of other phase-transfer agents such as tetrabutylammonium hydroxide or tetrabutylammonium bicarbonate. This modification has been incorporated into a commercially available synthesizer produced by Nuclear Interface (now part of GE Healthcare). The Nuclear Interface synthesis module is flexible in that it can be set up to utilize either tetrabutylammonium bicarbonate or Kryptofix [2.2.2] as the phase-transfer reagent. In addition, the module can perform the hydrolysis of the radiolabeled intermediate, 2-deoxy-2-[F-18]fluoro-1,3,4,6-tetra-O-acetyl-β-D-glucopyrranose, under either acidic or basic conditions. There are several other variations of this radiolabeling scheme. One variation is the use of an immobilized quaternary 4-aminopyridinium resin material for the isolation of the [F-18]fluoride and subsequent incorporation into the [F-18]-radiolabeled intermediate. In this process, the [F-18]fluoride solution is passed across the resin column where [F-18]fluoride is trapped and the bulk of the [O-18] enriched water is recovered downstream. The resin bound [F-18]fluoride is dried by passing anhydrous acetonitrile across the resin column while heating the column. A solution of the precursor in anhydrous acetonitrile is then passed over the heated resin column in either a slow single-pass or a reciprocating flow across the resin column. The solution containing the radiolabeled intermediate is then transferred to a hydrolysis vessel where the acetonitrile is removed. Following the acid hydrolysis, the [F-18]FDG is purified in an analogous manner to the original method described above.[25] It was this methodology that formed the basis of one commercially available synthesis unit (PETtrace FDG MicroLab, GE Medical Systems, Uppsala, Sweden). This unit uses a disposable cassette system for the reaction column, as well as transfer and addition lines which facilitates the set-up of the unit.

The substitution of a solid-phase-supported basic hydrolysis step[26] has been implemented in the FDG synthesizer marketed by Coincidence Technologies, Inc (now part of GE Healthcare). The basic hydrolysis conditions allow for a faster reaction time as compared to the standard acidic hydrolysis conditions with no evidence of epimerization under the conditions employed (2 minutes at room temperature). Using this system, over 7 Ci of FDG have been produced in a single production run.

The production of [F-18]FDG entails not only the generation of the radionuclide ([F-18]fluoride) and the radiosynthetic procedure, but also the quality control determination that ensures the final product formulation is suitable for human use administration. There are a variety of criteria that must be met for a radiopharmaceutical to be deemed suitable for human use. Routine quality control and release criteria for PET radiopharmaceuticals may include tests for radiochemical purity, chemical purity, stereochemical purity, radionuclidic identity, residual organic solvent contamination, pH, sterility, and apyrogenicity of the final formulation. The United States Pharmacopoeia (USP) Chapter < 823 >, *Radiopharmaceuticals for Positron Emission Tomography-Compounding, Investigational, and Research Uses*, provides a more detailed presentation of these concerns.[27] In addition, there are currently a number of USP monographs for individual PET radiotracers, including F-18 fludeoxyglucose ([F-18]FDG).

While the majority of the quality control issues mentioned above are relatively straightforward in their application to the routine quality control of [F-18]FDG, a few deserve some elaboration. One of these is the determination of residual volatile organic solvents. The two primary organic solvents in question are acetonitrile and ethanol with release limits of 0.04 and 0.5% by volume, respectively. It should be noted that these values are based on the *permitted daily exposure* values for the respective solvent(s) and the percent volume limits assume that no more than 10 mL of material will be administered in a given day at the maximum allowed limit. In addition, there are two chemical purity issues regarding the "standard" nucleophilic radiosynthetic method that utilizes

an acidic hydrolysis process. The first of these is the determination of residual Kryptofix [2.2.2] in the final product preparation of [F-18]FDG. A color spot test method has been reported in the literature for the detection of this impurity at the detection limit specified in the USP (50 µg/mL).[28] It should be noted that a false positive is possible with this test and that a confirmatory thin-layer chromatography test (USP method) should be performed to confirm the identity of the suspected impurity. In addition, the amount of 2-chloro-2-deoxy-D-glucose in the final product is to be determined (USP limit of 1 mg of 2-chloro-2-deoxy-D-glucose per total volume of final product formulation). The USP chapter < 823 > and the monograph Fludeoxyglucose F 18 Injection are the current regulatory framework under which the production of [F-18]FDG is to be carried out if its intended use is for research or investigational applications. The production of [F-18]FDG intended for clinical diagnostic uses (in the United States) is now regulated by the Food and Drug Administration under 21 CFR Part 212 (Current Good Manufacturing Practice for PET Drugs-CGMP).

2.4 Basic Modeling/Biology

The utility of [F-18]FDG for noninvasive in vivo imaging is based as much on the pharmacokinetics of the tracer as it is on the relative ease (at the present time) of production and delivery of [F-18]FDG to the end user. The general model for [F-18]FDG is the two-tissue compartmental model based on the work of Sokoloff et al using [C-14]-DG[29] and later adopted for use with [F-18]FDG. More detailed discussions of the modeling of [F-18]FDG can be found in several other publications, but a brief description follows.[30,31] The model consists of three compartments: $C_p(t)$, arterial plasma concentration; $C_f(t)$, unmetabolized or free FDG; and $C_m(t)$, metabolized FDG trapped as FDG-6-phosphate (▶ Fig. 2.4).

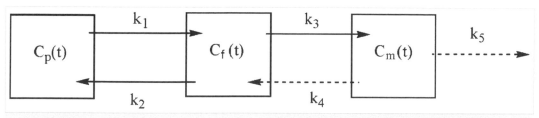

Fig. 2.4 Schematic representation of the two-tissue compartmental model for [F-18]FDG. For a more detailed description of C_P, C_F, C_M, and K_{1-5}, see the text.

K_1 represents the rate constant for transport from arterial plasma to the tissue compartment. The rate constant k_2 is defined as the rate constant for transport from the free tissue compartment to arterial plasma. The rate constant k_3 represents the rate of phosphorylation, which is a measure of hexokinase activity. The rate constant k_4 represents the rate of dephosphorylation and k_5 is the rate constant for further metabolism. In general, both k_4 and k_5 are ignored for [F-18]FDG as the rate of dephosphorylation is very low compared to phosphorylation, and further metabolism by glucose-6-phosphate dehydrogenase is not possible due to the lack of a hydroxyl group at C-2.

By definition, the metabolic rate of glucose is the net rate of the conversion of glucose to glucose-6-phosphate. However, in a PET study, one measures the rate constants not for glucose, but rather for [F-18]FDG, and through the use of a "lumped constant" that represents the ratio of metabolic rates of FDG and glucose, one then calculates the metabolic rate of glucose in absolute terms ($\mu mol/min/100$ g).

The kinetics of FDG allows for an even simpler approach that was ultimately based on the autoradiography work of Sokoloff et al using [C-14]DG.[29] This approach is based on the presumption that [F-18]FDG is trapped in the tissue following phosphorylation. The fraction of trapped radioactivity continually increases throughout a study, while clearance from tissue of the free component is relatively rapid. Consequently, a single static image at 40 to 60 minutes postinjection reflects, to a very close degree, the relative metabolic rate of glucose.

Phosphorylation by hexokinase corresponding to the rate constant k_3 is the rate-limiting step for FDG metabolism, and overexpression of hexokinase may account to a large extent for the increased signal seen in some lesions. However, the etiology of the signal seen on FDG PET images is multifactorial. FDG activity in a lesion may be largely dependent on blood flow in cases where perfusion is decreased. Cell density in the lesion also plays a factor in the amount of signal seen. Once the FDG reaches a lesion, it must be transported through the cell membrane. There are multiple facilitative mammalian glucose transporters (GLUT). The most important glucose transporter for FDG is GLUT1, which is expressed in almost all cell types. Overexpression of GLUT1 transporters is primarily responsible for the increased FDG signal seen in many lesions, and this may be independent of hexokinase activity. Another glucose transporter significant in FDG PET imaging is the GLUT4

transporter, which is insulin sensitive and present in the myocardium and skeletal muscle. Therefore, insulin will increase FDG uptake in the myocardium and skeletal muscle, with important implications for patient preparation for FDG PET studies and cardiac imaging with FDG (see Chapter 4). In general, the etiology of a hot spot seen on clinical FDG PET studies is a complex interaction of multiple factors, and interpreters should be cautious in ascribing the uptake to one specific physiological or molecular mechanism.

2.5 Conclusion

The development of high-yield, [O-18] enriched water targets for the production of [F-18]fluoride, the capabilities of current generation of cyclotrons to perform dual-target irradiations at relatively high target currents, and the availability of automated synthesis modules for the production of [F-18]FDG now make possible the production of multicurie amounts of [F-18]FDG in a single production run. This capability has significantly increased the utilization of [F-18]FDG and has led to the introduction of production facilities dedicated to the synthesis and distribution of FDG to end users with only imaging capabilities.

References

[1] Antonini A, Kazumata K, Feigin A, et al. Differential diagnosis of parkinsonism with [18F]fluorodeoxyglucose and PET. Mov Disord. 1998; 13(2):268–274

[2] Bar-Shalom R, Valdivia AY, Blaufox MD. PET imaging in oncology. Semin Nucl Med. 2000; 30(3):150–185

[3] Saab G, Dekemp RA, Ukkonen H, Ruddy TD, Germano G, Beanlands RS. Gated fluorine 18 fluorodeoxyglucose positron emission tomography: determination of global and regional left ventricular function and myocardial tissue characterization. J Nucl Cardiol. 2003; 10(3):297–303

[4] Fazekas F, Payer F. F-18 fluorodeoxyglucose positron emission tomography in neurology [in German]. Wien Med Wochenschr. 2002; 152(11)(–)(12):293–297

[5] Fowler JS, Ido T. Initial and subsequent approach for the synthesis of 18FDG. Semin Nucl Med. 2002; 32(1):6–12

[6] Beuthien-Baumann B, Hamacher K, Oberdorfer F, Steinbach J. Preparation of fluorine-18 labelled sugars and derivatives and their application as tracer for positron-emission-tomography. Carbohydr Res. 2000; 327(1)(–)(2):107–118

[7] Bessell EM, Courtenay VD, Foster AB, Jones M, Westwood JH. Some in vivo and in vitro antitumour effects of the deoxy-fluoro-D-glucopyranoses. Eur J Cancer. 1973; 9(7):463–470

[8] Machado de Domenech EE, Sols A. Specificity of hexokinases towards some uncommon substrates and inhibitors. FEBS Lett. 1980; 119(1):174–176

[9] Ido T, Wan C-N, Fowler JS, et al. Fluorination with F2. A convenient synthesis of 2-deoxy-2-fluoro-D-glucose. J Org Chem. 1977; 42:2341–2342

[10] Adam MJ. A rapid, stereoselective, high yielding synthesis of 2-deoxy-2-fluoro-D-hexopyranoses: Reaction of glycols with acetyl hypofluorite. J Chem Soc Chem Comm. 1982:730–732

[11] Ehrenkaufer RE, Potocki JF, Jewett DM. Simple synthesis of F-18-labeled 2-fluoro-2-deoxy-D-glucose: concise communication. J Nucl Med. 1984; 25(3):333–337

[12] Sood S, Firnau G, Garnett ES. Radiofluorination with xenon difluoride: A new high yield synthesis of [18F]2-fluoro-2-deoxy-D-glucose. J Nucl Med. 1983; 24:718–721

[13] Bida GT, Satyamurthy N, Barrio JR. The synthesis of 2-[F-18] fluoro-2-deoxy-D-glucose using glycals: a reexamination. J Nucl Med. 1984; 25(12):1327–1334

[14] Ruth T, Wolf AP. Absolute cross sections for the production of 18F via the 18O(p,n)18F reaction. Radiochim Acta. 1979; 26: 21–24

[15] Kilbourn MR, Hood JT, Welch MJ. A simple 18O water target for 18F production. Int J Appl Radiat Isot. 1984; 35(7):599–602

[16] Wieland B, Hendry G, Schmidt D, Bida G, Ruth T. Efficient small-volume 18O-water targets for producing 18F-fluoride with low energy protons. J Labelled Comp Radiopharm. 1986; 23:1205–1207

[17] Schlyer D, Bastos M, Wolf A. A quantitative separation of fluorine-18 fluoride from oxygen-18 water. J Nucl Med. 1987; 28:764

[18] Schlyer DJ, Bastos MA, Alexoff D, Wolf AP. Separation of [18F] fluoride from [18O]water using anion exchange resin. Int J Rad Appl Instrum [A]. 1990; 41(6):531–533

[19] Jewett DM, Toorongian SA, Mulholland GK, Watkins GL, Kilbourn MR. Multiphase extraction: rapid phase-transfer of [18F]fluoride ion for nucleophilic radiolabeling reactions. Int J Rad Appl Instrum [A]. 1988; 39(11):1109–1111

[20] Hamacher K, Coenen HH, Stöcklin G. Efficient stereospecific synthesis of no-carrier-added 2-[18F]-fluoro-2-deoxy-D-glucose using aminopolyether supported nucleophilic substitution. J Nucl Med. 1986; 27(2):235–238

[21] Alexoff DL, Casati R, Fowler JS, et al. Ion chromatographic analysis of high specific activity 18FDG preparations and detection of the chemical impurity 2-deoxy-2-chloro-D-glucose. Int J Rad Appl Instrum [A]. 1992; 43(11):1313–1322

[22] Padgett HC, Schmidt DG, Luxen A, Bida GT, Satyamurthy N, Barrio JR. Computer-controlled radiochemical synthesis: a chemistry process control unit for the automated production of radiochemicals. Int J Rad Appl Instrum [A]. 1989; 40(5): 433–445

[23] Mock BH, Vavrek MT, Mulholland GK. Back-to-back "one-pot" [18F]FDG syntheses in a single Siemens-CTI chemistry process control unit. Nucl Med Biol. 1996; 23(4):497–501

[24] Padgett H, Wilson D, Clanton J, Zigler S. Two for the price of one: single-vessel FDG syntheses using the CPCU- the PETNet Experience, RDS Users' Meeting, San Francisco, California, April 2-4; 1998

[25] Toorongian SA, Mulholland GK, Jewett DM, Bachelor MA, Kilbourn MR. Routine production of 2-deoxy-2-[18F]fluoro-D-glucose by direct nucleophilic exchange on a quaternary 4-aminopyridinium resin. Int J Rad Appl Instrum B. 1990; 17 (3):273–279

[26] Lemaire C, Damhaut Ph, Lauricella B, et al. Fast [18F]FDG synthesis by alkaline hydrolysis on a low polarity solid phase support. J Labelled Comp Radiopharm. 2002; 45(5):435–447

[27] United States Pharmacopeial Convention, Inc. Chapter <823> Radiopharmaceuticals for Positron Emission Tomography-Compounding, Investigational, and Research Uses in United States Pharmacopeia 35/National Formulary 30. Rockville, MD: The United States Pharmacopeial Convention, Inc.; 2012

[28] Mock BH, Winkle W, Vavrek MT. A color spot test for the detection of Kryptofix 2.2.2 in [18F]FDG preparations. Nucl Med Biol. 1997; 24(2):193–195

[29] Sokoloff L, Reivich M, Kennedy C, et al. The [14C]deoxyglucose method for the measurement of local cerebral glucose utilization: theory, procedure, and normal values in the conscious and anesthetized albino rat. J Neurochem. 1977; 28(5):897–916

[30] Reivich M, Kuhl D, Wolf A, et al. The [18F]fluorodeoxyglucose method for the measurement of local cerebral glucose utilization in man. Circ Res. 1979; 44(1):127–137

[31] Phelps ME, Huang SC, Hoffman EJ, Selin C, Sokoloff L, Kuhl DE. Tomographic measurement of local cerebral glucose metabolic rate in humans with (F-18)2-fluoro-2-deoxy-D-glucose: validation of method. Ann Neurol. 1979; 6(5):371–388

3 The Role of Glucose and FDG Metabolism in the Interpretation of PET Studies

Ronald L. Korn, Melissa Singer Pressman, and John Millstine

3.1 Introduction

Ask most physicians to recall the enzymatic pathways of glucose metabolism, and you will likely provoke memories of premedical or medical school biochemistry classes where the common dictum was, "Glucose metabolism? Why do I need to know this stuff? I will never use this information again!"

Fortunately, a few students of science and medicine have had the astuteness to realize that even the most mundane and obscure fact could someday come in handy. Such is the story of glucose metabolism and its relationship to [fluorine 18] fluorodeoxyglucose ([18F]FDG) positron emission tomography (PET) imaging. In 1924, Otto Warburg, a famous German biochemist, made a fundamental observation that would forever change the course of our understanding of the role of glucose metabolism in cancer biology. In an article published in the journal *Biochemische Zeitschrift*,[1] he and his colleagues noted that cancer cells consume more glucose and produce more lactic acid than normal (resting) cells. This straightforward observation, later termed the Warburg effect in his honor, was apparent even under aerobic conditions. Because of his pioneering work, Warburg was awarded the Nobel Prize for Medicine and is considered one of the central figures in PET imaging.

One glucose molecule metabolized in the presence of adequate oxygen can lead to the production of 36 adenosine triphosphate (ATP) molecules with CO_2 and H_2O as its byproducts (so-called tricarboxylic acid, or TCA, cycle). However, in hypoxic conditions and in many cancer cell types, only two ATPs are formed from glucose metabolism, with lactic acid (glycolysis) produced as its by-product. These observations have given rise to several theories about the survival and tenacity of cancer even under the most formidable conditions.[2,3,4,5,6,7,8] Yet it is the rather simplified pathway of glucose metabolism through the glycolytic pathway that has been responsible for the explosion of FDG PET imaging over the last few decades.

Although a detailed understanding of the role of glucose metabolism in the context of the critical changes that occur to transform a normal cell into a malignant one is beyond the scope of this chapter, we will briefly focus on the biology of FDG imaging in the framework of what the clinician needs to know for everyday interpretation of FDG PET studies. We will attempt to provide a basic understanding of the changes that occur at the molecular level that account for the increased glucose metabolism in cancer cells and other benign inflammatory conditions. It is hoped that this chapter will serve as a starting point for our readers to delve further into the complex biology of glucose and FDG metabolism and to begin to appreciate the central role of glucose metabolism as a molecular probe in oncology imaging. Furthermore, this chapter will focus almost exclusively on the biology of FDG oncology imaging, but it will not address the biological changes that occur in cardiac or neurologic diseases. Finally, we hope that this chapter will help answer the age-old question of "why you need to know this stuff."

3.2 The Breakdown of Glucose/FDG from Injection to Cell Entry

The importance of glucose metabolism in malignancy has provided a foundation for understanding cancer biology. A decisive advantage of FDG in oncology imaging is that it behaves in so many ways like glucose. For example, glucose metabolism in most organs like the brain, heart, and visceral structures is closely coupled to blood flow. In some malignancies, such as breast cancer,[9] there is an uncoupling of the flow-metabolism cycle with subsequent elevated glucose metabolism compared with surrounding normal tissue. This elevated glucose metabolic rate seems to be a vital mechanism needed to feed the various biological alterations that have transformed the host cell into a malignant one.

Sanjiv Gambhir, in his chapter on the quantitative assay development for PET,[10] directs his readers to pretend to be a molecule of FDG and then asks the readers to think about all of the different directions that they can go once they are injected into the body. If we play along with his thought experiment, we would begin our journey from the syringe into the bloodstream (plasma). Once in the blood, we would either leave the plasma space to enter the interstitium or travel in the blood to the kidneys, where we would be excreted because of our ^{18}F atom on the 2-carbon position of the deoxy-glucose molecule. If not excreted by the kidneys, we would be transported into the cell, and then we would proceed down the chemical reaction pathway of our journey. Once in the cell, most of us would be phosphorylated and chemically trapped by the glycolytic pathway and end up with our ^{18}F moiety decaying; some of us would be kicked back out of the cell into the interstitium, eventually migrating back into the bloodstream and kidneys. If we brought a PET scanner to take pictures of our journey, we would inevitably find that many of us are congregating in a tumor against a low background of FDG in host tissues due to the rapid clearance of FDG from the bloodstream and body.

When thought about in this way, we can begin to divide our journey into at least four different phases or spaces: (1) the vascular space, (2) the interstitial space, (3) the intracellular space, and (4) the FDG-6-phosphate (FDG-6-P) or glucose-6-phosphate (G-6-P) space. The concentration (or, more precisely, the mass) of FDG in each of these compartments can be accurately measured by the PET scanner through kinetic analysis for detailed quantitative PET imaging, a feature that is unique to this modality. As kinetic analysis is cumbersome in routine clinical practice, a semiquantitative estimate of FDG concentration also exists in the form of the standardized uptake value. The interested reader is referred to many excellent review articles on this subject.[11,12,13,14]

3.2.1 Similarities between Glucose and FDG

It is very fortunate, if not fortuitous, that FDG behaves very similarly, if not identically, to glucose in the first three phases or compartments of the journey. FDG is circulated in the blood like glucose (vascular space). It migrates from the plasma space into the interstitium similarly to glucose (interstitial space). It is transported into the cells (intracellular space) via facilitated transport (whether malignant or not) just like glucose, utilizing a family of glucose transport proteins (GLUT). Although there are approximately 13 GLUTs,[15] it is GLUT1 that is found in most noncardiac tissue, including tumors. This is important to remember because the translocation of GLUT1 from the cytosol to the cell membrane in tumors is an insulin-independent process, whereas GLUT4 (whose presence predominates on the cell membrane in myocytes) requires insulin for it to translocate on the cell membrane. This phenomenon helps explain why

one needs to either inject a patient with insulin to perform myocardial viability PET studies with FDG or give an exogenous glucose load (initiates a spike in endogenous insulin production) to drive the tracer into the myocytes; however, this is not required for oncology or neurology PET imaging.

Once glucose or FDG is internalized into the cell, it is acted upon by hexokinase II (HK II) in a similar way to glucose. HK II phosphorylates both glucose and FDG to G-6-P and FDG-6-P, respectively. Once in the G-6-P form, this moiety can be further degraded through the glycolysis or TCA cycle to produce ATP for cellular energy and metabolism. However, FDG-6-P cannot undergo further metabolism. Furthermore, the negative charge from the phosphate group on FDG-6-P serves to trap it in the cell. Because cancer cells metabolize more glucose than host cells, they will accumulate more FDG, thus paving the way for detection on PET (▶ Fig. 3.1).

This difference in glucose metabolism between host cells and cancer cells is not the only explanation for elevated FDG-6-P activity in the malignant cell. Some cells, such as hepatocytes, have increased glucose-6-phosphatase activity (G-6-Pase). This enzyme is responsible for dephosphorylating both G-6-P and FDG-6-P back into their respective native forms, which then allows them to diffuse back out of the cell. Indeed, some tumors, such as low-grade hepatocellular carcinomas, have increased G-6-Pase, which might account for their low metabolic potential (relative lack of FDG accumulation; see the next section).[16]

3.3 FDG Activity in Different Cells, Tissues, Organs, and Bodies

The presence of FDG in a particular cell, tissue, or organ—and even in the whole body—is dependent on multiple factors and cannot be simplified to a single mechanism. Much of the FDG uptake, however, is dependent on the balance of local factors and the metabolic behavior occurring at the organ and whole-body level.

3.3.1 Cellular Level

At the cellular level, the following components have been implicated in promoting elevated FDG uptake in malignant cells compared with host cells.
1. Increased vascular tumor flow → more tracer is available for uptake.
2. Increased GLUT1 on the cellular membrane → more FDG movement into the cell.

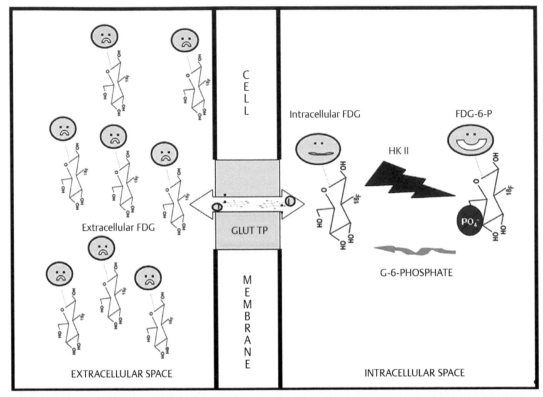

Fig. 3.1 Metabolism of [fluorine 18]fluorodeoxyglucose ([^{18}F]FDG). Cartoon depicts the metabolism of FDG at a very basic level. FDG (stick figure in cartoon with blue head and FDG backbone body) in the extracellular space is taken up by the cell via facilitated transport through the glucose transport protein (GLUT). There are at least 13 different types of GLUTs. GLUT1 is the prominent protein that is responsible for most of the FDG uptake in malignant and many inflammatory cells. Once in the cytosol, FDG is phosphorylated by hexokinase II [HK II] to form FDG-6-P. The FDG-6-P is essentially trapped in the cytosol of the cell and cannot either participate further in metabolism or diffuse out of the cell due to the negative charge on the phosphate group. A small fraction of the intracellular FDG-6-P can be dephosphorylated back to FDG by the action of glucose-6-phosphatase. This "free" fraction of FDG can diffuse back out of the cell via GLUT. It is the relative balance of these processes that determines the overall FDG activity in a cell.

3. More HK II → more FDG-6-P production, leading to metabolic trapping of FDG in cancer cells.
4. Reduced G-6-Pase → less intracellular dephosphorylation of FDG-6-P and less egress of FDG activity out of the malignant cell.

All these different mechanisms contribute to FDG uptake in tumors, making PET very sensitive for many tumor types; however, these processes also occur in nonmalignant tissues. For example, inflammatory cells also demonstrate increased GLUT1, which can simulate malignancy when associated FDG uptake is intense.[17] The inflammatory-type uptake has been especially noted in macrophages, neutrophils, histiocytes, and lymphocytes. As noted before, some tumors have higher than average G-6-Pase compared with other tumors, which favors egress of FDG activity out of the cell and, subsequently, diminished lesion conspicuity on the PET scan. In short, the mechanism for increased glucose metabolism can be different for different cells. Thus, FDG uptake can be dependent on blood flow (cardiac tissue), HK II activity (most tumors), and dephosphorylating activity (brain tissue and hepatocytes).[18,19]

3.3.2 Tissue Level

At the tissue level, FDG uptake is closely linked to the number of viable cells, proliferation activity, tissue perfusion (or neovascularity), hypoxia, and presence of inflammatory cells.[20,21,22] It is the balance of these factors that can control the overall

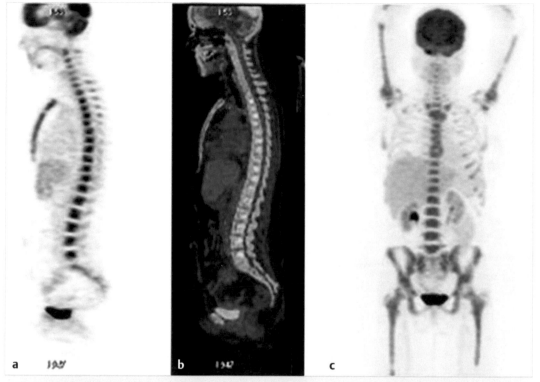

Fig. 3.2 Robust [fluorine 18]fluorodeoxyglucose ([18F]FDG) uptake in the marrow space due to stimulation from colony-stimulating factor therapy. This figure illustrates how FDG metabolism can be influenced at the organ level by multiple factors, including iatrogenically induced conditions. **(a)** A sagittal image showing the intense uptake of FDG activity in the bone marrow. **(b)** A positron emission tomography/computed tomography (PET/CT) fusion image. **(c)** A maximum intensity projection (MIP) of a whole-body scan. An MIP is a computer rendering technique that allows the interpreter to view the PET images in a three-dimensional fashion.

activity and even heterogeneity of FDG activity in the tissue. For example, some early studies demonstrated a significant FDG accumulation in macrophages and granulation tissue over the tumor cells in patients with non–small cell lung cancers.[23] Finally, there is some preliminary evidence that endothelial cells in tumor vessels can have enhanced FDG metabolism and account for some of the FDG activity observed on PET scans.[24]

3.3.3 Organ Level

At the organ level, the amount of FDG uptake is closely linked to organ perfusion, tumor volume, intrinsic glucose metabolism, and presence of inflammatory responses such as concurrent chemotherapy and radiation therapy or stimulated glucose metabolic activity from the use of medications (e.g., colony-stimulating factors) (▶ Fig. 3.2). In addition, some tumors, such as well-differentiated thyroid and prostate cancers, have FDG

uptake based on their endocrine responsiveness. As these tumors dedifferentiate, their hormone responsiveness decreases, while their FDG uptake increases and is an indicator of poor prognosis.[25,26]

3.3.4 Whole-Body Level

On a systemic or whole-body level, the amount of endogenous blood glucose can affect FDG uptake. For example, circulating glucose in the setting of hyperglycemia (blood glucose levels > 200 mg/dL) can effectively compete at the cellular level for FDG uptake, thus reducing the overall uptake of FDG.[27] Patients who have exercised within 24 hours of their scan, who recently consumed food or liquid calories, or who arrive in the PET centers intoxicated will have FDG uptake driven preferentially into the skeletal muscles rather than tumors, thus reducing the sensitivity of FDG PET. Also, diabetic patients who have administered short-acting insulin within 3 to 4 hours prior to FDG

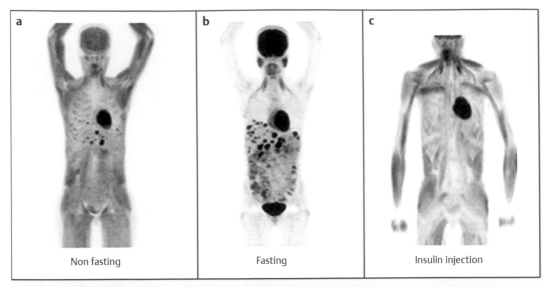

Fig. 3.3 The influence of glucose, insulin, and proper patient preparation on positron emission tomography (PET) scan quality. Maximum intensity projection (MIP) images from different patients are shown. PET scans **(a)** and **(b)** demonstrate two studies in the same patient obtained at different times 1 week apart. They show a 37-year-old with a stage IV gastrointestinal stroma tumor who claimed adherence to a 4-hour fast prior to [fluorine 18]fluorodeoxyglucose ([18F]FDG) **(a)**. On further questioning, the patient recalled eating 1 hour before arriving at the PET/CT center. **(b)** PET scan shows the MIP from the repeat study, with the patient having undergone a true 4-hour fast. On both occasions, the patient's blood glucose level was normal before FDG injection. Note that the MIP in **(a)** has extensive FDG uptake in the skeletal muscles and heart (presumably due to increased GLUT4 transport protein), with a relative paucity of activity in the brain, hepatic metastases, and urinary tract system compared with **(b)**. This case underlies the need for proper patient preparation for accurate interpretation and illustrates how endogenous insulin release from eating can quickly alter FDG uptake and metabolism. **(c)** MIP image from a separate patient who failed to tell the technologist that he self-administered 5 units of Humulin (Eli Lilly & Co., Indianapolis, IN) 1 hour prior to FDG injection. Notice how similar the MIP image in **(a)** is to **(c)**. Tumor metabolic uptake is reduced in this setting, rendering the study nondiagnostic. Current recommendations suggest at least a 3- to 4-hour hiatus between short-acting insulin dosing and FDG injection for oncologic imaging.

injection will have preferential uptake of activity in their muscles because of the stimulation of GLUT4 (▶ Fig. 3.3). In general, FDG administration should be delayed for about 3 to 4 hours post insulin administration to reduce this skeletal-dominant pattern of uptake for oncology PET scans. Cardiac activity can also be altered based on both dietary and fasting states and insulin levels. In particular, high protein and fat diets consumed the night before an exam can reduce cardiac activity by favoring fatty acid metabolism in the myocytes over glucose metabolism. Finally, the mental state of a patient or cold weather can drive FDG into brown fat deposits in the neck and chest and neuronally activated tissue along the spine.[28] Even in warm states like Arizona, brown fat uptake can be highly stimulated when a patient enters an air-conditioned, 72 °F imaging center environment after walking through 120 °F heat from the parking lot to the facility (▶ Fig. 3.4). An awareness of all of these variables can assist the clinician in optimizing PET scan acquisition parameters and interpretation.

Molecular Interactions in the Cellular and Tumor Microenvironment that Promote Glucose Metabolism and FDG Uptake

Cancer has a "molecular sweet tooth"[6] that can be traced to various biological changes that occur at the cellular level during host cell malignant transformation. In addition to activating the Warburg effect, these cellular alterations can result in a series of modifications in the biology of the tumor cell, which can assist tumor survival in a relatively hostile host environment, lead to

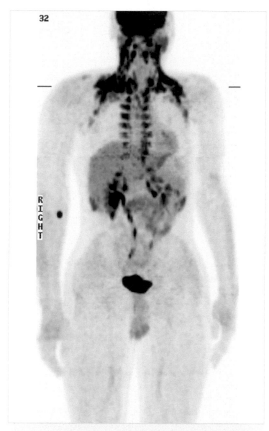

Fig. 3.4 Maximum intensity projection image showing fluorodeoxyglucose (FDG) uptake in brown fat. Note the extensive metabolism in the neck and paraspinal area from neuronal activation of brown fat deposits in these locations. The study was obtained in July when the outside temperature in Scottsdale, Arizona, was 116 °F, but ambient temperature was a pleasant 71 °F in the injection bay. Such climate changes can alter FDG uptake and metabolism. Keeping the patient warm and comfortable prior to injection can reduce such activity.

multidrug resistance and metastasis, and promote the suppression of programmed cellular death (apoptosis). In this section, we will provide an elementary understanding of the altered biological pathways, which will help explain why FDG is such an ideal tracer for tumor imaging. The reader is encouraged to consult an excellent review on this subject for more details.[29]

3.3.5 Hypoxic Environment

Many tumors exist in a relatively hostile environment of dysfunctional tumor perfusion, low pH, and hypoxia.[2] Their adaptation to this environment

is therefore critical for survival and metastasis. Central to tumor survival might be a protein called hypoxia induction factor 1 (HIF-1). HIF-1 is a heterodimer composed of two protein subunits—α and β. In hypoxic conditions, HIF-1α is stabilized, and the HIF-1 heterodimer is reinforced. This stabilization of the HIF-1 protein can lead to the direct production of GLUT1 and HK II. In addition, HIF-1 stimulates the manufacture of vascular endothelial growth factor, which promotes tumor neovascularity. As a result, glucose metabolism is increased by enhanced substrate delivery to the tumor via developing neovascularity, elevated glucose (or FDG) flux into the tumor cells due to transactivation of GLUT1, and ultimately higher metabolic activity because of greater HK II–dependent conversion of glucose to G-6-P (or FDG-6-P).[30] As elegant as this process sounds, it is clearly not the entire story and does not fully account for the Warburg effect.

3.3.6 Aerobic Glycolysis

For aerobic glycolysis to occur, oxidative phosphorylation in the mitochondria has to be reduced, and the metabolism of glucose into pyruvate and lactic acid needs to be enhanced, even when oxygen is plentiful. Many alterations in the transformed cell biology promote aerobic glycolysis by accentuating the effects of HIF-1. For example, several oncogene and/or tumor suppressor gene products help stabilize HIF-1, prevent its degradation, or increase its production. These include *Src* oncogene, *H-Ras*, phosphatidylinositol 3-kinase, *VHL*, *SDH*, and *FH* mutations. However, not all the changes that occur in a cancer cell favor the bolstering of HIF-1 protein. For example, activation of the serine-threonine kinase *AKT* can lead to increased aerobic glycolysis by affecting glucose transport and HK II activity directly, independent of HIF-1.

So, how does one explain the Warburg effect of aerobic glycolysis? Ultimately for this to occur, glucose metabolism will require a switchover from the TCA cycle to glycolysis. Although not fully understood, it appears that the *MYC* oncogene found in many tumors is key to this change: it enhances mitochondrial production, which eventually creates more reactive oxygen species or radicals. As a result, these oxygen radicals can induce local mitochondrial DNA damage, resulting in mitochondrial dysfunction. This process, compounded by the action of the p53 protein found in most tumor cells and several other enzymes involved in the TCA cycle, will favor a switch from oxidative phosphorylation to lactic acid production, leading to dwindling mitochondrial function. Thus, oncogene activation (*AKT*, *MYC*, *H-Ras*, etc.) along with HIF-1 stabilization can lead to the immortalization of the cancer cell and activate those changes that Warburg observed over 80 years ago.[6,7]

3.4 New Therapies Based on Glycolytic Metabolism

Altered cellular metabolism is one of the main hallmarks of cancer. Tumors can utilize a variety of catabolites to feed the demand for energy and reduction-oxidation (redox) control and to generate biomass. Beginning with Warburg's original speculations that tumorigenesis is the result of mitochondrial dysfunction to the current concepts of oncogenic and tumor suppression-guided activation of a variety of metabolic pathways, many investigators are refocusing their attention on disabling metabolism as a strategy to design cancer therapy. The details of the druggable targets are beyond the scope of this chapter but the reader is directed to an excellent review on cancer metabolism.[31] However, glucose metabolism is not the only target being considered. Among the intriguing approaches either currently in trials or under consideration is the use of biological agents that target the enzymes of glycolysis, lactate secretion and uptake, hydrogen ion excretions, TCA cycle, oxidative phosphorylation, glutamine metabolism, fatty acid oxidation, lipid synthesis, mevalonate pathways, pentose phosphate, and nucleic acid and amino acid metabolism. As a result of this molecularly driven approach to strangulate the energy supply, PET scans especially using FDG will continue to play a pivotal role in assessment of treatment responses for these novel therapies.

3.5 Summary

Aerobic glycolysis as observed by Otto Warburg in the 1930s has come full circle. The central role of FDG in probing this pathway has made it an almost ideal tracer for cancer detection in PET. Although several benign and inflammatory conditions share elevated glucose metabolism with tumor cells, FDG remains one of the best agents available for cancer imaging. The mechanism of FDG metabolism in tumor cells has been explored in this chapter in a most elementary fashion to give the clinician the flavor of the molecular sweet tooth of

a cancer cell and a basic understanding of the meaning of "hot spots" on FDG PET scans. Although aerobic glycolysis might not cause cellular malignant transformation, it is clear that it is necessary to facilitate the cancerous state. Such adaptive responses by the tumor to the host cell can trigger tumor survival, multidrug resistance, and suppression of programmed cell death. Strategies that disrupt the Warburg effect are therefore of top priority in the development of therapeutic agents that can target these survival mechanisms of a cancer cell.

References

[1] Warburg O, Posener K, Negelein E. VIII. The metabolism of cancer cells. Biochem Z. 1924; 152:129–169

[2] Gatenby RA, Gillies RJ. Why do cancers have high aerobic glycolysis? Nat Rev Cancer. 2004; 4(11):891–899

[3] Izuishi K, Kato K, Ogura T, Kinoshita T, Esumi H. Remarkable tolerance of tumor cells to nutrient deprivation: possible new biochemical target for cancer therapy. Cancer Res. 2000; 60(21):6201–6207

[4] Graeber TG, Osmanian C, Jacks T, et al. Hypoxia-mediated selection of cells with diminished apoptotic potential in solid tumours. Nature. 1996; 379(6560):88–91

[5] Gatenby RA, Gawlinski ET, Gmitro AF, Kaylor B, Gillies RJ. Acid-mediated tumor invasion: a multidisciplinary study. Cancer Res. 2006; 66(10):5216–5223

[6] Kim JW, Dang CV. Cancer's molecular sweet tooth and the Warburg effect. Cancer Res. 2006; 66(18):8927–8930

[7] Dang CV. Role of MYC and HIF in the Warburg effect and tumorigenesis. Paper presented at: American Association for Cancer Research Annual Meeting; April 14, 2007

[8] Bomanji JB, Costa DC, Ell PJ. Clinical role of positron emission tomography in oncology. Lancet Oncol. 2001; 2(3):157–164

[9] Tseng J, Dunnwald LK, Schubert EK, et al. 18F-FDG kinetics in locally advanced breast cancer: correlation with tumor blood flow and changes in response to neoadjuvant chemotherapy. J Nucl Med. 2004; 45(11):1829–1837

[10] Gambhir SS. Quantitative assay development for PET. In: Phelps ME, ed. PET: Molecular Imaging and Its Biological Applications. New York, NY: Springer-Verlag; 2004:125–216

[11] Weber WA, Schwaiger M, Avril N. Quantitative assessment of tumor metabolism using FDG-PET imaging. Nucl Med Biol. 2000; 27(7):683–687

[12] Keyes JW, Jr. SUV: standard uptake or silly useless value? J Nucl Med. 1995; 36(10):1836–1839

[13] Huang SC. Anatomy of SUV. Standardized uptake value. Nucl Med Biol. 2000; 27(7):643–646

[14] Mankoff DA, Muzi M, Krohn KA. Quantitative positron emission tomography imaging to measure tumor response to therapy: what is the best method? Mol Imaging Biol. 2003; 5 (5):281–285

[15] Wood IS, Trayhurn P. Glucose transporters (GLUT and SGLT): expanded families of sugar transport proteins. Br J Nutr. 2003; 89(1):3–9

[16] Torizuka T, Tamaki N, Inokuma T, et al. In vivo assessment of glucose metabolism in hepatocellular carcinoma with FDG-PET. J Nucl Med. 1995; 36(10):1811–1817

[17] Chung JH, Cho KJ, Lee SS, et al. Overexpression of Glut1 in lymphoid follicles correlates with false-positive (18)F-FDG

PET results in lung cancer staging. J Nucl Med. 2004; 45(6): 999–1003

[18] Phelps ME, Huang SC, Hoffman EJ, Selin C, Sokoloff L, Kuhl DE. Tomographic measurement of local cerebral glucose metabolic rate in humans with (F-18)2-fluoro-2-deoxy-D-glucose: validation of method. Ann Neurol. 1979; 6(5): 371–388

[19] Reivich M, Kuhl D, Wolf A, et al. The [18F]fluorodeoxyglucose method for the measurement of local cerebral glucose utilization in man. Circ Res. 1979; 44(1):127–137

[20] Brown RS, Leung JY, Fisher SJ, Frey KA, Ethier SP, Wahl RL. Intratumoral distribution of tritiated-FDG in breast carcinoma: correlation between Glut-1 expression and FDG uptake. J Nucl Med. 1996; 37(6):1042–1047

[21] Higashi K, Clavo AC, Wahl RL. Does FDG uptake measure proliferative activity of human cancer cells? In vitro comparison with DNA flow cytometry and tritiated thymidine uptake. J Nucl Med. 1993; 34(3):414–419

[22] Brown RS, Leung JY, Fisher SJ, Frey KA, Ethier SP, Wahl RL. Intratumoral distribution of tritiated fluorodeoxyglucose in breast carcinoma: I. Are inflammatory cells important? J Nucl Med. 1995; 36(10):1854–1861

[23] Kubota R, Yamada S, Kubota K, Ishiwata K, Tamahashi N, Ido T. Intratumoral distribution of fluorine-18-fluorodeoxyglucose in vivo: high accumulation in macrophages and granulation tissues studied by microautoradiography. J Nucl Med. 1992; 33(11):1972–1980

[24] Maschauer S, Prante O, Hoffmann M, Deichen JT, Kuwert T. Characterization of 18F-FDG uptake in human endothelial cells in vitro. J Nucl Med. 2004; 45(3):455–460

[25] Morris MJ, Akhurst T, Osman I, et al. Fluorinated deoxyglucose positron emission tomography imaging in progressive metastatic prostate cancer. Urology. 2002; 59(6):913–918

[26] Wang W, Larson SM, Tuttle RM, et al. Resistance of [18f]-fluorodeoxyglucose-avid metastatic thyroid cancer lesions to treatment with high-dose radioactive iodine. Thyroid. 2001; 11(12):1169–1175

[27] Lindholm P, Minn H, Leskinen-Kallio S, Bergman J, Ruotsalainen U, Joensuu H. Influence of the blood glucose concentration on FDG uptake in cancer–a PET study. J Nucl Med. 1993; 34(1):1–6

[28] Hany TF, Gharehpapagh E, Kamel EM, Buck A, Himms-Hagen J, von Schulthess GK. Brown adipose tissue: a factor to consider in symmetrical tracer uptake in the neck and upper chest region. Eur J Nucl Med Mol Imaging. 2002; 29(10):1393–1398

[29] Mankoff DA, Eary JF, Link JM, et al. Tumor-specific positron emission tomography imaging in patients: [18F] fluorodeoxyglucose and beyond. Clin Cancer Res. 2007; 13(12):3460–3469

[30] Bos R, van Der Hoeven JJ, van Der Wall E, et al. Biologic correlates of (18)fluorodeoxyglucose uptake in human breast cancer measured by positron emission tomography. J Clin Oncol. 2002; 20(2):379–387

[31] Martinez-Outschoorn UE, Peiris-Pagés M, Pestell RG, Sotgia F, Lisanti MP. Cancer metabolism: a therapeutic perspective. Nat Rev Clin Oncol. 2017; 14(1):11–31

Part II

Clinical Basics

4 Patient Preparation   28

5 Standardized Uptake Value   36

6 Quantitative Whole-Body PET/
   CT Imaging   42

7 Normal Variants and Benign
   Findings   51

8 Interpretation of FDG PET
   Studies   89

9 PET/CT   98

10 PET/MRI: Introduction to
   Clinical Applications   109

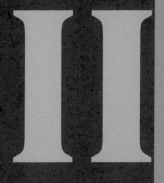

4 Patient Preparation

Eugene C. Lin

4.1 Introduction

Proper patient preparation prior to and during the positron emission tomography (PET) study is important to ensure maximum diagnostic yield. The most important factors are glucose level, minimizing effects of physiologic activity, and timing of the study.

4.2 Oncological PET Patient Preparation

4.2.1 Diet and Blood Glucose Levels

1. **Effects of elevated blood glucose levels**. Elevated blood glucose levels can potentially decrease FDG uptake in malignant tumors due to competitive saturation of glucose transporters by unlabeled glucose. In addition, increased insulin secondary to elevated blood glucose increases fludeoxyglucose (FDG) uptake in tissues with a high density of insulin-sensitive GLUT4 glucose transporter such as the skeletal muscle and heart, resulting in altered biodistribution of FDG and suboptimal image quality.
2. **Acceptable glucose levels**. There are no evidence-based standards for acceptable glucose levels prior to FDG PET/computed tomography (CT).
   a) In surveys,[1,2] the majority of institutions do not perform PET/CT at blood glucose levels above 200 mg/dL.
   European Association of Nuclear Medicine (EANM) guidelines[3] suggest that PET/CT should not be performed at blood glucose levels above 200 mg/dL.
   National Cancer Institute (NCI) guidelines[4] suggest a blood glucose cutoff of < 120 mg/dL for nondiabetic patients, and 150 to 200 mg/dL for diabetic patients.
3. **Acute hyperglycemia versus chronic hyperglycemia**. It should be noted that the effect of elevated blood glucose levels on FDG uptake has been demonstrated primarily in cases of acute hyperglycemia in nondiabetic patients. Chronic hyperglycemia in diabetic patients may have less of an effect on tumor

FDG uptake. Several studies[5,6,7,8] showed that chronic hyperglycemia and diabetes mellitus had minimal or no effect on tumor FDG uptake in most cases. Given these findings, higher glucose levels may be acceptable for diabetic patients undergoing FDG PET/CT compared to nondiabetic patients.
   a) Chronic hyperglycemia may have more effect on smaller lesions[7] and in posttreatment studies.[6]
   b) *Pancreatic adenocarcinoma*. Diabetes does decrease FDG uptake in patients with pancreatic adenocarcinoma, even in normoglycemic diabetics.[9]
   c) *Brain uptake*. In general, chronic hyperglycemia will decrease brain FDG uptake, and increase muscular FDG uptake, while FDG uptake in other organs is not significantly affected.[5,10] FDG uptake in the brain has an inverse relationship with plasma glucose levels, even in the normoglycemic range.[11]
4. **Diet**. The purpose of fasting is to ensure low blood glucose and insulin levels. The patient should be fasting, except for plain water, for at least 4 hours prior to the exam, although many sites recommend at least a 6-hour fast.[2]
   a) If there is known or suspected thoracic pathology, fasting for at least 12 hours is desirable to minimize cardiac activity.
   b) Many sites ask patients to follow a low-carbohydrate/high-protein diet prior to the exam. This diet should be followed for at least 24 hours before the exam. However, it is not known how effective this diet is in improving the quality or reproducibility of PET/CT studies.[2]
   c) Parenteral nutrition and intravenous fluids containing glucose should be discontinued for at least 4 hours before FDG injection.
   d) Many sites recommend that caffeine, nicotine, and alcohol should be avoided for 12 to 24 hours before the exam.
      • Caffeine can have a variable effect on cardiac uptake; it can increase uptake, or stimulate myocardial fatty acid metabolism and decrease FDG uptake.[12]
5. **Hydration**. Hydration, along with frequent voiding, reduces bladder radiation dose and may improve image quality by reducing urinary artifact. In addition, effective hydration can

reduce background FDG activity in the soft tissues.[13]

a) Oral prehydration (e.g., 1 liter of water in the 2 hours prior to the scan) and continued hydration after the scan is recommended.[3]

b) Intravenous hydration may be more useful but less frequently employed. If intravenous hydration is used, the fluid should not contain dextrose or lactose.

6. **Diabetic patients**. If needed, the physician managing the patient should be consulted for lowering blood glucose levels.

a) Type I diabetes and insulin-dependent type II diabetes. EANM guidelines[3] suggest three options:

- The patient should eat a normal breakfast and inject the normal amount of insulin, with nothing except water afterward, and the PET scan should be performed late morning or midday. FDG injection should occur at least 4 hours after subcutaneous injection of rapid-acting insulin or 6 hours after short-acting insulin. This protocol should not be used for intermediate or long-acting insulin.

- Patients receiving intermediate or long-acting insulin administered in the evening can be imaged early morning after an overnight fast, and then eat a normal breakfast and inject insulin after the scan. Ideally, this protocol should be performed with an intermediate-acting insulin, as a long-acting insulin still has the potential to interfere with the PET/CT scan.

- Patients on continuous insulin infusion should switch off the pump at least 4 hours prior to FDG administration, be scheduled early morning, and eat breakfast after the PET, switching the insulin infusion back on at that time.

b) *Type II diabetes controlled by oral medication*. Patients should continue to take oral medication and comply with normal fasting guidelines, and the PET should be performed, if possible, late morning.

7. **Insulin administration**. Insulin administration will increase FDG uptake in the heart, skeletal muscles, and liver (the same pattern is seen if the patient has eaten before FDG administration). This will degrade image quality and therefore the ability to detect lesions (▶ Fig. 4.1). However, insulin can be administered before PET/CT to lower blood glucose levels (e.g., in diabetics or in patients

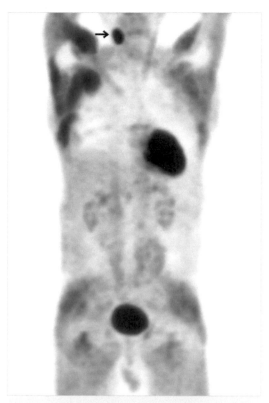

Fig. 4.1 Effects of insulin release on FDG uptake. A patient with lymphoma did not follow instructions and ate 1 hour before the exam. Increased uptake is present in the skeletal muscle and heart with minimal activity elsewhere. An abnormal cervical node is seen (*arrow*), but this exam should be repeated as disease elsewhere could be missed.

taking glucocorticoids) if there is a sufficient interval between insulin administration and FDG injection.

a) *Intravenous insulin*. Short-acting intravenous insulin can be administered before PET/CT to lower blood glucose, with an interval ranging from 30 to 90 minutes prior to FDG injection in different protocols.[14]

b) *Subcutaneous insulin*. EANM guidelines[3] suggest that if insulin administration is necessary, a rapid-acting insulin should be administered subcutaneously with an interval between insulin administration and FDG injection of at least 4 hours.

8. **Metformin**. Metformin treatment can increase bowel FDG uptake (▶ Fig. 4.2), primarily in the colon, with a lesser effect in the small bowel.

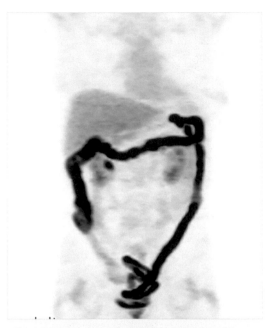

Fig. 4.2 Metformin-induced bowel uptake. MIP PET scan demonstrates intense colonic FDG uptake in a patient taking metformin.

This uptake can be diffused, multifocal, or nodular,[15] and could potentially mask a malignant lesion, or result in false-positive finding.

a) Discontinuing metformin 2 days prior to the study is effective in reducing the high intestinal uptake.[15] Discontinuation of metformin could interfere with optimal glycemic control prior to the study. However, in one study,[15] discontinuation of metformin 2 days prior to the PET study did not result in significant changes to blood glucose levels.

b) Bowel lavages are not effective in reducing the increased FDG uptake induced by metformin.[16]

9. Other antidiabetic drugs

a) Sulfonylureas lower plasma glucose primarily by stimulating insulin secretion and should not be taken the morning of the FDG PET/CT study. Another reason to avoid sulfonylureas the morning of the PET/CT study is that they can potentially cause hypoglycemia in fasting diabetic patients.

b) Insulin sensitizers, such as rosiglitazone and pioglitazone, should not affect FDG uptake since their mode of action is primarily

activation of peroxisome proliferator-activated receptors; they do not need to be withheld before a PET/CT study.[14]

4.2.2 Minimization of Physiologic Uptake

Physiologic uptake in muscle, brown fat, the urinary tract, and bowel can obscure or mimic disease.

1. **Muscle uptake.**

a) The patient should avoid strenuous exercise for at least 6 hours (preferably 24 hours) before the PET scan.

b) Muscle relaxants such as diazepam are helpful in reducing muscle uptake from stress. Note that diazepam may be helpful in reducing brown fat uptake as well.

- Pretreatment with diazepam could be considered for all patients with suspicion of cervical and supraclavicular nodal disease, because muscular uptake is most common in these regions.

c) Laryngeal muscle uptake can be minimized by instructing the patient not to talk 5 minutes before and 20 minutes after the injection.

2. **Brown fat uptake (see Chapter 7).** Brown fat uptake can be limited by decreasing adrenergic stimulation. This can be achieved by pharmacologic intervention and/or limiting patient exposure to cold temperatures.

a) Pharmacologic interventions

- *Diazepam.* Diazepam (e.g., 5 mg of intravenous diazepam administered 10 minutes prior to FDG) may decrease brown fat uptake (brown fat has benzodiazepine receptors, and in addition diazepam may decrease general sympathetic activity).
  - *Oral diazepam.* However, there have been several reports, including one randomized controlled trial,[17] that did not find a beneficial effect of oral diazepam. Intravenous diazepam[18] may be more effective.
- *Other drugs.* Administration of propranolol (20–80 mg of oral propranolol 1–2 hours before FDG administration)[14] has been shown to decrease brown fat uptake. Resperine has also been shown to decrease brown fat uptake.
  - Resperine and propranolol also decrease cardiac activity.

- *Drugs to avoid*: Drugs that stimulate the sympathetic nervous system (e.g., nicotine and ephedrine) can potentially increase brown fat uptake and should be avoided prior to the study if possible.

  b) **Minimizing exposure to cold temperature.** FDG uptake in brown fat is more common in the winter months, but has also been visualized on PET scans after cold exposures for short periods of time, ranging from 1 to 2 days to several hours before the scan.[19] Patients should dress warmly and avoid cold temperature for 48 hours before the scan. Also patients should be kept warm between injection and imaging.[20] Temperature control may be helpful even when pharmacologic intervention is unsuccessful.

3. **Urinary activity.** Reduction of urinary FDG activity can be helpful. The role of intervention to reduce urinary artifacts depends on the pathology being evaluated. Collecting system activity can mimic or obscure renal neoplasms (▶ Fig. 24.3). Reducing ureteral activity is helpful for evaluating retroperitoneal nodes (▶ Fig. 23.2). Reduction of bladder activity is important for evaluating pelvic pathology and nodes (▶ Fig. 24.9). However, in most circumstances, additional intervention is usually not necessary, particularly if the cancer being evaluated does not have a propensity for pelvic or retroperitoneal metastases.

   The easiest method to minimize bladder activity is to ask the patient to void prior to imaging and acquire the images caudocranially. This is adequate for most oncological PET applications. In specific cases (e.g., evaluation of pelvic nodes in patients with cervical cancer), specific interventions may be helpful. Two general methods are placement of a bladder catheter with or without bladder irrigation and a combination of a diuretic and hydration.

   a) ***Bladder catheterization***. Placement of a bladder catheter to drainage will greatly reduce bladder activity and decrease radiation dose to the bladder. However, even a small amount residual urine with intense activity can cause difficulty in interpretation near the bladder. If a double-lumen Foley catheter is used, warm normal saline can be injected into the bladder to dilute the radioactive urine. However, bladder irrigation can increase radiation to the staff and has a risk of infection.[21] Catheter placement has the disadvantage of adding an invasive component to a noninvasive study.

   b) ***Hydration/diuretics***. Hydration and diuretics dilute urine activity and also result in more frequent voiding. Diuretic administration has a potential additional advantage over hydration alone: both hydration and diuretics increase urine volume, but hydration can also increase FDG delivery to the bladder (potentially offsetting the value of increased voiding).[22] The most effective protocols combine intravenous hydration with furosemide administration.[13] However, oral hydration in combination with furosemide is still effective.[23]
   - Dosages of furosemide vary from 10 to 40 mg, with 10 to 20 mg the most common range.[13,23]
   - Patient tolerance may be improved if the furosemide is administered earlier (e.g., 15 minutes after FDG injection), rather than 15 minutes before imaging.[24]

4. **Bowel activity.** Bowel activity is primarily seen in the cecum, right colon, and rectosigmoid and to a lesser extent in the remaining colon and small bowel. Bowel activity is due to activity in both the wall and lumen. Diffuse bowel uptake typically does not present diagnostic difficulties as it is usually a normal variant if the corresponding CT images are normal. However, focal areas of physiologic bowel uptake can potentially mimic pathology. Several methods have been used to attempt to reduce bowel activity. However, many of these methods are of questionable effectiveness and some may be difficult to implement in practice.

   a) Bowel preparation may irritate the colon and lead to increased FDG uptake.[25,26]
   b) A low-residue diet does not decrease bowel activity.[26]
   c) There is conflicting evidence on the effectiveness of reducing bowel activity.[27,28]
   d) Administration of glucagon or oral spasmolytic medications (e.g., mebeverine) to decrease peristalsis is typically not helpful.[29]

4.2.3 PET Scan Timing

1. **Postbiopsy**: At least 1 week (▶ Fig. 4.3).
2. **Postsurgery**: 6 weeks (EANM guidelines)[3]
   a) Should be adjusted based on the invasiveness of the procedure.

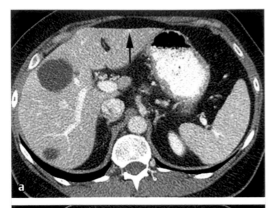

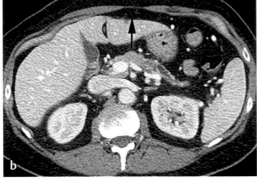

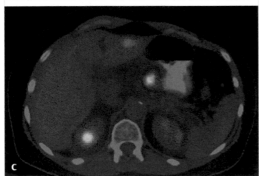

Fig. 4.3 Postbiopsy FDG uptake. **(a)** Axial contrast-enhanced CT in a patient with pancreatic adenocarcinoma demonstrates a tiny hypervascular lesion at the surface of the left lobe of the liver (*arrow*). This was surgically biopsied and was a small hemangioma. **(b)** Axial contrast-enhanced CT performed 15 days after the surgery demonstrates a small area of hypodensity in the region of the biopsy (*arrow*). **(c)** Axial PET/CT performed 15 days after the surgery demonstrates increased FDG uptake in the region of the biopsy.

3. **Postradiofrequency ablation**: 4 weeks.[30]
4. **Postchemotherapy**: 10 days (EANM guidelines)[3] to 2 weeks (NCI guidelines).[4]

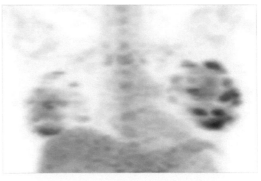

Fig. 4.4 FDG uptake in lactating breasts. MIP PET demonstrates increased FDG uptake in both breasts. This is related to suckling; however, there is little secretion of activity into breast milk.

5. **Postradiation**: 2 to 3 months (EANM guidelines)[3]
   a) Both chemotherapy and radiation can cause false-positive results (from inflammation) and false-negative results (from presumed "stunning" of viable tumor). Corticosteroids decrease the inflammatory response after chemotherapy.[31]
   b) Although the guidelines above can be used in general practice, it should be noted that there is a wide range of values in published literature, and false-positive/false-negative results have been reported up to 3 months postchemotherapy[32] and 5 months postradiation.[33] One study[34] suggests that PET can be accurately performed 1 month after radiotherapy of head and neck cancer. Baseline studies should be performed before initiation of chemotherapy because FDG uptake can be decreased even 1 day after start of chemotherapy.[35]
6. Post–granulocyte colony stimulating factor (G-CSF): At least 2 weeks (EANM guidelines)[3]
   a) The reported time interval after cessation of G-CSF necessary to avoid increased uptake due to the stimulation is variable, ranging from 5 days to 1 month (see hapter 7).[36,37]

4.2.4 Breast Feeding

1. There is high activity in the lactating breast related to suckling (▶ Fig. 4.4). However, most of the radiation dose to the baby from breastfeeding is from proximity to the mother as there is little FDG excretion into breast milk.[38]

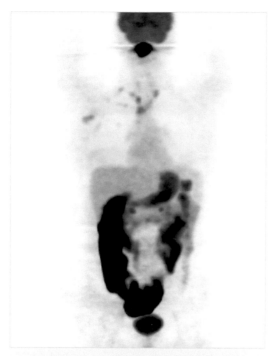

Fig. 4.5 Oral FDG administration. Coronal PET scan performed with oral FDG administration has substantial oral and bowel activity but adequate FDG uptake. (This image is provided courtesy of Bruce Higginbotham, MD, Seattle, WA.)

2. Contact between the mother and child should be limited for 12 hours after FDG injection. Breastfeeding should be withheld for 12 hours after injection to reduce the radiation dose from external exposure to radiation emitted by the mother. During this time, breast milk can be expressed and fed to the infant via bottle.[3]

4.2.5 Route of FDG Administration

FDG can be administered orally if intravenous access is not available (▶ Fig. 4.5). The same delay before imaging used with intravenous injection can be employed with oral administration.

4.3 Cardiac FDG PET Patient Preparation[39]

4.3.1 Myocardial Viability

The myocardium metabolizes free fatty acids in the fasting state. To image the myocardium specifically, the nutrient substrate must be switched to glucose. This can be achieved either by oral glucose loading or by hyperinsulinemic-euglycemic clamp. Another approach is to decrease myocardial fatty acid metabolism.

1. **Oral glucose loading**: 25 to 100 g of oral glucose can be administered prior to FDG injection.
   a) *Advantages*. Glucose loading is very easy to perform compared with the hyperinsulinemic-euglycemic clamp.
   b) *Disadvantages*. Image quality may be suboptimal, particularly in diabetic patients.
   c) *Diabetics*. Supplemental doses of short-acting insulin after oral glucose loading may be helpful in diabetic patients and patients with blood glucose > 110 mg/dL.
   d) *Glucose level*. Blood glucose level should be in the 100 to 130 mg/dL range at the time of FDG injection.
2. **Hyperinsulinemic-euglycemic clamp**: Insulin is infused for the duration of the study. Glucose is infused at the same time to maintain blood glucose at baseline levels (based on multiple blood glucose determinations).
   a) *Advantages*. Use of the clamp technique results in greater and more homogeneous myocardial uptake, particularly in diabetic patients.
   b) *Disadvantages*:
   • Time- and labor-intensive procedure.
   • Often requires supplemental potassium due to hypokalemia.
3. **Decreasing free fatty acid metabolism**: Niacin and acipimox (nicotinic acid derivatives) lower free fatty acid levels in plasma and therefore increase myocardial glucose uptake.
4. **General protocol**: Multisociety guidelines[40] suggest the following preparation protocol for cardiac viability studies:
   a) Patients should fast 6 to 12 hours. Blood glucose is checked. If fasting blood glucose is < 110 mg/dL and there is no known diabetes, an oral glucose load of 25 to 100 g is administered and glucose is monitored.
   b) Intravenous insulin is administered (ranging from 1 to 5 U depending on blood glucose) if fasting blood glucose is > 110 to 130 mg/dL, there is known diabetes, or blood glucose level 45 to 90 minutes after oral glucose loading is ≥ 130 mg/dL.
   c) Intravenous dextrose or 250 mg of oral acipimox can also be considered.

4.3.2 Sarcoidosis

FDG uptake in normal myocardium must be suppressed in order to accurately evaluate the myocardium for potential sarcoidosis. This can be achieved by lowering insulin levels to suppress glucose consumption by the myocardium, and/or increasing serum free fatty acids to promote myocardial free fatty acid consumption. Different methods have been used for patient preparation, including a high-fat, low-carbohydrate diet or low-carbohydrate diet followed by fasting of 4 to 12 hours, prolonged fasting (> 18 hours) with or without dietary restrictions, and increasing serum free fatty acids (e.g., by administering low-molecular-weight heparin). However, in one study[41] the use of heparin did not significantly reduce physiologic FDG uptake. In another report,[42] an 18-hour fast was more effective than a 12-hour fast with heparin loading in inhibiting myocardial uptake.

Japanese Society of Nuclear Cardiology guidelines[43] recommend a fasting time of at least 12 hours and a low-carbohydrate diet (less than 5 g) the night before the study. American multisociety guidelines[44] recommend avoidance of carbohydrates and at least two high-fat, high-protein meals beginning 24 hours prior to the test, with an overnight fast. This can potentially be combined with intravenous unfractionated heparin (10 IU/kg 30 minutes prior + 5 IU/kg 15 minutes prior or 50 IU/kg 15 minutes prior to radiotracer administration), although lower doses of intravenous heparin (15 IU/kg) may be effective. A systematic review[45] advocates at least two high-fat, no-carbohydrate meals followed by a fast of at least 4 hours. Intravenous heparin administered after at least one high-fat, no-carbohydrate meal and an overnight fast is likely as efficacious. Fasting alone was not recommended but at least 18 hours was suggested if the diet cannot be followed. Strategies such as verapamil administration and the addition of a high-fat drink within an hour of the scan were not recommended.

References

[1] Beyer T, Czernin J, Freudenberg LS. Variations in clinical PET/CT operations: results of an international survey of active PET/CT users. J Nucl Med. 2011; 52(2):303–310

[2] Graham MM, Badawi RD, Wahl RL. Variations in PET/CT methodology for oncologic imaging at U.S. academic medical centers: an imaging response assessment team survey. J Nucl Med. 2011; 52(2):311–317

[3] Boellaard R, Delgado-Bolton R, Oyen WJ, et al. European Association of Nuclear Medicine (EANM). FDG PET/CT: EANM procedure guidelines for tumour imaging: version 2.0. Eur J Nucl Med Mol Imaging. 2015; 42(2):328–354

[4] Shankar LK, Hoffman JM, Bacharach S, et al. National Cancer Institute. Consensus recommendations for the use of 18F-FDG PET as an indicator of therapeutic response in patients in National Cancer Institute Trials. J Nucl Med. 2006; 47(6):1059–1066

[5] Büsing KA, Schönberg SO, Brade J, Wasser K. Impact of blood glucose, diabetes, insulin, and obesity on standardized uptake values in tumors and healthy organs on 18F-FDG PET/CT. Nucl Med Biol. 2013; 40(2):206–213

[6] Haley M, Konski A, Li T, et al. Influence of diabetes on the interpretation of PET scans in patients with esophageal cancer. Gastrointest Cancer Res. 2009; 3(4):149–152

[7] Hara T, Higashi T, Nakamoto Y, et al. Significance of chronic marked hyperglycemia on FDG-PET: is it really problematic for clinical oncologic imaging? Ann Nucl Med. 2009; 23(7):657–669

[8] Oh DY, Kim JW, Koh SJ, et al. Does diabetes mellitus influence standardized uptake values of fluorodeoxyglucose positron emission tomography in colorectal cancer? Intest Res. 2014; 12(2):146–152

[9] Chung KH, Park JK, Lee SH, et al. Lower maximum standardized uptake value of fluorine-18 fluorodeoxyglucose positron emission tomography coupled with computed tomography imaging in pancreatic ductal adenocarcinoma patients with diabetes. Am J Surg. 2015; 209(4):709–716

[10] Lindholm H, Brolin F, Jonsson C, Jacobsson H. The relation between the blood glucose level and the FDG uptake of tissues at normal PET examinations. EJNMMI Res. 2013; 3(1):50–53

[11] Claeys J, Mertens K, D'Asseler Y, Goethals I. Normoglycemic plasma glucose levels affect F-18 FDG uptake in the brain. Ann Nucl Med. 2010; 24(6):501–505

[12] Cook GJ, Wegner EA, Fogelman I. Pitfalls and artifacts in 18FDG PET and PET/CT oncologic imaging. Semin Nucl Med. 2004; 34(2):122–133

[13] Ceriani L, Suriano S, Ruberto T, Giovanella L. Could different hydration protocols affect the quality of 18F-FDG PET/CT images? J Nucl Med Technol. 2011; 39(2):77–82

[14] Surasi DS, Bhambhvani P, Baldwin JA, Almodovar SE, O'Malley JP. 18F-FDG PET and PET/CT patient preparation: a review of the literature. J Nucl Med Technol. 2014; 42(1):5–13

[15] Oh JR, Song HC, Chong A, et al. Impact of medication discontinuation on increased intestinal FDG accumulation in diabetic patients treated with metformin. AJR Am J Roentgenol. 2010; 195(6):1404–1410

[16] Massollo M, Marini C, Brignone M, et al. Metformin temporal and localized effects on gut glucose metabolism assessed using 18F-FDG PET in mice. J Nucl Med. 2013; 54(2):259–266

[17] Sturkenboom MG, Hoekstra OS, Postema EJ, Zijlstra JM, Berkhof J, Franssen EJ. A randomised controlled trial assessing the effect of oral diazepam on 18F-FDG uptake in the neck and upper chest region. Mol Imaging Biol. 2009; 11(5):364–368

[18] Rakheja R, Ciarallo A, Alabed YZ, Hickeson M. Intravenous administration of diazepam significantly reduces brown fat activity on 18F-FDG PET/CT. Am J Nucl Med Mol Imaging. 2011; 1(1):29–35

[19] Skillen A, Currie GM, Wheat JM. Thermal control of brown adipose tissue in 18F-FDG PET. J Nucl Med Technol. 2012; 40(2):99–103

[20] Cohade C, Mourtzikos KA, Wahl RL. "USA-Fat": prevalence is related to ambient outdoor temperature-evaluation with 18F-FDG PET/CT. J Nucl Med. 2003; 44(8):1267–1270

[21] Agarwal KK, Roy SG, Kumar R. Diuretic 18F-fluorodeoxyglucose PET/computed tomography in evaluation of genitourinary malignancies. PET Clin. 2016; 11(1):39–46

[22] Moran JK, Lee HB, Blaufox MD. Optimization of urinary FDG excretion during PET imaging. J Nucl Med. 1999; 40(8):1352–1357

[23] Nayak B, Dogra PN, Naswa N, Kumar R. Diuretic 18F-FDG PET/CT imaging for detection and locoregional staging of urinary bladder cancer: prospective evaluation of a novel technique. Eur J Nucl Med Mol Imaging. 2013; 40(3):386–393

[24] Nijjar S, Patterson J, Ducharme J, Leslie WD, Demeter SJ. The effect of furosemide dose timing on bladder activity in oncology imaging with 18F-fluorodeoxyglucose PET/CT. Nucl Med Commun. 2010; 31(2):167–172

[25] Soyka JD, Strobel K, Veit-Haibach P, et al. Influence of bowel preparation before 18F-FDG PET/CT on physiologic 18F-FDG activity in the intestine. J Nucl Med. 2010; 51(4):507–510

[26] Tu DG, Chen CR, Wang YW, Tu CW, Huang YC. Bowel-cleansing methods affecting PET-CT image interpretation. Nucl Med Commun. 2011; 32(7):570–574

[27] Emmott J, Sanghera B, Chambers J, Wong WL. The effects of N-butylscopolamine on bowel uptake: an 18F-FDG PET study. Nucl Med Commun. 2008; 29(1):11–16

[28] Murphy R, Doerger KM, Nathan MA, Lowe VJ. Pretreatment with diphenoxylate hydrochloride/atropine sulfate (Lomotil) does not decrease physiologic bowel FDG activity on PET/CT scans of the abdomen and pelvis. Mol Imaging Biol. 2009; 11 (2):114–117

[29] De Barsy C, Daenen F, Benard F, Ishimori T. Is FDG bowel uptake modified by oral spasmolytic premedication? J Nucl Med. 2002; 43(5):203

[30] Okuma T, Matsuoka T, Okamura T, et al. 18F-FDG small-animal PET for monitoring the therapeutic effect of CT-guided radiofrequency ablation on implanted VX2 lung tumors in rabbits. J Nucl Med. 2006; 47(8):1351–1358

[31] Brepoels L, Stroobants S, Vandenberghe P, et al. Effect of corticosteroids on 18F-FDG uptake in tumor lesions after chemotherapy. J Nucl Med. 2007; 48(3):390–397

[32] Akhurst T, Kates TJ, Mazumdar M, et al. Recent chemotherapy reduces the sensitivity of [18F]fluorodeoxyglucose positron emission tomography in the detection of colorectal metastases. J Clin Oncol. 2005; 23(34):8713–8716

[33] Peng N, Yen S, Liu W, Tsay D, Liu R. Evaluation of the effect of radiation therapy to nasopharyngeal carcinoma by positron emission tomography with 2-. Clin Positron Imaging. 2000; 3(2):51–56

[34] Kim SY, Lee SW, Nam SY, et al. The feasibility of 18F-FDG PET scans 1 month after completing radiotherapy of squamous cell carcinoma of the head and neck. J Nucl Med. 2007; 48(3): 373–378

[35] Yamane T, Daimaru O, Ito S, et al. Decreased 18F-FDG uptake 1 day after initiation of chemotherapy for malignant lymphomas. J Nucl Med. 2004; 45(11):1838–1842

[36] Hollinger EF, Alibazoglu H, Ali A, Green A, Lamonica G. Hematopoietic cytokine-mediated FDG uptake simulates the appearance of diffuse metastatic disease on whole-body PET imaging. Clin Nucl Med. 1998; 23(2):93–98

[37] Kazama T, Swanston N, Podoloff DA, Macapinlac HA. Effect of colony-stimulating factor and conventional- or high-dose chemotherapy on FDG uptake in bone marrow. Eur J Nucl Med Mol Imaging. 2005; 32(12):1406–1411

[38] Hicks RJ, Binns D, Stabin MG. Pattern of uptake and excretion of (18)F-FDG in the lactating breast. J Nucl Med. 2001; 42(8): 1238–1242

[39] Takalkar A, Mavi A, Alavi A, Araujo L. PET in cardiology. Radiol Clin North Am. 2005; 43(1):107–119, xi

[40] Dorbala S, Di Carli MF, Delbeke D, et al. SNMMI/ASNC/SCCT guideline for cardiac SPECT/CT and PET/CT 1.0. J Nucl Med. 2013; 54(8):1485–1507

[41] Manabe O, Yoshinaga K, Ohira H, et al. The effects of 18-h fasting with low-carbohydrate diet preparation on suppressed physiological myocardial (18)F-fluorodeoxyglucose (FDG) uptake and possible minimal effects of unfractionated heparin use in patients with suspected cardiac involvement sarcoidosis. J Nucl Cardiol. 2016; 23(2):244–252

[42] Morooka M, Moroi M, Uno K, et al. Long fasting is effective in inhibiting physiological myocardial 18F-FDG uptake and for evaluating active lesions of cardiac sarcoidosis. EJNMMI Res. 2014; 4(1):1–4

[43] Ishida Y, Yoshinaga K, Miyagawa M, et al. Recommendations for (18)F-fluorodeoxyglucose positron emission tomography imaging for cardiac sarcoidosis: Japanese Society of Nuclear Cardiology recommendations. Ann Nucl Med. 2014; 28(4): 393–403

[44] Dilsizian V, Bacharach SL, Beanlands RS, et al. ASNC imaging guidelines/SNMMI procedure standard for positron emission tomography (PET) nuclear cardiology procedures. J Nucl Cardiol. 2016; 23(5):1187–1226

[45] Osborne MT, Hulten EA, Murthy VL, et al. Patient preparation for cardiac fluorine-18 fluorodeoxyglucose positron emission tomography imaging of inflammation. J Nucl Cardiol. 2017; 24(1):86–99

5 Standardized Uptake Value

Eugene C. Lin and Paul E. Kinahan

5.1 Introduction

The fluorodeoxyglucose (FDG) activity identified by positron emission tomography (PET) imaging is secondary to three components: phosphorylated intracellular FDG, nonphosphorylated intracellular FDG, and nonphosphorylated intravascular FDG. Only phosphorylated FDG is directly related to the metabolic activity of tumor cells. However, static measures of FDG uptake do not differentiate among the three components and may not correlate with glucose metabolic rates.

The basic concept underlying the standardized uptake value (SUV) is that activity concentration measured after a sufficiently long time (when plasma activity is low relative to tissue activity), if normalized for the injected dose and volume of distribution, is correlated linearly with net FDG phosphorylation.[1] The SUV is widely used in clinical studies as other techniques such as nonlinear regression analysis and simplified tracer kinetic approaches (e.g., Patlak–Gjedde analysis) are of very limited value in the clinical setting as both methods require dynamic imaging over a single bed position, and nonlinear regression analysis also utilizes arterial blood sampling.

5.2 Acronyms

1. SUR (standardized uptake ratio).
2. DUR (differential uptake value, dose uptake ratio).
3. DAR (differential absorption ratio, dose absorption ratio).

5.3 SUV Calculation

1. The SUV is the measured activity normalized for volume of distribution (body weight/surface area) and injected dose. As a reference, if the dose were uniformly distributed over entire body, the value everywhere would be SUV ~ 1.0. Thus, SUV is a relative uptake measure.[2]
2. **Formula**. Region of interest (ROI) activity (mCi/mL) × body weight(g)/injected dose (mCi)
   a) Although the above equation would have units of g/mL, SUV is unitless as it is typically defined over soft tissue with a mass density of approximately 1 g/mL.

b) Lean body mass or body surface area can be substituted for body weight. This will be more accurate for obese patients (see pitfalls section).

5.4 Pitfalls

The SUV is a semiquantitative measurement. Numerous factors can result in erroneous results.[3]
1. **Patient size**. The SUV has a strong positive correlation with weight if calculated using body weight.
   a) The SUVs in normal tissues of heavy patients can be up to twice those in lighter patients. This is secondary to the relatively low FDG uptake in fat. An obese patient who weighs 300 pounds will not have twice the glucose metabolizing mass of a patient weighing 150 pounds, as much of the additional weight is from fat. Thus, using 300 pounds in the SUV equation for an obese patient is inaccurate because the glucose metabolizing mass in this patient is substantially lower than 300 pounds.
   b) If the measured activity in an obese patient is multiplied by body weight, the SUV will be substantially overestimated.
   c) The overestimation of SUVs in obese patients can be avoided by using lean body mass or body surface area rather than weight in the calculation.
   d) The use of lean body mass or body surface area for SUV calculation is particularly important in patients whose weight changes substantially during therapy.
   e) SUVs calculated using lean body mass are typically lower than with body weight, but are relatively close, particularly in areas with low uptake. SUVs calculated with body surface area are typically much lower than with body weight.[4]
   f) The PET Response Criteria for Solid Tumors (PERCIST) criteria recommend the use of SUV corrected for lean body mass (called SUL).[5]
   g) *Lean body mass calculation*. Different formulas have been used to calculate lean body mass (LBM). The European Association of Nuclear Medicine guidelines[6] recommend the formulas below, as previously used formulas fail at weights greater than around 120 kg.

- LBM (male) = 9,270 × weight/ (6,680 + 216 × BMI)
- LBM (female) = 9,270 × weight/ (8,780 + 244 × BMI)

2. **Time of measurement**. FDG uptake in most lesions increases rapidly in the first 2 hours following the administration of FDG, and then increases slowly after that.[7]
   a) Imaging earlier provides low SUV results.
   b) Conversely, delayed scans provide high SUVs.
   c) Earlier scans are usually subject to greater measurement error because the SUV in lesions has not yet plateaued.
   d) The SUV plateaus earlier following therapeutic interventions.
   e) For therapy response assessment, the interstudy variability in the time between injection and imaging should be less than 10 minutes, as a difference of 10 minutes in the uptake period between baseline and response studies can result in significantly different SUV results.[8]

3. **Plasma glucose levels**. Elevated blood glucose levels can potentially decrease FDG uptake in malignant tumors due to competitive saturation of glucose transporters by unlabeled glucose. SUV can be corrected for plasma glucose levels by including the measured level as a multiplication factor in the SUV equation (e.g., SUV × glucose concentration/100 mg/dL). This assumes that FDG uptake is inversely proportional to the plasma glucose level. However, while this may be valid if glucose levels are close to normal, it is unclear whether this is accurate at very high glucose levels.[8] In addition, it is unclear whether glucose normalization is valid for malignant tumors, particularly in malignancies with unregulated glucose metabolic rates. There is no clear evidence that glucose normalization improves monitoring of therapy response or prediction of outcome compared to uncorrected SUV. Glucose normalization is primarily useful for serial monitoring in the same patient at the same institution, as test–retest variability may be improved,[8] but interstudy SUV variability in normal tissues will be increased. The PERCIST criteria[5] do not recommend glucose normalization.

4. **Partial volume effects**. Small lesions may have artifactually low SUVs from partial volume effects.
   a) Partial volume effects occur when lesions are less than 2 to 3 full width at half

maximum resolution of the scanner (5–10 mm in practice for most PET scanners).
   b) On standard PET scanners, partial volume effects will definitely occur below 2 cm. However, any lesion smaller than 3 cm can potentially demonstrate partial volume effects.
   c) Partial volume effects are more prominent for less compact tumors. "Compact" refers to the surface area for a given volume (spheric tumors are most compact). Thus, spheric tumors are least affected by partial volume effects.[9]
   d) *Partial volume correction*. Partial volume effect correction can be performed, which will result in an average SUVmax increase above 50%.[10] However, there are conflicting data on the clinical value of partial volume correction. In some studies, partial volume effect correction did not improve the predictive or prognostic effect of baseline FDG PET in lung cancer[11] or esophageal cancer[10] patients, but in other studies partial volume effect correction resulted in more accurate nodal staging in head and neck squamous cell carcinoma patients[12] and modified therapy response classification in breast cancer patients.[13]
   e) The PERCIST criteria[5] do not recommend partial volume effect correction, due to potential difficulties in the accurate computed tomography (CT) measurement of small lesions.

5. **Background activity**. Another partial volume effect is "spilling in" of background activity. A lung tumor with equal metabolic activity to a liver tumor may have a lower SUV due to less "spilling in" of background activity.[9]

6. **Dose extravasation**. Dose extravasation results in an underestimated SUV.
   a) If dose extravasation is known to have occurred, it is usually better to use a tumor-to-background ratio as this is not affected by dose extravasation.

7. **Reconstruction parameters**. Both reconstruction parameters and attenuation correction methods can affect SUV values.[14]
   a) *Filtered back versus interactive reconstruction*. SUVs from images reconstructed with filtered back-projection may be different from images reconstructed with iterative reconstruction.
   - *Number of iterations*. The SUV of "hot spots" will increase with more iterations. Most of the increase in average SUV will

occur in the first five iterations, with lesser degrees of increase with more iterations. The maximum SUV will increase steadily with more iterations. Thus, the number of iterations will affect the maximum SUV more than average SUV.[15]

b) The attenuation correction method can have more of an effect on SUV than the reconstruction method, particularly if there are artifacts introduced by the attenuation correction (e.g., due to patient motion).

8. **Computed tomography (CT-based attenuation correction)**. SUVs from CT attenuation–corrected studies may vary from those generated with radionuclide sources. In addition, SUV values on PET/CT may be erroneous due to misregistration or truncation artifact.

a) CT attenuation–corrected SUVs on early PET/CT scanners were reported to be 4 to 15% higher than those calculated by a germanium 68–corrected source.[16] However, there was no difference in SUVs between PET and PET/CT in a later study.[17]

- The largest difference is seen in the osseous structures.
  This may be related to errors associated with converting CT attenuation values to 511-keV positron annihilation values. Caution should be used when comparing SUVs between PET/CT and PET studies.

9. Measured SUVs can be erroneous due to acquiring CT and PET studies at different respiratory phases (see Chapter 8).

a) CT attenuation–corrected SUVs can vary up to 30% in areas of significant respiratory motion (e.g., the lung bases).[18]

10. Truncation artifact occurs due to differences in the field of view between PET and CT. Obese patients may have part of their anatomy outside the field of view of the CT scan. This truncated portion does not provide data for attenuation correction, resulting in artifactually low SUVs.

11. **Interpretation**. SUVs should be just one of many criteria used for interpretation, including visual uptake, lesion size relative to uptake, pattern of uptake, and clinical history. There is little evidence that SUVs in isolation are superior to visual interpretation for optimal diagnosis. Caution must be used when using SUV cutoffs from published literature in clinical practice.

a) The specifics of the data acquisition and analysis used to determine these SUV cutoffs are often not available in the published literature. As already noted, variations in data acquisition and analysis can have substantial effects upon measured SUVs. Also, the patient population varies from center to center.

b) In general, the reproducibility of SUV measurements between institutions is poor. In multicenter trials, the variation in FDG uptake in serial studies has been 30 to 40%.[19,20]

c) Given these factors, it is often advisable to use published SUV cutoffs with caution, if at all. Values substantially higher and lower than the cutoff are significant, but values close to the cutoff value may be of questionable value for diagnostic purposes. SUVs are most useful in primary diagnosis if the cutoff values were derived from data at the interpreting institution.

5.5 SUV Region of Interest[21]

Volumetric ROIs should be performed if possible. Two-dimensional ROIs can result in significant (> 25%) interobserver variability.[22] Maximum SUV uses maximum uptake over the entire tumor, while peak SUV uses a fixed size region. A fixed size ROI is useful for following tumors that have changed in size, to avoid partial volume effects related to the size change. Other ROI methods include manually defined tumor boundaries and semi-automated 2D and 3D region growing techniques involving the application of a fixed threshold or relative threshold to maximum uptake. In general, semi-automated methods will decrease variability. Semi-automatically generated 3D iso-contour-based ROIs at a percentage of the maximum pixel value are most accurate for noisy data and yield information on the metabolically active volume of tumor. These ROIs are typically used for calculation of metabolic tumor volume and total lesion glycolysis.[6,8]

5.6 Methods of SUV Measurement

The most commonly cited methods of SUV measurement are the maximum, mean, and peak SUV.

1. **Maximum SUV**. The primary advantage of using maximum SUV (SUVmax) is ease of measurement. For this reason, it is the most widely used method of SUV calculation.

SUVmax is the highest single voxel value with the ROI. As long as the highest lesion voxel value is included, and no higher nonlesion voxels are in the ROI, SUVmax should be independent of ROI definition. SUVmax can be calculated without interobserver variation.[23] Another potential advantage of SUVmax is that it is less sensitive to partial volume effects.[9] The major disadvantage of SUVmax is that the value from a single voxel is more affected by image noise, compared to other methods of SUV calculation. Image noise introduces a positive bias in SUVmax measurement, which results in an overestimation of metabolic activity which is more prominent with greater image noise and larger and more intense lesions with more counts. This positive bias can be increased when reconstruction methods and setting optimized for tumor detection are used (e.g., small voxel size, time-of-flight [TOF] imaging, and point spread function [PSF] reconstruction).[8,24] In one study,[24] the use of PSF and TOF increased the SUVmax by 43% and SUVmean by 32% in lymph node metastases, compared to standard ordered subset expectation maximization reconstruction. Thus, optimizing image quality for lesion detection may conflict with optimal quantification. The positive bias of SUVmax will increase as scan time decreases.[25] A negative bias is also possible secondary to motion, particularly in lung and liver lesions near the diaphragm. Motion can blur the target volume, resulting in reduction in the highest single-pixel value.[26] In a meta-analysis,[27] SUVmean had better test–retest repeatability than SUVmax, although both methods had poor repeatability for lesions with low FDG uptake.

2. **Mean SUV**. Mean SUV (SUVmean) is averaged over all the voxels in the ROI. The primary advantage of SUVmean is that it is less affected by image noise, resulting in better test–retest repeatability.[27] However, if the ROIs are drawn manually, SUVmean calculation is more time-consuming and particularly difficult for small lesions. Due to inconsistencies in ROI definition, interobserver variability is greater with SUVmean than with SUVmax.[23] In addition, areas of necrosis within the lesion can affect the SUVmean measurement. In one study, differences in tumor response were approximately twice as large when calculated with manual SUVmean, compared to SUVmax and automated SUVpeak.[28]

3. **Peak SUV**. The peak SUV (SUVpeak) is calculated by placing an approximately 1.2-cm sphere (1 cm^3 volume) ROI centered around the hottest uptake region in the tumor, and calculating an average SUV from this volume. This may correspond to the location (but not the value) of the SUVmax, but it is not always the case. This is the method recommended by the PERCIST criteria.[5] SUVpeak is less dependent on optimal lesion delineation than SUVmean. In addition, using the hottest uptake region in the tumor rather than the entire lesion avoids including areas of necrosis, which can lower the measured activity if SUVmean is employed. The SUVpeak is less affected by image noise than SUVmax, as it is an average over a larger area. The use of automated methods of SUVpeak calculation improves reproducibility. Although SUV measurement show variability with varying reconstruction methods, SUVpeak has the highest reproducibility in SUV quantification when comparing different reconstruction methods, especially in small lesions.[29]

5.7 Repeatability and Reproducibility

Repeatability of SUV measurement is particularly relevant for response assessment, where measurement variability must be differentiated from a real change in tumor metabolism. *Repeatability* is typically determined by repeat scanning of the same patient on the same scanner, with the same protocol, in a short time interval. A comprehensive review[30] indicates that tumor SUV has a within-subject coefficient of variation of approximately 10%, which would correspond to a repeatability coefficient of 28.5%. This value is close to the recommended values of 30% in PERCIST[5] and 25% in European Organization for Research and Treatment of Cancer (EORTC)[31] guidelines. However, a larger percentage change is needed to indicate a true metabolic change when the uptake increases, compared to decreasing uptake. For example, a decrease in SUV from 5 to 4 is a 20% change, and an increase in SUV from 4 to 5 is a 25% change, but the variability is the same in both cases. The review[30] indicates that SUV reductions of more than 25% and increases by more than 33% are unlikely to be due to measurement variability.

The *reproducibility* of SUV measurements (for studies performed in different settings) is more variable. In multicenter trials,[19,20] the variation in FDG uptake in serial studies has been 30 to 40%.

5.8 Dual Time Point Imaging[32, 33,34]

Imaging at two time points and evaluating SUV change between early and delayed imaging can improve accuracy. The disadvantage is decreased patient throughput, although this can be minimized if a limited scan is performed after completion of the whole-body scan. The rationale behind dual time point (DTP) PET/CT is that FDG tumor uptake and background clearance will increase on delayed images. Tissues with high glycolysis may continue to accumulate intracellular FDG-6-phosphate, while tissues with high glucose-6-phosphatase such as the liver will have an early peak in activity followed by a gradual decrease. In addition, blood pool and urinary tract activity clearance will increase over time.

DTP PET/CT is not recommended for routine clinical use, but can be helpful in specific situations. DTP PET/CT has been used to increase accuracy in discriminating between benign and malignant lesions with mixed results. In a meta-analysis of detection of mediastinal nodal metastasis in non–small cell lung cancer patients,[35] DTP PET/CT had a higher sensitivity than single time point (STP) PET/CT on a per-patient basis. In another meta-analysis of lymph node metastases in general,[36] the sensitivity of DTP PET/CT was higher on per-patient basis, but the specificity was lower. In a meta-analysis of DTP PET/CT for differential diagnosis of pulmonary nodules,[37] the accuracy of DTP and STP PET/CT was comparable, but DTP PET/CT was more specific.

Another technique is delayed time point imaging (a single acquisition after a longer time interval). Both DTP and delayed time point imaging may be useful in situations with potentially compromised lesion-to-background ratios, such as obese patients or patients with renal failure or poorly controlled diabetes.[38]

5.9 Pearls/Pitfalls

1. Active infection and inflammatory lesions can have higher FDG activity on delayed imaging, although chronic inflammatory lesions may show no significant change or a decline in activity on delayed images.[38]

2. A change in lesion configuration between early and delayed images may indicate a benign etiology.

3. The delay between early and delayed images should be 30 minutes or more.

References

[1] Allen-Auerbach M, Weber WA. Measuring response with FDG-PET: methodological aspects. Oncologist. 2009; 14(4): 369–377

[2] Thie JA. Understanding the standardized uptake value, its methods, and implications for usage. J Nucl Med. 2004; 45 (9):1431–1434

[3] Keyes JW, Jr. SUV: standard uptake or silly useless value? J Nucl Med. 1995; 36(10):1836–1839

[4] Maffione AM, Ferretti A, Vinjamuri S, Rubello D. The PERCIST criteria: an insightful appraisal. Nucl Med Commun. 2013; 34 (7):619–620

[5] Wahl RL, Jacene H, Kasamon Y, Lodge MA. From RECIST to PERCIST: evolving considerations for PET response criteria in solid tumors. J Nucl Med. 2009; 50 Suppl 1:122S–150S

[6] Boellaard R, Delgado-Bolton R, Oyen WJ, et al. European Association of Nuclear Medicine (EANM). FDG PET/CT: EANM procedure guidelines for tumour imaging: version 2.0. Eur J Nucl Med Mol Imaging. 2015; 42(2):328–354

[7] Hamberg LM, Hunter GJ, Alpert NM, Choi NC, Babich JW, Fischman AJ. The dose uptake ratio as an index of glucose metabolism: useful parameter or oversimplification? J Nucl Med. 1994; 35(8):1308–1312

[8] Boellaard R. Need for standardization of 18F-FDG PET/CT for treatment response assessments. J Nucl Med. 2011; 52 Suppl 2:93S–100S

[9] Soret M, Bacharach SL, Buvat I. Partial-volume effect in PET tumor imaging. J Nucl Med. 2007; 48(6):932–945

[10] Hatt M, Le Pogam A, Visvikis D, Pradier O, Cheze Le Rest C. Impact of partial-volume effect correction on the predictive and prognostic value of baseline 18F-FDG PET images in esophageal cancer. J Nucl Med. 2012; 53(1):12–20

[11] Ohtaka K, Hida Y, Kaga K, et al. Outcome analysis of (18)F-fluorodeoxyglucose positron-emission tomography in patients with lung cancer after partial volume correction. Anticancer Res. 2013; 33(11):5193–5198

[12] Fayad H, Le Pogam A, Lamare F, et al. Influence of partial volume correction in staging of head and neck squamous cell carcinoma using PET/CT. Q J Nucl Med Mol Imaging. 2014; 58 (3):319–328

[13] Stefano A, Gallivanone F, Messa C, Gilardi MC, Gastiglioni I. Metabolic impact of partial volume correction of [18F]FDG PET-CT oncological studies on the assessment of tumor response to treatment. Q J Nucl Med Mol Imaging. 2014; 58(4): 413–423

[14] Schöder H, Erdi YE, Chao K, Gonen M, Larson SM, Yeung HW. Clinical implications of different image reconstruction parameters for interpretation of whole-body PET studies in cancer patients. J Nucl Med. 2004; 45(4):559–566

[15] Jaskowiak CJ, Bianco JA, Perlman SB, Fine JP. Influence of reconstruction iterations on 18F-FDG PET/CT standardized uptake values. J Nucl Med. 2005; 46(3):424–428

[16] Nakamoto Y, Osman M, Cohade C, et al. PET/CT: comparison of quantitative tracer uptake between germanium and CT transmission attenuation-corrected images. J Nucl Med. 2002; 43(9):1137–1143

[17] Souvatzoglou M, Ziegler SI, Martinez MJ, et al. Standardised uptake values from PET/CT images: comparison with conventional attenuation-corrected PET. Eur J Nucl Med Mol Imaging. 2007; 34(3):405–412

[18] Erdi YE, Nehmeh SA, Pan T, et al. The CT motion quantitation of lung lesions and its impact on PET-measured SUVs. J Nucl Med. 2004; 45(8):1287–1292

[19] Frings V, van Velden FH, Velasquez LM, et al. Repeatability of metabolically active tumor volume measurements with FDG PET/CT in advanced gastrointestinal malignancies: a multicenter study. Radiology. 2014; 273(2):539–548

[20] Weber WA, Gatsonis CA, Mozley PD, et al. ACRIN 6678 Research team, MK-0646-008 Research team. Repeatability of 18F-FDG PET/CT in advanced non-small cell lung cancer: prospective assessment in 2 multicenter trials. J Nucl Med. 2015; 56(8):1137–1143

[21] Boellaard R, Krak NC, Hoekstra OS, Lammertsma AA. Effects of noise, image resolution, and ROI definition on the accuracy of standard uptake values: a simulation study. J Nucl Med. 2004; 45(9):1519–1527

[22] Marom EM, Munden RF, Truong MT, et al. Interobserver and intraobserver variability of standardized uptake value measurements in non-small-cell lung cancer. J Thorac Imaging. 2006; 21(3):205–212

[23] Huang YE, Chen CF, Huang YJ, Konda SD, Appelbaum DE, Pu Y. Interobserver variability among measurements of the maximum and mean standardized uptake values on (18)F-FDG PET/CT and measurements of tumor size on diagnostic CT in patients with pulmonary tumors. Acta Radiol. 2010; 51(7):782–788

[24] Akamatsu G, Mitsumoto K, Taniguchi T, Tsutsui Y, Baba S, Sasaki M. Influences of point-spread function and time-of-flight reconstructions on standardized uptake value of lymph node metastases in FDG-PET. Eur J Radiol. 2014; 83(1):226–230

[25] Akamatsu G, Ikari Y, Nishida H, et al. Influence of statistical fluctuation on reproducibility and accuracy of SUVmax and SUVpeak: a phantom study. J Nucl Med Technol. 2015; 43(3):222–226

[26] Ziai P, Hayeri MR, Salei A, et al. Role of optimal quantification of FDG PET imaging in the clinical practice of radiology. Radiographics. 2016; 36(2):481–496

[27] de Langen AJ, Vincent A, Velasquez LM, et al. Repeatability of 18F-FDG uptake measurements in tumors: a metaanalysis. J Nucl Med. 2012; 53(5):701–708

[28] Vanderhoek M, Perlman SB, Jeraj R. Impact of different standardized uptake value measures on PET-based quantification of treatment response. J Nucl Med. 2013; 54(8):1188–1194

[29] Brendle C, Kupferschläger J, Nikolaou K, la Fougère C, Gatidis S, Pfannenberg C. Is the standard uptake value (SUV) appropriate for quantification in clinical PET imaging? - Variability induced by different SUV measurements and varying reconstruction methods. Eur J Radiol. 2015; 84(1):158–162

[30] Lodge MA. Repeatability of SUV in Oncologic 18F-FDG PET. J Nucl Med. 2017; 58(4):523–532

[31] Young H, Baum R, Cremerius U, et al. European Organization for Research and Treatment of Cancer (EORTC) PET Study Group. Measurement of clinical and subclinical tumour response using [18F]-fluorodeoxyglucose and positron emission tomography: review and 1999 EORTC recommendations. Eur J Cancer. 1999; 35(13):1773–1782

[32] Döbert N, Hamscho N, Menzel C, Neuss L, Kovács AF, Grünwald F. Limitations of dual time point FDG-PET imaging in the evaluation of focal abdominal lesions. Nucl Med (Stuttg). 2004; 43(5):143–149

[33] Conrad GR, Sinha P. Narrow time-window dual-point 18F-FDG PET for the diagnosis of thoracic malignancy. Nucl Med Commun. 2003; 24(11):1129–1137

[34] Hustinx R, Smith RJ, Benard F, et al. Dual time point fluorine-18 fluorodeoxyglucose positron emission tomography: a potential method to differentiate malignancy from inflammation and normal tissue in the head and neck. Eur J Nucl Med. 1999; 26(10):1345–1348

[35] Shen G, Hu S, Deng H, Jia Z. Diagnostic value of dual time-point 18 F-FDG PET/CT versus single time-point imaging for detection of mediastinal nodal metastasis in non-small cell lung cancer patients: a meta-analysis. Acta Radiol. 2015; 56(6):681–687

[36] Shen G, Deng H, Hu S, Jia Z. Potential performance of dual-time-point 18F-FDG PET/CT compared with single-time-point imaging for differential diagnosis of metastatic lymph nodes: a meta-analysis. Nucl Med Commun. 2014; 35(10):1003–1010

[37] Zhang L, Wang Y, Lei J, Tian J, Zhai Y. Dual time point 18FDG-PET/CT versus single time point 18FDG-PET/CT for the differential diagnosis of pulmonary nodules: a meta-analysis. Acta Radiol. 2013; 54(7):770–777

[38] Cheng G, Torigian DA, Zhuang H, Alavi A. When should we recommend use of dual time-point and delayed time-point imaging techniques in FDG PET? Eur J Nucl Med Mol Imaging. 2013; 40(5):779–787

6 Quantitative Whole-Body PET/CT Imaging

Sina Houshmand, Ali Salavati, Abass Alavi, and Habib Zaidi

6.1 Introduction

Positron emission tomography/computed tomography (PET/CT) and, recently, PET/magnetic resonance imaging (MRI) are two rapidly developing and widely utilized imaging modalities in the whole world in the research and clinical settings. Qualitative, semiquantitative, and absolute quantitative methods are the three major categories for assessment of PET images. Qualitative measurement by the expert readers is the most subjective method. Semiquantitative parameters, which include standardized uptake value (SUV), lesion-to-background ratio (also known as target-to-background ratio), and some variants of SUV, are widely used in the clinic. Absolute quantitative techniques involve various mathematical models, Patlak–Gjedde graphical analysis, and nonlinear regression models for precise quantification of PET images. Absolute quantitative techniques are the most accurate and also most complicated, while the qualitative and semiquantitative techniques are the mostly used approaches due to their simplicity. However, the qualitative and semiquantitative techniques are prone to interreader and intrareader variability.

Qualitative visual assessment is still the mainstream technique for clinical use. Qualitative visual assessment relies on the contrast between high uptake areas of the PET image versus low uptake areas. The pitfall of the qualitative visual assessment is the lack of a definitive threshold to classify lesion vs. normal uptake and suboptimal intrareader and interreader agreement.[1]

A substantial amount of research has focused on development of optimal techniques and standardization of these methods across the world to enable comparability from center to center and machine to machine.[2] However, suboptimal quantification methods, hampering accurate evaluation of the disease extent and response to treatment and its widespread use, are a topic of debate in the literature.[3,4]

As the specific targeted molecular imaging probes used in the clinic are being introduced as validated approaches, there has been a growth in advanced quantitative PET imaging research and it is expected to continue in the near future as 8,441 PubMed entries have appeared in the literature since 1990, with more than 709 of them only from 2017 (▶ Fig. 6.1).

This chapter focuses on novel techniques being introduced to the clinic in addition to the different approaches of quantitative PET imaging tailored for clinical settings and their optimization methods.

6.2 Simplified versus Complex PET Quantification: Semiquantitative Metrics and Dynamic Imaging

Simplified PET quantification has been made possible by development of SUV. This quantification measure and its variants have been discussed in detail in Chapter 5. Here, we will discuss dynamic

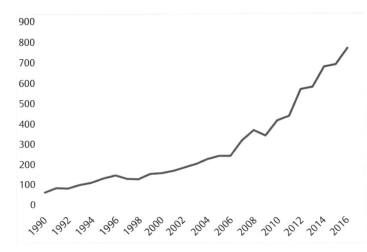

Fig. 6.1 The increase in the number of the peer-reviewed publications each year in the subject of PET quantification shows the increasing interest in this topic. The graph was generated using the results from the PubMed by using the following MeSH terms: ("PET" OR "positron emission tomography") AND ("quantification" OR "quantitation" OR "quantitative") for each year from 1990 to 2016.

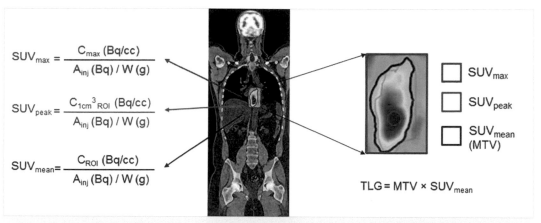

$$SUV_{max} = \frac{C_{max}\ (Bq/cc)}{A_{inj}\ (Bq)\ /\ W\ (g)}$$

$$SUV_{peak} = \frac{C_{1cm^3\ ROI}\ (Bq/cc)}{A_{inj}\ (Bq)\ /\ W\ (g)}$$

$$SUV_{mean} = \frac{C_{ROI}\ (Bq/cc)}{A_{inj}\ (Bq)\ /\ W\ (g)}$$

☐ SUV_{max}

☐ SUV_{peak}

☐ SUV_{mean} (MTV)

$$TLG = MTV \times SUV_{mean}$$

Fig. 6.2 Illustration of the basic foundations of PET quantification and the factors involved in the calculation of first- and second-order image-derived PET metrics used in clinical oncology

whole-body imaging, tracer kinetic modeling, and parametric whole-body imaging (▶ Fig. 6.2).

6.2.1 Static versus Dynamic Whole-Body PET Imaging

Static whole-body PET is the main imaging technique used in the clinic and SUV is the conventional metric for analysis of the static whole-body PET/CT studies owing to the relative simplicity of SUV calculation.

SUV cannot differentiate the metabolized and nonmetabolized concentrations of radiotracer, and the plasma dynamics is not considered in this parameter and is only used as a semiquantitative measure.[5,6,7]

To address this limitation, dynamic and parametric whole-body PET imaging has been developed.[8] In dynamic PET imaging, the time series of the radiotracer uptake is recorded, which is then used for estimation of physiologic parameters of interest by using tracer kinetic modeling. The approaches available for using dynamic PET data include region of interest (ROI)-based kinetic modeling, which uses the time–activity curves of defined ROIs, and voxel-based kinetic modeling (parametric imaging), which calculates the kinetic parameters of each voxel. Parametric imaging is more resource-consuming and more sensitive to noise.[8,9,10] The complexities related to the dynamic PET imaging have limited the use of this technique in the daily clinical use.[8]

Tracer kinetic analysis is another type of dynamic PET, which determines the absolute concentration

of substrate and product of glucose metabolism in the cells, giving more detailed information about the rate of glucose metabolism in the cells. This imaging technique uses dynamic data and therefore makes it less dependent on imaging time (as used for SUV calculation). However, tracer kinetic modeling is also time-consuming and cumbersome as it needs arterial blood sampling.

6.3 PET Image Segmentation

The calculation of a number of image-derived metrics (e.g., SUV_{mean}) requires a priori segmentation of PET images to derive the metabolic tumor volume (MTV). Segmentation of radiologic images involves the use of techniques implemented in image space to group voxels into sets of distinct tissue classes. Segmentation is currently being used for identification of normal tissues/organs and delineation of tumors, derivation of attenuation maps, and development of anthropomorphic models of different organs in addition to a number of other applications. However, the differentiation of malignant from benign tissue specifically in PET imaging can become challenging due to multiple reasons, including the high noise characteristics and limited spatial resolution of PET scanners. Therefore, manual delineation by human operators remains the most used option in the clinic. Considering the pitfalls of manual delineation including human error and inter/intraobserver variability, the need for sophisticated and reliable automatic techniques appears vital.

There is tremendous amount of research done for development of semi-automated and automated techniques for PET image segmentation.[11] Recently, the American Association of Physicists in Medicine (AAPM) mandated its task group no. 211 to issue an up-to-date comprehensive review of the state-of-the-art automatic segmentation and issued recommendations and guidelines for PET segmentation.[12] The survey provided detailed description of different categories of techniques, including thresholding, region growing, classifiers, clustering, edge detection, Markov random fields models, artificial neural networks, deformable models, and atlas-guided, which are few representative examples of the numerous techniques used for automatic segmentation of PET images.[12] The current trend is to move to fully automated or minimally interactive but still automated segmentation algorithms. The same task group reported on a standard benchmark tool for assessment and comparison of PET segmentation algorithms in order to provide a framework for simulation and experimental phantom studies and pathology-validated clinical datasets.[13] This and similar efforts will hopefully expedite the translation and usage of advanced segmentation approaches in clinical and research settings.

6.4 Texture Analysis and Radiomics

Regardless of the prevalent usage of the oversimplified PET metrics described in the previous sections, more innovative concepts involving advanced statistical approaches have been investigated over the years. A number of revolutionary studies confirmed evidence that important information can be extracted from molecular PET images documenting unequivocal and specific markers associated with tumor molecular and genetic profiles.[14] In this regard, radiogenomics[15] or radiomics[16] and texture analysis[13] emerged as promising concepts having the capability to circumvent the shortcomings of simplified approaches by bestowing consistent prognostic information with a high predictive power in many oncological indications.

Texture analysis is a newly introduced concept dealing with metabolic heterogeneity of malignant lesions enabling the clinicians to analyze the intratumoral heterogeneity in FDG uptake, which might be correlated with the degree of aggressiveness of the tumor.[17,18] These textural features derived from

PET images have been shown to be prognostic in certain tumors.[17] Over the past few years, some challenges have been faced about this technique which necessitates the need for further research to clarify the role of this new approach in clinic.[13]

In a study evaluating the correlation between therapy outcome and metrics derived by texture analysis in uterine cervix and head and neck cancer, a high predictive value for shape feature (solidity, extent, Euler's number) and texture features (energy, local homogeneity, entropy) outperforming the commonly used SUV-based parameters was described.[19] A statistical model for delineation of sarcoma, identifying spatial heterogeneity as the key feature for cancer staging and prediction of patient survival, has shown promising results.[20]

Radiomics is a new research domain, which increases the predictive power of the medical imaging by combining imaging techniques and the systems biology performed by extracting information from diagnostic images and correlating them with the biology of the tumor and the patients' clinical features.[19,21,22,23,24] Radiomics relies on the fundamental hypothesis of "tissues characteristics at the molecular level are reflected in macroscopic features of medical images and, therefore, an advanced quantitative analysis can infer genomics and proteomics patterns, possibly containing prognostic information."[25]

Despite the appealing theoretical foundations and robust mathematical framework of these advanced concepts, a number of shortcomings are worth mentioning. Overall, the results of the findings of the studies are difficult to compare due to lack of standardization, workflow for the calculation of textural features is complex, and the features are dependent on various factors such as acquisition, image reconstruction, preprocessing, functional volume segmentation, and methods of establishing and quantifying correspondences with genomic and clinical metrics of interest.[13] These techniques have not yet entered the clinical arena but are expected to gain importance and play a significant role in the future.

6.4.1 Parametric Whole-Body Imaging

Following its successful implementation in neurological and cardiovascular imaging typically requiring single-bed field-of-view (FOV) dynamic data acquisition and an appropriate kinetic model, parametric imaging was investigated in the

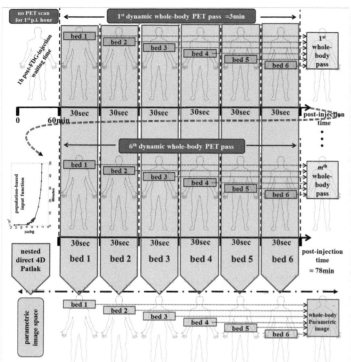

Fig. 6.3 Flowchart demonstrating a clinically feasible dynamic whole-body (WB) ^{18}F-FDG PET acquisition protocol performed at a standard-of-care acquisition window 60 minutes post ^{18}F-FDG injection for potential combined production of both K_i and noise-equivalent SUV WB PET images. The particular version consists of six WB passes, each consisting of six beds, each of 30-second acquisition, as optimized for the Siemens Biograph mCT TOF PET/CT system. (Reproduced with permission from Zaidi and Karakatsanis.[32])

context of clinical oncology to derive quantitative maps representing physiological parameters of interest. The approach has been first limited to single-bed FOV imaging owing to the limited axial FOV of current-generation PET scanners. Pioneering studies using this technique in combination with discriminant analysis demonstrated improved discrimination between benign and malignant metabolic abnormalities.[26] The main shortcoming of this approach is the region containing the suspected metabolic abnormalities need to be known a priori, thus limiting its aptitude to detect distant disease located far away from the primary tumor (e.g., lymph nodes, metastasis spread throughout the body). This weakness has been addressed by novel dynamic whole-body imaging protocols enabling the generation of quantitative maps representing relevant physiological parameters and facilitating their clinical translation.[27] Parametric imaging might provide additional information for both multiparametric assessment of malignant lesions across the body and improved reproducibility and treatment response monitoring. The protocol described in the above reference consists in acquiring an initial

6-minute dynamic study of 24 frames over the heart to extract the input function, followed by a sequence of a certain number of whole-body PET scans, each consisting of six to seven bed positions (45 seconds each) (► Fig. 6.3).[28] The acquired 4D PET data are then used to generate whole-body parametric PET images representing kinetic macroparameters of tracer uptake rate, Ki (slope) and blood volume – bv (intercept), at each voxel. This is achieved using ordinary least squares regression within the framework of Patlak linear graphical analysis modeling. Graphical Patlak analysis enables robust estimation of Ki parametric images through direct estimation of FDG net uptake rate from the time integral of the blood input function and the dynamic PET frames acquired at later times postinjection. This unique feature of dynamic whole-body imaging allows continuous temporal acquisition of a single bed after tracer injection, thus providing fine temporal sampling rate of the fast time-varying input function at this early time period. This is followed by a number of consecutive whole-body passes to adequately sample the late portion of the input function in addition to providing voxelwise FDG dynamics across the body. Thereafter, dynamic frames are fitted to the linear Patlak model to derive whole-body parametric K_i images. This can be achieved through either a postreconstruction analysis procedure by indirect fitting of the dynamic PET frames,[29] or through a direct procedure from the dynamic projection data by nesting the sPatlak model within each tomographic update step of the dynamic PET data.[30] Kinetic parameter estimation in dynamic PET imaging and potential improvement of the accuracy and precision of the estimates have been the subject of extensive research during the last decade, resulting in the development of a number of algorithms for direct parametric estimation using spatiotemporal image reconstruction.[31]

6.5 Concept of Global Disease Assessment and Volumetric Measures in Assessment of Diseases

6.5.1 Global Disease Burden: Assessing Global Metabolic Activity

The concept of global metabolic activity was introduced in the early 1990s Alzheimer's disease evaluation comparing the age-matched controls, where the segmented brain volume from MRI was multiplied to the mean cerebral metabolic rate of glucose obtained from PET.[33] The results of the study showed significant differences between the healthy volunteers versus patients with Alzheimer's disease. This concept resulted in introduction of a unique parameter named global disease burden or total lesion glycolysis (TLG). TLG is being increasingly used as a parameter for evaluation of entire cancerous lesions' metabolic response.[34,35,36]

TLG has shown to be reproducible and strongly prognostic for overall survival (OS) of cancer patients such as non–small cell lung cancer (NSCLC),[36] providing complementary information to conventional SUV and its variants. Recent image segmentation techniques have facilitated the delineation of different tissues, thus making the quantification of global disease possible.

With development of automated software packages providing clinicians a single number summing up the global disease activity of an individual patient with multiple lesions, disease monitoring and assessment of treatment response will be possible.

6.5.2 Examples of Global Disease Assessment in Various Clinical Settings

The value of global disease assessment has been successfully demonstrated in various conditions such as malignant mesothelioma,[37,38,39] adrenal malignancies,[40] breast cancer,[41] ovarian cancer,[42] gastric cancer,[43] colorectal cancer,[44] prostate cancer,[45] renal cell carcinoma,[46] hepatocellular carcinoma,[47] lymphoma[48] (▶ Fig. 6.4), and even inflammatory processes such as sarcoidosis,[49] Crohn's disease,[50] radiation pneumonitis,[51] and atherosclerosis.[52,53,54] Here, we will discuss some of them.

Cancer

Lung Cancer

In a cohort of 196 patients with inoperable stage IIB/III NSCLC, pretreatment whole-body and primary tumor volumetric FDG-PET parameters were independently prognostic of OS. In addition, MTV and TLG uniformly had a higher aread under the curve (t) (AUC(t)) in receiver operator curve analyses compared to SUV over all time points in time-dependent receiver operating characteristic analysis.[36]

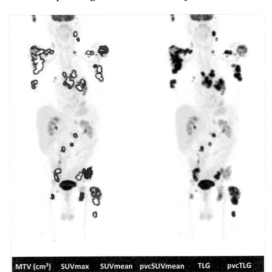

MTV (cm³)	SUVmax	SUVmean	pvcSUVmean	TLG	pvcTLG
265.9	21.1	8.4	12.86	2239.5	3541.2

Fig. 6.4 An example of global disease assessment in lymphoma. Segmented FDG-PET/CT images of a patient with non-Hodgkin's lymphoma showing FDG-avid lymph nodes. The quantitative measures including metabolic tumor volume (MTV), SUVmean, SUVmax, and total lesion glycolysis (TLG) are calculated with and without partial volume correction (pvc). (Reproduced with permission from Houshmand et al.[55])

Prognostic value of MTV and TLG was shown to be significant in a systematic review and meta-analysis of 13 studies including 1,581 patients with TNM stage I/II and stage III/IV NSCLC.[56] The findings of this study remained significant after subgroup analysis according to TNM stage.

Evaluation of disease-free survival and OS in surgical NSCLC patients using volumetric PET metrics versus SUV metrics was done in a systematic review and meta-analysis of 36 studies comprising 5,807 patients, which showed similar prognostic role for SUV_{max}, MTV, and TLG in this patient population, indicating higher risk of recurrence or death in patients with high values of SUV_{max}, MTV, and TLG.[57]

Malignant Mesothelioma

Baseline and interim PET evaluation for response assessment and outcome definition in malignant pleural mesothelioma (MPM) patients was performed in a retrospective study of 131 patients which showed correlation of baseline SUV_{max} and TLG with progression-free survival (PFS) and OS; ΔSUV_{max} and ΔTLG were correlated with disease control.[39]

Prognostic value of pretreatment volume-based quantitative FDG PET/CT in patients with MPM was retrospectively assessed in 201 patients with median follow-up of 15 months.[38] The results of the study showed shorter OS with high SUV_{max}, MTV, and TLG. TLG was an independent negative predictor in multivariate analysis.

Prostate Cancer

Prostate-specific membrane antigen (PSMA) ligands is a new tracer for imaging and therapy of patients with metastatic prostate cancer.[58] Schmuck et al[45] have shown that PSMA-derived volumetric parameters can be used as reasonable biomarkers for therapy monitoring by having a better correlation with PSA as a surrogate for tumor burden compared to traditional SUV_{mean} and SUV_{max}. Additionally, in their study, unlike SUV_{mean} and SUV_{max}, the response/failure of treatment was reflected in whole-body MTV and TLG.

Head and Neck Malignancies

The prognostic value of the volumetric PET parameters in head and neck cancer has been evaluated by Pak et al in a systematic review and meta-analysis comprising 13 studies (1,180 patients).[59] The primary outcome was event-free survival (EFS). The secondary end point was OS. The impact of MTV and TLG on survival was assessed by hazard ratio (HR). The combined HRs for adverse events were 3.06 (2.33–4.01, $p < 0.001$) and 3.10 (2.27–4.24, $p < 0.001$) with MTV and TLG, respectively. These findings suggest that tumors with higher volumetric parameters are associated with progression or recurrence. The pooled HRs for OS were 3.51 (2.62–4.72, $p < 0.001$) and 3.14 (2.24–4.40, $p < 0.001$) for MTV and TLG, respectively, suggesting worse overall survival for higher MTV and TLG. The I^2 heterogeneity of these measures was not statistically significant. This study concluded MTV and TLG, regardless of the various techniques used for measurement of these parameters in the studies, are good predictors of adverse events and death.

Gastrointestinal Tract Malignancies

The gastrointestinal tract malignancies have also been studied using the volumetric PET measures. As a representative, Park et al have evaluated the prognostic value of the volume-based PET parameters in gastric cancer based on the human epidural growth factor receptor 2 (HER2) gene status.[43] In their retrospective study of 124 patients with locally advanced or metastatic gastric cancer who had undergone baseline FDG PET/CT before the first-line chemotherapy, they measured various PET parameters including MTV and TLG with the threshold of ≥ 2.5 for the lesions and associated with the survival outcomes of these patient groups. They found higher SUV_{max} in HER2 positives ([median, 12.1; range, 3.4–34.6] compared to HER2 negative [7.4, 1.6–39.1, $p < 0.001$]), and in both HER2 positive and negatives, FDG PET/CT volumetric parameters had prognostic value. Whole-body TLG > 600, indicating high levels of metastatic burden, had worse PFS (HR, 2; range, 1.3–3.09; $p < 0.001$) and OS (HR, 3; range, 1.95–4.6; $p < 0.001$) compared to whole-body TLG of ≤ 600 in all patients. In the HER2-positive patients treated with trastuzumab, higher metabolic burden of the tumor was associated with worse OS only. Colorectal cancer[44] and hepatocellular carcinoma[35] have also showed similar favorable outcomes for utilization of volumetric measures. For example, measurement of TLG before and after treatment with regorafenib in metastatic colorectal cancer was able to predict treatment outcome,[44] or in patients with hepatocellular carcinoma after curative resection, volumetric PET parameters were able to predict the early intrahepatic recurrence-free survival[35] after resection. Additionally, another study[47] evaluated patients with very early and early hepatocellular carcinoma before the resection using volumetric PET parameters and has reported high preoperative MTV and TLG as independent prognostic factors for extrahepatic metastasis-free survival but not intrahepatic recurrence-free survival, making these parameters good predictors of extrahepatic metastasis before initiation of the treatment.

Bone Metastasis

In a novel approach, skeletal tumor burden was evaluated by using volumetric Na-F PET parameters[60] in 117 patients who underwent NaF PET/CT for bone metastasis detection. The whole-body NaF was calculated after filtering out the high uptake of the normal bone with cutoff of 10 and it was shown that the skeletal tumor burden moderately correlates with the variation of the tumor marker ($r = 0.67$, $p < 0.04$) after treatment in a subgroup of 61 breast cancer patients.

Global Assessment of Inflammatory Diseases

Atherosclerosis

Assessment of vascular wall inflammation and atherosclerosis was initially performed by qualitative and visual scoring systems before introduction of the semiquantitative and quantitative techniques (global inflammatory burden).[61] In quantitative technique, to measure the FDG uptake of the vessel wall, the regions of interest (ROI) are drawn around the outer boundaries of the vessel in transaxial plane of the PET/CT image and the FDG uptake and surface area of that particular slice is recorded.[61] By summing the recorded numbers of all the slices along the vessel, the total FDG uptake of a particular vessel also known as global inflammatory burden, atherosclerosis burden, or global metabolic activity is calculated, which has been suggested to be an early, accurate, and reliable biomarker for evaluation atherosclerosis burden.[61]

Lung Inflammation

Lung inflammation related to radiation pneumonitis is one of the side effects of radiation therapy. One of the proposed techniques for global assessment of lung inflammation in lung cancer patients includes segmentation of lung parenchyma using the CT portion of the PET/CT. The segmented lung is then used to compare the extent of FDG uptake before and after radiation therapy.[51] This pilot study showed an increase in lung parenchymal FDG uptake after radiation, presumably secondary to the inflammatory processes in the lung.[51] If proven, this technique could be a reliable biomarker for early prediction of radiation pneumonitis before clinical manifestations or be used for comparing different radiation therapy methods such as proton therapy versus photon therapy.[62]

Crohn's Disease

A study of 22 patients with Crohn's disease has proposed a novel technique for global Crohn's disease assessment and correlation with surrogate markers of disease activity.[50] Global Crohn's disease activity score, which has been described as a global marker of the FDG activity in the guts along with other PET parameters, was significantly correlated with clinical Crohn's disease activity score and Crohn's disease endoscopy index of severity.[50]

6.6 Concluding Remarks and Future Prospects

Hybrid PET/CT and newly introduced PET/MRI have enabled the combination of anatomy and morphology with functional and molecular processes.

The novel quantitative techniques described in this chapter are of great importance for enhancing the performance and accuracy of the modern hybrid imaging modalities, leading to improvement in the management and outcome of serious diseases and illnesses.

References

[1] Basu S, Zaidi H, Houseni M, et al. Novel quantitative techniques for assessing regional and global function and structure based on modern imaging modalities: implications for normal variation, aging and diseased states. Semin Nucl Med. 2007; 37(3):223–239

[2] Boellaard R. Optimisation and harmonisation: two sides of the same coin? Eur J Nucl Med Mol Imaging. 2013; 40(7): 982–984

[3] Basu S, Kwee TC, Torigian D, Saboury B, Alavi A. Suboptimal and inadequate quantification: an alarming crisis in medical applications of PET. Eur J Nucl Med Mol Imaging. 2011; 38 (7):1381–1382

[4] Lammertsma AA. Forward to the past: the case for quantitative PET imaging. J Nucl Med. 2017; 58(7):1019–1024

[5] Kim CK, Gupta NC. Dependency of standardized uptake values of fluorine-18 fluorodeoxyglucose on body size: compar-

ison of body surface area correction and lean body mass correction. Nucl Med Commun. 1996; 17(10):890–894

[6] Sadato N, Tsuchida T, Nakaumra S, et al. Non-invasive estimation of the net influx constant using the standardized uptake value for quantification of FDG uptake of tumours. Eur J Nucl Med. 1998; 25(6):559–564

[7] Zasadny KR, Wahl RL. Standardized uptake values of normal tissues at PET with 2-[fluorine-18]-fluoro-2-deoxy-D-glucose: variations with body weight and a method for correction. Radiology. 1993; 189(3):847–850

[8] Kotasidis FA, Tsoumpas C, Rahmim A. Advanced kinetic modelling strategies: towards adoption in clinical PET imaging. Clin Transl Imaging. 2014; 2(3):219–237

[9] Salavati A, Saboury B, Alavi A. Comment on: "Tumor aggressiveness and patient outcome in cancer of the pancreas assessed by dynamic 18F-FDG PET/CT". J Nucl Med. 2014; 55 (2):350–351

[10] Wang G, Qi J. Direct estimation of kinetic parametric images for dynamic PET. Theranostics. 2013; 3(10):802–815

[11] Zaidi H, El Naqa I. PET-guided delineation of radiation therapy treatment volumes: a survey of image segmentation techniques. Eur J Nucl Med Mol Imaging. 2010; 37(11):2165–2187

[12] Hatt M, Lee JA, Schmidtlein CR, et al. Classification and evaluation strategies of auto-segmentation approaches for PET: Report of AAPM task group No. 211. Med Phys. 2017; 44(6): e1–e42

[13] Berthon B, Spezi E, Galavis P, et al. Toward a standard for the evaluation of PET auto-segmentation methods following recommendations of AAPM task group No. 211: Requirements and implementation. Med Phys. 2017; 44(8):4098–4111

[14] O'Connor JP, Aboagye EO, Adams JE, et al. Imaging biomarker roadmap for cancer studies. Nat Rev Clin Oncol. 2017; 14(3): 169–186

[15] El Naqa I, Kerns SL, Coates J, et al. Radiogenomics and radiotherapy response modeling. Phys Med Biol. 2017; 62(16): R179–R206

[16] Yip SS, Aerts HJ. Applications and limitations of radiomics. Phys Med Biol. 2016; 61(13):R150–R166

[17] Cheng G, Alavi A, Lim E, Werner TJ, Del Bello CV, Akers SR. Dynamic changes of FDG uptake and clearance in normal tissues. Mol Imaging Biol. 2013; 15(3):345–352

[18] Orlhac F, Soussan M, Maisonobe JA, Garcia CA, Vanderlinden B, Buvat I. Tumor texture analysis in 18F-FDG PET: relationships between texture parameters, histogram indices, standardized uptake values, metabolic volumes, and total lesion glycolysis. J Nucl Med. 2014; 55(3):414–422

[19] El Naqa I, Grigsby P, Apte A, et al. Exploring feature-based approaches in PET images for predicting cancer treatment outcomes. Pattern Recognit. 2009; 42(6):1162–1171

[20] O'Sullivan F, Wolsztynski E, O'Sullivan J, Richards T, Conrad EU, Eary JF. A statistical modeling approach to the analysis of spatial patterns of FDG-PET uptake in human sarcoma. IEEE Trans Med Imaging. 2011; 30(12):2059–2071

[21] Aerts HJWL, Velazquez ER, Leijenaar RTH, et al. Decoding tumour phenotype by noninvasive imaging using a quantitative radiomics approach. Nat Commun. 2014; 5:4006

[22] Cook GJR, Siddique M, Taylor BP, et al. Radiomics in PET: principles and applications. Clin Transl Imaging. 2014; 2(3):269–276

[23] Kumar V, Gu Y, Basu S, et al. Radiomics: the process and the challenges. Magn Reson Imaging. 2012; 30(9):1234–1248

[24] Lambin P, Rios-Velazquez E, Leijenaar R, et al. Radiomics: extracting more information from medical images using advanced feature analysis. Eur J Cancer. 2012; 48(4):441–446

[25] Schaefer-Prokop C, Prokop M. New imaging techniques in the treatment guidelines for lung cancer. Eur Respir J Suppl. 2002; 35:71s–83s

[26] Dimitrakopoulou-Strauss A, Strauss LG, Heichel T, et al. The role of quantitative (18)F-FDG PET studies for the differentiation of malignant and benign bone lesions. J Nucl Med. 2002; 43(4):510–518

[27] Karakatsanis NA, Lodge MA, Tahari AK, Zhou Y, Wahl RL, Rahmim A. Dynamic whole-body PET parametric imaging: I. Concept, acquisition protocol optimization and clinical application. Phys Med Biol. 2013; 58(20):7391–7418

[28] Karakatsanis NA, Lodge MA, Yun Z, et al. Dynamic multi-bed FDG PET imaging: Feasibility and optimization. In: IEEE Nuclear Science Symposium and Medical Imaging Conference (NSS/MIC); 2011:3863–3870

[29] Karakatsanis NA, Lodge MA, Zhou Y, Wahl RL, Rahmim A. Dynamic whole-body PET parametric imaging: II. Task-oriented statistical estimation. Phys Med Biol. 2013; 58(20):7419–7445

[30] Karakatsanis NA, Casey ME, Lodge MA, Rahmim A, Zaidi H. Whole-body direct 4D parametric PET imaging employing nested generalized Patlak expectation-maximization reconstruction. Phys Med Biol. 2016; 61(15):5456–5485

[31] Rahmim A, Tang J, Zaidi H. Four-dimensional (4D) image reconstruction strategies in dynamic PET: beyond conventional independent frame reconstruction. Med Phys. 2009; 36(8): 3654–3670

[32] Zaidi H, Karakatsanis N. Towards enhanced PET quantification in clinical oncology. Br J Radiol. 2017

[33] Alavi A, Newberg AB, Souder E, Berlin JA. Quantitative analysis of PET and MRI data in normal aging and Alzheimer's disease: atrophy weighted total brain metabolism and absolute whole brain metabolism as reliable discriminators. J Nucl Med. 1993; 34(10):1681–1687

[34] Larson SM, Erdi Y, Akhurst T, et al. Tumor treatment response based on visual and quantitative changes in global tumor glycolysis using PET-FDG imaging. The visual response score and the change in total lesion glycolysis. Clin Positron Imaging. 1999; 2(3):159–171

[35] Lee JW, Hwang SH, Kim HJ, Kim D, Cho A, Yun M. Volumetric parameters on FDG PET can predict early intrahepatic recurrence-free survival in patients with hepatocellular carcinoma after curative surgical resection. Eur J Nucl Med Mol Imaging. 2017; 44(12):1984–1994

[36] Salavati A, Duan F, Snyder BS, et al. Optimal FDG PET/CT volumetric parameters for risk stratification in patients with locally advanced non-small cell lung cancer: results from the ACRIN 6668/RTOG 0235 trial. Eur J Nucl Med Mol Imaging. 2017; 44(12):1969–1983

[37] Basu S, Saboury B, Werner T, Alavi A. Clinical utility of FDG-PET and PET/CT in non-malignant thoracic disorders. Mol Imaging Biol. 2011; 13(6):1051–1060

[38] Kitajima K, Doi H, Kuribayashi K, et al. Prognostic value of pretreatment volume-based quantitative 18F-FDG PET/CT parameters in patients with malignant pleural mesothelioma. Eur J Radiol. 2017; 86:176–183

[39] Lopci E, Zucali PA, Ceresoli GL, et al. Quantitative analyses at baseline and interim PET evaluation for response assessment and outcome definition in patients with malignant pleural mesothelioma. Eur J Nucl Med Mol Imaging. 2015; 42(5): 667–675

[40] Ciftci E, Turgut B, Cakmakcilar A, Erturk SA. Diagnostic importance of 18F-FDG PET/CT parameters and total lesion glycolysis in differentiating between benign and malignant adrenal lesions. Nucl Med Commun. 2017; 38(9):788–794

[41] Jena A, Taneja S, Singh A, et al. Reliability of 18F-FDG PET metabolic parameters derived using simultaneous PET/MRI and correlation with prognostic factors of invasive ductal carcinoma: a feasibility study. AJR Am J Roentgenol. 2017; 209 (3):662–670

[42] Gallicchio R, Nardelli A, Venetucci A, et al. F-18 FDG PET/CT metabolic tumor volume predicts overall survival in patients with disseminated epithelial ovarian cancer. Eur J Radiol. 2017; 93:107–113

[43] Park JS, Lee N, Beom SH, et al. The prognostic value of volume-based parameters using 18F-FDG PET/CT in gastric cancer according to HER2 status. Gastric Cancer. 2018; 21:213–224

[44] Lim Y, Bang JI, Han SW, et al. Total lesion glycolysis (TLG) as an imaging biomarker in metastatic colorectal cancer patients treated with regorafenib. Eur J Nucl Med Mol Imaging. 2017; 44(5):757–764

[45] Schmuck S, von Klot CA, Henkenberens C, et al. Initial experience with volumetric 68Ga-PSMA I&T PET/CT for assessment of whole-body tumor burden as a quantitative imaging biomarker in patients with prostate cancer. J Nucl Med. 2017; 58 (12):1962–1968

[46] Hwang SH, Cho A, Yun M, Choi YD, Rha SY, Kang WJ. Prognostic value of pretreatment metabolic tumor volume and total lesion glycolysis using 18F-FDG PET/CT in patients with metastatic renal cell carcinoma treated with anti-vascular endothelial growth factor-targeted agents. Clin Nucl Med. 2017; 42(5):e235–e241

[47] Hwang SH, Lee JW, Cho HJ, Kim KS, Choi GH, Yun M. Prognostic value of metabolic tumor volume and total lesion glycolysis on preoperative 18F-FDG PET/CT in patients with very early and early hepatocellular carcinoma. Clin Nucl Med. 2017; 42(1):34–39

[48] Mikhaeel NG, Smith D, Dunn JT, et al. Combination of baseline metabolic tumour volume and early response on PET/CT improves progression-free survival prediction in DLBCL. Eur J Nucl Med Mol Imaging. 2016; 43(7):1209–1219

[49] Lee PI, Cheng G, Alavi A. The role of serial FDG PET for assessing therapeutic response in patients with cardiac sarcoidosis. J Nucl Cardiol. 2017; 24(1):19–28

[50] Saboury B, Salavati A, Brothers A, et al. FDG PET/CT in Crohn's disease: correlation of quantitative FDG PET/CT parameters with clinical and endoscopic surrogate markers of disease activity. Eur J Nucl Med Mol Imaging. 2014; 41(4):605–614

[51] Abdulla S, Salavati A, Saboury B, Basu S, Torigian DA, Alavi A. Quantitative assessment of global lung inflammation following radiation therapy using FDG PET/CT: a pilot study. Eur J Nucl Med Mol Imaging. 2014; 41(2):350–356

[52] Blomberg BA, de Jong PA, Thomassen A, et al. Thoracic aorta calcification but not inflammation is associated with increased cardiovascular disease risk: results of the CAMONA study. Eur J Nucl Med Mol Imaging. 2017; 44(2):249–258

[53] Bural GG, Torigian DA, Chamroonrat W, et al. Quantitative assessment of the atherosclerotic burden of the aorta by combined FDG-PET and CT image analysis: a new concept. Nucl Med Biol. 2006; 33(8):1037–1043

[54] Mehta NN, Torigian DA, Gelfand JM, Saboury B, Alavi A. Quantification of atherosclerotic plaque activity and vascular inflammation using [18-F] fluorodeoxyglucose positron emission tomography/computed tomography (FDG-PET/CT). J Vis Exp. 2012(63):e3777

[55] Houshmand S, Salavati A, Hess S, Werner TJ, Alavi A, Zaidi H. An update on novel quantitative techniques in the context of evolving whole-body PET imaging. PET Clin. 2015; 10(1):45–58

[56] Im HJ, Pak K, Cheon GJ, et al. Prognostic value of volumetric parameters of (18)F-FDG PET in non-small-cell lung cancer: a meta-analysis. Eur J Nucl Med Mol Imaging. 2015; 42(2):241–251

[57] Liu J, Dong M, Sun X, Li W, Xing L, Yu J. Prognostic value of 18F-FDG PET/CT in surgical non-small cell lung cancer: a meta-analysis. PLoS One. 2016; 11(1):e0146195

[58] Herrmann K, Bluemel C, Weineisen M, et al. Biodistribution and radiation dosimetry for a probe targeting prostate-specific membrane antigen for imaging and therapy. J Nucl Med. 2015; 56:855–861

[59] Pak K, Cheon GJ, Nam HY, et al. Prognostic value of metabolic tumor volume and total lesion glycolysis in head and neck cancer: a systematic review and meta-analysis. J Nucl Med. 2014; 55(6):884–890

[60] Lapa P, Marques M, Costa G, Iagaru A, Pedroso de Lima J. Assessment of skeletal tumour burden on 18F-NaF PET/CT using a new quantitative method. Nucl Med Commun. 2017; 38(4):325–332

[61] Gholami S, Salavati A, Houshmand S, Werner TJ, Alavi A. Assessment of atherosclerosis in large vessel walls: A comprehensive review of FDG-PET/CT image acquisition protocols and methods for uptake quantification. J Nucl Cardiol. 2015; 22(3):468–479

[62] Jahangiri P, Pournazari K, Torigian DA, et al. A prospective study of the feasibility of FDG-PET/CT imaging to quantify radiation-induced lung inflammation in locally advanced non-small cell lung cancer patients receiving proton or photon radiotherapy. Eur J Nucl Med Mol Imaging. 2018 [Epub ahead of print]. DOI: 10.1007/s00259-018-4154-5

7 Normal Variants and Benign Findings

Eugene C. Lin

7.1 General Principles

As a general rule, most inflammatory or infectious processes are visualized by positron emission tomography (PET) because activated white cells have increased glycolysis. Thus, it is not possible to exhaustively list all potential nonneoplastic causes of fludeoxyglucose (FDG) uptake. Correlation with clinical data and other imaging studies should alert the interpreter in many cases to potential false-positive findings in such settings. The discussion in this chapter will focus on the range of normal sites of FDG uptake and the common noninfectious/inflammatory causes of increased uptake. Artifacts specific to PET/computed tomography (CT) will be discussed in Chapter 9.

7.2 Brain

It is important that physicians who interpret PET brain scans review a large number of normal images before interpreting studies in patients with neuropsychiatric disorders.[1]

1. Normal pattern of uptake
   a) The normal brain has high FDG uptake in the gray matter, with a gray-to-white matter activity ratio ranging from 2:5 to 4:1.
   b) The basal ganglia usually have slightly more uptake than the cortex.
   c) The medial temporal cortices typically have less uptake than the other cortical areas.[2]
   d) Mild focal areas of increased activity can be seen normally in the[3]
      • Frontal eye fields.
      • Posterior cingulate cortex.
      • Wernicke's region (posterosuperior temporal lobe).
        Visual cortex (▶ Fig. 32.2).
2. **Age-related changes**. Cortical metabolism decreases with age, particularly in the frontal lobes. Other areas that can show decreased activity with aging are the insula, temporal lobes (lateral), parietal lobes, and anterior and middle cingulate cortices. The least altered regions during aging are the primary motor cortices, occipital cortices, precuneus, mesial temporal lobes, basal ganglia, and cerebellum.[2]
3. **Renal function**. Patients with renal failure have decreased FDG uptake in the cortex and white matter compared to those with normal renal function.[4]
4. **Symmetry of uptake**. There are often minimal asymmetries in uptake between areas in the left and right hemispheres. Asymmetric uptake should be interpreted with caution unless
   a) There is a significant difference between the two sides that correlates with clinical findings. For example, any level of asymmetry in the temporal lobes in a patient with epilepsy should be considered a potential focus for seizure activity. Quantitatively, a difference of 10 to 15% is often considered significant but clinical correlation is paramount.
   b) The asymmetry is fairly extensive and seen on multiple slices.
5. Comparison with single-photon emission computed tomography (SPECT).
   a) FDG uptake usually correlates with uptake of SPECT perfusion tracers, except in cases where metabolism and perfusion are uncoupled (e.g., luxury perfusion postinfarct).
   b) The magnitude of hypometabolism seen on PET is usually greater than that of hypoperfusion seen on SPECT.
   c) Cerebellar uptake of FDG is variable but in general is less than seen on SPECT. This differs from brain SPECT images, where consistently the cerebellum appears more active than other brain structures.
6. **Crossed cerebellar diaschisis**. The glucose metabolism in the cerebellar hemisphere contralateral to a supratentorial abnormality (tumor, infarct, or trauma) is frequently decreased (▶ Fig. 7.1) in the acute phase of the disease and may change over time. This does not indicate cerebellar pathology.
   a) Diaschisis is thought to be related to interruption of the corticopontocerebellar pathway.
   b) Ipsilateral pontine hypometabolism and preservation of metabolism in the contralateral dentate nucleus have been reported.[5]

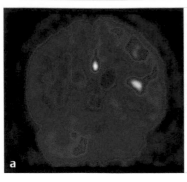
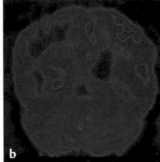

Fig. 7.1 Crossed cerebellar diaschisis. Coronal PET scans in a different patients demonstrate decreased activity in the left cerebellar hemisphere secondary to right cerebral infarct **(a)** and right-sided glioblastoma multiforme **(b)**.

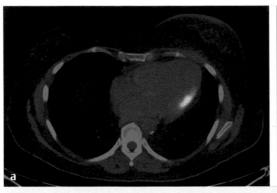
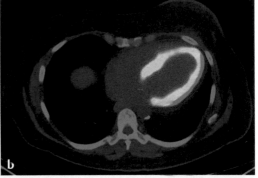

Fig. 7.2 Changing pattern of cardiac uptake. **(a)** Axial PET/CT demonstrates absent FDG uptake in the septum, anterior wall, and apex. This should not be interpreted as an infarct in the absence of a supporting clinical history and this patient did not have a history of cardiac disease. **(b)** Axial PET/CT in the same patient done at a later date demonstrates homogeneous myocardial uptake.

7.3 Spinal Cord

Spinal cord uptake is variable. Mild spinal cord uptake is normal.

7.4 Heart

1. Ventricular uptake
   a) ***Fasting state uptake***. For noncardiac PET studies done during fasting, myocardial metabolism shifts from utilizing glucose to utilizing fatty acids. Therefore, in theory myocardial uptake on fasting PET studies should be minimal. However, in many cases there will be substantial myocardial FDG uptake on fasting PET studies.
   Different patterns of normal myocardial uptake under fasting conditions have been described, specifically increased posterolateral wall uptake[6] and increased basal wall uptake.[7] However, one study has not found any discernable pattern of myocardial FDG uptake.[8] Decreased septal activity has been noted as a common normal variant in fasting patients (► Fig. 7.2). However, left bundle branch block can also cause decreased septal uptake.[9]
   b) Outpatients, men, younger patients, patients with heart failure, and patients receiving benzodiazepines tend to have more myocardial uptake.[10,11] However, one study[8] did not find any difference in myocardial uptake related to gender or age.
   c) Diabetic patients and patients receiving bezafibrate or levothyroxine tend to have less myocardial uptake.[10,12]
   d) The myocardial uptake pattern demonstrates a large spatial and temporal variability and a patient without cardiac disease can demonstrate substantially different patterns of myocardial FDG uptake on serial studies (► Fig. 7.3).[13]

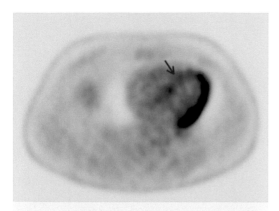

Fig. 7.3 Normal variant decreased septal uptake. Axial PET scan demonstrates decreased septal uptake (*arrow*), which is a normal variant in this patient. In the majority of cases, this finding is a normal variant, but an infarct or left bundle branch block could also cause this appearance and cannot be differentiated from normal variant decreased uptake without clinical history.

e) Heterogeneous myocardial uptake is more likely to be abnormal, and has been reported to be associated with sarcoidosis.[14]

f) *Insulin effect*. Increased myocardial activity is seen after insulin administration or insulin release secondary to a recent meal (myocardial glucose receptors are insulin sensitive). This is seen in conjunction with intense skeletal muscle uptake (▶ Fig. 4.1).

g) *Right ventricular uptake*. There is greater uptake in the left ventricle than the right ventricle. Typically, right ventricular uptake is minimal unless there is right ventricular pressure overload secondary to pulmonary hypertension or valvular disease.[15]

h) *Papillary muscle uptake*. Papillary muscle uptake is often seen in conjunction with uptake in the left ventricular wall. Occasionally, papillary muscle uptake can be seen in isolation (▶ Fig. 7.4).[16] In these cases, the uptake could mimic an intraventricular neoplasm or thrombus. Note that there are no septal left ventricular papillary muscles and left ventricular uptake arising from the septum cannot represent papillary muscle (▶ Fig. 7.4).

2. Atrial uptake
   a) Atrial uptake can be irregular and focal. Focal atrial FDG uptake can mimic a mediastinal node (▶ Fig. 7.5). This is particularly true on axial images in the subcarinal region.

Therefore, correlation with sagittal and coronal PET images and CT is necessary before diagnosing subcarinal nodal uptake on axial images.

b) Ringlike atrial wall uptake can mimic a large necrotic subcarinal node (▶ Fig. 7.6). This is easily differentiated by correlation with all imaging planes and CT.

c) Uptake in the atrial appendages can be seen due to overload physiology or thrombus. In addition, uptake can be seen in the crista terminalis, between the atrial appendage and the venous portion of the atrium.[17]

d) Increased right atrial wall uptake is associated with atrial fibrillation.[18,19,20] Left atrial wall uptake is less common and could be related to overload physiology.[15] Right atrial uptake (▶ Fig. 7.7) is usually more prominent.[19]

3. **Perfusion imaging**: If perfusion imaging is performed with nitrogen-13 ammonia, lateral wall activity is normally decreased compared to the septum.[21] This is of unknown etiology.

7.5 Head and Neck

1. **Normal uptake (sagittal)**. On sagittal images, there is normally an inverted "**C**" shape composed of the mylohyoid muscles and sublingual glands, soft palate, and tonsils (▶ Fig. 7.8). These are the most common areas of normal uptake.

2. **Mylohyoid muscles and sublingual glands (axial)**. On axial images, uptake in the mylohyoid muscles and/or sublingual glands can form an inverted "**V**" medial to the mandible. Due to their proximity, it is difficult to distinguish whether uptake is in the sublingual glands, mylohyoid muscles, or both. Sublingual uptake is more superior and focal (▶ Fig. 7.9), while mylohyoid uptake is more inferior and linear (▶ Fig. 7.8).

3. **Soft palate (axial)**. The soft palate can appear as a prominent focus of activity on axial images (▶ Fig. 7.10).
   a) Soft palate uptake is more prominent in males.[22]

4. **Tonsils (coronal)**. Normal uptake in the palatine and lingual tonsils (▶ Fig. 7.8, ▶ Fig. 7.11) forms two vertical linear bands of uptake on coronal images (▶ Fig. 7.11). This may be prominent in cold/temperate climates and is also prominent in children.

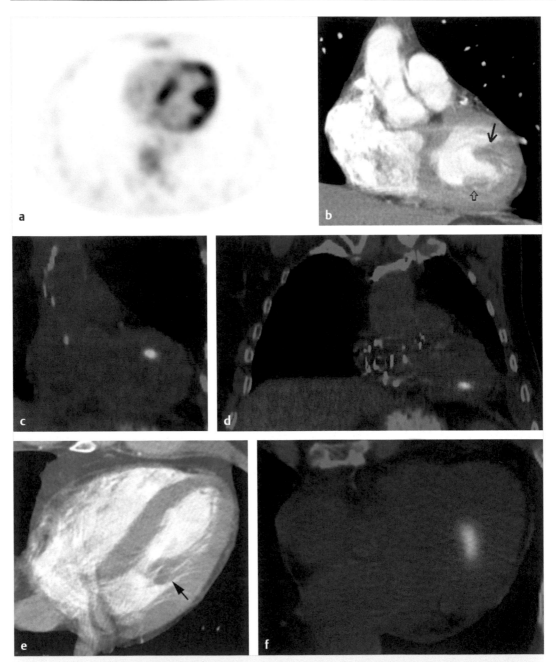

Fig. 7.4 Isolated papillary muscle uptake vs. cardiac metastasis. **(a)** Axial PET scan demonstrates uptake in the left ventricular myocardium and a papillary muscle. However, papillary muscle uptake is sometimes seen without myocardial uptake. **(b)** Coronal CT scan demonstrates the anterior lateral (*arrow*) and posterior medial (*open arrow*) papillary muscles. **(c)** Coronal PET/CT scan demonstrates isolated uptake in the anterior lateral papillary muscle. **(d)** Coronal PET/CT scan demonstrates isolated uptake in the posterior medial papillary muscle **(e)** Axial CT scan demonstrates the anterior lateral papillary muscle (*arrow*). **(f)** Axial PET/CT scan demonstrates isolated anterior lateral papillary muscle uptake. (*continued*)

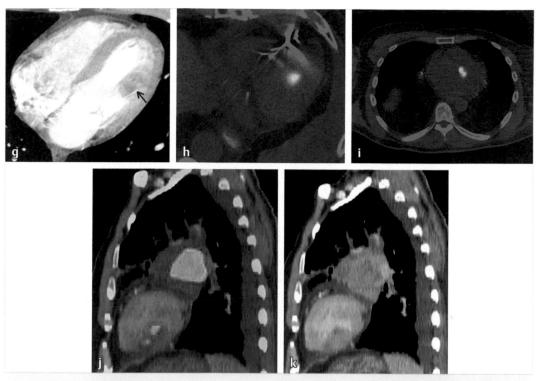

Fig. 7.4 *(continued)* **(g)** Axial CT scan demonstrates the posterior medial papillary muscle (*arrow*). **(h)** Axial PET/CT demonstrates isolated posterior medial papillary muscle uptake. **(i)** Focal uptake is noted in a left ventricular metastasis. Note that this cannot represent papillary muscle, as it arises from the septum and there are no left ventricular septal papillary muscles. **(j)** Sagittal PET/CT scan in a patient with lung cancer demonstrates uptake in a left perihilar mass and in a cardiac metastasis. Although this is in the region of the papillary muscle, the bilobed pattern of uptake would not be consistent with papillary muscle uptake. **(k)** Sagittal CT demonstrates an intraventricular mass corresponding to the FDG uptake. (Reproduced with permission from Lin.[16] (j) and (k) courtesy of Evan Sirc MD, Walnut Creek, CA.)

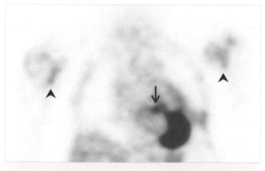

Fig. 7.5 Focal left atrial uptake mimicking nodal uptake and glenohumeral joint uptake. Coronal PET scan demonstrates focal increased uptake in the left atrium (*arrow*). This could mimic abnormal subcarinal node uptake on an axial slice through this focus. On the coronal image, the uptake can be seen to be contiguous with the left atrium. Increased glenohumeral joint uptake (*arrowheads*) is noted. While this can mimic adenopathy, it can be distinguished by its linear appearance and location immediately medial to the humeral heads.

a) Asymmetric physiologic tonsil uptake can be difficult to differentiate from tonsillar carcinoma. In one study,[23] a ratio of SUVmax between the tonsils (with a cutoff of 1.48) was effective in differentiating tonsillar cancer from asymmetric physiologic uptake.

b) There is less uptake with increasing age in the palatine tonsils.[22]

5. **Salivary glands**. Salivary gland uptake is more variable than tonsillar uptake.[22] Salivary gland uptake, if seen, is usually less than tonsillar uptake (▶ Fig. 7.11).

a) There is less uptake with increasing age in the sublingual glands.[22]

b) The submandibular glands are in close proximity to submandibular nodes and submandibular nodal uptake can be difficult to distinguish from normal glandular uptake even with PET/CT (▶ Fig. 7.12).

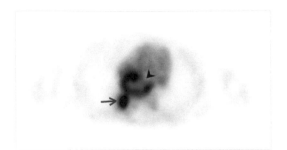

Fig. 7.6 Diffuse left atrial uptake mimicking a necrotic node. Axial PET scan in a patient with lung cancer (*arrow*) demonstrates a circular area of uptake medially suggestive of a necrotic mediastinal node. This is uptake in the left atrium which can be suspected given the lack of uptake in the region of the valve plane (*arrowhead*).

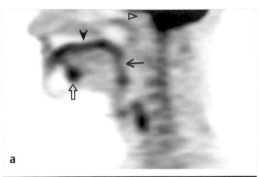

a

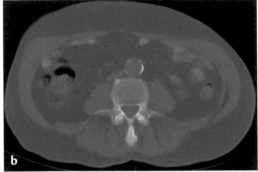

b

Fig. 7.8 (a,b) Normal sagittal head and neck. Sagittal PET scan demonstrates a typical inverted "**U**"-shaped pattern of uptake in the tonsils (*solid arrow*), soft palate (*arrowhead*), and mylohyoid muscle and sublingual glands (*open arrow*). Nasopharyngeal uptake (*open arrowhead*) is also seen.

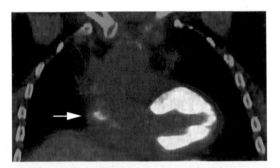

Fig. 7.7 Right atrial uptake. Coronal PET/CT scan demonstrates uptake in the right atrium (*arrow*).

6. **Nasopharyngeal uptake**. Nasopharyngeal uptake is sometimes seen as a normal variant (▶ Fig. 7.8), although larger degrees of uptake could be secondary to inflammation or tumor. Uptake in the lateral pharyngeal recess can be symmetric or asymmetric.
   a) *Asymmetric uptake.* Asymmetric uptake in the lateral pharyngeal recess (▶ Fig. 7.11), cervical nodal uptake, and asymmetric wall thickening in the lateral pharyngeal recess on CT are associated with nasopharyngeal carcinoma.[24]
      • However, in patient populations where nasopharyngeal carcinoma is less frequent, asymmetric uptake in the lateral pharyngeal recesses is often inflammatory.

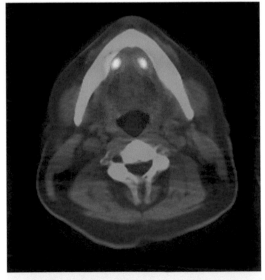

Fig. 7.9 Sublingual gland uptake. Axial PET/CT scan demonstrates normal inverted "**V**"-shaped uptake in the sublingual glands. Mylohyoid muscle uptake can have a similar appearance but is slightly inferior and more linear.

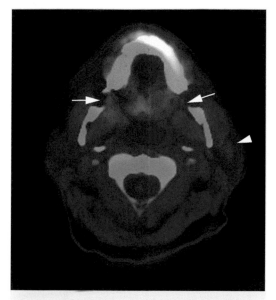

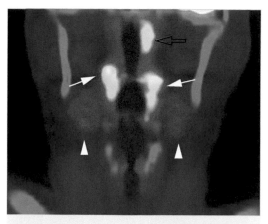

Fig. 7.11 Tonsil and submandibular gland uptake and nasopharyngeal carcinoma. Coronal PET/CT scan demonstrates typical vertical bands of tonsillar uptake (*arrows*). Mild submandibular gland uptake is seen (*arrowheads*). Tonsil uptake is usually greater than salivary gland uptake. There is asymmetric uptake in the left nasopharynx (*open arrow*) secondary to nasopharyngeal carcinoma. However, in populations where nasopharyngeal carcinoma is not endemic, asymmetric uptake is often inflammatory. If this uptake were symmetric, it could be a normal variant or secondary to inflammation.

Fig. 7.10 Soft palate, parotid gland, and spinal cord uptake. Axial PET/CT scan demonstrates normal soft palate uptake (*arrows*), which can appear very prominent on axial images. There is normal uptake in the left parotid gland (*arrowhead*). This is more prominent than right parotid uptake as this patient has more left parotid tissue at this level. Normal spinal cord uptake is also seen.

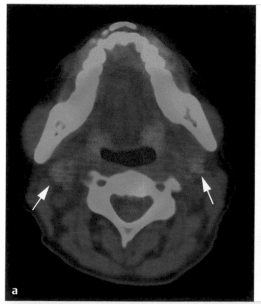

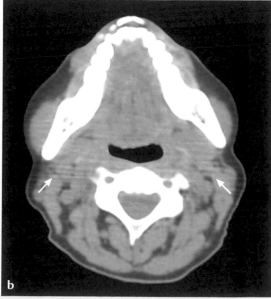

Fig. 7.12 Node or submandibular gland? (a) Axial PET/CT demonstrates bilateral uptake near the submandibular glands (*arrows*). It is difficult to determine whether this uptake is in nodes or the submandibular glands, particularly as the uptake is bilateral. However, the uptake is relatively posterior suggesting that it is not in the submandibular glands. (b) Corresponding axial CT demonstrates bilateral nodes (*arrows*) corresponding to the FDG uptake. Lower density submandibular glands are noted anterior to the nodes.

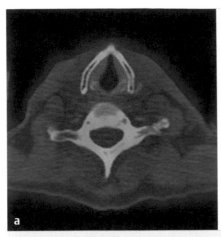
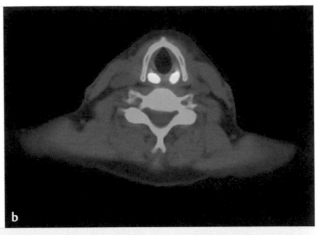

Fig. 7.13 Patterns of laryngeal uptake. (a) Axial PET/CT scan demonstrates an inverted "V"-shaped appearance of the laryngeal uptake secondary to uptake in both the vocal cords and cricoarytenoid muscles. (b) Axial PET/CT scan demonstrates two foci of posterior cricoarytenoid uptake. Note the absence of anterior cord uptake in this patient, which is a normal variant. If anterior cord uptake was greater than posterior uptake, this would be more worrisome for pathology.

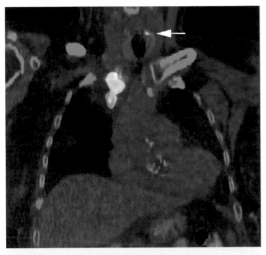

Fig. 7.14 Coronal PET/CT demonstrates unilateral uptake in the left vocal cord (arrow) secondary to right vocal cord paralysis caused by a right apical lung cancer.

b) An SUV cutoff of < 3.9 and a lateral pharyngeal recess-to-palatine tonsil uptake ratio of < 1.5 are helpful in differentiating benign from malignant lateral pharyngeal recess uptake.[24]

c) Uptake in the midline roof the nasopharynx could be secondary to uptake in adenoidal tissue or nasopharyngeal carcinoma. In one study,[25] an SUV level of less than 4.61 and a midline roof-to-palatine tonsil ratio of < 1.14 were helpful in differentiation, although there was still overlap between neoplastic and nonneoplastic uptake levels. Additional findings were necessary to increase the accuracy of PET. For example, associated increased FDG uptake in Waldeyer's ring and the salivary glands occurred in benign but not malignant lesions. Symmetric uptake in the lateral pharyngeal regions was associated with benign etiologies.

7. **Tongue**. Tongue uptake can occasionally be seen, particularly if the patient speaks after FDG injection. In children, adenoid tissues are commonly visualized at the base of the tongue.

8. **Laryngeal uptake**. Laryngeal muscle uptake is a normal variant, and is pronounced if the patient speaks soon after FDG administration. It can have a horseshoelike appearance with uptake in both the vocal cords and cricoarytenoid muscles, or can appear as two foci of posterior uptake in the cricoarytenoid muscles (▶ Fig. 7.13). Normal activity is most pronounced posteriorly.

a) It is better to use asymmetry of uptake rather than absolute uptake in the larynx as a criterion of abnormality.

b) However, laryngeal uptake may be asymmetric secondary to postoperative changes or vocal cord paralysis (▶ Fig. 7.14).

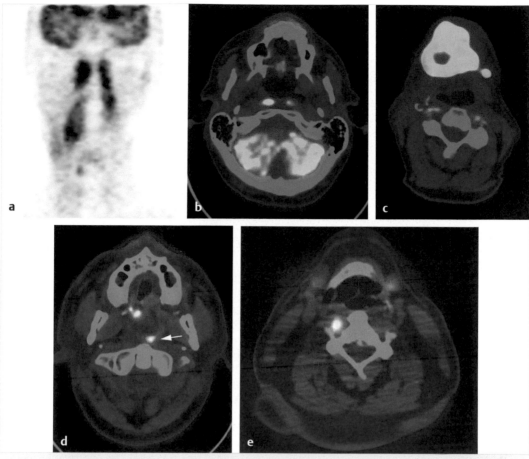

Fig. 7.15 Asymmetric longus colli uptake. **(a)** Coronal PET scan demonstrates bilateral uptake in the longus colli muscles. The longus colli muscles are located on the anterior surface of the vertebral column and arise from the anterior vertebral bodies of T1–T3 and the anterior tubercles of the transverse processes of C3–C7. They insert on the anterior arch of C1 and the C2–C4 vertebral bodies. Axial PET/CT images demonstrate uptake in the longus colli muscles superiorly **(b)** and inferiorly **(c)**. Asymmetric uptake is sometimes seen, which can mimic disease. Axial PET/CT images demonstrate asymmetric longus colli uptake (*arrow*) superiorly **(d)** and inferiorly **(e)**. (Reproduced with permission from Lin.[27])

c) Anterior uptake is more concerning than posterior uptake.

d) Injection of Teflon or calcium hydroxylapatite microspheres can result in increased FDG uptake.[26]

9. **Muscle uptake.** Muscular uptake is common, particularly in the sternocleidomastoids. Less commonly, uptake is seen in the longus colli muscles. This can be asymmetric and potentially mimic neoplasm (▶ Fig. 7.15).[27] However, before attributing uptake to asymmetric longus colli activity, retropharyngeal adenopathy (▶ Fig. 7.16) should be excluded as it can have a similar appearance on axial images.

7.6 Thyroid

1. **Diffuse uptake.** Mild diffuse thyroid uptake can be a normal variant. Greater degrees of diffuse uptake are seen in Graves' disease and chronic thyroiditis (▶ Fig. 7.17).[28,29] In particular, diffuse thyroid uptake is often associated with chronic lymphocytic (Hashimoto's) thyroiditis. This is not affected by thyroid hormone therapy. The SUV does not correlate with the degree of hypothyroidism.[30] Approximately 30% of patients with Graves' disease will have increased thyroid uptake.[31] However, Graves' disease is typically associated with sparse thyroid uptake and increased skeletal muscle and thymus uptake.

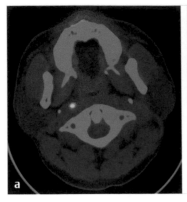
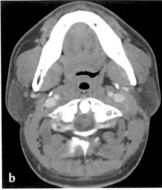

Fig. 7.16 Retropharyngeal node vs. longus colli uptake. **(a)** Axial PET/CT demonstrates focal uptake in the region of the right longus colli. This could mimic normal variant asymmetric longus colli uptake, but correlation with contrast-enhanced CT **(b)** demonstrates asymmetric soft tissue in this region. The uptake was in a retropharyngeal node.

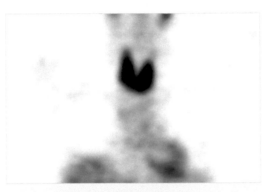

Fig. 7.17 Thyroiditis. Diffuse increased thyroid uptake is secondary to thyroiditis. Lesser degrees of diffuse uptake could be a normal variant.

a) *SUV*. The normal thyroid has an SUVmean of 1.25 ± 0.24 (age, 56 +)[32] and SUVmax of 1.5 ± 0.2.[30,33]

b) *Graves' disease*. Increased thyroid uptake in Graves' disease is relatively uncommon; increased skeletal muscle and thymus activity is actually more commonly seen in this disorder.[34]

2. **Focal uptake.** Focal uptake is nonspecific and can be seen in both benign and malignant nodules (see Chapter 15).

3. **Thyroid nodule mimics.** Correlation with anatomic imaging is necessary before diagnosing peripheral thyroid nodules on PET.

a) *Lymph node*. A medial lymph node adjacent to the thyroid can mimic a thyroid nodule (▶ Fig. 15.3).

b) *Parathyroid abnormality*. Both parathyroid adenomas and hyperplasia can cause focal increased uptake mimicking a thyroid nodule. The normal parathyroids are not visualized on FDG PET.

7.7 Axilla

1. **Glenohumeral joint.** Glenohumeral joint activity can mimic axillary adenopathy on axial and coronal images (▶ Fig. 7.18). It can be distinguished by its linear appearance and location immediately medial to the humeral head. This finding may not always be a normal variant as it is often associated with joint pain.

2. **Dose extravasation.** Extravasation at the injection site can cause ipsilateral axillary node uptake due to particle formation and phagocytosis at the draining lymph nodes (▶ Fig. 7.19).

7.8 Breast

1. **Premenopausal.** Diffuse low-grade uptake is seen in glandular breast tissue in premenopausal women (▶ Fig. 7.20). The SUV in dense breasts is higher than in nondense breasts; however, the uptake in dense breasts is still very low (SUV around 1).[35]

2. **Postmenopausal.** Postmenopausal women on hormone replacement therapy may also have glandular uptake. The breast uptake should be less than the liver in postmenopausal women who are not on hormonal therapy.[36]

3. **Lactation.** Prominent diffuse uptake is seen during lactation.

4. **Nipple.** Nipple uptake is commonly seen.

5. **Breast implants.** Mildly increased uptake can be seen around breast implants, which appear as negative defects.

6. **Focal uptake.** Focal uptake is seen due to a wide range of benign conditions but commonly represents malignancy (see Chapter 17).

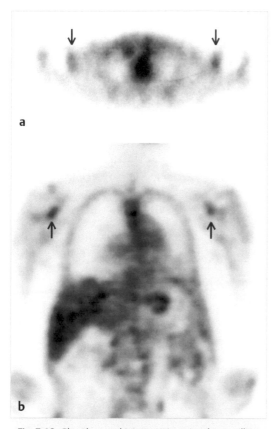

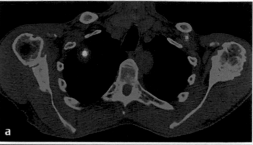

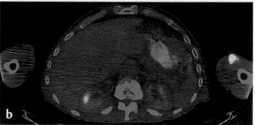

Fig. 7.19 Node uptake secondary to injection extravasation. **(a)** Axial PET/CT in a patient with increased FDG uptake in a malignant right lung nodule also demonstrates uptake in a left axillary node. This uptake is secondary to injection extravasation in the left antecubital fossa **(b)**.

Fig. 7.18 Glenohumeral joint activity mimicking axillary nodal uptake. **(a)** Axial PET scan through the upper thorax demonstrates bilateral glenohumeral joint uptake (*arrows*). **(b)** Coronal PET scan in the same patient demonstrates bilateral glenohumeral joint uptake (*arrows*). While this uptake could be confused with axillary nodal uptake, it can be distinguished by its linear appearance and location immediately medial to the humeral head.

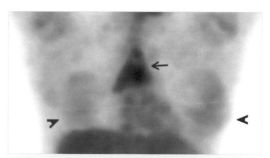

Fig. 7.20 Thymic hyperplasia and normal breast uptake. Coronal FDG scan demonstrates uptake in a hyperplastic thymus in a 35-year-old female. This should not be confused with mediastinal adenopathy as it has an inverted "**V**" shape and a horizontal photopenic cleft (*arrow*) characteristic of thymus. A photopenic cleft can sometimes be seen in the vertical direction. Normal uptake in premenopausal glandular breast tissue is seen (*arrowheads*).

7.9 Thymus

1. **Children**. Thymus uptake is a normal variant in children.
2. **Adults**. In adults, thymic uptake (▶ Fig. 7.20, ▶ Fig. 7.21) can be seen with thymic hyperplasia or if a substantial amount of normal thymic tissue remains after adolescence. The thymus can be distinguished from anterior mediastinal adenopathy by its characteristic inverted "**V**" shape. In addition, photopenic clefts are often seen extending through the thymic tissue.
    a) *Age*. While thymic uptake is usually seen in young adults, it has been reported in patients up to the 54 years old.[37]

    b) *Clinical scenarios*. Thymic uptake is occasionally seen soon after chemotherapy and is common following radioiodine treatment for thyroid cancer.
    c) *Malignancy*. If the uptake is focal or intense (greater than cerebellum or bladder or high SUV), or if the thymic shape is distorted, the

possibility of malignancy should be considered.

d) **SUV**[38]

- The average SUV in thymic hyperplasia is 1.9.[39] However, SUV measurements as high as 3.8 have been reported in thymic hyperplasia.
- Thymomas typically have higher SUVs than thymic hyperplasia.[39] However, the SUVs seen in thymic hyperplasia may overlap with those in thymoma.

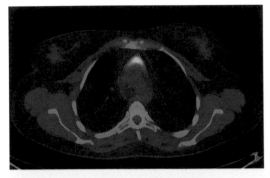

Fig. 7.21 Thymus uptake. Axial PET/CT scan demonstrates intense thymic uptake.

- Invasive thymomas do not have higher SUVs than noninvasive thymomas.
- Thymic carcinoma usually has higher SUVs than thymoma.
- SUV cutoffs to differentiate thymic carcinoma from thymoma are variable, ranging from 5 to 10.[40]
- Uptake in thymic carcinomas tends to be homogeneous, while uptake in thymomas is often heterogeneous.[40]

e) **Graves' disease.** Increased thymus uptake is common in Graves' disease. A clue to the diagnosis is seeing increased skeletal muscle uptake and thyroid uptake (less likely) in conjunction with the thymic uptake.[34]

f) **Density.** There is a positive correlation between the density of gland and the degree of FDG uptake.[41]

3. **Superior mediastinal activity.** A normal variant can be seen secondary to superior extension of the thymus (▶ Fig. 7.22).[42] In these cases, there is a soft tissue nodule anteromedial to the left brachiocephalic vein that can have increased FDG uptake, particularly in children and young adults who have thymic hyperplasia

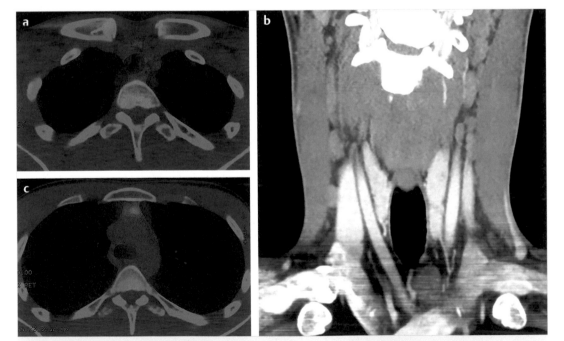

Fig. 7.22 Superior extension of the thymus. **(a)** Axial PET/CT demonstrates FDG activity in the superior mediastinum, which could potentially mimic nodal uptake. **(b)** Coronal contrast-enhanced CT demonstrates that this activity corresponds to soft tissue anteromedial to the left brachiocephalic vein, which is a typical location for cervical extension of thymic tissue. **(c)** Axial PET/CT at a more inferior level demonstrates FDG uptake in the thymus. Although a connection may not be seen to the superior thymic tissue, the degree of uptake should be comparable.

after chemotherapy. While this nodule may not be connected to the thymus, it should have a similar SUV.

7.10 Lung

1. **Normal gradient of activity**. The lungs typically have minimal or no activity on attenuation-corrected (AC) images. Lung activity increases from the anterior to the posterior and from the superior to the inferior segments, particularly if the lungs are not fully inflated. This is more prominently seen on non-AC images.
2. A wide range of infectious/inflammatory processes can cause diffuse or focal increased uptake. Some rare causes of uptake are
   a) ***Diffuse uptake***. Drug toxicity in cancer patients (▶ Fig. 7.23), radiation pneumonitis, acute respiratory distress syndrome.[43]
      • A neoplastic etiology of diffuse uptake is lymphangitic carcinomatosis (▶ Fig. 7.24).[44]
   b) ***Nodular uptake***.[45,46,47] Bronchiolitis obliterans organizing pneumonia, lung infarction, amyloidosis.
3. **Focal uptake without a CT correlate**. There should almost always be a correlative finding on CT for focal FDG uptake in the lung. If substantial motion artifact is present, small lung nodules may not be identified. If no correlative finding is identified on a CT without motion, a small focus of focal FDG uptake could represent a clot injected during FDG administration (▶ Fig. 7.25).
4. **Radiation pneumonitis**. Radiation pneumonitis can cause very intense uptake before radiographic changes are seen. This should be suspected in the proper clinical setting if the uptake has a linear margin (▶ Fig. 7.26). However, the lung is a relatively slow-reacting tissue to radiation, and radiation-induced elevation in FDG uptake typically does not occur until months after completion of radiotherapy.[48] Uptake (usually pleural) in the

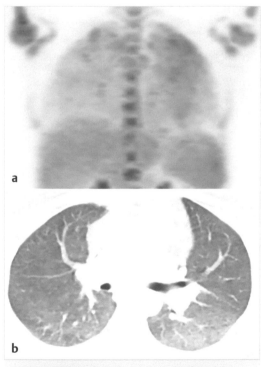

Fig. 7.23 Bleomycin lung toxicity. (a) Maximum intensity projection (MIP) PET in a patient with Hodgkin's disease demonstrates diffuse bilateral pulmonary uptake secondary to bleomycin toxicity. (b) Corresponding axial CT demonstrates diffuse ground glass opacities.

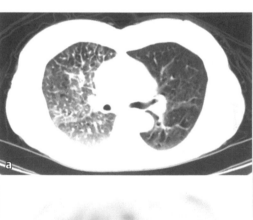
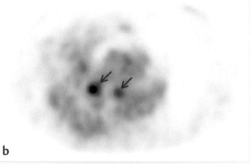

Fig. 7.24 Lymphangitic spread. (a) Axial CT scan demonstrates interstitial thickening in the right lung suspicious for lymphangitic spread. (b) Corresponding axial PET scan demonstrates diffuse right lung uptake secondary to lymphangitic spread. In addition, focal uptake (*arrows*) is present in right hilar and subcarinal nodal metastases.

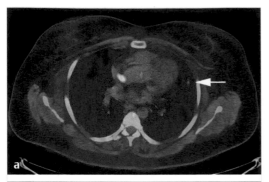

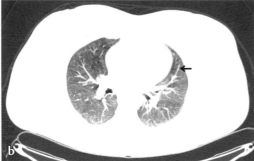

Fig. 7.25 Injected clot. **(a)** Axial PET/CT scan demonstrates focal uptake in the lingula (*arrow*). **(b)** Corresponding axial CT scan does not demonstrate a nodule in this region; however, this uptake appears to lie in a vessel (*arrow*). This uptake is likely secondary to injected clumped FDG.

contralateral shielded nonirradiated lung is common after radiation.[49]

5. **Atelectasis**. Atelectatic lung can have increased activity (▶ Fig. 7.27). There is a positive correlation between the density of the atelectatic lung and the degree of FDG activity.[50] However, PET is helpful in cases of postobstructive atelectasis, as the central obstructing tumor will have more uptake than the distal atelectasis (▶ Fig. 7.28).

6. Very rare causes of false-positive results are hamartoma, round atelectasis, and pleural fibrosis. In the majority of cases, these entities do not have significant uptake.[51]

7.11 Hila

1. Mild bilateral hilar nodal uptake is very common (▶ Fig. 7.29). This appearance is almost never associated with malignancy.

2. Uptake in a central pulmonary embolus could mimic hilar adenopathy.

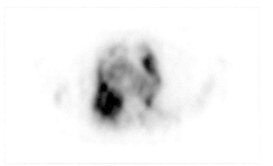

Fig. 7.26 Radiation pneumonitis. Axial PET scan demonstrates intense increased uptake around the mediastinum with linear margins corresponding to a radiation field. The appearance is typical for radiation pneumonitis.

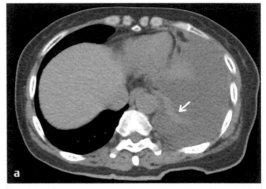

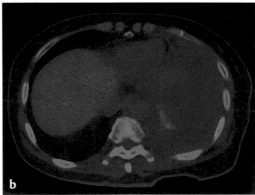

Fig. 7.27 Atelectasis. **(a)** Axial CT scan demonstrates a sliver of atelectatic lung (*arrow*) in a large left effusion. **(b)** Corresponding PET/CT scan demonstrates focal uptake in the atelectatic lung. This is commonly seen when the atelectasis is severe.

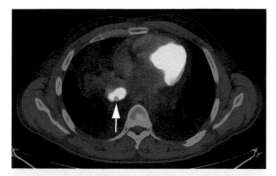

Fig. 7.28 Atelectasis secondary to obstructing tumor. Axial PET/CT scan demonstrates atelectasis secondary to a right hilar mass (*arrow*). The identification of an obstructing mass within an area of atelectasis is a particular strength of PET/CT as the mass often cannot be separated from the atelectasis by CT.

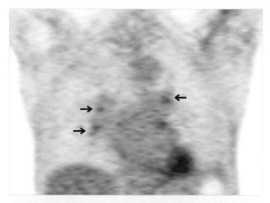

Fig. 7.29 Bilateral hilar uptake. Coronal PET scan demonstrates mild bilateral hilar uptake (*arrows*). This is a common finding on PET and may be related to granulomatous disease or smoking. This degree and pattern of uptake is almost never secondary to malignancy.

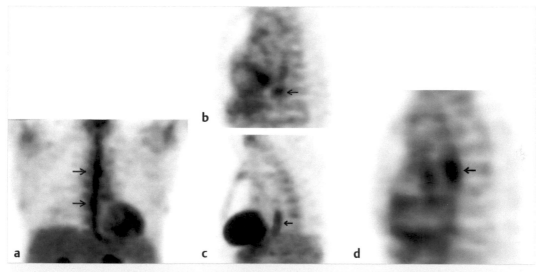

Fig. 7.30 Patterns of normal and abnormal esophageal uptake. **(a)** Normal esophagus. Uptake throughout the esophagus (*arrows*) on sagittal PET/CT scan is a normal variant in this patient, although esophagitis could also cause this appearance. **(b)** Normal gastroesophageal junction uptake. Sagittal PET scan demonstrates a small focus of normal variant uptake at the gastroesophageal junction (*arrow*). **(c)** Esophageal cancer. Increased uptake in the distal esophagus (*arrow*) on sagittal PET scan is secondary to esophageal carcinoma. This extends over a longer distance and is more intense than the normal uptake in **b**. **(d)** Esophageal cancer. Focal uptake in the mid-to-distal esophagus on sagittal PET/CT scan is secondary to esophageal carcinoma. Focal esophageal uptake not at the gastroesophageal junction is almost never normal. (Courtesy of Wengen Chen MD, Baltimore, MD.)

7.12 Esophagus

1. **Patterns of esophageal uptake** (▶ Fig. 7.30)
   a) Mild diffuse esophageal uptake is often a normal variant.
   b) Intense diffuse uptake can be noted secondary to esophagitis. Radiation therapy to the thorax can cause a limited area of diffuse intense esophageal uptake in the radiation port.

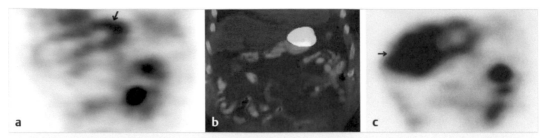

Fig. 7.31 Normal and abnormal gastric uptake. (a) Sagittal PET scan demonstrates normal stomach uptake, proximal (*arrow*) greater than distal with no focal uptake. (b) Coronal PET/CT scan demonstrates focal uptake in the fundus of the stomach secondary to gastric cancer. Even though this is proximal, it is abnormal because it is focal and the degree of intensity is much greater than the distal stomach. (c) Sagittal PET scan in a patient with gastric cancer demonstrates focal increased uptake in the distal stomach (*arrow*) greater than the normal uptake in proximal stomach. The distal uptake is abnormal because it is both focal and greater than the proximal uptake.

c) Minimal focal uptake is often seen at the gastroesophageal junction as a normal variant. However, greater degrees of activity at the gastroesophageal junction may warrant further evaluation with endoscopy. In two studies, SUV cutoffs of 3.5 or 4 differentiated pathological from nonpathological FDG uptake at the gastroesophageal junction.[52]

Focal esophageal activity not at the gastroesophageal junction is worrisome for neoplasm.

2. Esophageal uptake can be seen with esophageal spasm, reflux, and Barrett's esophagus.
3. **Brown fat mimic**. Brown fat uptake in the azygoesophageal recess can mimic focal esophageal uptake.[53]

7.13 Stomach

1. **Normal pattern of uptake**
   a) Moderate diffuse stomach uptake is a normal variant.
   b) Physiological gastric uptake is higher proximally (▸ Fig. 7.31).
2. **Abnormal uptake**. These patterns of uptake are abnormal and should raise suspicion for inflammatory or neoplastic processes (▸ Fig. 7.31, ▸ Fig. 7.32):
   a) Focal uptake (benign ulceration [▸ Fig. 7.32] as well as malignancy can cause focal uptake).[54]
   b) Diffuse intense uptake.
   c) If distal uptake is more prominent than proximal uptake, a malignancy should be suspected.[55]

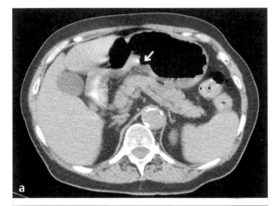

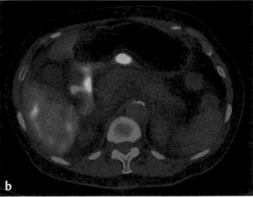

Fig. 7.32 Gastric ulcer. (a) Axial CT scan demonstrates a gastric ulcer (*arrow*). (b) Corresponding axial PET/CT scan demonstrates intense uptake in the ulcer. PET cannot differentiate between benign and malignant ulcers. This ulcer was benign. (Reproduced with permission from Lin.[54])

3. **Hiatal hernia**. Hiatal hernias can cause large foci of uptake at the expected region of the gastroesophageal junction, mimicking a distal esophageal neoplasm or node.

4. **SUV**[56]:

   a) *Without reflux*. In two studies, SUV cutoffs of 3.5 or 4 differentiated pathological from nonpathological FDG uptake at the gastroesophageal junction.[52]

   b) *Reflux disease*. Patients with reflux may have SUV values slightly higher than 4 at the gastroesophageal junction. However, reflux does not result in SUV values much greater than 4 and further workup should still be pursued in patients with reflux and very high levels of uptake.

7.14 Small and Large Bowel

1. Bowel activity can be a normal variant; contributors to bowel activity include bowel wall smooth muscle motility, lymphoid tissue, mucosal activity, and sloughed cells in the lumen. Constipation has been associated with increased bowel activity.[57] Medications, specifically metformin, can result in increased bowel activity. In addition, artifactual increased activity can be seen secondary to motion or attenuation correction artifact from dense contrast.

2. **Small bowel activity**. Small bowel activity is usually less than large bowel activity.

3. **Large bowel activity**. Large bowel activity is most prominent in the right colon, particularly the cecum (▶ Fig. 7.33), and the rectosigmoid. However, the pattern is unpredictable and at times the entire colon is visualized. Children often have minimal uptake in the large bowel.

   a) A nodular pattern of uptake is more often a normal variant in the ascending colon.[58]

   b) A segmental pattern of uptake is most commonly seen in the rectosigmoid colon (▶ Fig. 7.35).[58]

4. **Oral contrast**. Oral contrast can cause focal or diffuse increased colonic FDG uptake. This is not only secondary to the high CT density of the contrast (see Chapter 9), but also from accelerated physiologic reaction.[58]

5. **Focal and segmental uptake**. Focal or segmental areas of increased uptake are often pathologic. Segmental colonic activity suggests inflammation; focal colonic activity can be secondary to polyps (▶ Fig. 25.1) or colon cancer (▶ Fig. 25.2) (see Chapter 25).

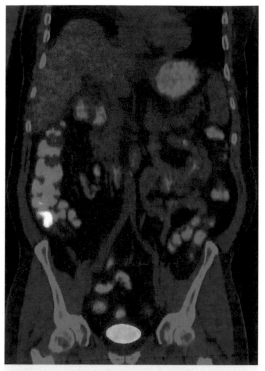

Fig. 7.33 Cecal uptake. Focal cecal uptake on a coronal PET/CT scan is a normal variant in this patient. Outside the cecum and ascending colon, focal uptake is more worrisome.

   a) However, focal uptake in the ascending colon is more often a normal variant. In particular, focal cecal uptake (▶ Fig. 7.34) is often normal. Focal uptake in the descending colon can be seen in constipated patients. Segmental uptake in the rectosigmoid is often a normal variant (▶ Fig. 7.35).[58]

   b) If there is a question whether a focal or segmental area of colonic uptake is abnormal, corresponding CT scans, if available, should be reviewed for an associated abnormality at the same site. A benign etiology is more likely if the "peristaltic segment sign" (any short segment expanded with air just before or after the uptake area) is identified.[59] Increased FDG uptake in conjunction with a CT abnormality is associated with a high incidence of cancerous or precancerous lesions.[60]

   c) Focal bowel uptake noted on PET/CT is associated with gastrointestinal tract

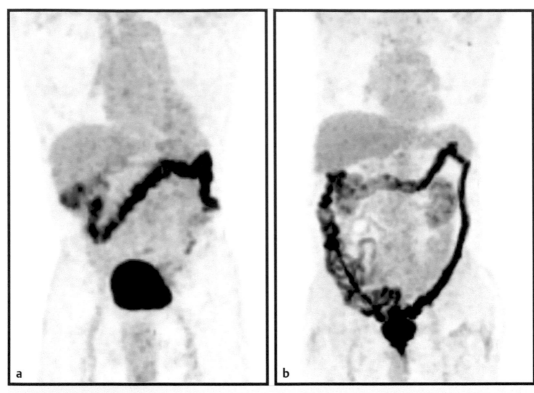

Fig. 7.34 Physiologic colonic uptake. Coronal PET images in two different patients demonstrates FDG uptake in the transverse colon **(a)** and throughout the colon **(b)**. (The image is provided courtesy of Gang Chen MD, Philadelphia, PA.)

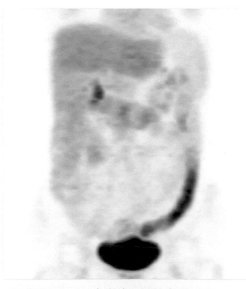

Fig. 7.35 Segmental uptake. Coronal PET scan demonstrates segmental distal descending and sigmoid colon uptake. This pattern is often a normal variant in this region.

pathology in approximately 70% of cases.[61,62] The incidence of false-positive results is substantially higher with PET alone.

d) **SUV**. While SUVs tend to be higher in true-positive findings than false-positive findings, SUVs cannot be used to differentiate physiologic from pathologic gastrointestinal tract uptake.[61,62]

7.15 Liver

1. **SUV**. The normal liver has an SUVmean of 2.18 ± 0.44 (age, 56 +)[32] and an SUVmax of 3.2 ± 0.8.[33]
2. **Noise artifact**. On AC images, the liver may appear to have substantial nonuniform uptake (more so than any other visceral organ) secondary to image noise. Therefore, it is possible that the noise associated with AC images could mimic or obscure liver lesions (▶ Fig. 11.5).

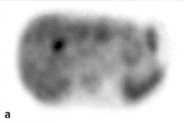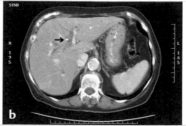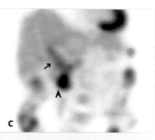

Fig. 7.36 Biliary tract uptake from stent placement. **(a)** Axial PET scan in a patient with pancreatic cancer demonstrates focal liver uptake suspicious for metastasis. **(b)** CT scan demonstrates this uptake to correspond to a biliary stent (*arrow*). **(c)** Coronal PET scan demonstrates the full extent of the biliary tract uptake (*arrow*). Uptake is also seen in the pancreatic head cancer (*arrowhead*). (Reproduced with permission from Lin EC, Studley M. Biliary tract FDG uptake secondary to stent placement. Clin Nucl Med 2003;28:318–319.)

3. **Insulin**. Insulin administration increases liver FDG uptake.[63]
4. Cholestasis and inflammatory biliary tract uptake (► Fig. 7.36) can cause false-positive liver lesions.

7.16 Gallbladder/Biliary Tree

1. No uptake is seen in the normal gallbladder wall or lumen.
2. **Gallbladder wall uptake**. Gallbladder wall uptake is seen in inflammatory conditions such as acute or chronic cholecystitis (► Fig. 8.8).
3. **Focal uptake**. Focal uptake in the gallbladder is seen with benign polyps, adenomyomatosis,[64] and gallbladder carcinoma. In polyps between 1 and 2 cm in size, FDG uptake is a strong risk factor for malignancy that can be used to determine the necessity of surgical intervention.[65]
4. Biliary tract uptake can be seen after recent stent placement (► Fig. 7.36).

7.17 Spleen

1. **SUV**. The normal SUVmean is 1.81 ± 0.32 (age, 56 +)[32] and the SUVmax is 2.4 ± 0.6.[33]
2. The uptake is usually equal to or less than that of the liver, and does not change with age. Splenic FDG uptake greater than the liver is usually abnormal.
3. Diffuse increased splenic FDG uptake is associated with malignancy, particularly lymphoma, but is more commonly associated with benign conditions such as a wide range of infectious and inflammatory processes,[66]

congestive splenomegaly, and anemia.[67] Granulocyte colony-stimulating factor (G-CSF) and interferon adjuvant therapy[68] are other cause of diffuse increased uptake.
4. **Granulocyte colony stimulating factorG-CSF**. Splenic uptake is seen in 53% of patients during or immediately after G-CSF treatment (► Fig. 7.37).[69] The degree of increased uptake is less intense than seen in bone marrow. Like bone marrow activity, the splenic activity declines after the G-CSF treatment stops, but is typically seen for at least 10 days.

7.18 Pancreas

1. **SUV**. The pancreas demonstrates minimal uptake, less than the liver or spleen. The uptake is difficult to visualize if normal. The normal SUVmean is 1.28 ± 0.36 (age, 56 +)[32] and the SUVmax is 2.0 ± 0.5.[33]
2. **Diffuse uptake**. Diffuse uptake is seen in acute or chronic pancreatitis (► Fig. 22.1).
3. **Focal uptake**. Focal uptake is seen in both benign and malignant lesions (see Chapter 22).

7.19 Adrenal

1. The adrenals are often not discretely identified on a normal PET scan. However, they are often visible on PET/CT studies with minimal uptake.
2. **Focal uptake**. Focal adrenal uptake is abnormal. Besides metastatic disease, other causes of focal adrenal uptake include
   a) Benign and malignant pheochromocytoma (malignant more likely).[70]

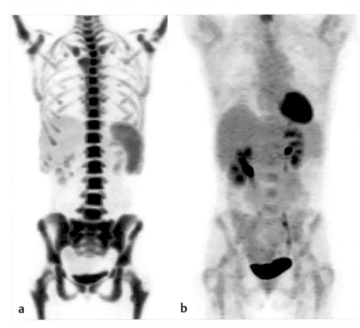

Fig. 7.37 Effects of G-CSF. **(a)** Maximum intensity projection (MIP) PET in a patient with diffuse large B-cell lymphoma on G-CSF therapy demonstrates diffuse increased bone marrow uptake as well as a lesser degree of increased splenic uptake. **(b)** MIP PET from a follow-up study approximately 2 months later demonstrates resolution of the bone marrow and splenic uptake.

a   b

b) Giant adrenal myelolipoma[70,71] (the majority of myelolipomas do not have uptake).

c) Adrenal carcinoma.

d) Adrenal hemorrhage.

Adrenal histoplasmosis.

3. **Bilateral uptake**. While bilateral adrenal uptake is worrisome for metastases, this can also be secondary to adrenal hyperplasia (▶ Fig. 7.38).

7.20 Genitourinary Tract

1. Unlike glucose, the kidneys excrete any filtered fluorodeoxyglucose. There is normally a large amount of activity in the renal collecting systems and bladder, and variable activity is seen in the ureters.

2. **Renal false positives**

a) Pooled activity in the renal collecting system can mimic a renal lesion (▶ Fig. 24.3).

b) Oncocytomas and angiomyolipomas have been reported to have increased uptake despite their benign nature (see Chapter 24).

3. **Ureteral false positives**

a) Focal activity in the ureters can mimic retroperitoneal nodal uptake (▶ Fig. 7.39, ▶ Fig. 7.40). This is easily differentiated on PET/CT but may be difficult to differentiate on PET. Correlation between three imaging planes can often localize this to the ureter.

b) Even if focal, ureteral activity is usually linear. In addition, the most common location for focal ureteral activity is in the superior pelvis where the ureter crosses the iliac vessels. These findings can aid in determining whether a focus of increased activity is ureteral in origin (▶ Fig. 7.39, ▶ Fig. 7.40).

7.21 Uterus

1. The uterus is usually not discretely identified on PET.

2. **Leiomyomas**. Leiomyomas are a common cause of focal uterine uptake. As there is no uptake in the remaining uterus, they are often difficult to identify as leiomyomas on PET alone and can mimic other pelvic masses. In a woman with a large focus of uptake above the bladder, a leiomyoma is a highly likely etiology (▶ Fig. 7.41, ▶ Fig. 7.42). Leiomyomas cannot be differentiated from leiomyosarcomas by PET.

a) Most leiomyomas demonstrate minimal FDG uptake, less than or equal to liver, but more substantial FDG uptake is noted in a minority of uterine leiomyomas, and is seen more commonly in premenopausal women. In one study,[72] FDG uptake was noted in 10.4 and 1.2% of leiomyomas in premenopausal and postmenopausal women, respectively.

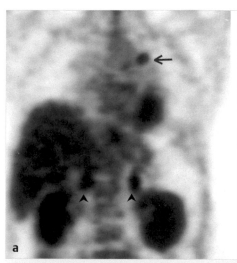
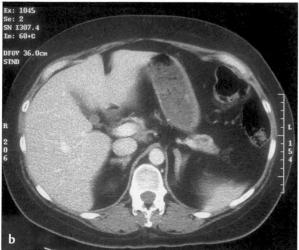

Fig. 7.38 Adrenal hyperplasia. **(a)** Coronal PET scan demonstrates uptake in the mediastinum (*arrow*) and both adrenals (*arrowheads*). While a primary lung cancer with bilateral adrenal metastases would be the first consideration, the adrenal uptake is symmetric, which would be unlikely for metastases. **(b)** CT scan demonstrates bilateral adrenal hyperplasia. The patient had Cushing's syndrome and adrenal hyperplasia secondary to a mediastinal paraganglioma. (Reproduced with permission from Lin EC, Helgans R. Adrenal hyperplasia in Cushing's syndrome demonstrated by FDG positron emission tomographic imaging. Clin Nucl Med 2002;27(7):516–517.)

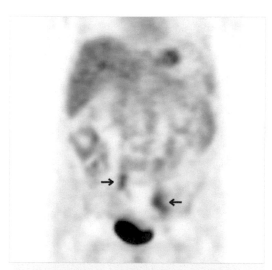

Fig. 7.39 Ureteral activity or node? Coronal PET scan in a lymphoma patient demonstrates two foci of uptake (*arrows*) in the course of the ureters. Unless these foci of uptake can be definitely linked to the ureters, they cannot be differentiated from nodal uptake without CT correlation. However, the linear nature of the uptake on the right suggests that it is ureteral and the more nodular uptake on the left suggests nodal uptake. In addition, the location of the right-sided activity in the superior pelvis (where the ureter crosses the iliacs) also suggests ureteral activity. In this case, the right-sided activity was ureteral and the left-sided activity was in a node.

b) It is unclear whether or not FDG uptake in leiomyomas depends upon menstrual cycle. In one report,[73] there was no correlation between intensity of uptake and menstrual cycle, but another report[72] found that changes in FDG uptake on serial studies were sometimes related to menstrual phases.

c) FDG uptake in leiomyomas can change on serial studies, and newly appearing FDG uptake does not necessarily mean malignant transformation.[72]

d) Leiomyomas with high T2 signal intensity on MRI, suggesting abundant cellularity, are substantially more likely to have FDG uptake.[72] FDG uptake in leiomyomas is also related to vascularity and tumor size.[73]

e) Uterine leiomyosarcomas usually have moderate to intense FDG uptake. While leiomyosarcomas typically have more uptake than leiomyomas,[74] there is some overlap and PET cannot accurately differentiate leiomyosarcomas from leiomyomas based on degree of FDG uptake.

3. **Endometrial uptake.** Endometrial uptake (▶ Fig. 7.43) is usually a normal variant in premenopausal women, most commonly seen during menstruation.[51]

a) Most prominent in the menstrual flow phase, followed by the ovulating phase.

b) Postmenopausal women can have very mild endometrial uptake, with a mean SUVmax of 1.7 in one report.[75] Hormonal therapy does not affect endometrial uptake. Substantial increased endometrial FDG in a postmenopausal woman is typically of clinical significance and should be further evaluated.

c) Intrauterine devices also cause endometrial uptake.

d) Scheduling PET a week before or a few days after the menstrual flow phase minimizes physiologic endometrial and ovarian uptake.[52]

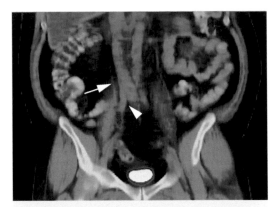

Fig. 7.40 Focal ureteral activity. Coronal PET/CT scan demonstrates focal linear activity in the right ureter. Note the characteristic location in the superior pelvis where the ureter crosses the right iliac vein (*arrowhead*). Unopacified ureter (*arrow*) is seen contiguous with the ureteral activity.

4. **Postpartum**. The postpartum uterus demonstrates intense diffuse uptake (▶ Fig. 7.44).[53]

7.22 Ovary

1. Normally, the ovaries are not visualized on PET.

2. Ovarian uptake can be seen in malignancy as well as in a wide range of benign conditions (see Chapter 23) (▶ Fig. 7.42). The most common cause are normally developed ovarian follicles and corpora lutea between the 10th and 25th days of the menstrual cycle.[76] Occasionally, the ovary can be confused with a pelvic lymph node (▶ Fig. 11.15).

3. **Premenopausal uptake**. In premenopausal women, physiologic ovarian uptake is most common around ovulation and during the early luteal phase of the menstrual cycle.[54] Physiologic uptake can be minimized by scheduling PET a week before or a few days after the menstrual flow phase.[52] However, physiologic ovarian uptake can be seen in women of reproductive age even after hysterectomy.[55]

4. **Chemotherapy**. Chemotherapy is associated with increased ovarian FDG uptake, often bilateral, in women less than 35 years old, with a negative relationship between the time elapsed from the end of chemotherapy and the incidence of uptake.[77]

5. **Postmenopausal uptake**. Ovarian uptake in the postmenopausal woman is much more worrisome than in a premenopausal woman, and malignancy should be considered.[51]

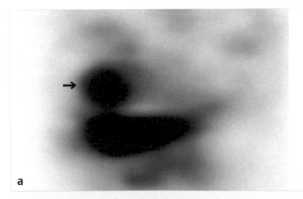
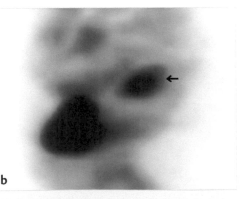

Fig. 7.41 Uterine leiomyomas. Sagittal PET scans demonstrate large foci of uptake (*arrows*) in uterine fundal leiomyomas in an anteverted (**a**) and a retroverted (**b**) uterus. When large foci of uptake are seen superior to the bladder, leiomyomas should be suspected, but correlation with anatomic imaging is necessary.

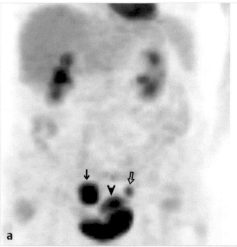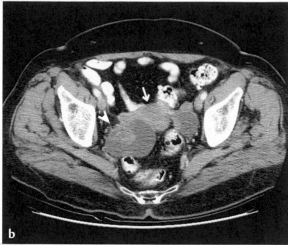

Fig. 7.42 Spectrum of pelvic uptake. **(a)** Coronal PET scan in a premenopausal woman demonstrates uptake In a right ovarian carcinoma (*arrow*), fibroid (*arrowhead*), and left ovarian follicular cyst (*open arrow*). The size and degree of the right ovarian uptake Is worrisome of malignancy. The left ovarian uptake would be equivocal without imaging correlation in a premenopausal woman. In a postmenopausal woman, the left ovarian uptake would be worrisome for malignancy. **(b)** Axial CT scan in the same patient demonstrates the right ovarian carcinoma and left ovarian follicular cyst. Most of the fibroid is inferior to this level but the top of the fibroid is seen as an area of minimal hypodensity (*arrow*). A solid component is seen in the right ovarian carcinoma (*arrowhead*).

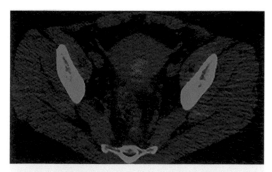

Fig. 7.43 Physiologic endometrial uptake. Axial PET/CT demonstrates physiologic endometrial uptake in premenopausal woman.

7.23 Testes

1. Symmetric testicular uptake is normal variant, which declines with age (▶ Fig. 8.1).
2. **SUV**. The normal testis can have an SUV as high as 5.7 (mean, 2.2).[56]

7.24 Bone and Bone Marrow

1. **Normal uptake**. Normal bone (without red marrow) has very minimal FDG uptake due to low metabolic activity. Red marrow activity is responsible for relatively increased FDG uptake in the axial skeleton.

2. **Benign fractures**. Benign fractures can have uptake (▶ Fig. 7.45, ▶ Fig. 7.46).
   a) **Amount of uptake**. Uptake in fractures is variable, and likely depends on the site and severity of the fracture. Some acute fractures may not have significant uptake.
   b) **Duration**. The duration of uptake in fractures is variable, but uptake has been reported up to 6 months after a fracture.[57] Most fractures do not have substantial uptake after 2 to 3 months.[11,37]
   c) **Insufficiency fractures**. Sacral insufficiency fractures can mimic pelvic bone metastases.[58] Usually, they do not have the classic "**H**"-shaped pattern of uptake seen on bone scans. The uptake is often linear, rather than nodular, which suggests the diagnosis. Vertebral insufficiency fractures can also have uptake in the more acute phase, which can mimic vertebral metastases. Like sacral insufficiency fractures, a linear appearance suggests the diagnosis (▶ Fig. 7.47).

3. **Granulocyte colony-stimulating factor (G-CSF**. Diffuse bone marrow uptake is seen in 87% of patients during and immediately after G-CSF

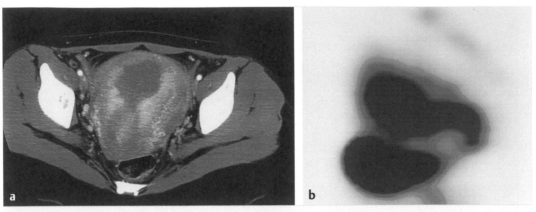

Fig. 7.44 Postpartum uterus. **(a)** CT of the pelvis demonstrates a heterogenous postpartum uterus with a prominent endometrial cavity. **(b)** Sagittal PET scan demonstrates intense diffuse FDG uptake in the uterus. (Reproduced with permission from Lin E. FDG PET appearance of a postpartum uterus. Clin Nucl Med 2006;31:159–160.)

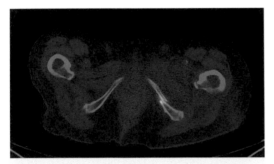

Fig. 7.45 Acute fracture FDG uptake: axial PET/CT scan demonstrates uptake in an acute pelvic fracture.

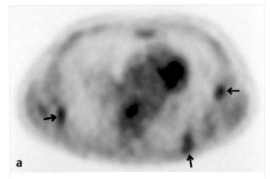

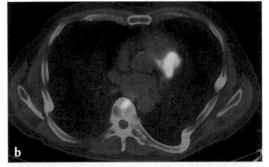

treatment (▶ Fig. 7.37).[59] The uptake declines after the end of treatment. The reported time interval after treatment necessary to avoid increased uptake is variable, ranging from 5 days to 1 month.[60] However, patients treated with high-dose chemotherapy followed by transplantation and G-CSF often do not have increased marrow uptake, possibly secondary to severely decreased marrow reserve. If marrow uptake is diffusely increased secondary to G-CSF, bone metastases (▶ Fig. 7.48) and benign bone lesions such as vertebral hemangiomas (▶ Fig. 7.49) can appear as photopenic defects relative to the hyperplastic marrow.[61,62]

a) **Chemotherapy.** Multiple cycles of chemotherapy may cause decreased bone marrow uptake.[60] Recovery of marrow

Fig. 7.46 Chronic fracture FDG uptake. **(a)** Axial PET scan demonstrates multiple foci of uptake in the peripheral thorax (*arrows*). PET has difficulty in localizing peripheral lesions such as these: it cannot be determined whether these foci are in the lungs, pleura, or ribs. Note that these foci are similar in appearance to the peripheral lung neoplasm in ▶ Fig. 16.1. **(b)** Axial PET/CT scan demonstrates that these foci of uptake correspond to old rib fractures. This degree of uptake in old fractures is unusual.

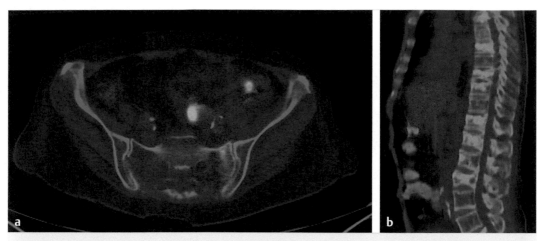

Fig. 7.47 Sacral and vertebral insufficiency fractures. **(a)** Axial PET/CT scan demonstrates linear uptake in a left sacral insufficiency fracture. **(b)** Sagittal PET/CT scan demonstrates multiple horizontal linear areas of uptake in the spine secondary to compression fractures. The location of the uptake is comparable to the location of the fracture lines sometimes seen by MRI in vertebral Insufficiency fractures.

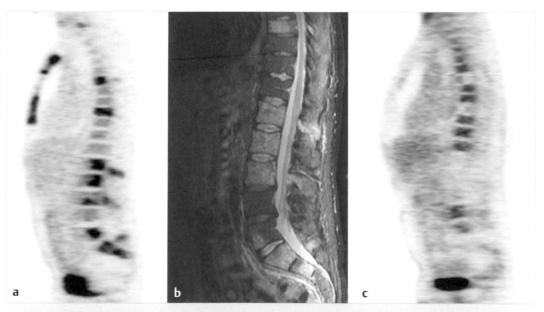

Fig. 7.48 Flip-flop phenomenon of treated bone marrow disease. **(a)** Sagittal PET scan demonstrates bone marrow infiltration from lymphoma involving the sternum, spine, and sacrum. **(b)** The areas of FDG uptake are seen as abnormal hyperintense signal on sagittal short TI inversion recovery (STIR) MRI. **(c)** Posttherapy scan demonstrates the previously noted areas of uptake to be photopenic. However, the normal marrow now appears to have increased uptake relative to the treated regions (this appearance could be accentuated by G-CSF or recovery from chemotherapy). If pretherapy studies are not available for comparison, these areas of normal marrow uptake could mimic disease. (Reproduced with permission from Lin EC. FDG PET/CT flip flop phenomenon in treated lymphoma of bone. Clin Nucl Med 2006;31:803–805.)

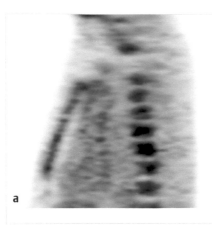
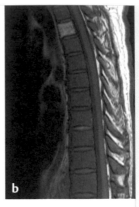

Fig. 7.49 Vertebral body hemangioma. **(a)** Sagittal PET scan in a patient with marrow hyperplasia demonstrates a single vertebral body in the upper thoracic spine which is relatively photopenic. **(b)** Sagittal T1-weighted MR demonstrates a hyperintense hemangioma in this photopenic vertebral body. The remaining marrow is hypointense consistent with marrow hyperplasia. Bone lesions which contain little or no red marrow may appear as areas of decreased FDG uptake in the setting of marrow hyperplasia.

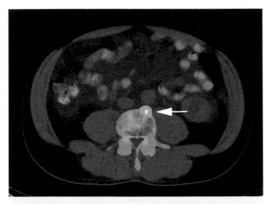

Fig. 7.50 Degenerative spur. Axial PET/CT scan demonstrates intense uptake in an anterior vertebral column spur (*arrow*).

following chemotherapy may cause a mild increase in bone marrow uptake, although this is not observed in some cases, possibly due to poor marrow reserve.

b) **Erythropoietin.** Erythropoietin can cause extensive diffuse increased uptake.

c) Pathological processes such as myelodysplastic syndromes, beta-thalassemia, and chronic myeloid leukemia can result in diffuse marrow uptake.[63,64,65]

4. **Arthritis.** There is often minimal or no uptake in arthritic joints (because of this, FDG PET is more specific than bone scan), unless there is an inflammatory component. In the spine, uptake can be seen corresponding to both degenerative disc and facet disease. The degree of uptake weakly correlates with the severity on CT.[66] Inflammatory arthritis can have

substantial uptake depending on the degree of inflammation.

a) Degenerative spurring in the spine can sometimes demonstrate substantial FDG uptake (▶ Fig. 7.50).

b) Subchondral cysts can have FDG uptake (▶ Fig. 7.51).

c) Uptake in joints affected by rheumatoid arthritis is much more likely than in those affected by osteoarthritis. In rheumatoid arthritis, there is usually uptake if the joint is clinically inflamed.[67]

5. **Specific joints.** Uptake is more common in these joints[18,19]:

a) Glenohumeral joints (▶ Fig. 7.18).

b) Sternoclavicular joints.

c) Costovertebral joints.

6. **Radiation effects.** Radiation therapy will cause reduced uptake corresponding exactly to the radiation field (▶ Fig. 7.52).

7. **Focal uptake.** Focal uptake in skeletal structures can be secondary to bone marrow metastases or primary bone lesions. Uptake in a bone lesion does not necessarily indicate malignancy as many benign primary bone lesions have FDG uptake (see Chapter 26).

8. **Intraspinous bursa uptake.** Uptake is often seen in the lower lumbar spine in the region of the posterior spinous processes. On axial images, this uptake often appears to be in the spinous process and mimics an osseous lesion, but on sagittal images it can be seen to lie between the spinous processes. This uptake is usually secondary to Baastrup's disease (kissing spine) where there is inflammation in the intraspinous bursa secondary to close approximation and contact between adjacent spinous processes (▶ Fig. 7.53).[68,69]

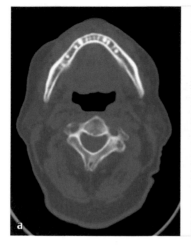
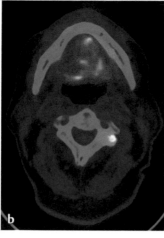

Fig. 7.51 Subchondral cyst. **(a)** CT scan demonstrates a subchondral cyst related to a cervical facet joint. **(b)** Axial PET/CT demonstrates FDG uptake in this subchondral cyst.

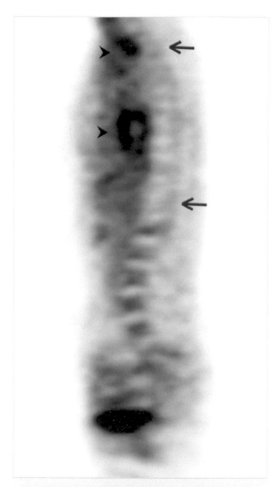

Fig. 7.52 Radiation effects on bone. Sagittal PET scan demonstrates a large area of decreased uptake in the thoracic spine (*arrows*) secondary to radiation for thoracic tumors (*arrowheads*).

7.25 Skeletal Muscle

1. Causes of increased skeletal muscle uptake
   a) ***Insulin***. Skeletal muscle uptake is diffusely increased after insulin administration or insulin release from recent ingestion of food (skeletal muscle glucose receptors are insulin sensitive) (▶ Fig. 4.1). This is seen in conjunction with increased myocardial uptake.
   b) ***Exercise***. Skeletal muscle uptake is increased after recent exercise.
   c) ***Anxiety***. Anxiety will increase skeletal muscle uptake. This is most prominent in the neck, supraclavicular region, and thoracic paravertebral muscles.
   d) ***Graves' disease***. Skeletal muscle uptake is often increased in Graves' disease.
      • Most common in the psoas and rectus abdominis muscles.
      • Usually seen in conjunction with increased thymic and, less commonly, thyroid uptake.
2. **Mimics**. Skeletal muscle can be difficult to differentiate from nodal and brown fat uptake.
   a) ***Nodal uptake***. Skeletal muscle uptake can usually be differentiated from nodal uptake by its linear appearance and symmetry.
      • Skeletal muscle uptake can occasionally be nodular and mimic the appearance of nodes. However, in these cases a symmetric appearance will suggest muscle as the site of uptake.
      As nodal disease can exist in conjunction with skeletal muscle uptake in the same

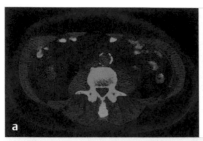 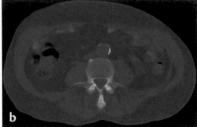 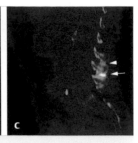

Fig. 7.53 Baastrup's disease. **(a)** Axial PET/CT demonstrates apparent uptake in a lumbar spinous process. **(b)** Corresponding axial CT demonstrates sclerosis, hypertrophy, and flattening involving this spinous process. **(c)** Sagittal PET/CT demonstrates that the uptake (*arrow*) lies between spinous processes. Minimal uptake is also noted between the spinous processes just above this level (*arrowhead*). Intraspinous bursal uptake can often appear to lie in the spinous process on axial images. As spinous process metastases are rare, close correlation with sagittal images is necessary. Although the CT findings suggest Baastrup's disease in this case, intraspinous bursal uptake on PET is often seen with a normal CT appearance of the spinous processes. (Reproduced with permission from Lin E. Baastrup's disease [kissing spine] demonstrated by FDG PET/CT. Skeletal Radiol 2008; 37:173–175.)

region, it is important to further evaluate all areas of asymmetry for possible disease. Correlation with anatomic imaging is very helpful in these cases (▶ Fig. 7.54).

b) ***Brown fat uptake***. Both brown fat (see Brown Fat section) and muscle uptake are usually symmetric. A linear appearance suggests muscle. Fat and muscle uptake often cannot be differentiated without PET/CT (▶ Fig. 7.54), but this is usually of no clinical significance.

3. **Specific muscles**
   a) Teres minor uptake can be seen, often unilaterally.[18]
   b) Extraocular muscle uptake is often seen due to eye movement.
   c) Diaphragmatic crus uptake can be seen with increased respiratory effort (▶ Fig. 7.55). The crus uptake can be diagnosed by its linear appearance. On coronal images, it appears as continuous vertical line. The right crus is larger and extends more inferiorly than the left crus (▶ Fig. 7.56). Occasionally, a retrocrural node can be difficult to distinguish from normal crural uptake (▶ Fig. 7.57).
   d) Diaphragmatic slips can also have increased uptake.
   e) Intercostal muscle uptake is more common in smokers and patient with chronic obstructive pulmonary disease.[30]
   f) The longus colli muscles in the neck often have asymmetric uptake (▶ Fig. 7.15).[10]

7.26 Vascular

1. **Vascular wall**
   a) ***Atherosclerosis***. Uptake in the vascular wall can be seen in atherosclerosis (▶ Fig. 7.58). This is common in the thoracic aorta and iliac and femoral arteries. It usually does not correspond to areas of calcification and may reflect metabolically active macrophages in the atherosclerotic plaques.[70]
   b) ***Vasculitis***. Vasculitis (▶ Fig. 7.59) is another cause of vascular wall uptake.

2. **Thrombosis**. Both acute and chronic benign thrombosis can demonstrate significant uptake (▶ Fig. 7.60). PET/CT also detects tumor thrombosis (▶ Fig. 7.61).
   a) Uptake in a central pulmonary embolus could mimic hilar adenopathy (▶ Fig. 7.62).

3. **Vascular grafts**. Mild linear uptake along a vascular graft usually does not indicate infection; focal uptake is suspicious for infection (▶ Fig. 7.63).[71]

4. **Perivascular tumor infiltration**. Tumor infiltration along the course of a vessel can have a linear appearance (▶ Fig. 7.64). While a linear appearance usually suggests a benign abnormality or normal variant, perivascular tumor infiltration is one exception.

7.27 Soft Tissues

Uptake is common at sites of intervention such as catheter insertion, ostomies, and surgical scars.

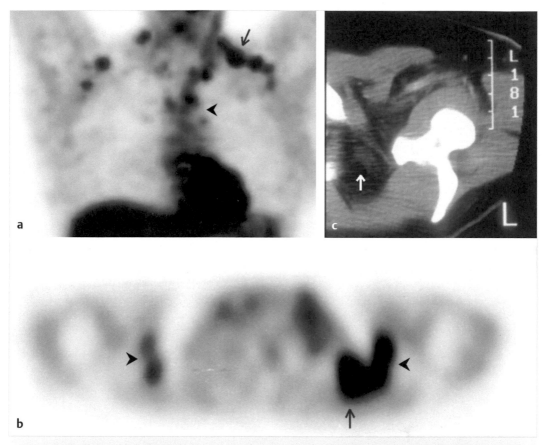

Fig. 7.54 Muscle/brown fat activity obscuring a lymph node. **(a)** Coronal PET scan in a patient with lymphoma demonstrates multiple foci of uptake in the superior mediastinum and supraclavicular region bilaterally. This was not a PET/CT study which makes evaluation more difficult, although a CT was available for correlation. The superior mediastinal activity is most consistent with brown fat as no nodes were seen in this region on CT and there should not be muscle uptake in the superior mediastinum. In addition, the mediastinal uptake does not extend below the aortic arch (*arrowhead*), which suggests brown fat uptake rather than nodal disease. The supraclavicular activity could either be brown fat or muscle; this could not be differentiated without CT fusion. However, there is an asymmetric focus of increased activity in the left supraclavicular region (*arrow*). Even if brown fat/muscle activity is known to be present, the images should be closely scrutinized for asymmetric activity. **(b)** Axial PET scan shows that the asymmetric focus (*arrow*) corresponds to a left supraclavicular node (*arrow*) seen on CT **(c)**. The bilateral uptake (*arrowheads*) could be in either the subscapularis muscles or the fat just medial to the muscles (fusion would be necessary to exactly localize the activity as side-by-side correlation is inadequate for this purpose). This case demonstrates the synergy of PET and CT. The supraclavicular node was not detected prospectively on CT. PET detected a potential but equivocal abnormality, and retrospective correlation with the CT was necessary to determine that a node was definitely present.

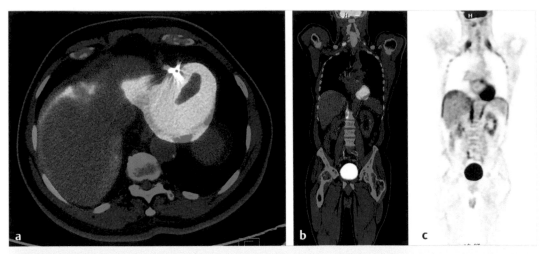

Fig. 7.55 Diaphragmatic muscle uptake. Muscle uptake in a 71-year-old patient with COPD and shortness of breath. There is significantly increased FDG uptake in the diaphragm, overlapping the dome of the liver or mimicking pleural based lesions **(a–c)**. The crural muscle uptake could be mistaken as retroperitoneal node activity and should be avoided. Also note increased uptake in accessory muscles of respiration in the neck **(b and c)**, and in the intercostal muscles **(c)**. (The images are provided courtesy of Gang Cheng MD, Philadelphia, PA.)

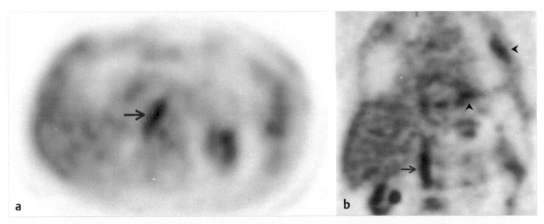

Fig. 7.56 Diaphragmatic crus uptake. **(a)** Axial PET scan demonstrates linear uptake in the right retroperitoneum (*arrow*). **(b)** Coronal PET scan demonstrates linear uptake corresponding to the right diaphragmatic crus (*arrow*). Typically, crus uptake is bilateral and secondary to hyperventilation. In this case, the unilateral uptake is likely secondary to decreased movement of the left hemidiaphragm related to left pleural metastases (*arrowheads*). (Reproduced with permission from Lin EC, Bhola R. Unilateral diaphragmatic crus uptake on FDG positron emission tomographic imaging. Clin Nucl Med 2001;26(5):479.)

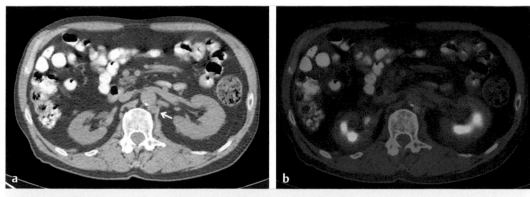

Fig. 7.57 Retrocrural node. (a) Axial CT scan demonstrates slight nodularity in the region of the left crus (*arrow*). Without intravenous contrast, it is difficult to differentiate this from the normal crus. (b) Corresponding axial PET/CT scan demonstrates focal uptake in a left retrocrural node.

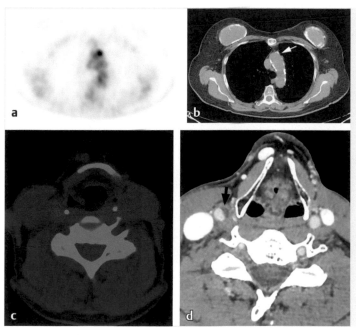

Fig. 7.58 Focal plaque uptake. (a) Intense focal uptake is noted on an axial PET scan (b) corresponding to an atherosclerotic aortic plaque (*arrow*) seen on CT. Uptake in aortic plaque can occasionally mimic adenopathy. (c) Axial PET/CT demonstrates increased uptake in the medial internal right carotid. (d) Axial contrast-enhanced CT demonstrates that this uptake corresponds to noncalcified plaque (*arrow*).

7.28 Brown Fat[72,73,74]

There are two types of fat in the human body: white and brown fat. White fat stores energy; brown fat generates heat in response to cold exposure. Brown fat can cause focal increased FDG uptake mimicking muscle activity or malignancy.

1. **Locations**
   a) Neck.
   b) Supraclavicular region.
   c) Axilla.
   d) Around the large vessels in the mediastinum.
   e) Interatrial septum (▶ Fig. 7.65).
   f) Azygoesophageal recess.
   g) Paraspinal (▶ Fig. 7.66).
   h) Intercostal spaces.
   i) Perinephric space.
   j) Paracolic and parahepatic spaces.
2. **Pearls**
   a) SUVs cannot differentiate brown fat uptake from malignancy as SUVs in brown fat can be very high.

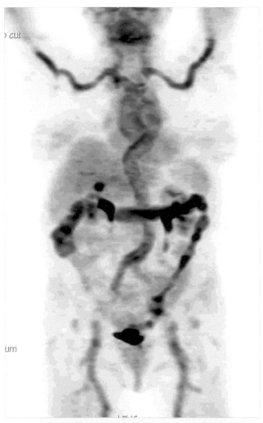

Fig. 7.59 Vasculitis. Coronal PET scan demonstrates extensive arterial FDG uptake secondary to vasculitis.

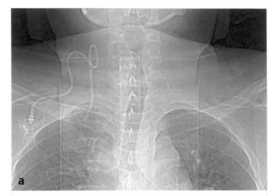

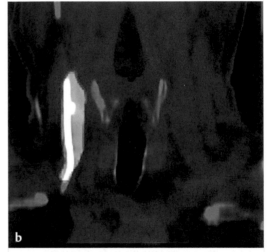

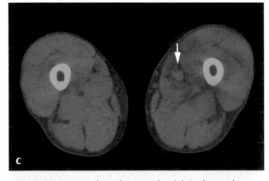

Fig. 7.60 Benign thrombus uptake. (a) Radiograph demonstrates a catheter coiled in the right internal jugular vein. (b) Coronal PET/CT demonstrates intense FDG uptake in thrombus around the catheter. (c) Axial PET/CT scan demonstrates uptake in a deep vein thrombus (*arrow*) in the left superficial femoral vein.

b) Neck/supraclavicular uptake is most common. There is usually uptake in the neck/supraclavicular region also when uptake in other brown fat areas is seen.

c) Brown fat uptake in the neck/supraclavicular regions is usually symmetric.

d) Uptake is more common in females and younger patients.
   • Low body mass index has been reported to increase uptake in some studies but not others.[38]

e) Uptake is more common with colder temperatures.

3. **Differential diagnosis**
   a) The diagnosis of brown fat uptake usually requires PET/CT. If PET/CT is not available, the diagnosis can still be suggested in many cases. The other entities that are in the differential diagnosis are muscle uptake and node uptake. Often two or three of these entities (brown fat, muscle, and nodes) exist in conjunction, which can further complicate interpretation (▶ Fig. 7.54, ▶ Fig. 7.67).

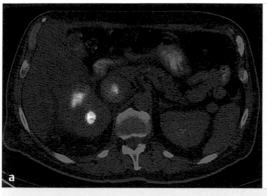
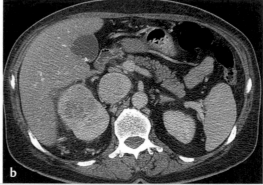

Fig. 7.61 Tumor thrombus. Axial PET/CT **(a)** and corresponding contrast-enhanced CT **(b)** demonstrate FDG uptake in tumor thrombus expanding the inferior vena cava, secondary to a right renal cell carcinoma.

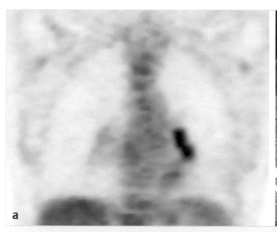
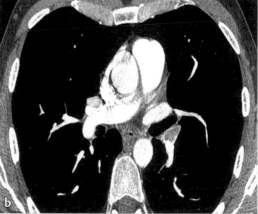

Fig. 7.62 Pulmonary embolus uptake. **(a)** Coronal PET demonstrates increased FDG uptake in the left hilum, corresponding to a segmental left lower lobe pulmonary embolism noted on a CT pulmonary angiogram **(b)**.

b) ***Neck/supraclavicular uptake***. Without PET/CT, brown fat uptake in the neck/supraclavicular region often cannot be differentiated from muscle uptake, but this is not clinically relevant. The usual symmetric appearance will suggest that the uptake is either in fat or in muscle rather than nodes. Any area of asymmetry should raise concern for nodal disease (▶ Fig. 7.54, ▶ Fig. 7.67). If no correlative finding is seen on CT images and there is asymmetric FDG uptake, a follow-up CT is helpful as adenopathy may be noted on subsequent CT exams (▶ Fig. 8.9).

c) ***Other areas***. Uptake outside the neck/supraclavicular region is rarely seen in isolation. Thoracic uptake is usually accompanied by neck/supraclavicular uptake. Infradiaphragmatic uptake is usually seen in conjunction with supradiaphragmatic uptake (in particular, suprarenal uptake is usually seen in conjunction with paravertebral uptake).[75,76]

d) ***Practical pointers***. In practice, the hardest area to differentiate from nodal disease without PET/CT is mediastinal fat uptake. Usually, there is also neck/supraclavicular uptake in addition, which suggests the diagnosis, but very rarely isolated mediastinal brown fat uptake is seen.

• A correlative CT is helpful even if fusion is not available. If no nodes are seen on CT, the uptake is likely in the mediastinal fat.

• A useful pattern for making the diagnosis of mediastinal brown fat is involvement of only the superior mediastinum. With brown fat, the uptake will usually not

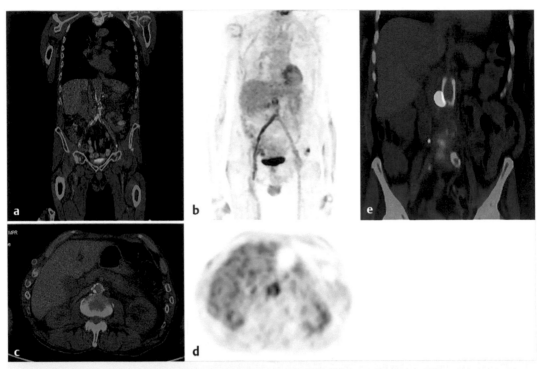

Fig. 7.63 Patterns of graft uptake. A 65-year-old male is status post aortobifemoral bypass, with lymphoma in remission. (**a**) and (**b**) are coronal images showing increased FDG uptake in the infrarenal abdominal aorta and in the right iliac artery. (**c**) and (**d**) are axial images showing increased FDG uptake in the abdominal aorta. This uptake is secondary to sterile inflammation. Coronal PET/CT (**e**) in a different patient demonstrates focal uptake adjacent to an aortic graft, consistent with infection. (Images **a–d** provided courtesy of Gang Cheng, Philadelphia, PA; image **e** courtesy of Wengen Chen, Baltimore, MD.)

extend below the aortic arch (▶ Fig. 7.54, ▶ Fig. 7.68), which would be an uncommon pattern for nodal disease.

e) If differentiation from disease is not possible, the study can be repeated with premedication (e.g., diazepam) and/or keeping the patient in a warm environment for 48 hours before the study is repeated.

7.29 Metallic Prosthesis

Artifactually increased uptake can be seen around a metallic prosthesis on AC images. This could potentially mimic prosthesis infection. In the head and neck, areas of increased activity adjacent to the metallic dental implants (▶ Fig. 9.1) could cause false-positive tumor localization.

1. This artifact is seen with both CT and radionuclide-based AC.[77] However, it is more prominent when CT-based AC is used, particularly in metallic dental implants.
2. The artifacts are enhanced by patient motion.

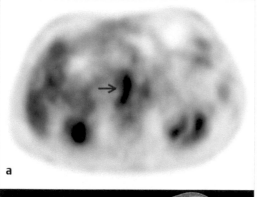

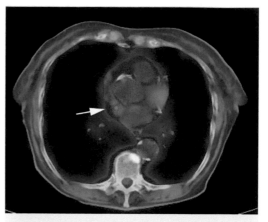

Fig. 7.65 Brown fat uptake in the interatrial septum. Axial PET/CT scan demonstrates uptake in the fat of the interatrial septum (*arrow*).

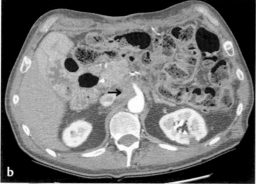

Fig. 7.64 Perivascular tumor uptake. **(a)** Axial PET scan demonstrates a linear area of uptake in the posterior abdomen (*arrow*). While a linear focus of uptake often suggests a benign or physiologic etiology, in this case the uptake was secondary to perivascular tumor infiltration from pancreatic cancer. Note the similarity in appearance of this uptake to the diaphragmatic crus uptake in ▶ Fig. 7.56. **(b)** Axial CT at the same level demonstrates tumor infiltration (*arrow*) around the celiac axis.

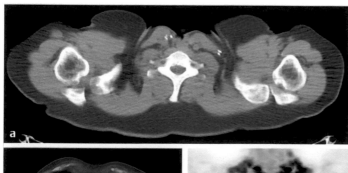

Fig. 7.66 Paraspinal brown fat uptake. Axial CT **(a)** and PET/CT **(b)** demonstrate uptake in paraspinal fat. **(c)** Maximum intensity projection (MIP) PET in another patient with lung cancer demonstrates a characteristic pattern of paraspinal and supraclavicular brown fat uptake.

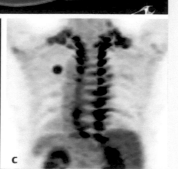

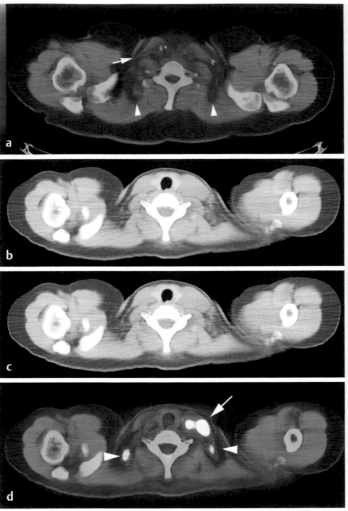

Fig. 7.67 Brown fat, muscle, and node uptake. Brown fat, muscle, and node uptake can have similar locations and appearances and occur in conjunction. CT (**a**) and PET/CT (**b**) exams demonstrate uptake in both brown fat (*arrowheads*) and muscle (*arrow*). The muscle uptake is atypical as it is unilateral and could have been a worrisome finding on PET alone; however, PET/CT localizes it to muscle. In another patient, CT (**c**) and PET/CT (**d**) demonstrate uptake in both brown fat (*arrowheads*) and nodes (*arrow*).

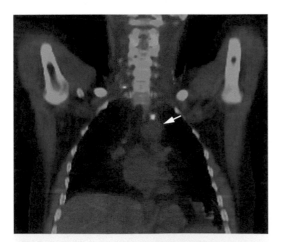

Fig. 7.68 Neck and mediastinal brown fat uptake. Coronal PET/CT scan demonstrates neck and mediastinal brown fat uptake. The mediastinal brown fat uptake does not extend below the top of the aortic arch (*arrow*).

References

[1] Bohnen N. Neurological applications. In: Wahl RL, ed. Principles and Practice of Positron Emission Tomography. Philadelphia, PA: Lippincott Williams & Wilkins; 2002:276–297

[2] Berti V, Mosconi L, Pupi A. Brain: normal variations and benign findings in fluorodeoxyglucose-PET/computed tomography imaging. PET Clin. 2014; 9(2):129–140

[3] Loessner A, Alavi A, Lewandrowski KU, Mozley D, Souder E, Gur RE. Regional cerebral function determined by FDG-PET in healthy volunteers: normal patterns and changes with age. J Nucl Med. 1995; 36(7):1141–1149

[4] Minamimoto R, Takahashi N, Inoue T. FDG-PET of patients with suspected renal failure: standardized uptake values in normal tissues. Ann Nucl Med. 2007; 21(4):217–222

[5] Fulham MJ, Brooks RA, Hallett M, Di Chiro G. Cerebellar diaschisis revisited: pontine hypometabolism and dentate sparing. Neurology. 1992; 42(12):2267–2273

[6] Gropler RJ, Siegel BA, Lee KJ, et al. Nonuniformity in myocardial accumulation of fluorine-18-fluorodeoxyglucose in normal fasted humans. J Nucl Med. 1990; 31(11):1749–1756

[7] Maurer AH, Burshteyn M, Adler LP, Gaughan JP, Steiner RM. Variable cardiac 18FDG patterns seen in oncologic positron emission tomography computed tomography: importance for differentiating normal physiology from cardiac and paracardiac disease. J Thorac Imaging. 2012; 27(4):263–268

[8] Thut DP, Ahmed R, Kane M, Djekidel M. Variability in myocardial metabolism on serial tumor (18)F-FDG PET/CT scans. Am J Nucl Med Mol Imaging. 2014; 4(4):346–353

[9] Zanco P, Desideri A, Mobilia G, et al. Effects of left bundle branch block on myocardial FDG PET in patients without significant coronary artery stenoses. J Nucl Med. 2000; 41(6): 973–977

[10] Israel O, Weiler-Sagie M, Rispler S, et al. PET/CT quantitation of the effect of patient-related factors on cardiac 18F-FDG uptake. J Nucl Med. 2007; 48(2):234–239

[11] Kaneta T, Hakamatsuka T, Takanami K, et al. Evaluation of the relationship between physiological FDG uptake in the heart and age, blood glucose level, fasting period, and hospitalization. Ann Nucl Med. 2006; 20(3):203–208

[12] Khandani AH, Isasi CR, Donald Blaufox M. Intra-individual variability of cardiac uptake on serial whole-body 18F-FDG PET. Nucl Med Commun. 2005; 26(9):787–791

[13] Inglese E, Leva L, Matheoud R, et al. Spatial and temporal heterogeneity of regional myocardial uptake in patients without heart disease under fasting conditions on repeated whole-body 18F-FDG PET/CT. J Nucl Med. 2007; 48(10):1662–1669

[14] Tahara N, Tahara A, Nitta Y, et al. Heterogeneous myocardial FDG uptake and the disease activity in cardiac sarcoidosis. JACC Cardiovasc Imaging. 2010; 3(12):1219–1228

[15] Lobert P, Brown RK, Dvorak RA, Corbett JR, Kazerooni EA, Wong KK. Spectrum of physiological and pathological cardiac and pericardial uptake of FDG in oncology PET-CT. Clin Radiol. 2013; 68(1):e59–e71

[16] Lin EC. Isolated papillary muscle uptake on FDG PET/CT. Clin Nucl Med. 2007; 32(1):76–78

[17] Maurer AH, Burshteyn M, Adler LP, Steiner RM. How to differentiate benign versus malignant cardiac and paracardiac 18F FDG uptake at oncologic PET/CT. Radiographics. 2011; 31(5): 1287–1305

[18] Cook GJ, Wegner EA, Fogelman I. Pitfalls and artifacts in 18FDG PET and PET/CT oncologic imaging. Semin Nucl Med. 2004; 34(2):122–133

[19] Fujii H, Ide M, Yasuda S, Takahashi W, Shohtsu A, Kubo A. Increased FDG uptake in the wall of the right atrium in people who participated in a cancer screening program with whole-body PET. Ann Nucl Med. 1999; 13(1):55–59

[20] Nguyen BD. PET demonstration of left atrial appendage in chronic atrial fibrillation. Clin Nucl Med. 2005; 30(3):177–179

[21] Beanlands RS, Muzik O, Hutchins GD, Wolfe ER, Jr, Schwaiger M. Heterogeneity of regional nitrogen 13-labeled ammonia tracer distribution in the normal human heart: comparison with rubidium 82 and copper 62-labeled PTSM. J Nucl Cardiol. 1994; 1(3):225–235

[22] Nakamoto Y, Tatsumi M, Hammoud D, Cohade C, Osman MM, Wahl RL. Normal FDG distribution patterns in the head and neck: PET/CT evaluation. Radiology. 2005; 234(3):879–885

[23] Davison JM, Ozonoff A, Imsande HM, Grillone GA, Subramaniam RM. Squamous cell carcinoma of the palatine tonsils: FDG standardized uptake value ratio as a biomarker to differentiate tonsillar carcinoma from physiologic uptake. Radiology. 2010; 255(2):578–585

[24] Chen YK, Su CT, Chi KH, Cheng RH, Wang SC, Hsu CH. Utility of 18F-FDG PET/CT uptake patterns in Waldeyer's ring for differentiating benign from malignant lesions in lateral pharyngeal recess of nasopharynx. J Nucl Med. 2007; 48(1):8–14

[25] Chen YK, Wang SC, Cheng RH, Yeh CL, Tsui CC, Chia-Hung K. Utility of 18F-FDG uptake in various regions of Waldeyer's ring to differentiate benign from malignant lesions in the midline roof of the nasopharynx. Nucl Med Commun. 2014; 35(9):922–931

[26] Halpern BS, Britz-Cunningham SH, Kim CK. Intense focal F-18 FDG uptake in vocal cord associated with injection of calcium hydroxylapatite microspheres. Clin Nucl Med. 2011; 36(11): e175–e177

[27] Lin EC. Focal asymmetric longus colli uptake on FDG PET/CT. Clin Nucl Med. 2007; 32(1):67–69

[28] Shreve PD, Anzai Y, Wahl RL. Pitfalls in oncologic diagnosis with FDG PET imaging: physiologic and benign variants. Radiographics. 1999; 19(1):61–77, quiz 150–151

[29] Shreve PD, Wahl RL. Normal variants in FDG PET imaging. In: Wahl RL, ed. Principles and Practice of Positron Emission Tomography. Philadelphia, PA: Lippincott Williams & Wilkins; 2002:111–136

[30] Karantanis D, Bogsrud TV, Wiseman GA, et al. Clinical significance of diffusely increased 18F-FDG uptake in the thyroid gland. J Nucl Med. 2007; 48(6):896–901

[31] Agrawal K, Weaver J, Ngu R, Krishnamurthy Mohan H. Clinical significance of patterns of incidental thyroid uptake at (18)F-FDG PET/CT. Clin Radiol. 2015; 70(5):536–543

[32] Wang Y, Chiu E, Rosenberg J, Gambhir SS. Standardized uptake value atlas: characterization of physiological 2-deoxy-2-[18F]fluoro-D-glucose uptake in normal tissues. Mol Imaging Biol. 2007; 9(2):83–90

[33] Zincirkeser S, Sahin E, Halac M, Sager S. Standardized uptake values of normal organs on 18F-fluorodeoxyglucose positron emission tomography and computed tomography imaging. J Int Med Res. 2007; 35(2):231–236

[34] Chen YK, Chen YL, Liao AC, Shen YY, Kao CH. Elevated 18F-FDG uptake in skeletal muscles and thymus: a clue for the diagnosis of Graves' disease. Nucl Med Commun. 2004; 25(2): 115–121

[35] Kumar R, Chauhan A, Zhuang H, Chandra P, Schnall M, Alavi A. Standardized uptake values of normal breast tissue with 2-deoxy-2-[F-18]fluoro-D: -glucose positron emission tomography: variations with age, breast density, and menopausal status. Mol Imaging Biol. 2006; 8(6):355–362

[36] Lin CY, Ding HJ, Liu CS, Chen YK, Lin CC, Kao CH. Correlation between the intensity of breast FDG uptake and menstrual cycle. Acad Radiol. 2007; 14(8):940–944

[37] Alibazoglu H, Alibazoglu B, Hollinger EF, et al. Normal thymic uptake of 2-deoxy-2[F-18]fluoro-D-glucose. Clin Nucl Med. 1999; 24(8):597–600

[38] Ferdinand B, Gupta P, Kramer EL. Spectrum of thymic uptake at 18F-FDG PET. Radiographics. 2004; 24(6):1611–1616

[39] El-Bawab H, Al-Sugair AA, Rafay M, Hajjar W, Mahdy M, Al-Kattan K. Role of flourine-18 fluorodeoxyglucose positron emission tomography in thymic pathology. Eur J Cardiothorac Surg. 2007; 31(4):731–736

[40] Sung YM, Lee KS, Kim BT, Choi JY, Shim YM, Yi CA. 18F-FDG PET/CT of thymic epithelial tumors: usefulness for distinguishing and staging tumor subgroups. J Nucl Med. 2006; 47 (10):1628–1634

[41] Nakahara T, Fujii H, Ide M, et al. FDG uptake in the morphologically normal thymus: comparison of FDG positron emission tomography and CT. Br J Radiol. 2001; 74(885): 821–824

[42] Smith CS, Schöder H, Yeung HW. Thymic extension in the superior mediastinum in patients with thymic hyperplasia: potential cause of false-positive findings on 18F-FDG PET/CT. AJR Am J Roentgenol. 2007; 188(6):1716–1721

[43] Jacene HA, Cohade C, Wahl RL. F-18 FDG PET/CT in acute respiratory distress syndrome: a case report. Clin Nucl Med. 2004; 29(12):786–788

[44] Digumarthy SR, Fischman AJ, Kwek BH, Aquino SL. Fluorodeoxyglucose positron emission tomography pattern of pulmonary lymphangitic carcinomatosis. J Comput Assist Tomogr. 2005; 29(3):346–349

[45] Kamel EM, McKee TA, Calcagni ML, et al. Occult lung infarction may induce false interpretation of 18F-FDG PET in primary staging of pulmonary malignancies. Eur J Nucl Med Mol Imaging. 2005; 32(6):641–646

[46] Lyburn ID, Lowe JE, Wong WL. Idiopathic pulmonary fibrosis on F-18 FDG positron emission tomography. Clin Nucl Med. 2005; 30(1):27

[47] Ollenberger GP, Knight S, Tauro AJ. False-positive FDG positron emission tomography in pulmonary amyloidosis. Clin Nucl Med. 2004; 29(10):657–658

[48] Kong FM, Frey KA, Quint LE, et al. A pilot study of [18F]fluorodeoxyglucose positron emission tomography scans during and after radiation-based therapy in patients with non small-cell lung cancer. J Clin Oncol. 2007; 25(21):3116–3123

[49] Hassaballa HA, Cohen ES, Khan AJ, Ali A, Bonomi P, Rubin DB. Positron emission tomography demonstrates radiation-induced changes to nonirradiated lungs in lung cancer patients treated with radiation and chemotherapy. Chest. 2005; 128 (3):1448–1452

[50] Gerbaudo VH, Julius B. Anatomo-metabolic characteristics of atelectasis in F-18 FDG-PET/CT imaging. Eur J Radiol. 2007; 64(3):401–405

[51] Asad S, Aquino SL, Piyavisetpat N, Fischman AJ. False-positive FDG positron emission tomography uptake in nonmalignant chest abnormalities. AJR Am J Roentgenol. 2004; 182(4):983–989

[52] Stagg J, Farukhi I, Lazaga F, et al. Significance of 18F-fluorodeoxyglucose uptake at the gastroesophageal junction: comparison of PET to esophagogastroduodenoscopy. Dig Dis Sci. 2015; 60(5):1335–1342

[53] Truong MT, Erasmus JJ, Munden RF, et al. Focal FDG uptake in mediastinal brown fat mimicking malignancy: a potential pitfall resolved on PET/CT. AJR Am J Roentgenol. 2004; 183 (4):1127–1132

[54] Lin E. F-18 fluorodeoxyglucose uptake in a benign gastric ulcer. Clin Nucl Med. 2007; 32(6):462–463

[55] Koga H, Sasaki M, Kuwabara Y, et al. An analysis of the physiological FDG uptake pattern in the stomach. Ann Nucl Med. 2003; 17(8):733–738

[56] Salaun PY, Grewal RK, Dodamane I, Yeung HW, Larson SM, Strauss HW. An analysis of the 18F-FDG uptake pattern in the stomach. J Nucl Med. 2005; 46(1):48–51

[57] Kim S, Chung JK, Kim BT, et al. Relationship between gastrointestinal F-18-fluorodeoxyglucose accumulation and gastrointestinal symptoms in whole-body PET. Clin Positron Imaging. 1999; 2(5):273–279

[58] Otsuka H, Graham MM, Kubo A, Nishitani H. The effect of oral contrast on large bowel activity in FDG-PET/CT. Ann Nucl Med. 2005; 19(2):101–108

[59] Yildirim D, Tamam MO, Sahin M, Ekci B, Gurses B. Differentiation of incidental intestinal activities at PET/CT examinations with a new sign: peristaltic segment sign. Rev Esp Med Nucl Imagen Mol. 2013; 32(2):86–91

[60] Kamel EM, Thumshirn M, Truninger K, et al. Significance of incidental 18F-FDG accumulations in the gastrointestinal tract in PET/CT: correlation with endoscopic and histopathologic results. J Nucl Med. 2004; 45(11):1804–1810

[61] Gutman F, Alberini JL, Wartski M, et al. Incidental colonic focal lesions detected by FDG PET/CT. AJR Am J Roentgenol. 2005; 185(2):495–500

[62] Israel O, Yefremov N, Bar-Shalom R, et al. PET/CT detection of unexpected gastrointestinal foci of 18F-FDG uptake: incidence, localization patterns, and clinical significance. J Nucl Med. 2005; 46(5):758–762

[63] Iozzo P, Geisler F, Oikonen V, et al. 18F-FDG PET Study. Insulin stimulates liver glucose uptake in humans: an 18F-FDG PET Study. J Nucl Med. 2003; 44(5):682–689

[64] Maldjian PD, Ghesani N, Ahmed S, Liu Y. Adenomyomatosis of the gallbladder: another cause for a "hot" gallbladder on 18F-FDG PET. AJR Am J Roentgenol. 2007; 189(1):W36–8

[65] Lee J, Yun M, Kim KS, Lee JD, Kim CK. Risk stratification of gallbladder polyps (1–2 cm) for surgical intervention with 18F-FDG PET/CT. J Nucl Med. 2012; 53(3):353–358

[66] Liu Y. Clinical significance of diffusely increased splenic uptake on FDG-PET. Nucl Med Commun. 2009; 30(10):763–769

[67] Nam HY, Kim SJ, Kim IJ, Kim BS, Pak K, Kim K. The clinical implication and prediction of diffuse splenic FDG uptake during cancer surveillance. Clin Nucl Med. 2010; 35(10):759–763

[68] Ridolfi L, Cangini D, Galassi R, et al. Reversible, PET-positive, generalized lymphadenopathy and splenomegaly during high-dose interferon-alpha-2b adjuvant therapy for melanoma. J Immunother. 2008; 31(7):675–678

[69] Sugawara Y, Zasadny KR, Kison PV, Baker LH, Wahl RL. Splenic fluorodeoxyglucose uptake increased by granulocyte colony-stimulating factor therapy: PET imaging results. J Nucl Med. 1999; 40(9):1456–1462

[70] Shulkin BL, Thompson NW, Shapiro B, Francis IR, Sisson JC. Pheochromocytomas: imaging with 2-[fluorine-18]fluoro-2-deoxy-D-glucose PET. Radiology. 1999; 212(1):35–41

[71] Ludwig V, Rice RH, Martin WH, Kelley MC, Delbeke D. 2-Deoxy-2-[18F]fluoro-D-glucose positron emission tomography uptake in a giant adrenal myelolipoma. Mol Imaging Biol. 2002; 4(5):355–358

[72] Nishizawa S, Inubushi M, Kido A, et al. Incidence and characteristics of uterine leiomyomas with FDG uptake. Ann Nucl Med. 2008; 22(9):803–810

[73] Lin CY, Ding HJ, Chen YK, Liu CS, Lin CC, Kao CH. F-18 FDG PET in detecting uterine leiomyoma. Clin Imaging. 2008; 32 (1):38–41

[74] Tsujikawa T, Yoshida Y, Mori T, et al. Uterine tumors: pathophysiologic imaging with 16alpha-[18F]fluoro-17beta-estradiol and 18F fluorodeoxyglucose PET–initial experience. Radiology. 2008; 248(2):599–605

[75] Lerman H, Metser U, Grisaru D, Fishman A, Lievshitz G, Even-Sapir E. Normal and abnormal 18F-FDG endometrial and ovarian uptake in pre- and postmenopausal patients: assessment by PET/CT. J Nucl Med. 2004; 45(2):266–271

[76] Liu Y. Benign ovarian and endometrial uptake on FDG PET-CT: patterns and pitfalls. Ann Nucl Med. 2009; 23(2):107–112

[77] Navve D, Kaidar-Person O, Keidar Z. Physiological (18)F-FDG uptake patterns in female reproductive organs before and after chemotherapy treatments: assessment by PET/CT. Med Oncol. 2013; 30(2):598–0598

8 Interpretation of FDG PET Studies

Eugene C. Lin

8.1 Introduction

Optimal fluorodeoxyglucose positron emission tomography (FDG PET) interpretation requires attention to many details, both before and after the exam is performed.

8.2 Appropriate Indication

PET has a wide range of potential applications, with varying degrees of scientific evidence for the efficacy of each application. It is helpful to have a process for screening less common requests for PET. Knowledge of PET is somewhat variable among referring physicians, and it is not uncommon to receive requests for indications for which PET would be unlikely to provide the expected answers. In cases where PET is of marginal value, the referring physician should be made aware of the potential limitations before the examination if performed. This is important to avoid generalization of the information provided in these settings to the overall role of the test in other indications. Screening unusual requests will avoid situations where the referring physician believes that PET will provide specific information that it is unlikely to provide based on available knowledge. Possible limitations of PET are

1. **Limited/inadequate evidence**
   a) *Limited accuracy*. There are disease processes where PET has either poor sensitivity or specificity, or both (e.g., FDG PET for detection of metastatic prostate cancer).
   b) *Limited management effect/cost-effectiveness*. PET may not change management for some potential applications regardless of the results, or may not be cost-effective relative to other options (e.g., PET is not cost-effective in differentiating benign from malignant thyroid nodules, and does not change management as it is not accurate enough to preclude biopsy).
   c) *Limited evidence*. There are many potential applications for which the literature is limited at this time. In these cases, PET may be potentially useful but it may be unclear what additive benefit PET would have over conventional imaging techniques.
2. **Technical limitations**. PET is limited in evaluation of small lesions. In some cases, PET

may be limited for lesions below 1 cm. This can be used as a threshold, but is not a definite cutoff. Lesions below 1 cm are detectable but with lower sensitivity. Detectability of lesions in the 5- to 7-mm range has been reported in clinical studies, and in our experience lesions below 5 mm in size can be detected if they metabolically active and if they are in locations where motion and background activity are limited.

   a) Lesion detectability is dependent, in large part, on location. Lesion detectability is increased in areas with minimal motion (e.g., the retroperitoneum, neck, and extremities) and minimal background physiologic activity (e.g., the lungs and retroperitoneum). It is often possible to easily detect uptake in lesions < 1 cm in certain locations. Areas with large amounts of physiologic activity (e.g., the liver) will have decreased detection rates for small lesions. In the lungs, background activity is low, but respiratory motion decreases detection particularly in the lung bases. Respiratory misregistration artifact specific to PET/CT exams would further limit lesion detection in the lung bases.
   b) PET is sometimes requested for evaluation of equivocal lesions that may be too small to detect by PET. It is optimal to evaluate larger lesions, but lesions smaller than 1 cm in size could be considered for evaluation depending on the location. In these cases, the referring physician should be made aware that false-negative results are possible and only positive results are reliable. The PET study may be very helpful if positive, as this is very specific for malignancy in small lesions. Standardized uptake values (SUVs) will likely be of limited value due to partial volume effects.
3. **Patient limitations**. Patient factors such as recent chemotherapy or radiation or inability to lie still may limit optimal examination. In most cases, these situations can be resolved with further communication with the referring physician and instituting measures such as delaying the exam or sedation.

8.3 Interpretation

In general, FDG PET is a very sensitive but less specific modality (although PET can be very specific in

certain settings). Therefore, an approach to optimal interpretation is to maximize specificity. Specificity can be maximized by
- Correlation with clinical data.
- Correlation between all available PET data.
- Correlation with anatomic imaging.

8.3.1 Clinical Data

It is essential that pertinent information about the history of the illness and relevant ancillary studies are collected before interpreting PET. This is especially true for PET compared to other imaging modalities, given the numerous potential pitfalls. Although the interpreting physician may choose to review the images initially without benefit of patient history, the final interpretation should take into consideration all available and pertinent data related to the disease process. Clinical pretest probability is often useful in the interpretation of PET findings.

1. If the pretest probability of disease is low (e.g., the incidence of mediastinal metastases in peripheral lung cancer or residual disease after treatment of early-stage Hodgkin's disease), then a negative PET is highly predictive of lack of disease and a positive PET is more likely to be false-positive.
2. If the pretest probability of disease is high (e.g., a spiculated lung nodule), a negative PET is more likely to be false-negative and a positive PET is highly predictive of disease.

8.3.2 Correlation between All PET Data

For typical PET scans, three sets of data are provided: maximum intensity projection (MIP), non-attenuation-corrected (NAC), and attenuation-corrected (AC). The NAC and AC images are typically reconstructed in axial, sagittal, and coronal planes. Findings on all data sets should be closely correlated.

1. **MIP images.** The MIP image is reviewed in a rotating format and allows review of the entire volume imaged in different projections. In general, MIP images are less sensitive than the tomographic sets, but they allow a complete overview of the extent of disease and help define relationships of the abnormalities to each other and to anatomical sites.
2. **NAC images.** NAC images can be distinguished from AC images (▸ Fig. 8.1) by
   a) High skin activity.
   b) High lung activity.
   c) Decreased central activity (e.g., low activity in the deep structures of the mediastinum and abdomen).
3. **NAC advantages**
   Overall, there is a similar accuracy and lesion detection for NAC versus AC PET[1]; however, the AC and NAC images are complementary, with NAC images superior for superficial lesions and small lung lesions, and AC images superior for deep lesions.[2,3]
   a) *Low noise.* AC adds noise to the study, which can cause false-positive results. In addition, dense areas can cause artifacts on AC images if computed tomography (CT) is used for AC (see Chapter 9). Review of NAC images may be vital to identify these false-positive findings.
   b) If a potential lesion is seen on AC images but not on NAC images, the possibility of a false-positive secondary to artifact (noise or dense

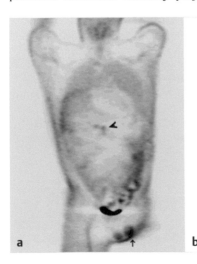
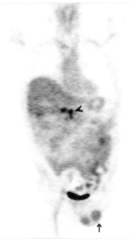

Fig. 8.1 Differences between non-attenuation-corrected and attenuation-corrected images. **(a)** Coronal non-attenuation-corrected image demonstrates increased skin activity, increased lung activity, and central decreased activity including a photopenic mediastinum. Note that the superficial testes (*arrow*) appear more intense than central abdominal nodes (*arrowhead*). **(b)** Coronal attenuation-corrected image at the same level demonstrates that the central nodes (*arrowhead*) are actually more intense than the testes (*arrow*).

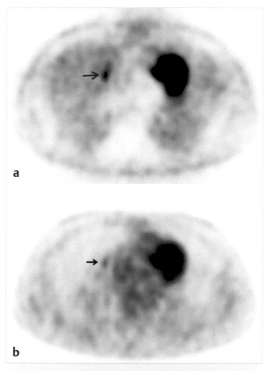

Fig. 8.2 Lung nodule detection: attenuation-corrected vs. non-attenuation-corrected. A right lung nodule (*arrow*) which is much better visualized on a non-attenuation-corrected axial PET scan (a) than an attenuation-corrected scan (b).

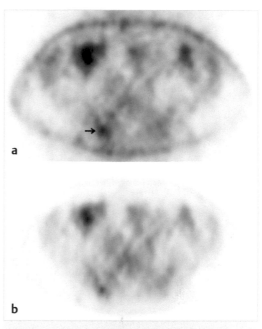

Fig. 8.3 Bone lesion detection: attenuation-corrected vs. non-attenuation-corrected. A bone metastasis to the sacrum (*arrow*) is seen on a non-attenuation-corrected axial PET scan (a), but was not identified prospectively on an attenuation-corrected scan (b).

material) should be considered. This is more of a consideration if the lesion is peripheral (because a central lesion may not be visualized on NAC images secondary to attenuation).

c) ***Detectability***. It is possible that some lesions are only detected on NAC images. In the author's experience, detection of lung (▶ Fig. 8.2), bone (▶ Fig. 8.3), or superficial lesions may be superior on NAC images.

- A clinical study suggests that NAC may be superior for lung lesion detection,[4] but a phantom study suggests that NAC may be superior for abdominal lesions and inferior for lung lesions.[5] A clinical PET/CT study[6] did not demonstrate a difference between AC and NAC images in detection of pulmonary metastases.
- Lesions in areas of uniform attenuation (e.g., the abdomen), will demonstrate greater contrast on NAC images, but lesions in areas of nonuniform attenuation (e.g.,

the thorax) will demonstrate greater contrast on AC images.[5]

- Superficial lesions may be better visualized on NAC images due to the increased activity of peripheral structures. However, if these lesions are close to the intense skin activity on NAC images, they may be obscured.

4. **AC images.** AC images are the standard format for review of PET studies, but AC images should not be reviewed alone without also reviewing the NAC data.

a) AC Advantages[7]

- Anatomic localization. Without AC, it is often difficult to localize lesions accurately. In particular, AC is very helpful for side-by-side CT correlation.
- *SUV measurement*. AC must be performed if SUV is measured (otherwise the measured SUV would depend on the amount of attenuation).
- *Lesion detection*. Although there is no published evidence that AC images detect more lesions in most clinical settings, NAC images can potentially miss deeply seated lesions secondary to attenuation.

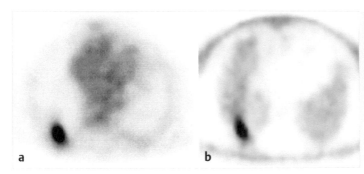

Fig. 8.4 Distortion of lesion shape on non-attenuation-corrected images. **(a)** Axial attenuation-corrected image demonstrates a right lung nodule. **(b)** Axial non-attenuation-corrected image of the same nodule demonstrates that nodule appears smaller in the horizontal dimension due to more attenuating tissue in this direction. The overall shape of the nodule is more elongated.

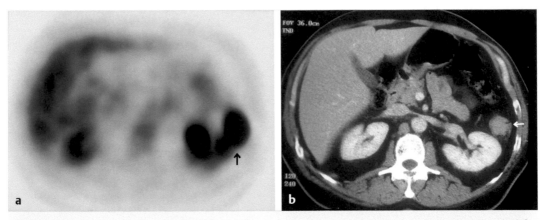

Fig. 8.5 Colon cancer found incidentally. **(a)** Axial PET scan shows an intense focus of uptake (*arrow*) lateral to the left kidney. This was thought initially to be exophytic from the kidney. **(b)** CT scan at the same level demonstrates soft-tissue filling the colonic lumen (*arrow*). This was not seen prospectively on the CT as there was no associated colonic wall thickening or pericolonic abnormality. Both PET and CT were necessary to make this diagnosis: the lesion was obvious on PET but not seen on CT; however, the initial anatomic localization on PET was incorrect and retrospective correlation with CT was necessary to correctly localize the uptake.

- *Accurate lesion size/shape.* NAC images will distort lesion size and shape (the lesion is elongated in the direction with the least attenuation) (▶ Fig. 8.4).
b) AC Disadvantages.
- *Image noise.* AC images are noisier than NAC images.
- *Additional time.* Generating an attenuation map for AC takes additional time. This is less of an issue with CT-based AC.
- *Artifacts.* Typically, these artifacts are created at areas of high density (barium, iodine, metal) and appear with falsely high intensity; they are most pronounced with CT-based AC (see Chapters 7 and 9). Misregistration artifacts are specific to the use of CT for AC (see Chapter 9).

8.3.3 Anatomic Correlation

Correlation with cross-sectional modalities such as CT and magnetic resonance imaging (MRI) can be very helpful in improving the specificity of PET. This can be done visually, with image fusion, or with a dedicated PET/CT scanner.

1. It is important not to rely on reports but to actually view the anatomic images in all cases even if the anatomic study was interpreted as negative. The contrast between the lesion and background is usually much greater with PET than with other imaging modalities. As a result, many abnormalities on anatomic images will be seen only retrospectively, after attention is directed to the specific region by a positive PET scan (▶ Fig. 8.5).

2. Anatomic correlation is primarily helpful in
   a) **Localizing lesions**. In many cases, anatomic correlation is necessary to localize a lesion seen on PET correctly to a specific site (▸ Fig. 8.5). This is particularly true with lesions that are peripheral in location (▸ Fig. 7.46; ▸ Fig. 16.1).
   b) **Identifying false-positives**. Many false positive sources of uptake can be identified as such after anatomic correlation.
   c) **Confirming equivocal PET findings/ increasing interpretation confidence**. Interpreter confidence in a PET finding improves considerably by identifying a corresponding abnormality on anatomic imaging (which is often seen only retrospectively). Although both the PET and CT findings may be equivocal in isolation when combined, they can be confidently interpreted as a positive finding (▸ Fig. 8.6).

8.3.4 Pearls

1. Lesion size. Lesion size on anatomic imaging should influence how the PET findings are interpreted.
   a) *Small lesions*. PET has decreased sensitivity but increased specificity in small lesions.
      - A small lesion (e.g., < 1 cm) with increased uptake is more likely to be malignant. Any definite uptake should be considered worrisome for malignancy because visible increased uptake in a small focus suggests a highly hypermetabolic lesion (▸ Fig. 25.3).
      - SUVs in small lesions should be interpreted with caution because SUVs are often low even in malignancy secondary to partial volume effects. Similarly, the degree of uptake as judged by visual criteria may be relatively minimal and of limited value in a small malignant lesion.
      - A small lesion with no uptake may be falsely negative. A small malignant focus with a mild-to-moderate degree of uptake may go undetected due to confounding factors such as motion and partial volume effects.
   b) *Large lesions*. PET has increased sensitivity but possibly decreased specificity in large lesions.
      - A large lesion with a negative PET study is more likely to be benign. A malignant focus large enough to result in a substantial structural abnormality should be

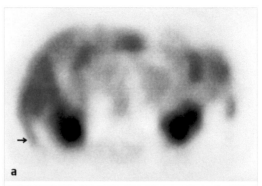

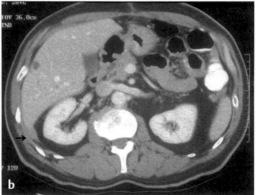

Fig. 8.6 Peritoneal metastasis from colon cancer. **(a)** Axial FDG PET scan shows a vertical linear area of uptake posterior to the right liver (*arrow*). This was detected on initial review of the PET but would be difficult to call definitively abnormal as it is not different in intensity than the liver (potentially it could represent an unusual configuration of the liver). **(b)** CT scan at the same level shows abnormal soft tissue with the same linear configuration (*arrow*) as seen on PET. This was not detected prospectively on CT but in conjunction with the PET findings is definitely abnormal as there should be no normal soft tissue in this location. The CT correlation in this case greatly increases interpreter confidence in the PET finding.

detectable on PET if it is metabolically active. Note that this may not apply to mildly enlarged lesions (e.g., a 1.5-cm lymph node); in these cases, the amount of tumor burden causing the mild enlargement may not be substantial, and a negative PET in these situations should still raise concern for false-negative results. A large lesion with a positive PET study may be falsely positive. Infectious or inflammatory processes severe enough to cause substantial anatomic enlargement may have substantial FDG uptake.

2. **Lesion location**. The value of CT correlation often depends on the location of the lesion. A true-positive PET finding may have no anatomic correlate in some areas, and almost always have a correlate in other areas. Two questions to consider are

a) What are the potential etiologies for the positive PET finding?

b) Would these potential etiologies be detected by CT?

- In certain anatomical sites, it is very unlikely that a true-positive PET finding would have no CT correlate. A focal area of mediastinal uptake should have a CT correlate (e.g., a normal sized node on CT). If correlation is accurate, a node large enough to cause PET uptake should be detected by CT, unless it is in an area where small nodes may be difficult to visualize (e.g., the hilum). For example, an area of increased uptake in the mediastinum without a corresponding node, localizing to mediastinal fat, can be interpreted as mediastinal brown fat uptake.

- In other anatomical sites, there may be no CT correlate for true-positive PET findings. For example, unexplained focal PET uptake in the abdomen is often due to colonic adenomas or less likely peritoneal metastases. Colonic adenomas are not usually detected on CT, and detection of peritoneal metastases by CT is limited. In these cases, further workup is usually necessary.[8]

8.3.5 Pitfalls

There are several potential pitfalls when correlating PET and anatomical imaging studies:

1. **Motion**. Because PET is performed during free breathing, whereas CT may be acquired during a breath-hold, inaccurate localization of lesions may result. Other structures such as the head and breast may also change in position between the CT and PET exams. This is predominately a factor during PET/CT exams, but may affect side-by-side PET and CT interpretation as well.

2. **Importance of correlation with recent studies**. Correlation with old examinations can result in interpretive error, particularly in posttherapy states (▶ Fig. 8.7).

3. **Delayed resolution of PET findings**. It is common for inflammatory processes to have increased FDG uptake weeks or months after resolution of the process on anatomic images. This may result in an apparent discrepancy between PET and recent anatomical imaging. Thus, if a current anatomical study does not demonstrate a corresponding finding, it is important to review preceding anatomical studies as well (▶ Fig. 8.8).

4. **Difficulty in correlation**. In the head and neck and pelvis, visual correlation of PET and CT can be difficult due to lack of anatomic landmarks or physiologic activity (e.g., bladder). In these cases, PET/CT or fusion imaging is usually necessary. Accurate correlation in the abdomen and pelvis is often possible with side-by-side reading of PET and CT.

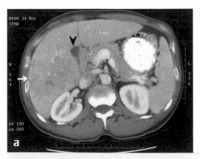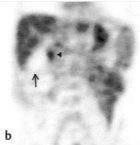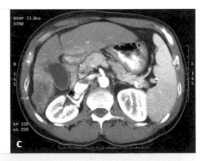

Fig. 8.7 False-positive from correlation with old exam: hepatocellular carcinoma status post radiofrequency (RF) ablation. **(a)** CT scan demonstrates a large mass in the right lobe of the liver (*arrow*). The gallbladder (*arrowhead*) is small. The patient underwent RF ablation of the mass after this CT. **(b)** Coronal PET scan performed 3 months after the ablation demonstrates a large photopenic area (*arrow*) with a focus of uptake at the medial margin (*arrowhead*). As a recent CT was not available, correlation was made by the CT in **(a)**. The photopenic area was initially thought to represent the ablated mass with the medial activity representing residual tumor. **(c)** However, CT performed a day after the PET scan demonstrates that the right lobe of the liver has greatly decreased in size post ablation (*arrow*). The gallbladder is much larger than on the previous CT. The photopenic area on PET is actually the gallbladder and the medial activity thought to represent residual tumor is in the duodenum (*arrowhead*).

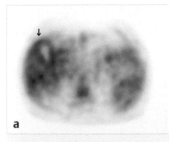 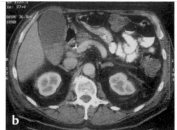 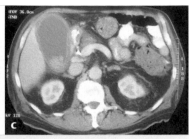

Fig. 8.8 Gallbladder wall inflammation. **(a)** Axial FDG PET scan shows increased uptake in the gallbladder wall (*arrow*). **(b)** CT scan at the same level done 1 day before the PET shows sludge in the gallbladder but a normal-appearing gallbladder wall. **(c)** CT scan done 1 month before shows a thickened gallbladder wall. Inflammatory processes will often resolve on anatomic imaging before PET imaging.

8.4 Reporting

1. **SUV**. For oncological patients with lesions, it is important to report SUVs of index lesions, even if these measurements are not used for interpretation of the current study. If the patient is restudied at a later date, the SUVs will be necessary to assess the course of the disease and response to treatment. In addition, it may be helpful to report the method of SUV calculation and the time of imaging after injection, as these factors may be helpful for comparison of SUVs if the patient is evaluated at another institution in the future.
2. The impression should state clearly about any potential limitations of PET for the specific disease process in question. For example, if there is a small lesion seen on CT that could potentially be missed on PET due to size, the report should state that a negative PET study does not exclude active disease due to the limited resolution of this modality.
3. The relevance of PET findings should be stated explicitly. For example, if the patient has had a recent CT with a nonspecific 1.5-cm hypodense liver lesion, rather than reporting that no abnormal liver uptake is identified, it is more helpful to report "the 1.5-cm hypodense liver lesion seen on CT does not demonstrate increased uptake on PET, suggesting that it is most likely a benign lesion. However, a low-grade hepatocellular carcinoma may appear hypometabolic on PET imaging."
4. Lesion size is not well evaluated by PET as the apparent size is largely dependent on the intensity of uptake (▸ Fig. 25.3). Unless obvious changes are present, comments about changes

in lesion size evaluated by PET alone should be avoided.

8.5 Follow-up

The first step toward follow-up of abnormalities noted on PET should include correlation with recent or concurrent (PET/CT) anatomical imaging studies. Often, findings seen with the superior contrast resolution of PET can be seen retrospectively on other imaging studies. If no recent anatomic imaging studies are available, they should be requested.

1. **Unexpected findings**. Findings that are not clearly related to the known disease process for which PET is requested are not uncommon. These findings often represent clinically undiagnosed malignant or premalignant disorders, and in most cases should be pursued further.[9]
2. **PET finding without imaging correlate**. In the authors' experience, the majority of true-positive PET findings have a corresponding structural abnormality, which is often seen in retrospect. If no corresponding abnormalities are seen, further workup might depend on the location of the abnormality and clinical history (see Pearls section). A PET finding without imaging correlate could be false-positive or represent a pathology that is usually not visible anatomically at an early stage. In one report,[10] FDG-avid lesions without a CT correlate were malignant in 41% of cases, with lesions in lymph node locations and in the bones having the highest rate of malignancy. In some cases, a follow-up CT at a short interval can be helpful because some processes seen on PET that are

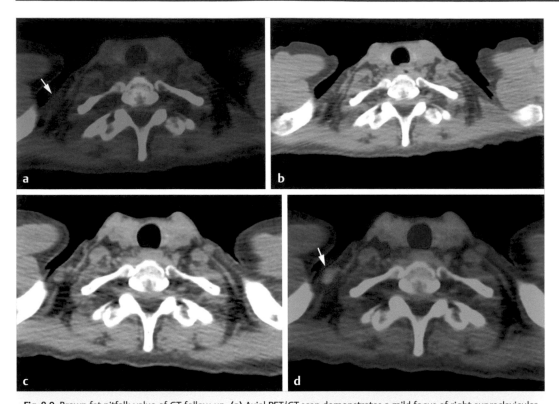

Fig. 8.9 Brown fat pitfall: value of CT follow-up. (**a**) Axial PET/CT scan demonstrates a mild focus of right supraclavicular uptake (*arrow*). (**b**) Corresponding axial CT scan does not demonstrate a lesion in this location. This was initially thought to represent brown fat uptake. However, no other brown fat uptake was identified. (**c**) Axial PET/CT scan at a later date demonstrates more intense uptake in the previously noted area of right supraclavicular uptake. (**d**) Corresponding axial CT scan demonstrates interval development of a node in this region (*arrow*). Initially, this case presents a diagnostic dilemma as a single focus of supraclavicular brown fat uptake would be very rare but the initial absence of a corresponding CT abnormality would also be very unusual. In these cases, close interval follow-up with CT is helpful as PET positive abnormalities initially invisible on CT may manifest on follow-up CT exams.

not visualized on initial CT may be visualized on follow-up CT (▶ Fig. 8.9).

- **Example**. Focal lung uptake without a corresponding finding on chest CT is very unlikely to represent a lung neoplasm. One possibility might be false-positive activity from a radiolabeled clot.[11] On the other hand, a diffuse pattern of uptake can represent radiation pneumonitis or even early pneumonia with a negative CT. In the former situation, no further imaging or follow-up is necessary. In the latter situation, a follow-up CT exam at a short interval may be helpful.

References

[1] Joshi U, Raijmakers PG, Riphagen II, Teule GJ, van Lingen A, Hoekstra OS. Attenuation-corrected vs. nonattenuation-corrected 2-deoxy-2-[F-18]fluoro-D-glucose-positron emission tomography in oncology: a systematic review. Mol Imaging Biol. 2007; 9(3):99–105

[2] Houseni M, Chamroonrat W, Basu S, et al. Usefulness of non attenuation corrected 18F-FDG-PET images for optimal assessment of disease activity in patients with lymphoma. Hell J Nucl Med. 2009; 12(1):5–9

[3] Huang YE, Pu YL, Huang YJ, et al. The utility of the nonattenuation corrected 18F-FDG PET images in the characterization of solitary pulmonary lesions. Nucl Med Commun. 2010; 31 (11):945–951

[4] Bleckmann C, Dose J, Bohuslavizki KH, et al. Effect of attenuation correction on lesion detectability in FDG PET of breast cancer. J Nucl Med. 1999; 40(12):2021–2024

[5] Bai C, Kinahan PE, Brasse D, et al. An analytic study of the effects of attenuation on tumor detection in whole-body PET oncology imaging. J Nucl Med. 2003; 44(11):1855–1861

[6] Reinhardt MJ, Wiethoelter N, Matthies A, et al. PET recognition of pulmonary metastases on PET/CT imaging: impact of attenuation-corrected and non-attenuation-corrected PET images. Eur J Nucl Med Mol Imaging. 2006; 33 (2):134–139

[7] Wahl RL. To AC or not to AC: that is the question. J Nucl Med. 1999; 40(12):2025–2028

[8] Pandit-Taskar N, Schöder H, Gonen M, Larson SM, Yeung HW. Clinical significance of unexplained abnormal focal FDG uptake in the abdomen during whole-body PET. AJR Am J Roentgenol. 2004; 183(4):1143–1147

[9] Agress H, Jr, Cooper BZ. Detection of clinically unexpected malignant and premalignant tumors with whole-body FDG PET: histopathologic comparison. Radiology. 2004; 230(2): 417–422

[10] Kumar R, Hawkins RA, Yeh BM, Wang ZJ. Focal fluorine-18 fluorodeoxyglucose-avid lesions without computed tomography correlate at whole-body positron emission tomography-computed tomography in oncology patients: how often are they malignant? Nucl Med Commun. 2011; 32(9):802–807

[11] Ha JM, Jeong SY, Seo YS, et al. Incidental focal F-18 FDG accumulation in lung parenchyma without abnormal CT findings. Ann Nucl Med. 2009; 23(6):599–603

9 PET/CT

Eugene C. Lin and Paul E. Kinahan

9.1 Introduction

Positron emission tomography combined with computed tomography (PET/CT) has tremendous potential as it combines the most sensitive imaging modality (PET) to the highest resolution cross-sectional imaging modality (CT). In a meta-analysis,[1] PET/CT had a higher sensitivity (95%) than PET alone (85%) or CT alone (80%), with similar specificity. The addition of fused CT to PET images has numerous advantages over PET alone, but the interpreter should be aware of potential pitfalls introduced by the process of CT fusion and attenuation correction in PET.

9.2 Advantages

1. **Increased accuracy**. PET/CT adds a substantial incremental benefit compared to using PET alone, and a lesser extent compared to side-by-side reading of PET and CT. In one study,[2] only 52% of pathologic lesions were accurately characterized (localization and infiltration of adjacent structures) by PET alone. The remaining 48% required either side-by-side CT reading or combined PET/CT. However, many of the cases which may require CT correlation can be accurately interpreted with side-by-side reading of PET and CT. In approximately 6 to 12%[2,3] of total PET cases, side-by-side reading is not adequate for either accurate lesion localization or characterization, and combined PET/CT may be needed for these purposes. In tumor staging, PET/CT has an incremental 8% increase in accuracy relative to PET and side-by-side CT interpretation and a 20% increase relative to PET interpretation alone.[4]

2. **Specific advantages**. PET/CT provides the same advantages that can be achieved by correlating any type of functional and structural imaging techniques (see Chapter 9). PET/CT maximizes these advantages by providing the most accurate correlation. The improved accuracy achieved is noted in
   a) Localizing lesions (▶ Fig. 9.1).
   b) Identifying false-positive findings (▶ Fig. 9.2).
   c) Determining the nature of subtle or equivocal PET findings and therefore improving the degree of certainty of the results (▶ Fig. 9.3).

PET/CT usually enhances the specificity rather than sensitivity compared to PET alone. Many sources of false-positive finding are easily identified by PET/CT. However, sensitivity can also improve with PET/CT. For example, areas that may be thought to definitely or questionably represent physiologic activity on PET alone can be shown to localize to a pathologic sites on the fused CT scan. The color images used to interpret PET/CT can also make some lesions more conspicuous.

3. **Contemporaneous correlation**. Although side-by-side CT correlation is often adequate, the CT studies are often not contemporaneous. This can result in errors (▶ Fig. 8.7) from changes that have taken place during the time interval between acquiring the CT and the PET scan. This issue is obviated with PET/CT.

4. **CT-based attenuation correction for PET**. The CT scan can be used for attenuation correction of PET data,[5] allowing for decreased scan time as the CT is completed more quickly than a radionuclide source scan. In addition, PET image noise is reduced due to the decreased noise of the CT relative to a radionuclide source scan and the lack of postemission contamination on transmission images.

9.3 Disadvantages

The only disadvantages of combined PET/CT relative to PET alone are the artifacts specific to PET/CT. These artifacts are primarily related to three factors[6]:
a) Misregistration due to differences in position of structures between PET and CT.
b) Artifacts due to differences in attenuation of structures between PET and CT.
c) Truncation artifacts related to the CT field-of-view diameter (typically 50 cm) differing from the larger PET field-of-view diameter (typically 70 cm). All manufacturers are addressing this issue by allowing for reconstruction of an extended CT field of view.

9.3.1 Misregistration

Misregistration artifacts are most prominent in areas of greatest respiratory motion—the lung bases and diaphragmatic region. Misregistration results in two basic artifacts:

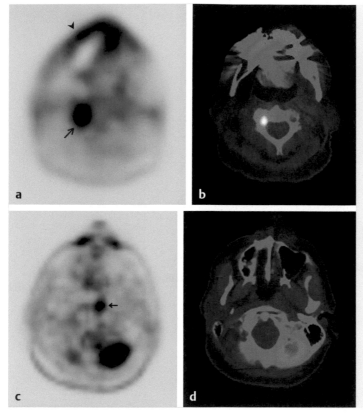

Fig. 9.1 Head and neck localization with PET/CT. Localization of FDG uptake is usually the hardest in the head and neck region due to lack of anatomic landmarks in this region on PET. **(a)** Axial PET scan demonstrates focal uptake in the right base of skull region (*arrow*). This cannot be localized on PET. Note the artifact (*arrowhead*) around photopenic dental hardware. **(b)** Axial PET/CT localizes this activity to the cervical spine (bone metastasis). **(c)** Axial PET in a different patient demonstrates focal uptake in the left base of skull region (*arrow*). This also cannot be localized on PET. **(d)** Axial PET/CT localizes this activity to the nasopharynx (nasopharyngeal carcinoma).

a) ***Incorrect uptake levels***. Motion between PET and CT results in inaccurate attenuation correction as the region on CT used for attenuation correction does not correspond exactly to the region on PET. This can result in artifactually decreased or increased visual levels of uptake and inaccurate calculation of standardize uptake value (SUV).

b) ***Mislocalization***. Lesions can be localized to the wrong location on fused PET/CT images.

1. ***Type of respiration***. In a combined PET/CT study, the CT scan can be acquired during free (shallow) breathing, maximum inspiration, and normal expiration. The PET scan must be acquired during free breathing due to the length of the scan. The type of breathing during the CT will affect the incidence of artifacts.[7] Mislocalizations from respiration will usually be in the superior to inferior dimension.

   a) *Normal expiration*. This will usually result in the most accurate fusion as most of the breathing cycle is spent in expiration. This may be the preferred protocol with fast CT scanners. Scanning in normal expiration is preferred but may not be possible, as some patients may not be able to breath-hold in normal expiration for the duration of the CT.

   b) *Inspiration*. Inspiratory maneuvers, whether a small or regular breath in, will typically result in the most significant misalignment of PET and CT at the diaphragm and heart.[8] Inspiration can cause photopenic curvilinear artifacts at the lung–diaphragm interface (▶ Fig. 9.4). This occurs because measured attenuation in this region is too low (there is only lung in this region on the maximum inspiration CT, whereas subdiaphragmatic structures are present in the same region on PET) leading to undercorrection of the detected activity in this region. Photopenic artifact can also be seen at the interface between the heart and the lungs (▶ Fig. 9.5).

   c) *Free breathing*. Free breathing can also cause photopenic curvilinear artifacts at the lung–diaphragm interface if the peridiaphragmatic area is scanned during inspiration. However, image coregistration with shallow breathing is typically superior to that with inspiration.[8]

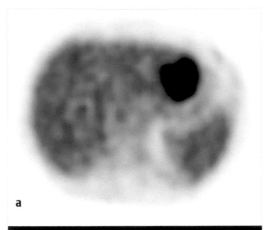

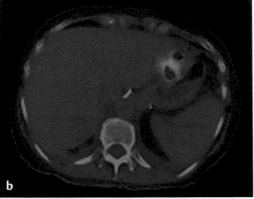

Fig. 9.2 Abscess mimicking gastric cancer. (a) Axial PET scan demonstrates intense uptake in the stomach region worrisome for gastric carcinoma. (b) Axial PET/CT scan at the same level shows the activity to lie in an abscess medial to the stomach.

2. Corrections for respiratory misregistration

 a) *Respiratory averaged low-dose CT scanning.* For some PET/CT scanners, this method uses cine-CT acquisition to form a respiratory-blurred CT-based attenuation correction image. This potentially reduces the mismatch with the respiratory-blurred PET image.[9] The low-dose respiratory-blurred CT image is not viewed, and care must be taken to use as low CT technique factors as possible to avoid excessive radiation dose to the patient.

 b) *Respiratory gating.* Four-dimensional PET/CT protocols with respiratory gating can improve the spatial matching between PET and CT but often require long acquisition and postprocessing times. Other protocols[10] have been developed which might improve

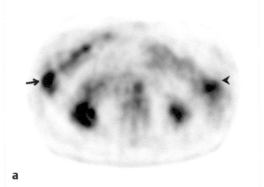

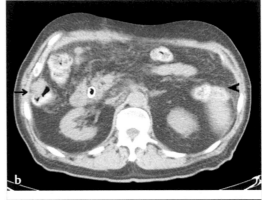

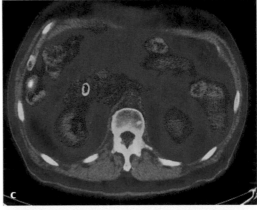

Fig. 9.3 Bowel vs. peritoneal disease. (a) Axial PET in a patient with cholangiocarcinoma demonstrates focal areas of increased uptake in the right (*arrow*) and left abdomen (*arrowhead*). It cannot be determined whether these are normal bowel uptake or peritoneal disease on PET alone. Correlation with CT (b) and PET/CT (c) demonstrates that the focus of the uptake on the right is a peritoneal lesion (*arrow*) and the focus on the left is bowel activity (*arrowhead*).

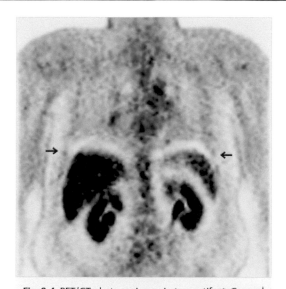

Fig. 9.4 PET/CT photopenic respiratory artifact. Coronal PET scan done with CT attenuation correction demonstrates curvilinear photopenic artifacts at the lung diaphragm interface bilaterally (*arrows*). This artifact is usually seen if the CT scans this region during inspiration (either during an inspiratory breath-hold or free breathing) resulting in a mismatch with the PET scan which is primarily in expiratory phase of the respiratory cycle.

registration with minimal acquisition and postprocessing time and effort.

3. ***Nonrespiratory motion***. This is most commonly seen in the head and neck where motion between the CT and PET scans results in mislocalization mostly in the medial to lateral dimension (▸ Fig. 9.6, ▸ Fig. 9.7). Another area where it is commonly seen is the breast (▸ Fig. 9.8). On some systems, this can be corrected (on the scanner console) by realignment tools.

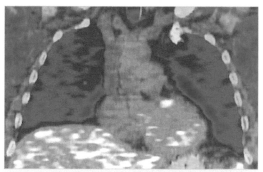

Fig. 9.5 Cardiac misregistration artifact. Coronal PET/CT scan demonstrates photopenic artifact around the heart.

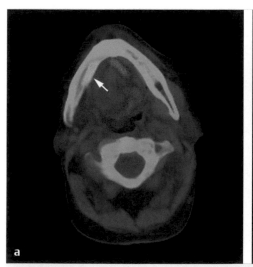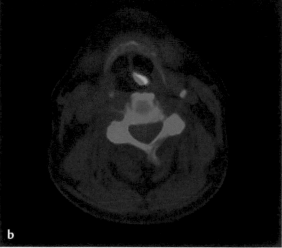

Fig. 9.6 Head and neck mislocalization. Mislocalizations in the head and neck usually result from motion of the head between the CT and PET studies. Mislocalizations are usually in the medial to lateral direction. **(a)** Axial PET/CT demonstrates mislocalization of linear mylohyoid uptake to the right, with the right mylohyoid uptake (*arrow*) overlapping the mandible. **(b)** More inferior axial PET/CT slice from the same study demonstrates that uptake from a left epiglottic neoplasm appears to be centered medial to the epiglottis, and normal cervical cord activity is in the right spinal canal. Submandibular gland uptake is localized slightly to the right of the submandibular glands. However, the mislocalization did not result in a diagnostic error in this case.

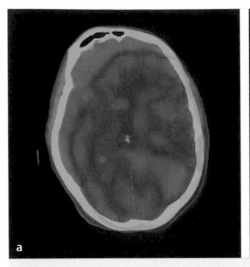
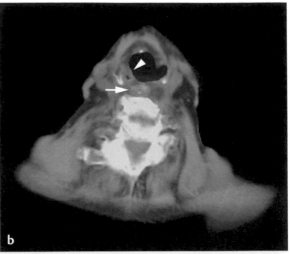

Fig. 9.7 Head and neck mislocalization. Sometimes mislocalizations can result in diagnostic errors. **(a)** Axial PET/CT study demonstrates severe mislocalization at the brain level. Review of this image suggests that mislocalization will cause activity to localize posteriorly and to left of the actual location. **(b)** Axial PET/CT scan demonstrates a focus of activity localizing to the esophagus (*arrow*). However, mislocalization would occur posteriorly and to the left based on image **a**, and the focus of activity is actually in the right piriform sinus (*arrowhead*), which demonstrates abnormal soft-tissue thickening on the CT.

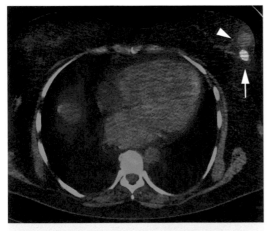

Fig. 9.8 Breast lesion misregistration. Axial PET/CT scan demonstrates a left breast lesion (*arrowhead*). FDG uptake (*arrow*) appears posterior to the lesion secondary to misregistration between the PET and CT studies.

4. **SUV**. Areas of artifactually decreased and increased activity and therefore inaccurate SUV measurements have been described in the lung bases and bowel. This can result in both false-positive and false-negative interpretation of the resulting images.

a) *Lung bases.* The SUV can be altered by up to 30%.

b) *Bowel.* Differences in bowel motion between PET and CT from peristalsis and respiration can result in areas of falsely increased or decreased activity and SUVs on CT attenuation-corrected imaging. This could result in reduced sensitivity for detecting adjacent malignant peritoneal implants and nodes, or false-positive findings (▶ Fig. 9.9). Areas of artifactually reduced activity are more common than those with increased activity.[11]

5. **Mislocalizations**. Significant mislocalizations can occur in the lung bases and the liver dome (e.g., a liver lesion localized to the lung) (▶ Fig. 9.10).[12]

a) *Thorax.* Error in lung nodule location is in the range of 7 to 10 mm on average, and is more pronounced in both the lung bases and left lung.[13]

b) *Abdomen.* There is usually less than 1-cm discrepancy noted, but discrepancy can be > 2 cm at the upper liver margin and the lower splenic margin.

6. **Differences between PET and CT**. The visceral organs may be in different positions and have different sizes on PET compared to CT due to normal physiologic motion.[14]

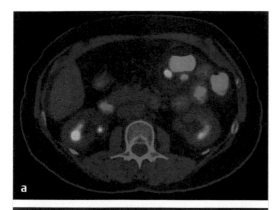

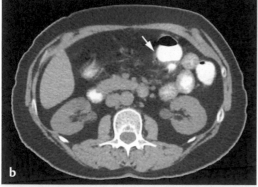

Fig. 9.9 (a,b) Misregistration. Sagittal PET/CT demonstrates misregistration between the PET and CT data sets, best seen at the inferior margin of the liver and kidney. Note that bowel activity (*arrow*) appears to localize to the mesentery.

a) *Liver.* The liver is slightly larger in size and superior and lateral in position on PET compared to CT.
b) *Spleen.* The spleen is slightly smaller in size and is positioned superior and posterior on PET compared to CT.
c) *Kidneys.* The kidneys are slightly smaller in size and superior, posterior, and rightward in position on PET compared to CT.

9.3.2 Attenuation Artifacts Secondary to Dense Material

Due to the method used to scale the CT image for PET attenuation correction, dense or high-atomic-number materials can cause artifactually increased activity on the PET image. With the 511-keV energy of positron emitters, the attenuation of gamma rays by barium and iodine solutions is not greatly different than that from soft tissues.

However, there is a significant difference in attenuation between barium/iodine solutions and soft tissue on CT. As a result, the 511-keV photon attenuation is overestimated in areas containing dense material when CT is used. In these areas, the visualized activity and SUVs will be artifactually elevated due to incorrect (too high) attenuation values provided by CT. The activity on the PET image is incorrectly increased to correct for attenuation which is not present. Roughly, the SUV error is about 0.1% per HU. In other words, a contrast enhancement of 100 HU causes a 10% error in PET SUV.[6] On some PET/CT scanners, it is possible to process the attenuation-corrected PET images by assuming that regions on the CT image with high HU value correspond to contrast agents, and not bone. This will lead to PET images with correct SUVs in soft tissue, even if significant contrast enhancement is present in the CT image. It should be noted, however, that any FDG uptake in bone may be incorrect as a result of this type of processing, and the original PET image should be used for the bone uptake values.

1. ***Oral contrast.*** The amount of artifactually increased activity will depend on the density of contrast used. High-density barium can cause substantial artifactual increased values (▶ Fig. 9.11). There is conflicting evidence on the impact of low-density oral contrast agents,[15,16] but the bulk of the evidence indicates that the degree of artifactual increase from the low-density barium used in CT is minimal, and generally not clinically significant[17] as long as there is not increased concentration secondary to water resorption.[18]
   a) On average, the SUV error will be less than 5%, and at the most slightly greater than 10%.
   b) Oral contrast agents that have been proposed include low-density barium and water with 2.5% mannitol and 0.2% locust bean gum. Negative oral contrast (e.g., water with 2.5% mannitol and 0.2% locust bean gum) can be used to avoid artifacts.[19]
   If artifactual increased activity is present, it can appear either in the area containing the contrast medium or as a ring of increased activity around the contrast medium. Larger areas of contrast material produce the ring artifacts.[15]
2. ***Intravenous contrast.*** The concentration of the intravenous contrast will not affect the degree of FDG activity.[20] However, FDG activity does differ between different phases of enhancement (e.g., activity is lower in the liver on arterial

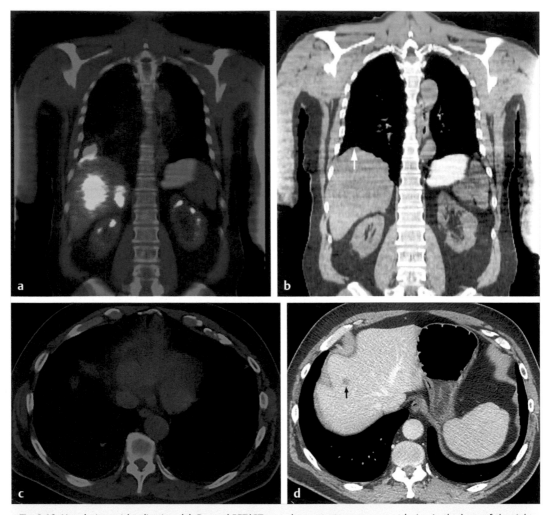

Fig. 9.10 Liver lesion mislocalization. **(a)** Coronal PET/CT scan demonstrates an apparent lesion in the base of the right lung. **(b)** Coronal CT scan at the same level does not demonstrate a lung lesion in this location. The apparent lung uptake is secondary to mislocalization of the lesion in the liver dome. A bulge in the contour of the liver dome (*arrow*) is seen secondary to this lesion (which is not otherwise seen on this noncontrast study). **(c)** Axial PET/CT demonstrates apparent increased uptake in the right lower lobe in a patient with rectal adenocarcinoma. **(d)** Axial contrast-enhanced CT demonstrates that the uptake corresponds to a liver metastasis (*arrow*), which was misregistered on the PET/CT.

phase images).[21] Intravenous contrast can also cause artifactually increased activity. As for oral contrast agents, the higher the density of intravenous contrast material, the greater the artifactually increased activity.[22]

a) *Thoracic veins.* Artifact is most prominent in the thoracic veins containing undiluted contrast from injection (▶ Fig. 9.12).[23]

b) *Urinary tract.* Artifact from urinary contrast excretion is also prominent in the kidneys, ureters, and bladder, where the percentage error can be greater than 25%.

c) *Arterial phase imaging.* Artifacts from dense vessels will be more pronounced on CT arterial phase imaging compared to the portal venous phase.

d) *Normal tissue.* The amount of increase in normal tissue is minimal, most prominent in the liver, spleen, and aorta, where the maximum SUV increases 5 to 7%.[24]

e) *Pathologic tissues.* Pathologic tissue usually enhances due to neovascularity and/or increased perfusion. Increases in maximum SUV are variable but are usually minimal (4% average increase).[24]

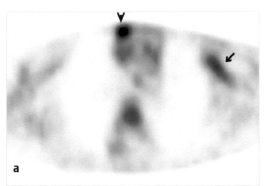

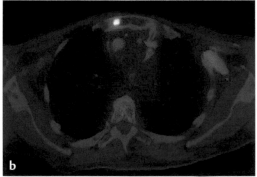

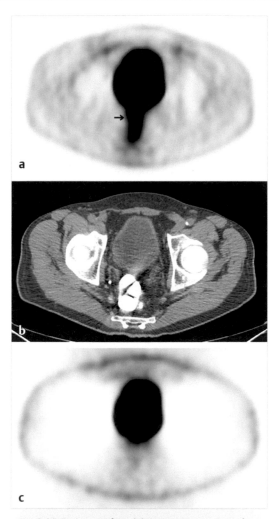

Fig. 9.11 Barium artifact. **(a)** Attenuation-corrected axial PET scan demonstrates intense activity in the rectum (*arrow*). **(b)** Corresponding axial CT scan demonstrates dense barium in this region. **(c)** Non-attenuation-corrected axial PET scan does not demonstrate increased activity in this region.

Fig. 9.12 Intravenous contrast artifact. **(a)** Axial PET with CT attenuation correction demonstrates increased activity in the left axilla (*arrow*) and right parasternal region (*arrowhead*). The right parasternal activity could represent sternal or internal thoracic nodal uptake on PET. **(b)** Axial PET/CT demonstrates that the activity on PET in the left axilla is artifactual from dense intravenous contrast and the parasternal uptake is in the bone.

f) *Liver and mediastinum activity.* If the liver and mediastinal activity are used as references sites to compare to tumor activity, contrast may cause errors as FDG uptake in the liver and mediastinum could be overestimated by 10 to 15%.[25]

g) *CT protocol.* Artifact from contrast in the thoracic veins can be minimized by scanning caudocranially with a biphasic contrast injection.[26]

3. *Calcified lesions*. Calcified lesions usually are not dense enough to result in artifactually increased activity. However, non-attenuation-corrected (NAC) images should always be reviewed if activity is noted in a calcified lesion (▶ Fig. 26.7) to determine that the activity is not artifactual.

4. *Metallic/dense material artifact*. Metallic and dense foreign material can cause artifactually increased activity and decreased activity. Areas of dark streak artifact result in an underestimation of activity.[27] High-density metallic implants such as hip prostheses will also attenuate the PET 511-kEV photons, resulting in no emission data in the implant region and a cold area.[28] Examples include

a) Metallic dental prostheses, orthopaedic implants, cements.

b) Cardiac leads and central venous line reservoirs.[29]

- In cardiac PET/CT, there are often significant artifacts seen with implantable cardioverter defibrillator leads, but pacemaker leads usually do not cause noticeable artifact.[30]

9.3.3 Truncation Artifact

Truncation artifact occurs due to differences in the field of view between PET and CT. Obese patients may have part of their anatomy outside the field of view of the CT scan. This truncated portion does not provide data for attenuation correction, resulting in artifactually low SUVs. Some PET/CT scanners provide methods for estimating the truncated regions of the CT images. While these enlarged field-of-view CT images may not always be suitable for diagnostic CT interpretation, they provide accurate attenuation correction for the PET images.

9.4 Interpretation

Interpretation of PET/CT is similar to that of PET alone with CT correlation (see Chapter 9), but the interpreter must be aware of the potential artifacts that are associated with combined PET/CT imaging. Some issues specific to PET/CT interpretation are
1. **Registration**. Before review of fused PET/CT images, it should be first determined whether the fused images are accurately registered.
2. **Non-attenuation corrected (NAC) images**. Review of NAC images is more essential in interpretation of combined PET/CT than in PET alone. Most of the PET/CT-specific artifacts are related to the use of CT-based attenuation correction. Therefore, the absence of a PET/CT abnormality on the NAC images would suggest the possibility of a PET/CT artifact.
3. **Lungs**
   a) *Lung nodules*. If PET/CT is performed in shallow breathing, small lung nodules are often not detected.[31] Thus, PET/CT performed in shallow breathing cannot completely replace breath-hold chest CT in cancer staging. The addition of an additional low-dose chest CT to the PET/CT exam may be helpful.[32]
   b) *Lung bases*. Caution must be employed in the interpretation of potential abnormalities in the lung bases given the high incidence of PET/CT misregistration artifacts in this region. In particular, the degree of uptake in distal esophageal and lung base lesions may be artifactually decreased if misregistration artifact is present.

4. **SUV**
   a) SUVs can be artifactually decreased or increased secondary to motion as described in the Disadvantages section.
   b) One study suggests that SUVs may be slightly higher on CT-attenuation-corrected PET compared to SUVs generated by germanium-corrected PET (see Chapter 5),[33] but another study suggests there is no difference.[34] Caution should be used when comparing PET/CT and PET SUV values.

9.5 Patient Preparation

Patient preparation for PET/CT is the same as for PET. However, factors specific to PET/CT are
1. **Patient position**. For standard PET scans, patients may be scanned with their arms at the sides for comfort. For PET/CT, it is preferable to scan the patient with the arms above the head if tolerated to avoid beam hardening artifacts, which will degrade images of the upper abdomen. The exception is head and neck where the arms should be down. The increased speed of PET/CT makes arms-up scanning tolerable for most patients.
2. **Oral contrast**. The choice of whether to use oral contrast may depend on the indication. For tumors that are unlikely to have peritoneal/mesenteric spread (e.g., lung cancer), oral contrast is unlikely to be helpful. Oral contrast may be very helpful for tumors with a propensity for peritoneal and/or mesenteric nodal spread. However, while oral contrast may allow differentiation between bowel and adjacent peritoneal disease, the increased density of the contrast could accentuate areas of artifactually increased and decreased activity due to bowel motion (see Disadvantages section). The key is to minimize the density of the contrast used. In addition, the physiologic effects of oral contrast may increase bowel activity independent of the effects of increased density.
3. **Intravenous contrast**. Intravenous contrast will improve the diagnostic quality of the CT but may introduce artifacts (see Disadvantages section). While some studies have indicated that contrast-enhanced PET/CT is not significantly more accurate than nonenhanced PET/CT,[35,36,37] the majority of reports indicate there is additional value in performing contrast-enhanced PET/CT. Additional value has been noted in staging and 3D conformal radiotherapy planning in advanced non–small cell lung

cancer,[38] definition of regional nodal status in rectal cancer,[39] detection and characterization of liver lesions in colorectal cancer,[40] staging pancreatic cancer,[41] assessing colorectal cancer recurrence,[42] pancreatic cancer reccurence,[43] uterine cancer recurrence,[44] ovarian cancer recurrence,[45] and local recurrence of head and neck cancer.[46]

Factors to consider in deciding whether to employ intravenous contrast:

a) Contrast enhancement of visceral organs will slightly increase the measured physiologic activity. This could potentially decrease visualization of pathologic lesions in these organs.

b) Pathologic lesions which enhance may have artifactually increased SUV values.

c) More intense activity in the thoracic veins and urinary tract from undiluted or concentrated contrast may obscure adjacent pathologic lesions.
- This can be minimized by scanning before renal contrast excretion and scanning caudocranially to minimize thoracic vein activity.

d) The patient may have contrast-enhanced CT studies before or after the PET exam. In many cases, review of the fused PET/noncontrast CT and the separate contrast-enhanced CT in conjunction can be comparable to review of a PET/contrast CT study, but without the possible artifacts.

4. **Respiration**. The phase of respiration during the CT scan may affect the type and incidence of artifacts (see Disadvantages section). The choice is often dependent on the degree of patient cooperation.

9.6 "True" Whole-Body PET/CT

"True" whole-body PET/CT refers to additional inclusion of the lower extremities and skull to the standard "eyes to thighs" PET/CT. There is conflicting evidence on the value of "true" whole-body PET/CT. While a few reports[47,48] support the use of this protocol, the majority of studies suggest that it is of low yield and unlikely to change clinical management.[47,49,50,51,52,53,54] In patients with melanoma, it has been suggested that "true" whole-body PET/CT should only be performed if the melanoma arises in the lower extremities.[53] In one report,[54] patients with melanoma, lymphoma, multiple myeloma, sarcomas, and stage IV lung, breast, prostate, bladder, testicular, and renal cancer were most likely to have findings outside the standard skull base to upper thighs field of view.

References

[1] Gao G, Gong B, Shen W. Meta-analysis of the additional value of integrated 18FDG PET-CT for tumor distant metastasis staging: comparison with 18FDG PET alone and CT alone. Surg Oncol. 2013; 22(3):195–200

[2] Reinartz P, Wieres FJ, Schneider W, Schur A, Buell U. Side-by-side reading of PET and CT scans in oncology: which patients might profit from integrated PET/CT? Eur J Nucl Med Mol Imaging. 2004; 31(11):1456–1461

[3] Pelosi E, Messa C, Sironi S, et al. Value of integrated PET/CT for lesion localisation in cancer patients: a comparative study. Eur J Nucl Med Mol Imaging. 2004; 31(7):932–939

[4] Antoch G, Saoudi N, Kuehl H, et al. Accuracy of whole-body dual-modality fluorine-18-2-fluoro-2-deoxy-D-glucose positron emission tomography and computed tomography (FDG-PET/CT) for tumor staging in solid tumors: comparison with CT and PET. J Clin Oncol. 2004; 22(21):4357–4368

[5] Kinahan PE, Townsend DW, Beyer T, Sashin D. Attenuation correction for a combined 3D PET/CT scanner. Med Phys. 1998; 25(10):2046–2053

[6] Kinahan PE, Hasegawa BH, Beyer T. X-ray-based attenuation correction for positron emission tomography/computed tomography scanners. Semin Nucl Med. 2003; 33(3):166–179

[7] Goerres GW, Burger C, Kamel E, et al. Respiration-induced attenuation artifact at PET/CT: technical considerations. Radiology. 2003; 226(3):906–910

[8] Gilman MD, Fischman AJ, Krishnasetty V, Halpern EF, Aquino SL. Optimal CT breathing protocol for combined thoracic PET/CT. AJR Am J Roentgenol. 2006; 187(5):1357–1360

[9] Pan T, Mawlawi O, Nehmeh SA, et al. Attenuation correction of PET images with respiration-averaged CT images in PET/CT. J Nucl Med. 2005; 46(9):1481–1487

[10] Nehmeh SA, Erdi YE, Meirelles GS, et al. Deep-inspiration breath-hold PET/CT of the thorax. J Nucl Med. 2007; 48(1):22–26

[11] Nakamoto Y, Chin BB, Cohade C, Osman M, Tatsumi M, Wahl RL. PET/CT: artifacts caused by bowel motion. Nucl Med Commun. 2004; 25(3):221–225

[12] Osman MM, Cohade C, Nakamoto Y, Marshall LT, Leal JP, Wahl RL. Clinically significant inaccurate localization of lesions with PET/CT: frequency in 300 patients. J Nucl Med. 2003; 44(2):240–243

[13] Cohade C, Osman M, Marshall LN, Wahl RN. PET-CT: accuracy of PET and CT spatial registration of lung lesions. Eur J Nucl Med Mol Imaging. 2003; 30(5):721–726

[14] Nakamoto Y, Tatsumi M, Cohade C, Osman M, Marshall LT, Wahl RL. Accuracy of image fusion of normal upper abdominal organs visualized with PET/CT. Eur J Nucl Med Mol Imaging. 2003; 30(4):597–602

[15] McKeown C, Dempsey MF, Gillen G, Paterson C. Quantitative analysis shows that contrast medium in positron emission tomography/computed tomography may cause significant artefacts. Nucl Med Commun. 2012; 33(8):864–871

[16] Otero HJ, Yap JT, Patak MA, et al. Evaluation of low-density neutral oral contrast material in PET/CT for tumor imaging: results of a randomized clinical trial. AJR Am J Roentgenol. 2009; 193(2):326–332

[17] Cronin CG, Prakash P, Blake MA. Oral and IV contrast agents for the CT portion of PET/CT. AJR Am J Roentgenol. 2010; 195(1):W5–W13

[18] Dizendorf E, Hany TF, Buck A, von Schulthess GK, Burger C. Cause and magnitude of the error induced by oral CT contrast agent in CT-based attenuation correction of PET emission studies. J Nucl Med. 2003; 44(5):732–738

[19] Antoch G, Kuehl H, Kanja J, et al. Dual-modality PET/CT scanning with negative oral contrast agent to avoid artifacts: introduction and evaluation. Radiology. 2004; 230(3):879–885

[20] Prechtel HW, Verburg FA, Palmowski M, et al. Different intravenous contrast media concentrations do not affect clinical assessment of 18F-fluorodeoxyglucose positron emission tomography/computed tomography scans in an intraindividual comparison. Invest Radiol. 2012; 47(9):497–502

[21] Rebière M, Verburg FA, Palmowski M, et al. Multiphase CT scanning and different intravenous contrast media concentrations in combined F-18-FDG PET/CT: Effect on quantitative and clinical assessment. Eur J Radiol. 2012; 81(8):e862–e869

[22] Nakamoto Y, Chin BB, Kraitchman DL, Lawler LP, Marshall LT, Wahl RL. Effects of nonionic intravenous contrast agents at PET/CT imaging: phantom and canine studies. Radiology. 2003; 227(3):817–824

[23] Antoch G, Freudenberg LS, Egelhof T, et al. Focal tracer uptake: a potential artifact in contrast-enhanced dual-modality PET/CT scans. J Nucl Med. 2002; 43(10):1339–1342

[24] Yau YY, Chan WS, Tam YM, et al. Application of intravenous contrast in PET/CT: does it really introduce significant attenuation correction error? J Nucl Med. 2005; 46(2):283–291

[25] Barrington SF, Mikhaeel NG, Kostakoglu L, et al. Role of imaging in the staging and response assessment of lymphoma: consensus of the International Conference on Malignant Lymphomas Imaging Working Group. J Clin Oncol. 2014; 32(27):3048–3058

[26] Beyer T, Antoch G, Bockisch A, Stattaus J. Optimized intravenous contrast administration for diagnostic whole-body 18F-FDG PET/CT. J Nucl Med. 2005; 46(3):429–435

[27] Shimamoto H, Kakimoto N, Fujino K, et al. Metallic artifacts caused by dental metal prostheses on PET images: a PET/CT phantom study using different PET/CT scanners. Ann Nucl Med. 2009; 23(5):443–449

[28] Sureshbabu W, Mawlawi O. PET/CT imaging artifacts. J Nucl Med Technol. 2005; 33(3):156–161, quiz 163–164

[29] Halpern BS, Dahlbom M, Waldherr C, et al. Cardiac pacemakers and central venous lines can induce focal artifacts on CT-corrected PET images. J Nucl Med. 2004; 45(2):290–293

[30] DiFilippo FP, Brunken RC. Do implanted pacemaker leads and ICD leads cause metal-related artifact in cardiac PET/CT? J Nucl Med. 2005; 46(3):436–443

[31] Allen-Auerbach M, Yeom K, Park J, Phelps M, Czernin J. Standard PET/CT of the chest during shallow breathing is inadequate for comprehensive staging of lung cancer. J Nucl Med. 2006; 47(2):298–301

[32] Juergens KU, Weckesser M, Stegger L, et al. Tumor staging using whole-body high-resolution 16-channel PET-CT: does additional low-dose chest CT in inspiration improve the detection of solitary pulmonary nodules? Eur Radiol. 2006; 16(5):1131–1137

[33] Nakamoto Y, Osman M, Cohade C, et al. PET/CT: comparison of quantitative tracer uptake between germanium and CT transmission attenuation-corrected images. J Nucl Med. 2002; 43(9):1137–1143

[34] Souvatzoglou M, Ziegler SI, Martinez MJ, et al. Standardised uptake values from PET/CT images: comparison with conventional attenuation-corrected PET. Eur J Nucl Med Mol Imaging. 2007; 34(3):405–412

[35] Kitajima K, Suzuki K, Senda M, et al. Preoperative nodal staging of uterine cancer: is contrast-enhanced PET/CT more accurate than non-enhanced PET/CT or enhanced CT alone? Ann Nucl Med. 2011; 25(7):511–519

[36] Pfluger T, Melzer HI, Schneider V, et al. PET/CT in malignant melanoma: contrast-enhanced CT versus plain low-dose CT. Eur J Nucl Med Mol Imaging. 2011; 38(5):822–831

[37] Chiaravalloti A, Danieli R, Caracciolo CR, et al. Initial staging of Hodgkin's disease: role of contrast-enhanced 18F FDG PET/CT. Medicine (Baltimore). 2014; 93(8):e50

[38] Pfannenberg AC, Aschoff P, Brechtel K, et al. Low dose non-enhanced CT versus standard dose contrast-enhanced CT in combined PET/CT protocols for staging and therapy planning in non-small cell lung cancer. Eur J Nucl Med Mol Imaging. 2007; 34(1):36–44

[39] Tateishi U, Maeda T, Morimoto T, Miyake M, Arai Y, Kim EE. Non-enhanced CT versus contrast-enhanced CT in integrated PET/CT studies for nodal staging of rectal cancer. Eur J Nucl Med Mol Imaging. 2007; 34(10):1627–1634

[40] Cantwell CP, Setty BN, Holalkere N, Sahani DV, Fischman AJ, Blake MA. Liver lesion detection and characterization in patients with colorectal cancer: a comparison of low radiation dose non-enhanced PET/CT, contrast-enhanced PET/CT, and liver MRI. J Comput Assist Tomogr. 2008; 32(5):738–744

[41] Yoneyama T, Tateishi U, Endo I, Inoue T. Staging accuracy of pancreatic cancer: comparison between non-contrast-enhanced and contrast-enhanced PET/CT. Eur J Radiol. 2014; 83(10):1734–1739

[42] Kitajima K, Murakami K, Yamasaki E, et al. Performance of integrated FDG PET/contrast-enhanced CT in the diagnosis of recurrent colorectal cancer: Comparison with integrated FDG PET/non-contrast-enhanced CT and enhanced CT. Eur J Nucl Med Mol Imaging. 2009; 36(9):1388–1396

[43] Kitajima K, Murakami K, Yamasaki E, et al. Performance of integrated FDG-PET/contrast-enhanced CT in the diagnosis of recurrent pancreatic cancer: comparison with integrated FDG-PET/non-contrast-enhanced CT and enhanced CT. Mol Imaging Biol. 2010; 12(4):452–459

[44] Kitajima K, Suzuki K, Nakamoto Y, et al. Low-dose non-enhanced CT versus full-dose contrast-enhanced CT in integrated PET/CT studies for the diagnosis of uterine cancer recurrence. Eur J Nucl Med Mol Imaging. 2010; 37(8):1490–1498

[45] Kitajima K, Ueno Y, Suzuki K, et al. Low-dose non-enhanced CT versus full-dose contrast-enhanced CT in integrated PET/CT scans for diagnosing ovarian cancer recurrence. Eur J Radiol. 2012; 81(11):3557–3562

[46] Suenaga Y, Kitajima K, Ishihara T, et al. FDG-PET/contrast-enhanced CT as a post-treatment tool in head and neck squamous cell carcinoma: comparison with FDG-PET/non-contrast-enhanced CT and contrast-enhanced CT. Eur Radiol. 2016; 26(4):1018–1030

[47] Osman MM, Chaar BT, Muzaffar R, et al. 18F-FDG PET/CT of patients with cancer: comparison of whole-body and limited whole-body technique. AJR Am J Roentgenol. 2010; 195(6):1397–1403

[48] Nguyen NC, Chaar BT, Osman MM. Prevalence and patterns of soft tissue metastasis: detection with true whole-body F-18 FDG PET/CT. BMC Med Imaging. 2007; 7:8

[49] Niederkohr RD, Rosenberg J, Shabo G, Quon A. Clinical value of including the head and lower extremities in 18F-FDG PET/CT imaging for patients with malignant melanoma. Nucl Med Commun. 2007; 28(9):688–695

[50] Kawata S, Imaizumi M, Kako Y, Oku N. Clinical impact of "true whole-body" (18)F-FDG PET/CT: lesion frequency and added benefit in distal lower extremities. Ann Nucl Med. 2014; 28 (4):322–328

[51] Tan JC, Chatterton BE. Is there an added clinical value of "true"whole body(18)F-FDG PET/CT imaging in patients with malignant melanoma? Hell J Nucl Med. 2012; 15(3):202–205

[52] Querellou S, Keromnes N, Abgral R, et al. Clinical and therapeutic impact of 18F-FDG PET/CT whole-body acquisition including lower limbs in patients with malignant melanoma. Nucl Med Commun. 2010; 31(9):766–772

[53] Lazaga FJ, Oz OK, Adams-Huet B, Anderson J, Mathews D. Comparison of whole-body versus limited whole-body 18F-FDG PET/CT scan in malignant cutaneous melanoma. Clin Nucl Med. 2013; 38(11):882–884

[54] Sebro R, Mari-Aparici C, Hernandez-Pampaloni M. Value of true whole-body FDG-PET/CT scanning protocol in oncology: optimization of its use based on primary diagnosis. Acta Radiol. 2013; 54(5):534–539

10 PET/MRI: Introduction to Clinical Applications

Ali Salavati, Sina Houshmand, Cory Daignault, Abass Alavi, and Drew Torigian

10.1 Introduction

The combination of sequentially acquired data from magnetic resonance imaging (MRI) with molecular information from positron emission tomography (PET) has long been conducted by side-by-side analysis of the images or software-based image coregistration. However, after successful incorporation of PET/computed tomography (CT) scanners, several investigators developed techniques to make hybrid PET/MRI scanner a clinical reality.[1] In 2007, the feasibility of simultaneous PET/MRI of the human brain was demonstrated.[2] In 2010, the first clinical sequential whole-body PET/MRI scanners were installed at Geneva University Hospital in Switzerland and at Mount Sinai Medical Center in the United States. In 2011, the first fully integrated whole-body simultaneous PET/MRI scanner received U.S. Food and Drug Administration (FDA) approval and became commercially available for clinical use.[3,4] Since then, clinical PET/MRI systems have been receiving increasing attention, and over 80 institutions have installed clinical PET/MRI scanners around the world. Currently, two companies offer clinical simultaneous (concurrent) PET/MRI systems: Biograph mMR (Siemens Healthcare GmbH, Erlangen, Germany) and Signa PET/MRI (GE Healthcare, Waukesha, WI).

10.2 Advantages and Disadvantages of PET/MRI (Relative to PET/CT)

10.2.1 Advantages

a) Improved soft-tissue contrast. The use of MRI in place of CT is particularly useful for improved evaluation of the brain and spinal cord,[5] heart,[6] abdominal and pelvic organs,[7] breasts, and musculoskeletal structures (including muscles, tendons, ligaments, cartilage, and bone marrow).[8,9] Compared to CT, MRI leads to improved sensitivity, specificity, and accuracy of disease detection and diagnosis in many organs and improves the delineation of the internal architecture of organs and tissues.[1]

b) Functional imaging capability. In addition to structural imaging capability, MRI provides functional imaging capability that may further improve the diagnostic performance of PET/MRI relative to PET/CT.[5,10] Some of the available functional imaging methods afforded by MRI include diffusion-weighted imaging (DWI), diffusion-tensor imaging, functional MRI (fMRI), magnetic resonance elastography,[11] magnetic resonance spectroscopy, and perfusion-weighted imaging.[1]

c) Decreased radiation exposure. Use of PET/MRI can reduce radiation exposure, and is therefore important to consider for use in children,[12] women of child-bearing age, and for patients undergoing multiple serial diagnostic imaging examinations.[13]

10.2.2 Disadvantages

a) Decreased sensitivity for lung lesions. The sensitivity of MRI for detection of solid pulmonary nodules (particularly when < 5 mm in size) and subsolid pulmonary nodules is less than that of CT.[14,15,16,17,18,19] This is due to the presence of susceptibility artifacts created by air in the lungs, a low signal-to-background ratio of aerated lung, and the presence of respiratory motion artifacts.[20]

b) Slower examination times. In general, PET/MRI acquisition times are longer than those for PET/CT, ranging from 30 to 120 minutes depending on the specific clinical question to be addressed, the anatomic region of coverage, and the number and types of MRI sequences that are acquired.

c) More demands on imaging-center infrastructure. PET/MRI scanners have higher instrumentation costs and higher operational costs, as well as greater logistical and space requirements. Furthermore, physicians and staff utilizing PET/MRI require safety training related to the use of radioactivity and powerful magnetic fields.

d) Additional contraindications. In general, certain metallic or electronic objects in the body such as some cerebral aneurysm clips, orbital metallic foreign bodies, transvenous pacemakers, implantable cardioverter defibrillators, neurostimulators, and cochlear implants are contraindications for MRI due to risks of device malfunction, movement, or heating with tissue injury. However, some patients with newer MRI-compatible versions of implanted metallic or electronic devices may be able to undergo PET/MRI.

10.3 Patient Preparation

Patient preparation for the PET portion of the PET/MRI is the same as for PET/CT, which is discussed in detail in Chapter 4. However, there are specific MRI-related factors that should be considered for PET/MRI scans:

a) Patient screening. As mentioned earlier, there are several conditions that may prevent the patient from having an MRI or that require particular modification of the MRI scanning protocol. These may include (but are not limited to) claustrophobia, a history of intravenous gadolinium-based contrast allergy, a history of shrapnel or bullet wounds, a history of metal working (e.g., welding) which could cause metal fragments in the orbit, and the presence of various devices such as cardiac pacemakers or defibrillators, implanted drug infusion devices (i.e., insulin pumps), metallic implants and prostheses, neurostimulators (i.e., transcutaneous electrical nerve stimulation), artificial heart valves, cerebral aneurysm clips, cochlear implants, dorsal column stimulators, programmable ventriculoperitoneal shunts, and vascular stents or stent grafts. Therefore, patients must be comprehensively screened for the presence of metallic or electronic devices and assessed for their MRI compatibility before entering the PET/MRI room, in order to prevent potential patient injury as well as to minimize image artifacts. This is performed with a patient screening form and physical screening with metal detectors or radiography/CT as needed. For comprehensive details regarding patient screening and safety issues relevant to MRI, please see www.mrisafety.com.

b) Image acquisition. Depending on the type of PET/MRI scanner that is utilized, PET and multiplanar MR images may be obtained either sequentially or concurrently. Surface coils are typically placed over the body regions to be scanned in order to improve signal-to-noise ratio and spatial resolution of the MR images. A fast MRI scan is initially performed using a T1-weighted gradient recalled echo (GRE) for the purpose of PET image attenuation correction. Depending on the body regions and the type of patient to be scanned (e.g., pediatric vs. adult), particular MRI sequences can be utilized. The MR images may be acquired during breath-holding, during respiratory gating or triggering, or during free breathing.

c) Contrast materials. Oral contrast material is not typically utilized for most MRI studies. The one exception is MR enterography, in which case oral contrast agent is typically administered in advance of the study to distend and opacify the bowel lumen with fluid. This is done to improve the detection and characterization of bowel pathology such as inflammatory bowel disease. If the clinical indication requires use of intravenous gadolinium-based contrast material, then assessment of estimated glomerular filtration rate (eGFR) is performed, particularly in patients with risk factors for renal function impairment such as older age, a history of renal disease, or a history of diabetes mellitus. Gadolinium-based intravenous contrast material is generally not administered when the eGFR is < 30 mL/min/1.73 m^2 in order to prevent the rare but serious complication of nephrogenic systemic fibrosis. In addition, assessment for a history of allergy to gadolinium-based contrast material (including assessment of the type and severity of reaction) should be performed prior to the PET/MRI study so that a corticosteroid preparation can be administered in advance if indicated. Also, intravenous gadolinium-based contrast material is not administered to women who are pregnant or potentially pregnant unless there are exceptional clinical circumstances that warrant its use, since gadolinium-based contrast agents pass through the placental barrier and may potentially be harmful to the fetus. For further detailed information about contrast materials, please see the American College of Radiology (ACR) contrast manual https://www.acr.org/Quality-Safety/Resources/Contrast-Manual.

d) Ear protection. Earplugs or headphones are provided to patients while in the scanner to protect their hearing from MRI system–related noise, as the MRI portion of the PET/MRI scanner often produces loud noises during image acquisition.

10.4 Interpretation (Brief Review of Various MRI Sequences and Their Utility)

Interpretation of PET/MRI is similar to that of PET alone in correlation with MRI alone. However, the reader must be aware of the basic MRI sequences that are available when interpreting hybrid PET/MRI studies. There are many MRI sequences that can be used as a part of PET/MRI scan, which are briefly introduced in the following paragraphs.

10.4.1 Basic MRI Sequences

a) In-phase (IP) and out-of-phase (OOP) T1-weighted GRE. These sequences are short enough to be acquired during breath-holding and are useful for assessment of overall anatomy and for tissue characterization. Low signal intensity cancellation artifacts will be present at all intra-voxel fat–water interfaces on OOP T1-weighted images. The presence of microscopic lipid within a tissue, such as with hepatic steatosis or in a lipid-containing adrenal adenoma, leads to loss of signal intensity on OOP T1-weighted images relative to IP T1-weighted images. The presence of iron, such as with hemochromatosis or chronic hemorrhage (containing hemosiderin), or metal, will lead to loss of signal intensity on IP T1-weighted images relative to OOP T1-weighted images. Macroscopic fat, proteinaceous fluid, subacute hemorrhage, dilute gadolinium-based contrast material, and other paramagnetic substances have high T1-weighted signal intensity relative to skeletal muscle. Iron, metal, gas, cortical bone, and fibrous structures (such as ligaments and tendons) have low T1-weighted signal intensity relative to skeletal muscle.

b) T2-weighted Rapid Acquisition with Refocused Echoes (RARE) (also called fast spin echo or turbo spin echo [TSE] on different systems). These relatively long sequences are acquired during respiratory-gating or triggering and are useful to assess the internal architecture of the central nervous system, the musculoskeletal system, and smaller organs such as the uterus, cervix, prostate gland, seminal vesicles, and testes. These are also useful to detect and characterize lesions, particularly when fat suppression is applied. If fluid is seen to have very high signal intensity on an MR image, then it is likely T2-weighted, whereas if it has low signal intensity, then it is likely T1-weighted. Iron, metal, gas, cortical bone, fibrous structures, and fast flow in vessels have low T2-weighted signal intensity relative to skeletal muscle.

c) Heavily T2-weighted RARE. This sequence can be acquired during breath-holding, and is useful for assessment of overall anatomy, fluid-filled anatomical structures (thecal sac, pancreatic duct, biliary tree, gallbladder, bowel, ureters, bladder, etc.), and fluid collections. Cysts, hemangiomas, fluid collections, and simple fluid within normal structures have very high heavily T2-weighted signal intensity relative to skeletal muscle. Magnetic resonance cholangiopancreatography (MRCP) is a very heavily T2-weighted imaging sequence where only fluid-filled structures have high signal intensity relative to background tissues.

d) Diffusion-weighted (DW) and apparent diffusion coefficient (ADC) map images. DW images are acquired with a modified T2-weighted imaging sequence with diffusion-sensitizing gradients using low and high b values (where high b value images are more diffusion-weighted than low b value images). ADC map images are then mathematically calculated from the DW images. Tissues that restrict water molecule diffusion will have high signal intensity on low and high b value DW images relative to background, and will have low signal intensity on ADC map images. The lower the signal intensity of a tissue on an ADC map image, the more restricted the water molecule diffusion is within the tissue. DW and ADC map images are useful to improve the detection of metastatic lesions, as well as to improve the characterization of lesions, given that malignant lesions tend to restrict diffusion more than normal tissues. Some benign neoplastic lesions and some nonneoplastic lesions (e.g., acute cerebrovascular infarction, abscess, hematoma) may also restrict diffusion. In addition, DW and ADC map images are sensitive to motion and susceptibility artifacts.

e) Precontrast and postcontrast fat-suppressed T1-weighted sequences. It is important to acquire precontrast and postcontrast images with the same image acquisition parameters, so that one can reliably determine whether enhancement is present or absent in a tissue of interest. This is because tissue signal intensities between precontrast and postcontrast images will change just by altering the image acquisition parameters, making it difficult (if not impossible) to determine whether an observed increase in tissue signal intensity on postcontrast images relative to precontrast images is due to true enhancement or is instead artifactual in nature. Precontrast fat-suppressed T1-weighted images are also useful to confirm the presence of macroscopic fat, as high signal intensity fat on non-fat-suppressed T1-weighted images will become low in signal intensity on fat-suppressed T1-weighted images. Postcontrast fat-suppressed T1-weighted images are typically acquired dynamically through one body region of interest during the arterial and venous phases of enhancement, followed by delayed phase images through one or more body regions. Postcontrast images are useful to improve the detection and characterization of lesions, as well as to assess for abnormalities of the arterial and venous structures. Vascularized solid tissues will enhance, whereas nonvascularized cystic or necrotic tissues will not enhance.

10.4.2 Other Considerations

- PET and MR image registration. Before review of the fused PET/MR images, it is important to first determine whether the fused images are accurately registered. Various sources of motion, including bulk patient motion and physiologic motion (e.g., cardiac, respiratory, peristaltic), may lead to misalignment between PET and MR images, introduce image artifacts, and lead to inaccuracies in standardized uptake value (SUV) measurement. Various PET and MRI motion correction strategies are available to mitigate these problems.
- MR images. The MR images should be reviewed (in conjunction with the PET images) to detect and characterize lesions that may be present. It is important to note that as signal intensity is not calibrated to a reference standard, one must always describe the signal intensity of a tissue or lesion of interest seen on a particular imaging sequence in comparison to another reference tissue such as skeletal muscle or liver. As an example, hepatic hemangiomas are high in signal intensity relative to liver parenchyma on T2-weighted images, and yet are simultaneously low in signal intensity relative to cerebrospinal

fluid on T2-weighted images. Simply put, signal intensity is relative.

10.5 MR-Based Attenuation Correction and PET Quantification

Since the signal intensity of a tissue is not correlated with its electron density, the conversion of signal intensities to attenuation coefficients (and therefore MRI-guided attenuation correction of PET images) is complex, potentially leading to discrepancies in SUV measurement based on PET/MRI compared to PET/CT. Tissues such as bone and lung that are associated with heterogeneous changes in tissue attenuation are among the most challenging, potentially leading to SUV underestimation on PET/MRI relative to that on PET/CT.

Over the last decade, multiple MRI-based attenuation correction methods have been proposed by different groups. However, they generally can be categorized into three groups[21,22]: (1) segmentation-based methods, which are more widely used and in which MR images are segmented into different tissue classes (e.g., background air, adipose tissue, soft tissue, lung tissue, and in some methods cortical and spongy bone tissues), and then a predefined linear attenuation coefficient is assigned for each tissue class (▶ Fig. 10.1)[23]; (2) template/atlas-based and machine learning methods, in which a priori knowledge of anatomy and a coregistered MR–CT atlas dataset are used to provide a pseudo-CT image and/or to extract an attenuation map that predicts the pseudo-CT image from the MR image of the patient; and (3) reconstruction-based methods, where attenuation map and activity simultaneously reconstruct from PET data based on maximum-likelihood using either time-of-flight (TOF) information[21] or non-TOF information.[24]

Each category of attenuation correction methods has its own advantages and limitations. For example, segmentation-based methods are prone to PET quantification inaccuracy caused by MR truncation, MR susceptibility artifact, and bone/air and lung segmentation errors although they are simple and robust. Atlas-based methods are time-consuming and require high computational capacity, registration errors or interpatient anatomical variability can cause quantification inaccuracy, and additional dedicated atlases for pediatric patients are usually needed.[21] Reconstruction-based methods use the PET radiotracer biodistribution. They

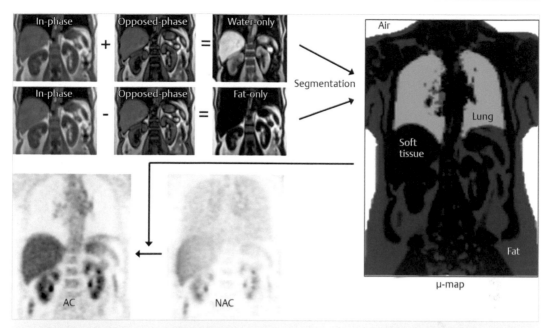

Fig. 10.1 One approach to MRI-based segmentation-based attenuation correction utilizes the Dixon method, which employs algebraic operations on in-phase and out-of-phase images to generate water-only and fat-only images. These images are then utilized in a segmentation algorithm that classifies components of the imaged anatomy as soft tissue, fat, lung, or air. The visual representation of these segmentation results is called a µ-map. Based on the known densities of these various tissue types, the µ-map information can be applied to the reconstruction algorithm, thereby generating attenuation-corrected PET images (AC). The non-attenuation-corrected (NAC) PET images are shown for comparison. The µ-map should be reviewed during Image interpretation to help identify potential AC errors due to incorrect segmentation. (Reproduced with permission from Fraum et al.[23])

particularly depend on the nonspecific accumulation of ^{18}F-fluorodeoxyglucose (FDG) in the skin, whereas other radiotracers may not accumulate sufficiently in the skin to provide enough signal for PET-based contour detection. The technical details of these methods are beyond the scope of this chapter, but the articles by Mehranian et al,[21] Catana et al,[25] Rausch et al,[26] and Beyer et al[27] are recommended for interested readers.

Currently, the vendor-implemented attenuation correction method in Philips Ingenuity TF PET/MR system employs a multistack T1-weighted spoiled GRE sequence to segment the MRI into three tissue classes (air, lung, soft tissue).[27] Siemens Biograph mMR scanners employs a dedicated Dixon-volume interpolated breath-hold excitation (VIBE) sequence to segment the MRI into four tissue classes (air, lung, soft tissue, fat) and, more recently, five tissue classes.[21,22,27] GE Signa PET/MRI scanners employ a three-dimensional dual-echo spoiled GRE sequence

(LAVA-Flex) to segment MRI into four tissue classes (air, lung, soft tissue, fat). For the head, it coregisters a CT-based atlas to acquired MR images to approximate the size and location of the bones and air cavities.[22,27]

Given the simplicity and robustness of segmentation-based methods, they are almost always the main method implemented in commercial PET/MRI systems. However, the most accurate correction method will likely be achieved by hybrid techniques combining the three methods to take advantage of each method in different parts of the body and in various clinical situations.[21]

The quantification accuracy of current attention correction methods implemented in commercial PET/MRI scanners is currently suboptimal, and is reported to underestimate SUV measurements by up to 25%, particularly in osseous lesions and in cortical brain regions.[21] However, for the majority of clinical scenarios, this is clinically irrelevant.[21,22,28]

10.6 Potential Clinical Applications of PET/MRI

PET/MRI is not presently covered for reimbursement by insurance agencies in the United States for clinical use, and clinical indications for PET/MRI have yet to be established. However, PET/MRI may play a future role for the following clinical applications listed below.

10.6.1 Oncologic Applications

As expected for a new evolving imaging modality, there is a significant heterogeneity among clinical studies using PET/MRI for evaluation of patients with cancer. As a result, there is only a limited number of meta-analyses that combine data from multiple institutions. Shen et al[29] performed a meta-analysis of 38 studies including 753 patients and 4,234 lesions to assess the diagnostic performance of PET/MRI in the staging of various cancers. They included studies involving both integrated PET/MRI and software-fused PET/MRI, and used histopathologic results and/or clinical and imaging follow-up as reference standards. On a per-patient level, the pooled sensitivity, specificity, positive likelihood ratio, negative likelihood ratio, and diagnostic odds ratio with 95% confidence intervals (CIs) of PET/MRI compared to reference standard were 0.93 (0.90–0.95), 0.92 (0.89–0.95), 6.67 (4.83–9.19), 0.12 (0.07–0.21), and 75.08 (42.10–133.91), respectively. On a per-lesion level, the corresponding estimates were 0.90 (0.88–0.92), 0.95 (0.94–0.96), 10.91 (6.79–17.54), 0.13 (0.08–0.19), and 102.53 (59.74–

175.97), respectively. In the subgroup analysis, they found integrated PET/MRI had a higher sensitivity than software-fused PET/MRI. In another meta-analysis[30] of 10 studies including 421 patients with head and neck carcinoma who underwent software-fused PET/MRI or integrated PET/MRI, the per-lesion pooled sensitivity and specificity with 95% CIs were 0.91 (0.89–0.93) and 0.63 (0.60–0.66), respectively. In subgroup analysis, the pooled specificity of integrated PET/MRI studies was higher than software-fused studies (0.87 vs. 0.53, respectively). However, the results of this meta-analysis should be interpreted with caution, given the significant heterogeneity among included studies and different reference standards used in included studies.

Given the established role of PET/CT in the management of oncology patients, the diagnostic performance of PET/MRI in the clinical assessment of different types of cancer is compared to PET/CT in the following section. As mentioned earlier, given the limited number of available studies and significant heterogeneity among them, pooled diagnostic indices were not discussed.

Head and Neck Malignancies

In 369 patients with head and neck cancer from 7 studies (2 retrospective and 5 prospective),[31] the diagnostic accuracies of PET/CT and PET/MRI for staging were comparable. Yet, one study[32] demonstrated superior lesion discernibility and improved lesion delineation for PET/MRI without a significant change in the patient management (▶ Fig. 10.2).[33] In 266 of the patients who underwent restaging,

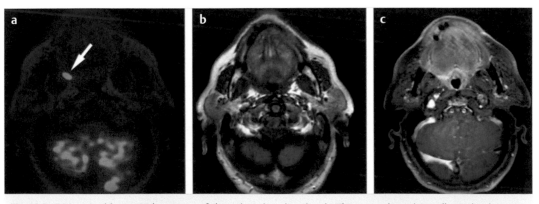

Fig. 10.2 A 70-year-old man with a tumor of the right palatoglossal arch. The tumor (*arrow*) is well visualized on transverse combined FDG PET/MR image (**a**), but is not visible on transverse T1-weighted MR image (**b**) or on transverse contrast-enhanced fat-suppressed T1-weighted MR image (**c**). (Reproduced with permission from Platzek.[33])

the diagnostic performances of PET/CT and PET/MRI for restaging were equivalent.[31] However, PET/MRI and PET/CT were superior to standalone MRI.

Thoracic Malignancies

Lung Cancer

For TNM staging, three studies[34,35,36] involving 117 non–small cell lung cancer patients reported that FDG-PET/MRI diagnostic performance was similar to that of FDG-PET/CT, with a lower estimated radiation dose. However, in a separate study of 10 patients[37] with clinical suspicion of lung cancer (8 with definite lung cancer), T and N staging were inconsistent between PET/MRI and PET/CT in 3 patients although without an associated change in therapeutic approach. Differences in T staging in 3 out of 15 patients with non–small cell lung cancer were also observed.[38] In summary, PET/MRI and PET/CT showed similar staging results in larger studies, whereas small patient series showed some discrepancies in T and N staging.

Pulmonary Nodules

A total of 503 patients with different primary cancers were included in 6 studies,[14,15,16,17,18,19] which reported that detection of pulmonary nodules was superior on FDG-PET/CT compared to FDG-PET/MRI (detection rates of 70.3 vs. 53.3%, respectively). The low sensitivity of PET/MRI in detecting very small pulmonary nodules was considered as the underlying cause. Two of the studies for which PET/MRI had missed small nodules and in which serial imaging was performed found that the majority of the nodules were benign although some were malignant.[18,19]

In summary, PET/MRI appeared to have similar diagnostic accuracy to that of PET/CT in the identification of FDG-avid thoracic lesions. However, its diagnostic performance is limited in the detection of non-FDG-avid lung nodules that are smaller than 5 to 10 mm in size.[14,15]

Central Nervous System Tumors

Standard imaging modalities for brain tumor evaluation are contrast-enhanced CT and MRI. FDG-PET does not generally add much value beyond CT and MRI for detection of metastatic disease in the brain.[39] However, FDG-PET is useful to characterize morphologically similar appearing contrast-enhancing brain lesions detected on MRI due to the typically higher FDG uptake in metastases compared to that seen in gliomas and benign

lesions.[39] FDG-PET can also help distinguish residual tumor from necrosis with great accuracy, which may be difficult to do on MRI alone.[39] Given the high physiologic uptake of FDG in the gray matter of the brain, other PET radiotracers have also been developed and studied for research purposes.[40,41] Since the brain is confined to the skull and is relatively resistant to motion artifacts, software coregistration and fusion has been utilized in studies even before the emergence of integrated PET/MRI devices. Therefore, integrated PET/MRI can be considered as the natural extension of such studies.

O-^{18}F-fluoroethyl-L-tyrosine (FET)-PET/MRI has been used for evaluation of brain tumor amino acid metabolism, structure, and blood volume.[42] Initial studies have shown a correlation between brain tumor amino acid metabolism and blood volume as measured by MRI, although spatial congruence was suboptimal and the two imaging modalities did not provide same information in their mixed sample of treated glioma patients, suggesting that the information was complementary. FET-PET/MRI for initial tumor grading showed improvement in the sensitivity and specificity for low-grade versus high-grade glioma detection. PET/MRI has been used in radiotherapy for more targeted treatment and improved tumor/normal tissue differentiation. For example, ^{68}Ga-DOTA-TOC-PET/MRI has been used for intensity-modulated radiation therapy treatment planning for meningioma, and dynamic contrast-enhanced MRI and DWI have been used for differentiation of residual tumor from postradiation changes.[43]

Afshar-Oromieh et al[44] compared ^{68}Ga-DOTA-TOC-PET/CT and PET/MRI in cranial meningioma patients, and showed the feasibility of image fusion without artifacts and comparability of results with PET/CT, although they noted that special attention should be paid for comparing SUV measurements (▶ Fig. 10.3).

Boss et al[45] compared PET/MRI to PET/CT in meningioma and glial tumors using ^{11}C-methyl-L-methionine or ^{68}Ga-DOTATOC, respectively. PET/MRI images were equivalent in diagnostic value. The tumor-to-reference tissue ratios in PET/MRI and PET/CT had 98% correlation. Fraioli et al[46] performed simultaneous acquisition of ^{18}F-fluoroethylcholine-PET and fMRI in patients with pediatric astrocytic brain tumors, which were shown to be concordant.

Gastrointestinal Tract Malignancies

Esophageal cancer: In a pilot study of 19 patients,[47] PET/MRI, PET/CT, endoscopic ultraso-

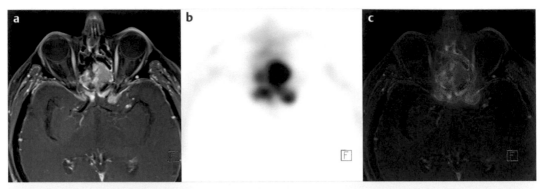

Fig. 10.3 Hybrid ^{68}Ga-DOTATOC-PET/MRI of a 72-year-old man with extensive and inhomogeneous meningioma infiltrating the nasal cavity despite previous treatments (surgery and external beam radiotherapy). ^{68}Ga-DOTATOC-PET can distinguish between viable meningioma and other tissues such as postoperative scarring or reactive tissue. **(a)** Transverse contrast-enhanced fat-suppressed T1-weighted MR image. **(b)** Transverse ^{68}Ga-DOTATOC-PET image 2 hours after radiotracer administration. **(c)** Fused PET/MR image from **a** and **b**. (Images courtesy of Ali Afshar-Oromieh, MD; Uwe Haberkorn, MD, from University Hospital Heidelberg; and Heinz-Peter Schlemmer, MD, from German Cancer Research Center, Heidelberg, Germany.)

nography (US), and CT were evaluated for their diagnostic efficacy in preoperatively staging esophageal cancer. In particular, the accuracy of PET/MRI for N staging was 83.3%, whereas the accuracies of endoscopic US, PET/CT, and CT were 75.0, 66.7, and 50.0%, respectively. Endoscopic US had the best accuracy for T staging.

Gastric cancer: In a study of 42 patients,[48] the ^{18}F-FDG-PET/MRI was compared to diagnostic CT for preoperative staging. They found a superior diagnostic accuracy of PET/MRI for M staging and resectability of gastric cancer compared to diagnostic CT; however, the corresponding PET/CT data results were not reported.

Colorectal cancer: In two studies including 27 patients with colorectal cancer,[49,50] PET/MRI was compared to PET/CT. In one study on 12 patients,[49] 2 patients underwent preoperative staging and 10 patients underwent restaging. Only PET/MRI provided accurate preoperative T stage. On a per-patient basis, with both patient groups combined for the evaluation, the sensitivity of PET/MRI was 6/7 (86%) and that of PET/CT was 5/7 (71%), with an equal specificity of 5/5 (100%) for both PET/MRI and PET/CT. On a per-lesion basis, PET/CT only detected 90% (26/29) of tumor lesions that were correctly detected by PET/MRI.[49] In another study in the lesion-based analysis study of 15 patients,[50] PET/MRI utilizing DWI showed a slightly higher, but not statistically significant, overall diagnostic accuracy compared to PET/CT (69 vs. 66%, respectively). However, PET/MRI had statistically significant higher diagnostic accuracy in the detection of

37 liver lesions compared to PET/CT (74 vs. 56%, respectively).

In summary, PET/MRI, including DWI, is comparable to PET/CT for evaluation of colorectal cancer metastases, and PET/MRI may have an advantage for T staging, N staging, and detection of metastatic colorectal cancer to the liver relative to PET/CT in the setting of gastrointestinal tract malignancies.

Liver metastases: In three studies including 330 liver lesions in 157 patients with different primary tumors, FDG PET/MRI was compared to PET/CT.[51,52,53] In the first study,[51] 120 liver lesions in 55 patients were evaluated by FDG PET/MRI and contrast-enhanced FDG PET/CT evaluated as the standard of reference. PET/MRI with T1-weighted and T2-weighted sequences had similar diagnostic accuracy to CE-PET/CT and better than routine noncontrast-enhanced PET/CT. When they used follow-up imaging as reference in patients with false-positive results in the first PET/MRI (CE PET/CT negative lesions which were positive in PET/MRI), additional metastases were detected in five patients on PET/MRI, using DWI and dynamic enhanced sequences. These additional lesions had potential impact on management in 10% (5/55) of the patients. As such, they concluded PET/MRI has a diagnostic impact on clinical decision making. In the second study by Beiderwellen et al, 97 liver lesions were evaluated in 70 patients using ^{18}F-FDG PET/MRI and PET/CT.[52] Although all 10 patients with liver metastasis were identified by both modalities, PET/MRI resulted in significantly ($p < 0.001$) higher diagnostic confidence. In addition,

PET/CT did not identify nine benign liver lesions. In another study by Beiderwellen et al, 32 patients with solid malignancies were evaluated with FDG-PET/CT and subsequent PET/MRI.[53] Imaging follow-up and/or histopathological specimen served as standards of reference. The PET/MRI showed higher sensitivity (92.2 vs. 67.8%), accuracy (96.1 vs. 82.4%), and negative predictive value (NPV) (95.1 vs. 82%) than PET/CT in the detection of 113 liver lesions. Utilization of PET/MRI also resulted in significantly ($p < 0.001$) higher lesion conspicuity and diagnostic confidence. PET/MRI detected additional PET-negative metastases.

In summary, PET/MRI appeared to have superior diagnostic accuracy compared to PET/CT for the detection of metastatic liver lesions. Its utilization also results in significantly higher interpreter diagnostic confidence and lesion conspicuity and has a diagnostic impact on clinical decision making.

Prostate Cancer

Four studies including 114 patients compared PET/CT to PET/MRI using [11]C- or ^{18}F-labeled choline and ^{68}Ga-prostate-specific membrane antigen (PSMA) radiotracers.[54,55,56,57] In these studies, PET/MRI was not superior to PET/CT for prostate lymph node detection or for bone lesion localization. However, PET/MRI was more accurate for lesion localization within the prostate gland, which has implications for biopsy or radiation therapy planning (▶ Fig. 10.4). One study[56] also showed that the visibility of lymph nodes was significantly greater on MRI using the postcontrast fat-suppressed T1-weighted, fat-suppressed T2-weighted, and DWI.

Neuroendocrine Tumors

Two prospective studies[58,59] involving 34 patients compared ^{68}Ga-DOTATOC-PET/CT to ^{68}Ga-DOTA-TOC-PET/MRI. Both studies found that PET/MRI outperformed PET/CT in detection of liver metastases, mainly due to the contribution of the MRI component. The diagnostic performance of PET/CT and PET/MRI for extrahepatic lesions was comparable. There was a robust correlation between SUVmax values measured by PET/CT and PET/MRI.

Bladder Cancer

FDG-PET/CT is historically known to be inaccurate for the assessment of localized bladder cancer, because of the high concentration of excreted FDG in the bladder lumen that obscures FDG-avid mural lesions. However, in recent years, FDG-PET/CT with a forced diuresis protocol has been reported to effectively clear excreted FDG from the bladder lumen to allow for evaluation of FDG-avid lesions in patients with bladder cancer.[60] In one study of six patients,[61] hybrid simultaneous PET/MRI with a forced diuresis protocol showed substantially improved coregistration of the bladder wall and slightly improved pelvic lymph node and bladder mass coregistration (▶ Fig. 10.5). Yet, more studies are needed to establish the role of diuretic PET/MRI and PET/CT in patients with bladder cancer.

Gynecological Malignancies

MRI is often utilized for disease staging/treatment planning and restaging in patients with endometrial, cervical, or ovarian cancer, and PET/CT is often used when metastatic disease is suspected.[62] The diagnostic performance of PET/MRI for staging and restaging was compared to PET/CT in three studies involving a total of 69 patients.

In a study by Beiderwellen et al[63] involving 19 patients with recurrent gynecologic cancer, both PET/MRI and PET/CT correctly identified all 58 malignant lesions (including 4 lung metastases measuring 7–10 mm). However, interpreter diagnostic confidence on PET/MRI (based on a 3-point scale) was significantly higher than that on PET/CT for both malignant and benign lesions. In another study by Queiroz et al[64] of 26 patients with suspicious or proven advanced gynecological cancers, although both modalities performed identically in the identification of all primary and recurrent tumors and abdominal metastases, the accuracy of PET/MRI for primary tumor delineation was statistically higher than that of PET/CT, particularly in patients with cervical and endometrial cancers. In 24 patients with suspected gynecologic tumor recurrence,[65] tumor relapse was correctly identified in 20 of 21 patients by both PET/CT and PET/MRI, using histopathology and imaging follow-up as reference standards.

In summary, PET/MRI appeared to have superior performance to PET/CT for primary tumor delineation and interpreter diagnostic confidence in the setting of gynecological malignancies, although its diagnostic accuracy is equivalent to that of PET/CT for the identification of local or distant metastases.

Breast Cancer

PET/MRI was compared with PET/CT in three studies involving a total of 106 patients. In the first study involving 36 patients with 74 lesions, Pace

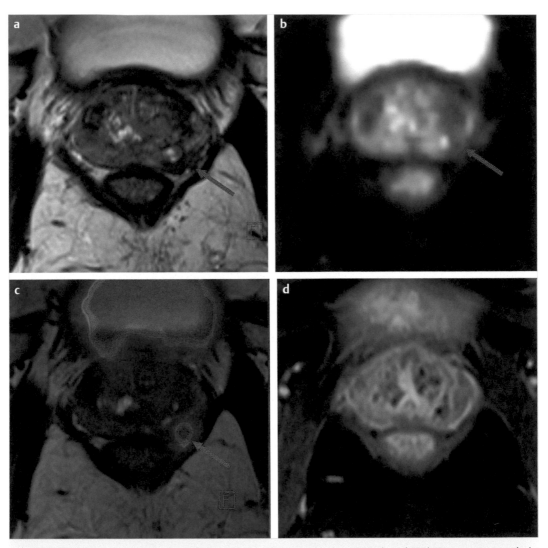

Fig. 10.4 ⁶⁸Ga-PSMA-11 PET/MRI of a 72-year-old man with prostate cancer. PSMA-ligand PET/MRI represents an ideal combination of high sensitivity/specificity (PET) with the best possible morphological visualization (MRI) of prostate cancer. (a) Transverse T2-weighted MR image, (b) transverse diffusion-weighted MR image, (c) transverse fused PET/MR image, and (d) transverse contrast-enhanced fat-suppressed T1-weighted image show focal prostate cancer (*arrows*) in left peripheral zone prostatic midgland. (Images courtesy of Ali Afshar-Oromieh, MD; Uwe Haberkorn, MD, from University Hospital Heidelberg; and Heinz-Peter Schlemmer, MD, from German Cancer Research Center, Heidelberg, Germany.)

et al[66] reported that all FDG-positive lesions were visualized by both modalities. There was also a robust correlation between the SUVmax and SUVmean measurements obtained by PET/MRI and PET/CT. In another study[67] involving 49 patients with 83 lesions, no significant difference was observed in N staging between PET/MRI and PET/CT. However, the diagnostic accuracy of PET/MRI was significantly higher than that of PET/CT for T staging (82 vs. 68%, respectively). PET/CT also missed a synchronous carcinoma in the contralateral breast in one patient. In a third study,[68] the diagnostic yield of PET/MRI was compared to PET/CT in 21 patients with suspected tumor recurrence. Both modalities correctly detected the 17 patients with tumor recurrence. However, in the

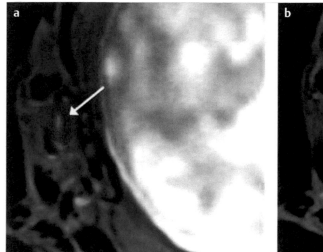
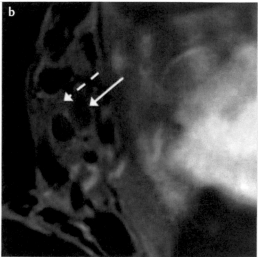

Fig. 10.5 FDG-PET/MRI of a 52-year-old man with muscle-invasive high-grade bladder cancer. (a) Small field-of-view PET/MR image from simultaneously acquired transverse T2-weighted MR image and transverse FDG-PET image demonstrates small FDG-avid right pelvic sidewall lymph node (*solid arrow*). Registration of the lymph node on the two images is excellent. Also note excreted FDG within the partially visualized urinary bladder. (b) Fused PET/MR image from sequentially obtained transverse T2-weighted MR and PET imaging demonstrates misregistration between lymph node on MRI (*solid arrow*) and PET (*dashed arrow*). Also note improved coregistration of bladder wall in (a). (Reproduced with permission from Rosenkrantz et al.[61])

per-lesion analysis, PET/MRI outperformed PET/CT while correctly characterizing 98.5 versus 94.8% of the lesions, respectively.

In summary, PET/MRI appeared to be better than PET/CT in the T staging of breast cancer, with equivalent diagnostic performance with PET/CT in N and M staging. However, it is worth mentioning that MRI alone is the diagnostic modality of choice for breast cancer T staging.

Osseous Metastases

FDG-PET/MRI was compared to FDG-PET/CT in four studies involving 346 patients with suspected osseous metastases. PET/MRI was able to detect more osseous metastases in 109 patients with breast cancer compared to PET/CT (100 vs. 88%, respectively). PET/MRI was able to detect osseous metastases in 12% of PET/CT-negative patients, changing the therapeutic plan.[69] In another study[70] of 67 patients with a variety of cancers including 25 with melanoma, 12 with breast cancer, 10 with non–small cell lung cancer, 4 with colorectal cancer, and 16 with other cancers, PET/MRI outperformed PET/CT (100 vs. 94%, respectively) in the detection of osseous metastases. Eiber et al[71] compared PET/MRI (using only T1-weighted

Dixon-VIBE images for attenuation correction and coronal T1-weighted TSE images) and PET/CT in 119 patients with cancer, and did not find statistically significant differences between the two groups in osseous metastasis detection. However, regarding the lesion delineation rating, T1-weighted TSE imaging performed significantly better than CT ($p < 0.0001$). In a prospective study of 51 patients with breast cancer,[72] PET/MRI with DWI and contrast-enhanced sequences had statistically significant higher sensitivity for detection of osseous metastases on a lesion-based analysis.

In summary, although further studies are still required to determine the appropriate MRI sequences for an accurate and reasonably long PET/MRI study for patients with suspected osseous metastases, it seems that FDG-PET/MRI has better diagnostic accuracy than FDG-PET/CT and can change the therapeutic plan.

It is worth noting that ^{18}F-sodium fluoride (Na[18]F)-PET/CT has been reported to have better sensitivity and specificity[73,74,75] than bone scanning with single-photon emission computed tomography (SPECT) using [99mTc] radiolabeled phosphonates for the detection of osseous metastases in patients with prostate cancer. Yet, DWI has been found to have higher specificity with lower sensitivity compared to Na[18]F-PET/CT.[76] Hybrid Na[18]F-PET/MRI with DWI sequences may prove to be the most accurate imaging modality in this context by combining the superior sensitivity of Na[18]F-PET with the superior specificity of DWI.

Lymphoma

Four studies involving 141 patients have compared FDG-PET/MRI to FDG-PET/CT. Heacock et al[77] studied 28 patients with various types of lymphoma. Staging by both modalities was concordant in 27 (96.4%) patients. However, PET/MRI increased disease stage in one patient by identifying a bone marrow lesion that was subsequently confirmed histopathologically (▶ Fig. 10.6). They also showed that both PET/CT and PET/MRI were more sensitive than DWI on a lesion-based analysis. In another study involving 34 patients,[78] Giraudo et al found that PET/MRI and PET/CT had comparable diagnostic performances. However, PET/MRI with DWI outperformed PET/CT, mainly due to the higher sensitivity of DWI for mucosa-associated lymphoid tissue (MALT) lymphomas. There was a robust correlation between SUVmax

and SUVmean measurements from PET/MRI and PET/CT, but no significant correlation between ADCmin and SUVmax measurements or between ADCmean and SUVmean measurements. Another study[79] involving 18 patients did not show a significant difference between the diagnostic accuracies of PET/CT and PET/MRI with DWI. They also did not find any correlation between ADCmin and SUVmax from PET/MRI. In one other study of 61 patients,[80] PET/MRI was compared to PET/CT and whole-body DWI. While PET/CT and PET/MRI had similar diagnostic performances, both outperformed whole-body DWI for staging, restaging, and evaluation of low-grade and high-grade lymphomas. Some investigators also explored the use of potential alternatives for gadolinium in FDG PET/MRI of lymphoma patients (▶ Fig. 10.7).

In summary, FDG-PET/MRI including DWI sequences seems to be the most accurate study in lymphoma, particularly when there is a concern for MALT lymphomas. It is worth reemphasizing that the current studies did not show correlations between ADCmin and SUVmax or between ADCmean and SUVmean, which may indicate that measurements of tumor water molecule diffusivity

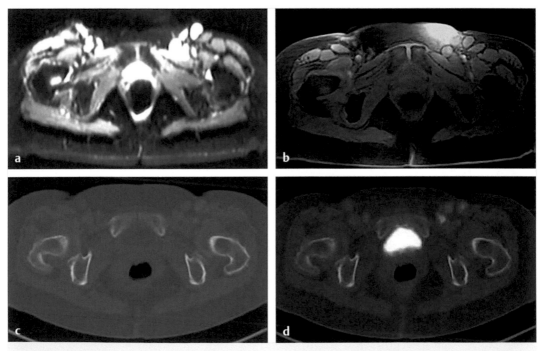

Fig. 10.6 FDG-PET/MRI of patient with lymphoma. **(a)** Transverse diffusion-weighted MR image shows a right femoral neck lesion with restricted diffusion. **(b)** Fused PET/MR image shows increased FDG uptake within the lesion. **(c)** Transverse CT image does not reveal presence of the lesion, and **(d)** transverse PET/CT image demonstrates subtle FDG uptake in the lesion which is more difficult to visualize than with PET/MRI. Right femoral neck lymphoma involvement was confirmed on bone biopsy. (Reproduced with permission from Heacock et al.[77])

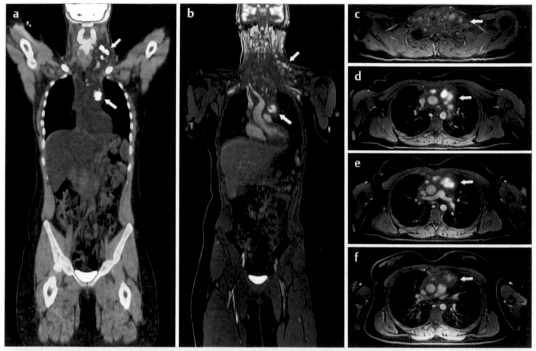

Fig. 10.7 FDG-PET/CT and FDG-PET/MRI of a 15-year-old female with Hodgkin's lymphoma demonstrating concordant findings. **(a)** Coronal PET/CT image shows mediastinal and left cervical FDG-avid lymphadenopathy (*arrows*). Corresponding coronal **(b)** and axial **(c–f)** T1-weighted LAVA sequence (TR/TE/Flip angle: 4.2/1.7/15) after intravenous ferumoxytol injection with superimposed PET images again reveal multiple enlarged FDG-avid lymph nodes in the mediastinum and left neck (*arrows*). (Images courtesy of Hossein Nejadnik, MD, PhD; and Heike Daldrup-Link MD, PhD, from Stanford University.)

from DWI and measurements of tumor FDG uptake from PET may have independent prognostic value.

Pediatric Malignancies

Given the greater concern regarding radiation exposure in the pediatric patient population, PET/MRI may play an important role in pediatric oncology.[12]

In three studies involving 86 patients, PET/MRI was compared to PET/CT. In 18 patients with various types of neoplasms,[81] PET/MRI provided almost identical diagnostic accuracy compared to PET/CT, while its estimated radiation dose was significantly reduced (by 73%) compared to PET/CT. In another study of nine patients undergoing lymphoma restaging,[82] there was complete concordance and very strong correlation between PET/MRI and PET/CT for lesion detection and SUV measurements. Use of PET/MRI resulted in an average of 39% radiation dose reduction. Another prospective study on 25 lymphoma patients[83] showed no statistically significant differences between PET/MRI and PET/CT in lesion classification, lesion detection rates, or Ann Arbor staging. A robust correlation between PET/MRI and PET/CT SUV measurements was reported, although PET/MRI provided systematically lower SUV measurements. PET/MRI offered an average of 45% radiation dose reduction compared to PET/CT.

In summary, PET/MRI appeared to perform similarly or slightly better (in the identification of soft-tissue lesions) compared to PET/CT in the pediatric patient population (▶ Fig. 10.8) while offering a significant reduction of radiation dose. Further studies are warranted to establish the role of PET/MRI in pediatric oncology.

10.6.2 Nononcologic Applications

Although nononcologic applications of PET are mostly limited to research studies at the present time, given the lower radiation dose in PET/MRI relative to PET/CT, PET/MRI can potentially be

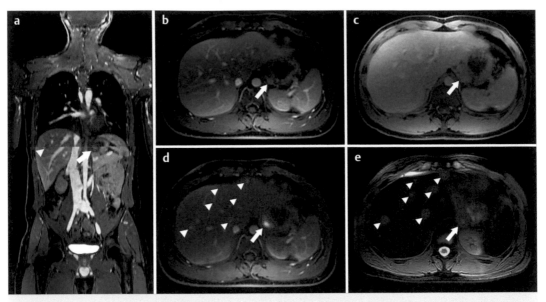

Fig. 10.8 FDG-PET/MRI of a 17-year-old male with gastrointestinal stromal tumor (GIST). **(a)** Coronal T1-weighted LAVA sequence (TR/TE/Flip angle: 4.2/1.7/15) MR image after intravenous ferumoxytol injection with superimposed PET image shows FDG-avid primary tumor in stomach (*arrow*) and a liver metastasis (*arrowhead*). **(b)** Transverse contrast-enhanced fat-suppressed T1-weighted MR image after intravenous ferumoxytol injection and **(c)** transverse contrast-enhanced fat-suppressed T1-weighted MR image after intravenous gadolinium chelate injection again show primary tumor in stomach (*arrow*), whereas liver metastases are not visualized. **(d)** Transverse contrast-enhanced fat-suppressed T1-weighted PET/MR image and **(e)** transverse contrast-enhanced fat-suppressed T2-weighted PET/MR image show superior delineation of primary tumor (*arrow*) and multiple hepatic metastases (*arrowheads*). (Images courtesy of Hossein Nejadnik, MD, PhD; and Heike Daldrup-Link, MD, PhD, from Stanford University.)

utilized in many clinical scenarios including inflammatory or infectious diseases. In the following, we discuss some potential clinical applications of PET/MRI in noncancer-related disorders.

Cardiovascular Disease

MRI and PET have clinically established roles[84,85] in the evaluation of benign and malignant cardiovascular diseases. PET/MRI can provide complementary strength of these modalities in a single scan, particularly for benign diseases including cardiac sarcoidosis,[86,87] myocarditis,[6] and atherosclerotic plaque imaging[6,88] when there is more concern regarding radiation exposure.

Neurologic Disease

As mentioned earlier, integrated PET/MRI can be considered as the natural extension of software coregistration of PET and MRI, since brain tissue is confined in the skull and is relatively resistant to motion artifacts. Given the availability of a wide variety of PET radiotracers, such as β-amyloid, tau, or α-synuclein binding radiotracers, as well as new MRI techniques, there is a great but mostly unexplored potential for evaluation of neurodegenerative,[5] cerebrovascular disorders,[89] atherosclerotic plaque evaluations,[90] epilepsy,[91,92] and inflammatory diseases of central nervous system.[5,93]

Musculoskeletal Disease

MRI is a standard imaging modality that is used for the diagnosis and follow-up of the majority of infectious, inflammatory, congenital, and posttraumatic musculoskeletal disorders, because it provides excellent soft-tissue contrast for anatomical assessment of muscles, ligaments, tendons, cartilaginous structures, bone marrow, peripheral nerves, and fat. However, the accuracy of MRI can be limited in certain situations such as when artifacts are induced by presence of postoperative hardware. The combination of excellent soft-tissue contrast from MRI and the molecular information provided by various PET radiotracers may make

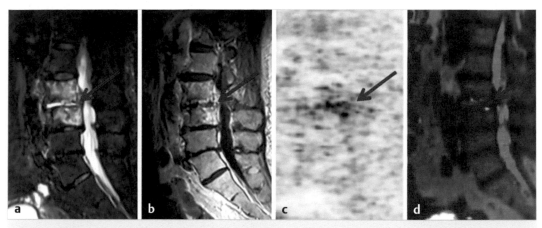

Fig. 10.9 FDG-PET/MRI of a 71-year-old woman with infectious spondylodiscitis. **(a)** Sagittal short tau inversion recovery T2-weighted MR image demonstrates increased signal intensity of a lumbar spine intervertebral disc (*arrow*) along with increased signal intensity of the surounding vertebral body bone marrow. **(b)** Sagittal T1-weighted MR image shows associated enhancement adjacent to the intervertebral disc space (*arrow*). Sagittal PET image **(c)** and sagittal fused PET/MR image **(d)** show focally increased FDG uptake in the affected intervertebral disc (*arrow*) (SUVmax, 8.14; SUVmean, 3.99), in keeping with active infection. (Reproduced with permission from Fahnert et al.[8])

PET/MRI the optimal imaging modality for diagnosis and response assessment of various musculoskeletal conditions. Although several studies have shown the complementary role of PET and MRI for clinical evaluation of nonneoplastic musculoskeletal conditions such as osteomyelitis, Charcot neuroarthropathy, the diabetic foot, and joint pain after arthroplasty, there are few clinical studies that have investigated the utility of hybrid PET/MRI for such disorders.

Spondylodiscitis

Spondylodiscitis is a rare but serious destructive infection of the intervertebral disc spaces and adjacent vertebrae, which is commonly seen in immunocompromised or elderly patients with chronic degenerative disease or with a history of prior spinal surgery or instrumentation. In a prospective study by Fahnert et al,[8] 30 patients suspected to have spondylodiscitis with previous inconclusive MRI results underwent FDG-PET/MRI including precontrast and postcontrast MRI sequences. They used histopathology or clinical follow-up as the reference standards. Review of the MR images alone resulted in sensitivity, specificity, positive predictive value, and NPV of 50, 71, 54, and 67%, respectively. However, after also reviewing the PET images, all diagnostic parameters significantly increased, with sensitivity, specificity, positive predictive value, and NPV of 67, 100, 88, and 100%, respectively. Therefore, they recommended the use of FDG-PET/MRI for all patients suspected to have spondylodiscitis who have inconclusive clinical or MRI findings (▶ Fig. 10.9).

Gastrointestinal Disease

In one study of 35 patients[94] with small bowel Crohn's disease (CD), patients were evaluated preoperatively by same-day FDG-PET/CT enterography and FDG-PET/MR enterography. PET/MR enterography showed significantly higher accuracy in the identification of extraluminal disease and conditions affecting bowel segments distant from those involved by CD, which resulted in management modification and reduced operative times. PET/MR enterography also demonstrated superior accuracy in the detection of fibrotic components compared to PET/CT enterography or MR enterography. In another study of 19 patients with Crohn's disease who were evaluated preoperatively,[95] a combined PET/MR enterography biomarker ADC x SUVmax was found to be the best discriminator between pure fibrotic and mixed or inflammatory strictures. This imaging biomarker had sensitivity, specificity, and accuracy values of 0.67, 0.73, and 0.71, respectively.

References

[1] Torigian DA, Zaidi H, Kwee TC, et al. PET/MR imaging: technical aspects and potential clinical applications. Radiology. 2013; 267(1):26–44

[2] Schlemmer HP, Pichler BJ, Schmand M, et al. Simultaneous MR/PET imaging of the human brain: feasibility study. Radiology. 2008; 248(3):1028–1035

[3] Drzezga A, Souvatzoglou M, Eiber M, et al. First clinical experience with integrated whole-body PET/MR: comparison to PET/CT in patients with oncologic diagnoses. J Nucl Med. 2012; 53(6):845–855

[4] U.S. Food and Drug Administration. FDA clears new system to perform simultaneous PET, MRI scans. 2017. Available at: https://wayback.archive-it.org/7993/20170114063438/http://www.fda.gov/NewsEvents/Newsroom/PressAnnouncements/ucm258700.htm

[5] Catana C, Drzezga A, Heiss WD, Rosen BR. PET/MRI for neurologic applications. J Nucl Med. 2012; 53(12):1916–1925

[6] Rischpler C, Nekolla SG, Kunze KP, Schwaiger M. PET/MRI of the heart. Semin Nucl Med. 2015; 45(3):234–247

[7] Gavra M, Syed R, Fraioli F, Afaq A, Bomanji J. PET/MRI in the upper abdomen. Semin Nucl Med. 2015; 45(4):282–292

[8] Fahnert J, Purz S, Jarvers JS, et al. The use of simultaneous 18F-FDG-PET/MRI for the detection of spondylodiscitis. J Nucl Med. 2016; 57(9):1396–1401

[9] Lecouvet FE, Whole-Body MR. Imaging: musculoskeletal applications. Radiology. 2016; 279(2):345–365

[10] Jadvar H, Colletti PM. Competitive advantage of PET/MRI. Eur J Radiol. 2014; 83(1):84–94

[11] Trout AT, Serai S, Mahley AD, et al. Liver stiffness measurements with MR elastography: agreement and repeatability across imaging systems, field strengths, and pulse sequences. Radiology. 2016; 281(3):793–804

[12] Pearce MS, Salotti JA, Little MP, et al. Radiation exposure from CT scans in childhood and subsequent risk of leukaemia and brain tumours: a retrospective cohort study. Lancet. 2012; 380(9840):499–505

[13] Brenner DJ, Hall EJ. Computed tomography–an increasing source of radiation exposure. N Engl J Med. 2007; 357(22): 2277–2284

[14] Chandarana H, Heacock L, Rakheja R, et al. Pulmonary nodules in patients with primary malignancy: comparison of hybrid PET/MR and PET/CT imaging. Radiology. 2013; 268(3): 874–881

[15] Rauscher I, Eiber M, Fürst S, et al. PET/MR imaging in the detection and characterization of pulmonary lesions: technical and diagnostic evaluation in comparison to PET/CT. J Nucl Med. 2014; 55(5):724–729

[16] Lee KH, Park CM, Lee SM, et al. Pulmonary nodule detection in patients with a primary malignancy using hybrid PET/MRI: is there value in adding contrast-enhanced MR imaging? PLoS One. 2015; 10(6):e0129660

[17] Sawicki LM, Grueneisen J, Buchbender C, et al. Comparative performance of 18F-FDG PET/MRI and 18F-FDG PET/CT in detection and characterization of pulmonary lesions in 121 oncologic patients. J Nucl Med. 2016; 57(4):582–586

[18] Raad RA, Friedman KP, Heacock L, Ponzo F, Melsaether A, Chandarana H. Outcome of small lung nodules missed on hybrid PET/MRI in patients with primary malignancy. J Magn Reson Imaging. 2016; 43(2):504–511

[19] Sawicki LM, Grueneisen J, Buchbender C, et al. Evaluation of the outcome of lung nodules missed on 18F-FDG PET/MRI compared with 18F-FDG PET/CT in patients with known malignancies. J Nucl Med. 2016; 57(1):15–20

[20] Boiselle PM, Nensa F, Ohno Y, Torigian DA. Expert opinion: which cardiothoracic imaging applications of PET/CT are most likely to be replaced by PET/MRI? J Thorac Imaging. 2014; 29(1):3

[21] Mehranian A, Arabi H, Zaidi H. Vision 20/20: Magnetic resonance imaging-guided attenuation correction in PET/MRI: Challenges, solutions, and opportunities. Med Phys. 2016; 43 (3):1130–1155

[22] Ladefoged CN, Law I, Anazodo U, et al. A multi-centre evaluation of eleven clinically feasible brain PET/MRI attenuation correction techniques using a large cohort of patients. Neuroimage. 2017; 147:346–359

[23] Fraum TJ, Fowler KJ, McConathy J, et al. PET/MRI for the body imager: abdominal and pelvic oncologic applications. Abdom Imaging. 2015; 40(6):1387–1404

[24] Benoit D, Ladefoged CN, Rezaei A, et al. Optimized MLAA for quantitative non-TOF PET/MR of the brain. Phys Med Biol. 2016; 61(24):8854–8874

[25] Catana C. Principles of simultaneous PET/MR imaging. Magn Reson Imaging Clin N Am. 2017; 25(2):231–243

[26] Rausch I, Quick HH, Cal-Gonzalez J, Sattler B, Boellaard R, Beyer T. Technical and instrumentational foundations of PET/ MRI. Eur J Radiol. 2017; 94:A3–A13

[27] Beyer T, Lassen ML, Boellaard R, et al. Investigating the state-of-the-art in whole-body MR-based attenuation correction: an intra-individual, inter-system, inventory study on three clinical PET/MR systems. MAGMA. 2016; 29(1):75–87

[28] Schulz V, Torres-Espallardo I, Renisch S, et al. Automatic, three-segment, MR-based attenuation correction for whole-body PET/MR data. Eur J Nucl Med Mol Imaging. 2011; 38(1): 138–152

[29] Shen G, Hu S, Liu B, Kuang A. Diagnostic performance of whole-body PET/MRI for detecting malignancies in cancer patients: a meta-analysis. PLoS One. 2016; 11(4):e0154497

[30] Xiao Y, Chen Y, Shi Y, Wu Z. The value of fluorine-18 fluorodeoxyglucose PET/MRI in the diagnosis of head and neck carcinoma: a meta-analysis. Nucl Med Commun. 2015; 36(4): 312–318

[31] Spick C, Herrmann K, Czernin J. 18F-FDG PET/CT and PET/ MRI perform equally well in cancer: evidence from studies on more than 2,300 patients. J Nucl Med. 2016; 57(3):420–430

[32] Kuhn FP, Hüllner M, Mader CE, et al. Contrast-enhanced PET/ MR imaging versus contrast-enhanced PET/CT in head and neck cancer: how much MR information is needed? J Nucl Med. 2014; 55(4):551–558

[33] Platzek I. (18)F-fluorodeoxyglucose PET/MR imaging in head and neck cancer. PET Clin. 2016; 11(4):375–386

[34] Heusch P, Buchbender C, Köhler J, et al. Thoracic staging in lung cancer: prospective comparison of 18F-FDG PET/MR imaging and 18F-FDG PET/CT. J Nucl Med. 2014; 55(3):373–378

[35] Fraioli F, Screaton NJ, Janes SM, et al. Non-small-cell lung cancer resectability: diagnostic value of PET/MR. Eur J Nucl Med Mol Imaging. 2015; 42(1):49–55

[36] Lee SM, Goo JM, Park CM, et al. Preoperative staging of non-small cell lung cancer: prospective comparison of PET/MR and PET/CT. Eur Radiol. 2016; 26(11):3850–3857

[37] Schwenzer NF, Schraml C, Müller M, et al. Pulmonary lesion assessment: comparison of whole-body hybrid MR/PET and PET/CT imaging–pilot study. Radiology. 2012; 264(2):551–558

[38] Heusch P, Köhler J, Wittsack HJ, et al. Hybrid [18F]-FDG PET/ MRI including non-Gaussian diffusion-weighted imaging (DWI): preliminary results in non-small cell lung cancer (NSCLC). Eur J Radiol. 2013; 82(11):2055–2060

[39] Buchbender C, Heusner TA, Lauenstein TC, Bockisch A, Antoch G. Oncologic PET/MRI, part 1: tumors of the brain, head and neck, chest, abdomen, and pelvis. J Nucl Med. 2012; 53 (6):928–938

[40] Henriksen OM, Marner L, Law I. Clinical PET/MR imaging in dementia and neuro-oncology. PET Clin. 2016; 11(4):441–452

[41] Fraum TJ, Fowler KJ, McConathy J. PET/MRI: emerging clinical applications in oncology. Acad Radiol. 2016; 23(2):220–236

[42] Henriksen OM, Larsen VA, Muhic A, et al. Simultaneous evaluation of brain tumour metabolism, structure and blood volume using [(18)F]-fluoroethyltyrosine (FET) PET/MRI: feasibility, agreement and initial experience. Eur J Nucl Med Mol Imaging. 2016; 43(1):103–112

[43] Varoquaux A, Rager O, Dulguerov P, Burkhardt K, Ailianou A, Becker M. Diffusion-weighted and PET/MR imaging after radiation therapy for malignant head and neck tumors. Radiographics. 2015; 35(5):1502–1527

[44] Afshar-Oromieh A, Wolf MB, Kratochwil C, et al. Comparison of 68Ga-DOTATOC-PET/CT and PET/MRI hybrid systems in patients with cranial meningioma: Initial results. Neuro-oncol. 2015; 17(2):312–319

[45] Boss A, Bisdas S, Kolb A, et al. Hybrid PET/MRI of intracranial masses: initial experiences and comparison to PET/CT. J Nucl Med. 2010; 51(8):1198–1205

[46] Fraioli F, Shankar A, Hargrave D, et al. 18F-fluoroethylcholine (18F-Cho) PET/MRI functional parameters in pediatric astrocytic brain tumors. Clin Nucl Med. 2015; 40(1):e40–e45

[47] Lee G, i H, Kim SJ, et al. Clinical implication of PET/MR imaging in preoperative esophageal cancer staging: comparison with PET/CT, endoscopic ultrasonography, and CT. J Nucl Med. 2014; 55(8):1242–1247

[48] Lee DH, Kim SH, Joo I, Hur BY, Han JK. Comparison between 18F-FDG PET/MRI and MDCT for the assessment of preoperative staging and resectability of gastric cancer. Eur J Radiol. 2016; 85(6):1085–1091

[49] Paspulati RM, Partovi S, Herrmann KA, Krishnamurthi S, Delaney CP, Nguyen NC. Comparison of hybrid FDG PET/MRI compared with PET/CT in colorectal cancer staging and restaging: a pilot study. Abdom Imaging. 2015; 40(6):1415–1425

[50] Brendle C, Schwenzer NF, Rempp H, et al. Assessment of metastatic colorectal cancer with hybrid imaging: comparison of reading performance using different combinations of anatomical and functional imaging techniques in PET/MRI and PET/CT in a short case series. Eur J Nucl Med Mol Imaging. 2016; 43(1):123–132

[51] Reiner CS, Stolzmann P, Husmann L, et al. Protocol requirements and diagnostic value of PET/MR imaging for liver metastasis detection. Eur J Nucl Med Mol Imaging. 2014; 41 (4):649–658

[52] Beiderwellen K, Gomez B, Buchbender C, et al. Depiction and characterization of liver lesions in whole body [18F]-FDG PET/MRI. Eur J Radiol. 2013; 82(11):e669–e675

[53] Beiderwellen K, Geraldo L, Ruhlmann V, et al. Accuracy of [18F]FDG PET/MRI for the detection of liver metastases. PLoS One. 2015; 10(9):e0137285

[54] Afshar-Oromieh A, Haberkorn U, Hadaschik B, et al. PET/MRI with a 68Ga-PSMA ligand for the detection of prostate cancer. Eur J Nucl Med Mol Imaging. 2013; 40(10):1629–1630

[55] Souvatzoglou M, Eiber M, Takei T, et al. Comparison of integrated whole-body [11C]choline PET/MR with PET/CT in patients with prostate cancer. Eur J Nucl Med Mol Imaging. 2013; 40(10):1486–1499

[56] Freitag MT, Radtke JP, Hadaschik BA, et al. Comparison of hybrid (68)Ga-PSMA PET/MRI and (68)Ga-PSMA PET/CT in the evaluation of lymph node and bone metastases of prostate cancer. Eur J Nucl Med Mol Imaging. 2016; 43(1):70–83

[57] Wetter A, Nensa F, Schenck M, et al. Combined PET imaging and diffusion-weighted imaging of intermediate and high-risk primary prostate carcinomas with simultaneous [18F] choline PET/MRI. PLoS One. 2014; 9(7):e101571

[58] Hope TA, Pampaloni MH, Nakakura E, et al. Simultaneous (68)Ga-DOTA-TOC PET/MRI with gadoxetate disodium in patients with neuroendocrine tumor. Abdom Imaging. 2015; 40 (6):1432–1440

[59] Gaertner FC, Beer AJ, Souvatzoglou M, et al. Evaluation of feasibility and image quality of 68Ga-DOTATOC positron emission tomography/magnetic resonance in comparison with positron emission tomography/computed tomography in patients with neuroendocrine tumors. Invest Radiol. 2013; 48 (5):263–272

[60] Nayak B, Dogra PN, Naswa N, Kumar R. Diuretic 18F-FDG PET/CT imaging for detection and locoregional staging of urinary bladder cancer: prospective evaluation of a novel technique. Eur J Nucl Med Mol Imaging. 2013; 40(3):386–393

[61] Rosenkrantz AB, Balar AV, Huang WC, Jackson K, Friedman KP. Comparison of coregistration accuracy of pelvic structures between sequential and simultaneous imaging during hybrid PET/MRI in patients with bladder cancer. Clin Nucl Med. 2015; 40(8):637–641

[62] Khiewvan B, Torigian DA, Emamzadehfard S, et al. An update on the role of PET/CT and PET/MRI in ovarian cancer. Eur J Nucl Med Mol Imaging. 2017; 44(6):1079–1091

[63] Beiderwellen K, Grueneisen J, Ruhlmann V, et al. [(18)F]FDG PET/MRI vs. PET/CT for whole-body staging in patients with recurrent malignancies of the female pelvis: initial results. Eur J Nucl Med Mol Imaging. 2015; 42(1):56–65

[64] Queiroz MA, Kubik-Huch RA, Hauser N, et al. PET/MRI and PET/CT in advanced gynaecological tumours: initial experience and comparison. Eur Radiol. 2015; 25(8):2222–2230

[65] Grueneisen J, Schaarschmidt BM, Heubner M, et al. Implementation of FAST-PET/MRI for whole-body staging of female patients with recurrent pelvic malignancies: A comparison to PET/CT. Eur J Radiol. 2015; 84(11):2097–2102

[66] Pace L, Nicolai E, Luongo A, et al. Comparison of whole-body PET/CT and PET/MRI in breast cancer patients: lesion detection and quantitation of 18F-deoxyglucose uptake in lesions and in normal organ tissues. Eur J Radiol. 2014; 83(2):289–296

[67] Grueneisen J, Nagarajah J, Buchbender C, et al. Positron emission tomography/magnetic resonance imaging for local tumor staging in patients with primary breast cancer: a comparison with positron emission tomography/computed tomography and magnetic resonance imaging. Invest Radiol. 2015; 50(8):505–513

[68] Sawicki LM, Grueneisen J, Schaarschmidt BM, et al. Evaluation of 18F-FDG PET/MRI, 18F-FDG PET/CT, MRI, and CT in whole-body staging of recurrent breast cancer. Eur J Radiol. 2016; 85(2):459–465

[69] Catalano OA, Nicolai E, Rosen BR, et al. Comparison of CE-FDG-PET/CT with CE-FDG-PET/MR in the evaluation of osseous metastases in breast cancer patients. Br J Cancer. 2015; 112(9):1452–1460

[70] Beiderwellen K, Huebner M, Heusch P, et al. Whole-body [18F]FDG PET/MRI vs. PET/CT in the assessment of bone lesions in oncological patients: initial results. Eur Radiol. 2014; 24(8):2023–2030

[71] Eiber M, Takei T, Souvatzoglou M, et al. Performance of whole-body integrated 18F-FDG PET/MR in comparison to PET/CT for evaluation of malignant bone lesions. J Nucl Med. 2014; 55(2):191–197

[72] Melsaether AN, Raad RA, Pujara AC, et al. Comparison of whole-body (18)F FDG PET/MR imaging and whole-body (18)F FDG PET/CT in terms of lesion detection and radiation dose in patients with breast cancer. Radiology. 2016; 281(1): 193–202

[73] Even-Sapir E, Metser U, Mishani E, Lievshitz G, Lerman H, Leibovitch I. The detection of bone metastases in patients with high-risk prostate cancer: 99mTc-MDP Planar bone scintigraphy, single- and multi-field-of-view SPECT, 18F-fluoride PET, and 18F-fluoride PET/CT. J Nucl Med. 2006; 47(2):287–297

[74] Leung D, Krishnamoorthy S, Schwartz L, Divgi C. Imaging approaches with advanced prostate cancer: techniques and timing. Can J Urol. 2014; 21(2) Supp 1:42–47

[75] Langsteger W, Rezaee A, Pirich C, Beheshti M. 18F-NaF-PET/CT and 99mTc-MDP bone scintigraphy in the detection of bone metastases in prostate cancer. Semin Nucl Med. 2016; 46(6):491–501

[76] Mosavi F, Johansson S, Sandberg DT, Turesson I, Sörensen J, Ahlström H. Whole-body diffusion-weighted MRI compared with (18)F-NaF PET/CT for detection of bone metastases in patients with high-risk prostate carcinoma. AJR Am J Roentgenol. 2012; 199(5):1114–1120

[77] Heacock L, Weissbrot J, Raad R, et al. PET/MRI for the evaluation of patients with lymphoma: initial observations. AJR Am J Roentgenol. 2015; 204(4):842–848

[78] Giraudo C, Raderer M, Karanikas G, et al. 18F-fluorodeoxyglucose positron emission tomography/magnetic resonance in lymphoma: comparison with 18F-fluorodeoxyglucose positron emission tomography/computed tomography and with the addition of magnetic resonance diffusion-weighted imaging. Invest Radiol. 2016; 51(3):163–169

[79] Atkinson W, Catana C, Abramson JS, et al. Hybrid FDG-PET/MR compared to FDG-PET/CT in adult lymphoma patients. Abdom Radiol (NY). 2016; 41(7):1338–1348

[80] Herrmann K, Queiroz M, Huellner MW, et al. Diagnostic performance of FDG-PET/MRI and WB-DW-MRI in the evaluation of lymphoma: a prospective comparison to standard FDG-PET/CT. BMC Cancer. 2015; 15:1002

[81] Schäfer JF, Gatidis S, Schmidt H, et al. Simultaneous whole-body PET/MR imaging in comparison to PET/CT in pediatric oncology: initial results. Radiology. 2014; 273(1):220–231

[82] Ponisio MR, McConathy J, Laforest R, Khanna G. Evaluation of diagnostic performance of whole-body simultaneous PET/MRI in pediatric lymphoma. Pediatr Radiol. 2016; 46(9): 1258–1268

[83] Sher AC, Seghers V, Paldino MJ, et al. Assessment of sequential PET/MRI in comparison with PET/CT of pediatric

lymphoma: a prospective study. AJR Am J Roentgenol. 2016; 206(3):623–631

[84] Chalian H, O'Donnell JK, Bolen M, Rajiah P. Incremental value of PET and MRI in the evaluation of cardiovascular abnormalities. Insights Imaging. 2016; 7(4):485–503

[85] Gholami S, Salavati A, Houshmand S, Werner TJ, Alavi A. Assessment of atherosclerosis in large vessel walls: a comprehensive review of FDG-PET/CT image acquisition protocols and methods for uptake quantification. J Nucl Cardiol. 2015; 22(3):468–479

[86] Schneider S, Batrice A, Rischpler C, Eiber M, Ibrahim T, Nekolla SG. Utility of multimodal cardiac imaging with PET/MRI in cardiac sarcoidosis: implications for diagnosis, monitoring and treatment. Eur Heart J. 2014; 35(5):312

[87] Wada K, Niitsuma T, Yamaki T, et al. Simultaneous cardiac imaging to detect inflammation and scar tissue with 18F-fluorodeoxyglucose PET/MRI in cardiac sarcoidosis. J Nucl Cardiol. 2016; 23(5):1180–1182

[88] Ripa RS, Knudsen A, Hag AM, et al. Feasibility of simultaneous PET/MR of the carotid artery: first clinical experience and comparison to PET/CT. Am J Nucl Med Mol Imaging. 2013; 3 (4):361–371

[89] Werner P, Saur D, Zeisig V, et al. Simultaneous PET/MRI in stroke: a case series. J Cereb Blood Flow Metab. 2015; 35(9): 1421–1425

[90] Hyafil F, Schindler A, Sepp D, et al. High-risk plaque features can be detected in non-stenotic carotid plaques of patients with ischaemic stroke classified as cryptogenic using combined (18)F-FDG PET/MR imaging. Eur J Nucl Med Mol Imaging. 2016; 43(2):270–279

[91] Salamon N, Kung J, Shaw SJ, et al. FDG-PET/MRI coregistration improves detection of cortical dysplasia in patients with epilepsy. Neurology. 2008; 71(20):1594–1601

[92] Chandra PS, Salamon N, Huang J, et al. FDG-PET/MRI coregistration and diffusion-tensor imaging distinguish epileptogenic tubers and cortex in patients with tuberous sclerosis complex: a preliminary report. Epilepsia. 2006; 47(9):1543–1549

[93] Barthel H, Schroeter ML, Hoffmann KT, Sabri O. PET/MR in dementia and other neurodegenerative diseases. Semin Nucl Med. 2015; 45(3):224–233

[94] Pellino G, Nicolai E, Catalano OA, et al. PET/MR Versus PET/CT Imaging: Impact on the Clinical Management of Small-Bowel Crohn's Disease. J Crohn's Colitis. 2016; 10(3):277–285

[95] Catalano OA, Gee MS, Nicolai E, et al. Evaluation of Quantitative PET/MR Enterography Biomarkers for Discrimination of Inflammatory Strictures from Fibrotic Strictures in Crohn Disease. Radiology. 2016; 278(3):792–800

Part III

Oncologic Applications

11 Oncological PET by Anatomic
Region   *128*

12 Therapy Response   *142*

13 Brain Neoplasms   *150*

14 Head and Neck Cancer   *157*

15 Thyroid Cancer   *169*

16 Thoracic Neoplasms   *177*

17 Breast Cancer   *195*

18 Gastric, Esophageal, and
Gastrointestinal Stromal
Tumors   *208*

19 Lymphoma   *220*

20 Melanoma   *232*

21 Hepatobiliary Tumors   *238*

22 Pancreatic Cancer   *245*

23 Gynecological Tumors   *253*

24 Urological Tumors   *264*

25 Colorectal Cancer   *280*

26 Musculoskeletal Tumors   *291*

27 ^{18}F Sodium Fluoride PET/CT in
Bone   *303*

28 ^{68}Ga-Based Imaging Techniques   *311*

III

11 Oncological PET by Anatomic Region

Eugene C. Lin

11.1 General Principles

The primary attribute of positron emission tomography (PET) imaging is its greater contrast resolution compared to anatomic imaging techniques. Because of this contrast resolution, in oncologic imaging PET has substantial advantages over anatomic techniques in the early detection of disease in staging and recurrence, and accurate evaluation of therapy response. In general, the disadvantages of PET are related to its relatively poor resolution relative to anatomic imaging techniques and the numerous sources of nonneoplastic uptake of fluorodeoxyglucose (FDG). However, many of the disadvantages of PET are greatly mitigated with the use of combined PET/CT imaging (see Chapter 9).

1. **Advantages.** The advantages of PET over conventional imaging techniques in assessing cancer are found in two areas:
   a) PET can detect early disease before gross anatomic changes (▶ Fig. 11.1). PET can detect disease in areas that would be interpreted as normal on anatomic imaging techniques due to lack of structural changes.
   b) There is a greater contrast-to-noise ratio of abnormal-to-normal structures on PET compared to that of the anatomic modalities (▶ Fig. 11.2). Due to this fact, abnormalities clearly seen on PET are often not prospectively detected on anatomic imaging techniques. In many cases, these abnormalities can be retrospectively detected after attention is specifically directed to the abnormal area by PET.
2. **Disadvantages:**
   a) *Limited sensitivity for small lesions:* In general, the sensitivity of PET is low for lesions smaller than 1 cm. PET (or any other gross imaging modality) cannot detect micrometastases.
   b) *False positives:* Potential false-positive results can be seen from a wide range of inflammatory/infectious processes or other benign etiologies.
   c) *Anatomic localization:* Occasionally, it is difficult to localize lesions to their exact anatomic sites based on PET, particularly in the head and neck and pelvic sites. This is largely remedied by combined PET/CT,

although misregistration is sometimes encountered with this approach.
   d) *Low sensitivity in specific areas:* PET has poor sensitivity for brain and lung metastases and sclerotic bone lesions.
   e) *Decreased sensitivity for specific tumors:* PET has poor sensitivity for specific tumors such as prostate cancer, adenocarcinoma in situ in the lung, and mucinous adenocarcinoma.
3. **Metastatic disease demonstrated by PET will often alter patient management.** Given the possibility of false-positive findings, confirmation with anatomic imaging techniques or biopsy should be strongly considered for PET findings that will alter patient management. This is particularly true if there is a solitary lesion demonstrated on PET that will potentially alter patient management.

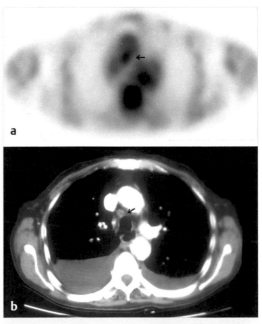

Fig. 11.1 FDG uptake in a benign-appearing but malignant node. **(a)** CT scan in a lung cancer patient demonstrates a nonenlarged mediastinal node with fatty hilum (*arrow*). This is a sign of a benign node on CT. **(b)** There is increased uptake (*arrow*) on axial PET scan corresponding to this node, consistent with malignancy.

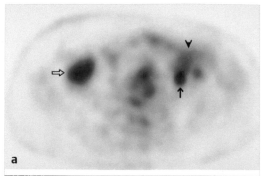

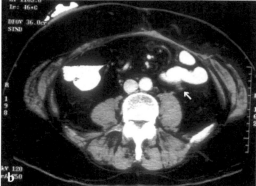

Fig. 11.2 Peritoneal metastasis from colon cancer. **(a)** Axial PET scan shows focal uptake (*arrow*), adjacent to small bowel (*arrowhead*). While mild diffuse small bowel uptake is usually normal, focal areas of uptake greater than the surrounding small bowel are usually not normal. It is normal to have substantially greater uptake in the right colon (*open arrow*) than the small bowel. **(b)** CT scan at the same level demonstrates a small focus of abnormal soft tissue (*arrow*) adjacent to small bowel. This was not seen prospectively on the CT, and was present only on one slice. The contrast-to-noise ratio of the abnormality on PET is much greater than on CT.

11.2 Liver

1. **Liver metastases.** PET is very sensitive for detecting liver metastases which are above 1 cm in size. In a meta-analysis[1] of patients with colorectal liver metastases, PET had a slightly lower sensitivity than MRI and CT on both a patient-based and lesion-based analysis, but was more specific than MRI and CT. Liver MRI performed with specific liver imaging agents such as superparamagnetic iron oxide[2] or mangafodipir trisodium[3] is also more sensitive than PET.

2. **Differentiation of benign from malignant lesions.** Focal uptake in a liver lesion is very specific for malignancy, and may represent either metastases, hepatocellular carcinoma (HCC), or cholangiocarcinoma.[4]

    a) Benign lesions such as hemangiomas, focal nodular hyperplasia, and hepatic adenomas typically do not have increased FDG uptake.

    b) There are several reports of hepatic adenomas with increased FDG uptake (▶ Fig. 11.3).[5] There is a single report of a focal nodular hyperplasia with increased FDG uptake.[6]

    c) **False positives.** Hepatic abscess, nodular lymphoid hyperplasia (pseudolymphoma), inflammatory pseudotumor, sarcoidosis.[7,8]

    d) **False negative.** Low-grade HCC (▶ Fig. 21.1), metastasis from mucinous primary.

3. **Evaluation of small liver lesions.** Although FDG PET has a limited sensitivity for liver lesions smaller than 1 cm in size, it still has a high specificity. This is particularly useful when CT detects liver lesions smaller than 1 cm, but cannot further characterize the nature of these

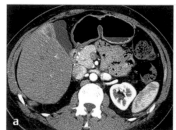

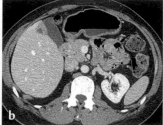

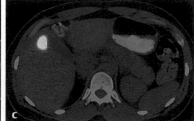

Fig. 11.3 Hepatic adenoma. Axial contrast-enhanced arterial **(a)** and portal-phase **(b)** contrast-enhanced CT demonstrate a lesion with mild peripheral arterial-phase hyperenhancement with washout. **(c)** Axial PET/CT demonstrates substantial increased FDG uptake in this lesion. In this patient with breast cancer, this was suspicious for a metastasis but was diagnosed as a hepatic adenoma with biopsy. Both the CT appearance and the FDG uptake are atypical for hepatic adenoma.

lesions. Statistically, these lesions most likely represent small cysts or hemangiomas, but in the setting of primary malignancy elsewhere it is not possible to determine noninvasively the true nature of these lesions. Given the low sensitivity, PET should not be used primarily for evaluating these small liver lesions, but PET is indicated for assessing for disease activity elsewhere. If focal FDG uptake is noted in these small lesions, they are almost certainly metastatic (► Fig. 11.4). However, even if there is no increased uptake seen on PET, these lesions cannot be diagnosed as benign, as they could be malignant and not detected on PET due to their small size.

4. **Artifacts.** The liver is often heterogeneous due to image noise on attenuation-corrected images. Image noise is more prominent in the liver than in any other organ. Due to the normal heterogeneity of the liver, caution must be exercised before interpreting subtle findings as liver metastases (► Fig. 11.5).

5. **How should one interpret subtle foci of uptake in the liver?** Most metastases in the liver will demonstrate greatly increased activity relative to normal liver. A subtle focus of activity in the liver on attenuation-corrected images may be due to image noise rather than a lesion. Before interpreting a subtle focus as a lesion:

   a) Review the nonattenuation corrected (NAC) images: If the focus is seen on the less noisy NAC images, the level of confidence for a lesion is greatly increased. If the focus is not detected on NAC images, it may be artifactual secondary to image noise. Note that this method may be less helpful for central lesions which may not be seen on NAC images due to attenuation.

   b) Correlation with CT must be performed. CT is very sensitive for detecting small liver lesions, but often cannot characterize these lesions. It is likely that if a focus seen on PET is a true lesion, it will be recognized on a contrast-enhanced CT, often in retrospect. Rarely, true positive lesions may not be seen on CT, particularly if the liver is fatty infiltrated and/or imaged in only one phase of enhancement (► Fig. 11.4, ► Fig. 11.6). However, if a noncontrast CT is obtained as part of a PET/CT exam, many true positive liver lesions identified on PET will not be detected on the noncontrast CT.

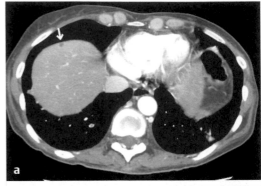

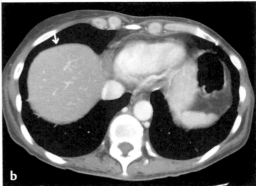

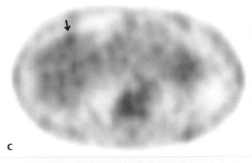

Fig. 11.4 Subtle liver metastasis. A metastasis in the dome of the liver (*arrow*) is much better seen on an arterial phase axial CT scan (**a**) than on a portal-phase scan (**b**). This lesion has mild FDG uptake on an axial PET scan (**c**). This lesion might be interpreted as artifactual secondary to image noise on the PET alone, or if correlated with the portal-phase CT. Correlation with arterial-phase CT was necessary. The lesion itself is nonspecific in appearance on CT, but the presence of visible FDG uptake in this small lesion is consistent with metastatic disease.

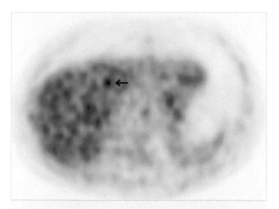

Fig. 11.5 Liver noise mimicking a lesion. Multiple foci of increased activity in the liver are present. It is difficult to differentiate whether these are secondary to lesions or image noise. One focus (*arrow*) is slightly more intense and was suspicious for a possible lesion. Note that this does not appear substantially different from the true positive liver lesion in ▶ Fig. 11.4. However, this was a false-positive finding as no lesion was identified by either CT or MRI in this region.

11.3 Spleen

There are limited data on PET/CT imaging for the evaluation of solid splenic masses.[9]
1. Known FDG avid malignancy:
   a) **PET/CT.** Sensitivity 100%, specificity 100%.
   b) **SUV.** A SUV of 2.3 is useful for differentiating benign from malignant lesions.
2. No known malignancy:
   a) **PET/CT.** Sensitivity 100%, specificity 83%.
   b) *PET* has a high negative predictive value in this setting.
      • However, a non-FDG avid primary tumor should be excluded before diagnosing the splenic mass as a benign process.
   c) An FDG avid splenic mass is likely (80%) to be malignant even without a known primary.
      • Possible false positives include infection, sarcoidosis, and hyalinized nodules.[10]

11.4 Peritoneum

1. Peritoneal metastases are most common in ovarian and gastrointestinal cancers. PET is more accurate than CT in detecting peritoneal metastases, but will not detect very small implants (thus, it will not replace second-look laparotomy). PET is particularly helpful when intraperitoneal fluid is present—it can detect

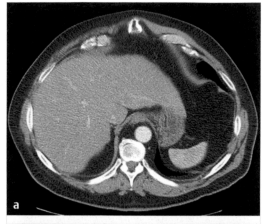

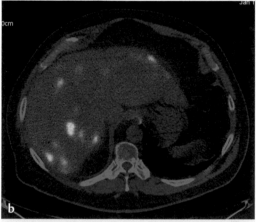

Fig. 11.6 Liver metastases seen by PET only. **(a)** Axial CT scan does not demonstrate any liver lesions. **(b)** Corresponding PET/CT scan demonstrates multiple hepatic metastases. This is a rare finding as the majority of liver metastases seen on PET can be visualized by contrast-enhanced CT. However, liver metastases are occasionally not visualized on portal-phase CT scans. The fatty infiltration of the liver in this case may contribute to the lack of visualization of the metastases. An arterial-phase CT was not done in this case; so, it is unclear whether the metastases would have been visualized in a different phase of contrast enhancement.

malignant ascites, or small solid implants (▶ Fig. 11.7).

2. **Patterns of spread.** It is important to understand the classic patterns of peritoneal spread. Specific attention should be directed to these areas (▶ Fig. 11.8):
   a) Serosal surfaces of the liver and spleen (note that when correlating with CT, splenic serosal metastases can appear cystic).

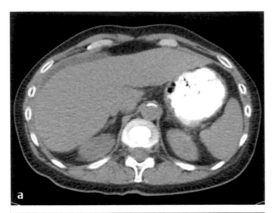

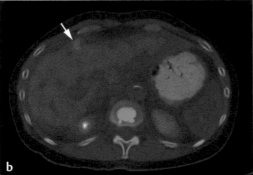

Fig. 11.7 Ascites and solid serosal implant. **(a)** Axial CT demonstrates free fluid over the liver. **(b)** A solid serosal implant (*arrow*) is identified in this free fluid on the corresponding PET/CT.

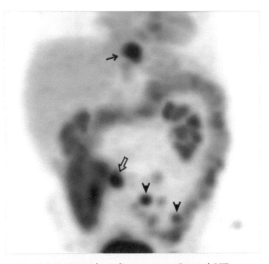

Fig. 11.8 Peritoneal seeding pattern. Coronal PET scan demonstrates multiple foci of peritoneal seeding medial to the cecum (*open arrow*) and on the sigmoid mesocolon (*arrowheads*) from a gastroesophageal carcinoma (*arrow*). This is a classic pattern of peritoneal spread. (Reproduced with permission from Lin EC, Lear J, Quaife RA. Metastatic peritoneal seeding patterns demonstrated by FDG positron emission tomographic imaging. Clin Nucl Med 2001;26(3):249–250.)

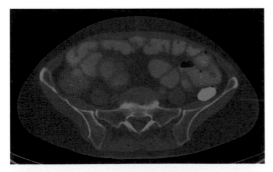

Fig. 11.9 Peritoneal implant. Axial PET/CT demonstrates focal uptake in a peritoneal implant on the surface of the medial cecum. This is difficult to distinguish from physiologic cecal activity. The eccentric location of the uptake is helpful in differentiating this from physiologic uptake.

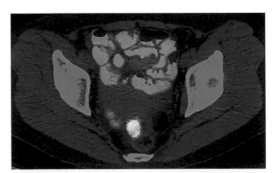

Fig. 11.10 Peritoneal metastasis. Axial PET/CT in a patient with colon cancer demonstrates increased uptake in a peritoneal metastasis in the retrouterine pouch (pouch of Douglas).

b) Omentum.

c) Paracolic gutters, particularly on the right.

d) Medial to the cecum (this must be differentiated from normal physiologic cecal uptake) (▶ Fig. 11.9).

e) Sigmoid mesocolon.

f) Pelvis—particularly between the bladder and uterus and between the uterus and rectum (▶ Fig. 11.10).

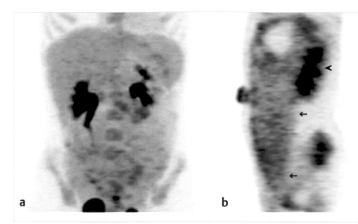

Fig. 11.11 Diffuse peritoneal carcinomatosis. **(a)** Coronal PET scan in a patient with ovarian cancer demonstrates diffuse increased peritoneal uptake (note that the inferior border of the liver is not visualized). **(b)** On sagittal PET, there is a straight line (*arrows*) caused by increased intensity of the peritoneum relative to the retroperitoneum. Normally, there is no demarcation between the peritoneum and retroperitoneum. Kidney activity (*arrowhead*) lies in the retroperitoneum.

3. **Distinguishing peritoneal metastasis from bowel activity.** It is sometimes difficult to differentiate peritoneal metastasis from bowel activity without PET/CT.
   a) The focus should be reviewed in all three planes with an attempt to link the activity to a segment of bowel in at least one plane. Often foci that appear outside the bowel in one plane are clearly visualized in the bowel on another plane.
   b) Outside the right colon, cecum, and rectosigmoid where normal intense areas of uptake are often noted, it is unusual to see foci of bowel activity which are substantially more intense than the surrounding structures—this is particularly true in the small bowel (▶ Fig. 11.2).
   c) CT correlation is very helpful as peritoneal metastases are often identified retrospectively with this modality after attention is directed to the area of abnormality by PET.
   d) **SUV.** A SUV cutoff of 5.1[11] may be helpful for the diagnosis of peritoneal carcinomatosis.
   e) **PET/CT.** While PET/CT can often allow for differentiation of bowel activity from peritoneal disease, PET/CT has the potential disadvantage of causing areas of artifactually increased and decreased uptake in the bowel (see Chapter 9). Potential peritoneal disease should be interpreted with caution on PET/CT, as bowel motion between the CT and PET scans can result in both false-positive and false-negative findings. NAC images should always be reviewed in conjunction with the corrected scans.
4. **Diffuse peritoneal carcinomatosis.** Diffuse peritoneal carcinomatosis can result in diffuse peritoneal uptake which may be difficult to clearly define as no focal lesions are seen in this setting.[12] Clues to identifying diffuse disease are as follows (▶ Fig. 11.11)[13]:
   a) **Liver border.** The liver border is poorly visualized as peritoneal activity is close in intensity to that of liver.
   b) **Straight line sign.** On sagittal and axial images, the retroperitoneum is less intense than the peritoneum in peritoneal carcinomatosis (normally the peritoneum and retroperitoneum are of comparable intensity). This results in a straight line demarcating the peritoneum and retroperitoneum on sagittal images.

11.5 Lymph Nodes

1. PET is more sensitive than CT in detecting lymph node metastases. Malignant nodes can be detected by PET before nodal enlargement (> 1 cm) on CT.
2. **Size.** The sensitivity of PET for metastatic deposits in nodes measuring 6 to 10 mm is 83%, while it drops to 23% for those ≤ 5 mm.[14] As PET will not detect micrometastases, it is not a substitute for sentinel node imaging for axillary nodal staging in breast cancer and local nodal staging in melanoma
3. **Inflammatory versus malignant lymph nodes.** A common problem is differentiating benign from malignant nodal uptake.
   a) **SUV.** In general, malignant nodes have higher SUV values (usually > 2.5) compared to inflammatory nodes. However, small nodes with metastases, due to partial volume effects, may have a low SUV and low uptake by visual interpretation.

b) **CT correlation.** Theoretically, there should be a detectable node by CT in any region of FDG uptake. The lack of a detectable node on CT suggests that the uptake may be related to a nonnodal structure. Although PET commonly detects metastases in normal-appearing nodes on CT, it is unlikely that a metastatic node would not be seen at all on CT. Note that this does not apply to areas where small nodes may be difficult to visualize (e.g., the hila). In addition, mediastinal nodes can sometimes be "flat" in shape and may be difficult to detect on CT (▶ Fig. 11.12).

- Substantial uptake in a normal-size node is very specific for malignancy, as inflammatory nodes would most likely be enlarged with the same amount of uptake. For example, definite positive uptake in a 5-mm mediastinal node in lung cancer is highly likely a true positive finding for metastasis.
- Nodes are typically considered benign if a fatty hilum is seen on CT. However, if the node has substantial FDG uptake, malignancy should be suspected as PET may detect disease before the fatty hilum is fully replaced by tumor (▶ Fig. 11.1).
- FDG uptake in a mediastinal or hilar node can be suspected as false positive if[15] the nodes are calcified or have high attenuation (see discussion on "lymph node density").

c) **Location and pattern.** The location and pattern of nodal uptake is often useful in differentiating between benign and malignant processes.

- For example, a left upper lobe lung carcinoma will spread first to the aortopulmonary window, and thus lack of aortopulmonary window uptake with nodal uptake elsewhere suggests a benign etiology.
- If multiple nodes are seen, the node in the first drainage area is usually the most intense if the etiology is metastatic disease (▶ Fig. 11.13).
- Symmetric low-grade uptake (such as bilateral hilar) is usually benign (▶ Fig. 11.14).

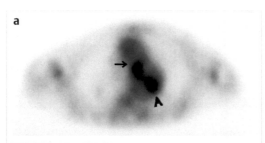

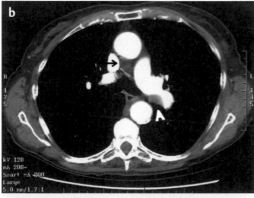

Fig. 11.12 Flat node missed by CT but detected on PET. (a) Axial PET scan in a patient with lung cancer demonstrates uptake in central mediastinal (*arrow*) and left hilar (*arrowhead*) nodes. (b) CT scan at the same level demonstrates the left hilar node (*arrowhead*). A less dense node (*arrow*) is seen corresponding to the central mediastinal uptake seen on PET. This is a "flat" node and was seen only on one slice of the CT. This was not prospectively called abnormal on CT because it resembles the superior pericardial recess which is a normal variant.

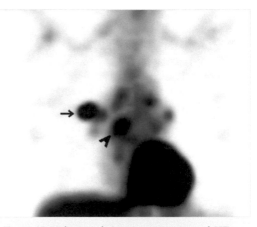

Fig. 11.13 Malignant drainage pattern. Coronal PET scan in a patient with a right upper lobe lung cancer (*arrow*) demonstrates activity in multiple nodes with the most intense uptake in the first nodal basin (*arrowhead*). This is a typical drainage pattern for a right upper lobe carcinoma which spreads first to lymph nodes along the medial surface of the right mainstem bronchus (seen as a linear photopenic area between the node and tumor). These nodes are known as the lymphatic sump of Borrie.

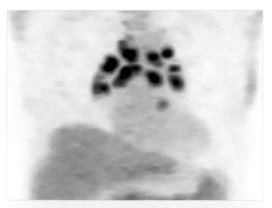

Fig. 11.14 Sarcoidosis. Coronal PET scan demonstrates a symmetric pattern of hilar and mediastinal uptake in a patient with sarcoidosis.

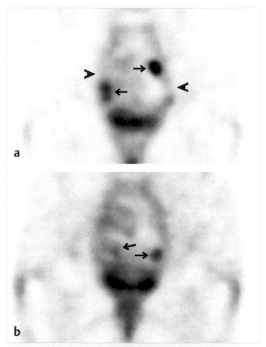

a

b

Fig. 11.15 Ovarian FDG uptake diagnosed using ureteral landmarks. **(a)** Coronal PET scan in a patient with lymphoma demonstrated two foci of pelvic uptake (*arrows*). While iliac lymphadenopathy is a concern, the iliac nodes are extraperitoneal and should lie lateral to the ureters (*arrowheads*). The intraperitoneal ovaries lie medial to the ureters. While ureteral activity is typically a confounding factor the ureters can be used as a landmark to differentiate ovarian uptake from iliac nodal uptake. CT did not demonstrate any nodes in the region. **(b)** The patient had a follow-up PET which demonstrates the two foci (*arrows*) to have moved and decreased in intensity, consistent with ovarian uptake. (Reproduced with permission from Lin EC, Siegal J. Pelvic anatomic localization using ureteral activity on FDG positron emission tomography. Clin Nucl Med 2003;28(10):836–837.)

d) ***Lymph node density.*** Lymph node density has been evaluated primarily in the context of mediastinal nodes in patients with non-small cell lung cancer. Malignant lymph nodes will typically be higher in density than benign lymph nodes, although very high densities can be seen in benign nodes. Lymph node density can be helpful in the evaluation of lymph nodes with intermediate degrees of FDG uptake (2.0 < SUVmax ≤ 4.0). In one report,[16] 71% of malignant lymph nodes had median Hounsfield units (HU) between 25 and 45. By using additional density criteria (median HU: 25–45) in lymph nodes with intermediate FDG uptake, the sensitivity improved from 70 to 88%. Other reports have used cutoff values of 7.5 and 20 HU[17,18] to distinguish between benign and malignant lymph nodes. A 20 HU cutoff may be useful specifically to exclude a benign etiology, as in one report[18] > 99% of benign lymph nodes were below the 20 HU cutoff.

e) ***Pelvic lymph nodes:***

- If pelvic lymph nodes are of clinical concern, it is important to reduce urinary activity (see Chapter 4).
- Ovarian activity is a common mimic of iliac nodal disease, as the ovaries are usually close to the iliac nodes. If the ureters are visualized on PET, they can be helpful in distinguishing ovarian from pelvic nodal activity.[19] The pelvic ureters are at the boundary of the intraperitoneal space medially and extraperitoneal space laterally. Ovaries are intraperitoneal and will be medial to the ureters (▶ Fig. 11.15). Iliac nodes are extraperitoneal and will be lateral to the ureters.

11.6 Lungs

1. **Lung metastases.** The primary value of PET in the lung parenchyma is in evaluating solitary pulmonary nodules rather than detecting lung metastases. Sensitivity for lung metastases < 1 cm is poor. Thus, PET does not replace CT to detect lung metastases.

a) **PET/CT versus CT**: PET/CT, if performed with shallow breathing, does not replace a breath-hold chest CT for the detection of lung metastases. PET/CT performed in shallow breathing often does not detect small lung nodules.[20] The addition of an additional low-dose breath-hold chest CT to the PET/CT exam may be helpful.[21]

b) **Small nodules with minimal or no uptake.** In patients with nonthoracic malignancies, small lung nodules (≤ 1 cm) with minimal or no FDG uptake turn out to be malignant approximately one-fifth of the time.[22]

- These small nodules are more likely to be malignant when no other benign pulmonary lesions can be identified.
- Small nodules with no visible uptake are not less likely to be malignant than those with minimal uptake.

2. If there are known lung lesions in a cancer patient, PET can be helpful in differentiating these lesions from benign etiologies if the lesions are > 1 cm. The interpretation of FDG PET in small subcentimeter pulmonary nodules is similar to that of the interpretation of subcentimeter liver lesions. A positive result is very useful, indicating that metastatic disease is likely, but a negative result is less helpful as the nodule could be malignant and not detectable by PET.

3. SUV values should be used with caution in the evaluation of potential pulmonary metastases.

A SUV cutoff of 2.5 may have value in this setting,[23] but this is not well established (as is the case for solitary pulmonary nodules).

11.7 Bone Marrow Metastases

1. The mechanism of uptake in bone marrow metastases is different on FDG PET than on bone scan. The bone marrow metastasis is positive on PET because the tumor itself has increased FDG uptake, while the metastasis will be positive on bone scan due to increased reactive uptake around the tumor (▶ Fig. 11.16).

2. **Lytic versus sclerotic metastasis.** FDG PET is sensitive for lytic bone metastases (▶ Fig. 11.16) but less sensitive for sclerotic metastasis (▶ Fig. 11.17).[24] Thus, the sensitivity of PET for bone metastases depends on the primary tumor. However, many sclerotic metastases without FDG uptake may represent treated metastases (▶ Fig. 11.18)—in these cases, the lack of FDG uptake in the sclerotic treated metastasis is an accurate finding. In one report,[25] there was no difference in the detection rate of osteolytic and osteoblastic metastases between FDG PET and bone scan; however, the mean SUVmax was higher for osteolytic lesions. Osteoblastic lesions that are FDG avid may be more resistant to treatment.[26]

3. **PET versus bone scan.** Although the CT portion of a PET/CT study may detect some bone metastases missed on PET, it is unclear

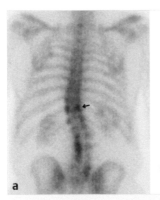
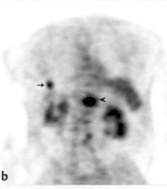
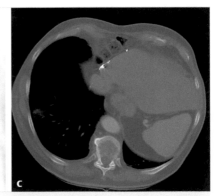

Fig. 11.16 Lytic bone metastases from lung cancer detected by PET only. **(a)** Whole body bone scan in a lung cancer patient demonstrates peripheral uptake at the T11 vertebral body (*arrow*). This appearance is not typical for metastasis. This was initially interpreted as negative for metastasis. **(b)** Coronal PET scan demonstrates intense uptake in the T11 vertebral body (*arrowhead*). Uptake is also seen in the primary right lower lobe lung cancer (*arrow*). This case illustrates the difference in uptake between PET and bone scan: uptake on PET is in the lesion itself, while bone scan uptake is in reactive bone around the lesion. The minimal peripheral bone scan uptake is in reactive bone around the central FDG avid lesion. **(c)** CT scan demonstrates a central lytic vertebral body metastasis. Note that there is still intact bone seen around the lesion which accounts for the peripheral uptake seen on bone scan.

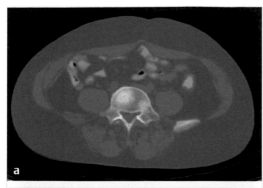

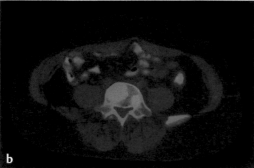

Fig. 11.17 Sclerotic bone metastases. **(a)** CT scan demonstrates sclerotic lumbar vertebral body metastases. **(b)** Axial PET/CT does not demonstrate increased uptake in the large right anterior vertebral body metastasis. There is minimal peripheral uptake in the smaller left posterior vertebral body metastasis.

currently whether the combination of the PET and CT data can replace bone scan. Compared to bone scan, FDG PET/CT will usually miss lesions that are outside the field-of-view, but additional sites of osseous metastatic disease are usually present in the field-of-view.[27] Lesions missed on bone scan but detected on PET/CT are often in the pelvis and spine.[27]

In particular, the fact that PET/CT has a substantial advantage in accuracy over bone scan is in the detection of osteolytic metastases in the spine.[28] The relative value of PET, bone scan, and MRI depend on the primary neoplasm being evaluated (see the specific chapters for each neoplasm), but neoplasms for which meta-analyses are available are listed as follows:

a) **Head and neck cancer.** In a meta-analysis,[29] PET/CT had a higher sensitivity and comparable specificity to bone scan.

b) **Lung cancer.** In three meta-analyses,[30,31,32] PET/CT had a higher sensitivity and

specificity than bone scan. In one meta-analysis,[32] FDG PET/CT had a higher sensitivity and specificity than MRI for the diagnosis of bone metastases in patients with lung cancer. In another meta-analysis in patients with lung cancer,[31] FDG PET/CT had a higher sensitivity and specificity than MRI on a per-patient basis; however, on a per-lesion basis, PET/CT had a higher sensitivity but lower specificity than MRI.

c) **Breast cancer.** In an early meta-analysis,[33] it was inconclusive whether FDG PET or bone scan was superior, but FDG PET had a higher specificity. In another meta-analysis,[34] FDG PET had a lower sensitivity and higher specificity than bone scan on a per-lesion basis, but on per-patient basis there was no difference in sensitivity. In a meta-analysis[35] of PET/CT specifically, FDG PET/CT had a higher sensitivity and accuracy than bone scan. Compared to MRI, FDG PET had a lower sensitivity but comparable specificity on a per-patient basis.[34]

4. PET and CT correlation:

a) There will be no correlative finding on CT in approximately 50% of bone metastases detected by PET (▶ Fig. 11.19).[36] Thus, the absence of a correlative CT finding in the presence of osseous FDG uptake does not exclude a lesion.

b) The positive predictive value (PPV) of PET/CT for bone malignancy is 98% when the results of PET and CT are concordant. However, if PET is positive and CT is negative, the PPV is 61%. If the lesion is solitary in this scenario, the PPV is 43%.[37] Therefore, confirmation with additional tests such as MRI is often necessary for bone lesions identified by PET but not by CT, particularly if solitary.

c) Bone lesions that are positive on CT but negative on PET have a PPV of 17% for malignancy.[37]

d) The sensitivity of PET is substantially superior to bone scan for lesions which are invisible on CT.[38]

e) FDG PET better reflects tumor activity of bone metastases than does CT. Radiographic changes vary widely after treatment and do not correlate well with the presence of active tumor.[26] Prior chemotherapy does not affect the PPV of PET, but decreases the PPV of CT.[37] Treated bone metastases tend to be blastic on CT and PET negative (▶ Fig. 11.18).[39]

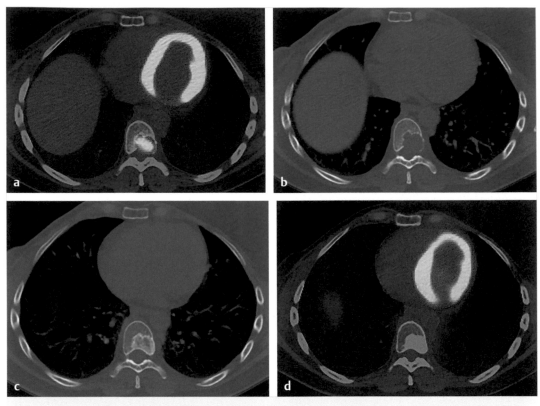

Fig. 11.18 Treated bone metastasis. **(a)** Axial PET/CT in a patient with breast cancer demonstrates increased uptake in a bone metastasis which is lytic on the corresponding CT **(b)**. After therapy, the lesion is now sclerotic **(c)** with resolution of the FDG uptake **(d)**.

5. PET is more specific than bone scan, as degenerative joint disease typically does not have substantial uptake (although there can be substantial uptake with an inflammatory component).

6. Although standard PET protocols image only from the face to upper thighs, this is not a major drawback given the low risk of solitary bone metastases to the skull and lower extremities.[40]

7. Radiographic correlation is necessary if single bone lesions are seen in cancer patients, as benign primary bone lesions can often have increased uptake (see Chapter 26).

11.8 Brain

1. The primary value of PET is in primary brain tumors rather than brain metastases. The overall sensitivity of PET for brain metastases is approximately 60%. Because most metastases are at the gray-white matter junction, detection is limited by high normal cortical brain activity (▶ Fig. 11.20). Smaller metastases are less well detected, with sensitivity for 1 cm lesions of approximately 40%.[41]

2. If brain imaging is added to the imaging protocol for patients with non-CNS malignancies, management is changed in < 1% of patients.[42]

11.9 Adrenals

FDG PET is useful in detecting unsuspected adrenal metastases (▶ Fig. 11.21) and evaluating equivocal adrenal masses seen on CT or MRI.

11.9.1 Accuracy/Comparison to Other Modalities

1. *PET and PET/CT for characterization of adrenal masses* (meta-analysis). Sensitivity 97%, specificity 91%.[43]

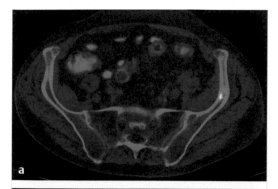

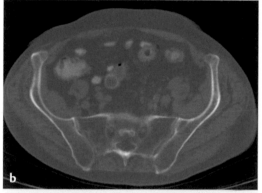

Fig. 11.19 Invisible metastasis. A left iliac bone metastasis seen on axial PET/CT scan (a) is not visualized on the corresponding CT scan (b).

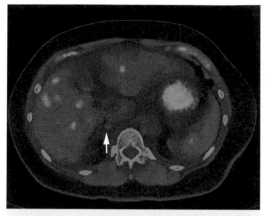

Fig. 11.21 Adrenal metastasis. Axial PET/CT scan demonstrates a small right adrenal metastasis (arrow).

2. The diagnostic accuracy of PET/CT for adrenal masses is comparable to that of CT and chemical shift MRI.[44] The highest accuracies—more accurate than any technique used in isolation— are achieved when the results of PET/CT are combined with specific CT techniques such as histogram analysis or Hounsfield unit measurement[45] or contrast-enhanced adrenal protocol CT.[46]

11.9.2 Pearls/Pitfalls

1. **SUV and visual analysis.** Adenomas can have a mild degree of FDG uptake. Several methods have been used to differentiate adrenal metastases from benign adenomas. These include visual analysis (uptake greater than the liver), SUV ratio (ratio of SUVmax in the adrenal lesion to SUVmean in the liver), and SUVmax.
   a) Published SUVmax cutoffs have ranged from 2.31 to 5.2.[47,48]
   b) Published SUV ratio cutoffs have ranged from 1.0 to 2.5.[47,49]
   c) In one study,[50] SUV ratio had a higher accuracy than SUVmax. In another study,[48] accuracy was comparable, but only SUV ratio was an independent predictor of malignancy.
   d) Adrenal uptake more than twice that of the liver[51] can be used to differentiate metastases

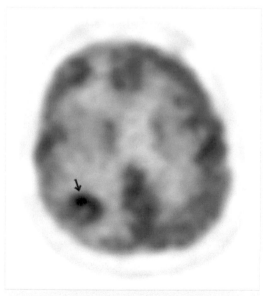

Fig. 11.20 Brain metastasis. Axial PET scan demonstrates a right parietal metastasis at the gray-white junction (arrow).

from adenomas. Most benign adrenal lesions have uptake less than liver.[51]

e) In a meta-analysis,[43] quantitative and qualitative analysis had comparable accuracy, but quantitative analysis had a higher sensitivity and lower specificity. A single-institution analysis[52] also found a slightly higher sensitivity and lower specificity for quantitative analysis, but accuracy was higher with qualitative analysis.

f) FDG uptake does not differ between lipid-rich and lipid-poor adenomas.[53] Thus, PET is accurate in cases where noncontrast CT is equivocal.[53]

2. *Nonmetastatic causes of adrenal uptake*

a) Adrenal hyperplasia can have FDG uptake, mimicking bilateral adrenal metastases (▶ Fig. 7.38).

b) Adrenal neoplasms other than metastases have FDG uptake (see Chapter 7), but these can usually be differentiated from metastasis by CT or MRI imaging.

c) Adrenal hemorrhage and histoplasmosis can have FDG uptake.[54,55]

d) Approximately 5% of adrenal adenomas will have substantial FDG uptake.[40]

3. *False-negative results.* False-negative results can be seen in lesions < 1 cm, metastases from primary tumors with low FDG avidity (e.g., carcinoid,) and in lesions with hemorrhage and necrosis.[36,40]

References

[1] Maffione AM, Lopci E, Bluemel C, Giammarile F, Herrmann K, Rubello D. Diagnostic accuracy and impact on management of (18)F-FDG PET and PET/CT in colorectal liver metastasis: a meta-analysis and systematic review. Eur J Nucl Med Mol Imaging. 2015; 42(1):152–163

[2] Rappeport ED, Loft A, Berthelsen AK, et al. Contrast-enhanced FDG-PET/CT vs. SPIO-enhanced MRI vs. FDG-PET vs. CT in patients with liver metastases from colorectal cancer: a prospective study with intraoperative confirmation. Acta Radiol. 2007; 48(4):369–378

[3] Sahani DV, Kalva SP, Fischman AJ, et al. Detection of liver metastases from adenocarcinoma of the colon and pancreas: comparison of mangafodipir trisodium-enhanced liver MRI and whole-body FDG PET. AJR Am J Roentgenol. 2005; 185(1):239–246

[4] Delbeke D, Martin WH, Sandler MP, Chapman WC, Wright JK, Jr, Pinson CW. Evaluation of benign vs malignant hepatic lesions with positron emission tomography. Arch Surg. 1998; 133(5):510–515, discussion 515–516

[5] Nakashima T, Takayama Y, Nishie A, et al. Hepatocellular adenoma showing high uptake of (18)F-fluorodeoxyglucose (FDG) via an increased expression of glucose transporter 2 (GLUT-2). Clin Imaging. 2014; 38(6):888–891

[6] Aznar DL, Ojeda R, Garcia EU, et al. Focal nodular hyperplasia (FNH): a potential cause of false-positive positron emission tomography. Clin Nucl Med. 2005; 30(9):636–637

[7] Kawamura E, Habu D, Tsushima H, et al. A case of hepatic inflammatory pseudotumor identified by FDG-PET. Ann Nucl Med. 2006; 20(4):321–323

[8] Guglielmi AN, Kim BY, Bybel B, Slifkin N. False-positive uptake of FDG in hepatic sarcoidosis. Clin Nucl Med. 2006; 31(3):175

[9] Metser U, Miller E, Kessler A, et al. Solid splenic masses: evaluation with 18F-FDG PET/CT. J Nucl Med. 2005; 46(1):52–59

[10] Choi AY, Wax BN, Yung E. Focal F-18 fluorodeoxyglucose positron emission tomography uptake in a hyalinized nodule as a false positive splenic metastasis in a patient with breast cancer and metastatic thyroid cancer. Clin Nucl Med. 2005; 30(12):799–800

[11] Suzuki A, Kawano T, Takahashi N, et al. Value of 18F-FDG PET in the detection of peritoneal carcinomatosis. Eur J Nucl Med Mol Imaging. 2004; 31(10):1413–1420

[12] Turlakow A, Yeung HW, Salmon AS, Macapinlac HA, Larson SM. Peritoneal carcinomatosis: role of (18)F-FDG PET. J Nucl Med. 2003; 44(9):1407–1412

[13] Lin EC. "Straight line" sign of diffuse peritoneal carcinomatosis on sagittal FDG positron emission tomographic images. Clin Nucl Med. 2002; 27(10):735–736

[14] Crippa F, Leutner M, Belli F, et al. Which kinds of lymph node metastases can FDG PET detect? A clinical study in melanoma. J Nucl Med. 2000; 41(9):1491–1494

[15] Shim SS, Lee KS, Kim BT, et al. Non-small cell lung cancer: prospective comparison of integrated FDG PET/CT and CT alone for preoperative staging. Radiology. 2005; 236(3):1011–1019

[16] Lee JW, Kim EY, Kim DJ, et al. The diagnostic ability of 18F-FDG PET/CT for mediastinal lymph node staging using 18F-FDG uptake and volumetric CT histogram analysis in non-small cell lung cancer. Eur Radiol. 2016; 26(12):4515–4523

[17] Flechsig P, Frank P, Kratochwil C, et al. Radiomic analysis using density threshold for FDG-PET/CT-based N-staging in lung cancer patients. Mol Imaging Biol. 2017; 19(2):315–322

[18] Giesel FL, Schneider F, Kratochwil C, et al. Correlation between SUVmax and CT radiomic analysis using lymph node density in PET/CT-based lymph node staging. J Nucl Med. 2017; 58(2):282–287

[19] Lin EC, Siegal J. Pelvic anatomic localization using ureteral activity on FDG positron emission tomography. Clin Nucl Med. 2003; 28(10):836–837

[20] Allen-Auerbach M, Yeom K, Park J, Phelps M, Czernin J. Standard PET/CT of the chest during shallow breathing is inadequate for comprehensive staging of lung cancer. J Nucl Med. 2006; 47(2):298–301

[21] Juergens KU, Weckesser M, Stegger L, et al. Tumor staging using whole-body high-resolution 16-channel PET-CT: does additional low-dose chest CT in inspiration improve the detection of solitary pulmonary nodules? Eur Radiol. 2006; 16(5):1131–1137

[22] O JH, Yoo IeR, Kim SH, Sohn HS, Chung SK. Clinical significance of small pulmonary nodules with little or no 18F-FDG uptake on PET/CT images of patients with nonthoracic malignancies. J Nucl Med. 2007; 48(1):15–21

[23] Hsu WH, Hsu NY, Shen YY, Yen RF, Kao CH. Differentiating solitary pulmonary metastases in patients with extrapulmonary neoplasmas using FDG-PET. Cancer Invest. 2003; 21(1):47–52

[24] Cook GJ, Fogelman I. The role of positron emission tomography in skeletal disease. Semin Nucl Med. 2001; 31(1):50–61

[25] Sahin E, Zincirkeser S, Akcan AB, Elboga U. Is (99m)Tc-MDP whole body bone scintigraphy adjuvant to (18)F-FDG-PET for the detection of skeletal metastases? J BUON. 2014; 19(1): 291–296

[26] Tann M, Sandrasegaran K, Jennings SG, Skandarajah A, McHenry L, Schmidt CM. Positron-emission tomography and computed tomography of cystic pancreatic masses. Clin Radiol. 2007; 62(8):745–751

[27] Chang CY, Gill CM, Joseph Simeone F, et al. Comparison of the diagnostic accuracy of 99 m-Tc-MDP bone scintigraphy and 18 F-FDG PET/CT for the detection of skeletal metastases. Acta Radiol. 2016; 57(1):58–65

[28] Zhang L, Chen L, Xie Q, et al. A comparative study of 18F-fluorodeoxyglucose positron emission tomography/computed tomography and (99m)Tc-MDP whole-body bone scanning for imaging osteolytic bone metastases. BMC Med Imaging. 2015; 15:7

[29] Yi X, Fan M, Liu Y, Zhang H, Liu S. 18 FDG PET and PET-CT for the detection of bone metastases in patients with head and neck cancer. A meta-analysis. J Med Imaging Radiat Oncol. 2013; 57(6):674–679

[30] Chang MC, Chen JH, Liang JA, et al. Meta-analysis: comparison of F-18 fluorodeoxyglucose-positron emission tomography and bone scintigraphy in the detection of bone metastasis in patients with lung cancer. Acad Radiol. 2012; 19(3):349–357

[31] Liu T, Xu JY, Xu W, Bai YR, Yan WL, Yang HL. Fluorine-18 deoxyglucose positron emission tomography, magnetic resonance imaging and bone scintigraphy for the diagnosis of bone metastases in patients with lung cancer: which one is the best?–a meta-analysis. Clin Oncol (R Coll Radiol). 2011; 23(5):350–358

[32] Qu X, Huang X, Yan W, Wu L, Dai K. A meta-analysis of 18FDG-PET-CT, 18FDG-PET, MRI and bone scintigraphy for diagnosis of bone metastases in patients with lung cancer. Eur J Radiol. 2012; 81(5):1007–1015

[33] Shie P, Cardarelli R, Brandon D, Erdman W, Abdulrahim N. Meta-analysis: comparison of F-18 fluorodeoxyglucose-positron emission tomography and bone scintigraphy in the detection of bone metastases in patients with breast cancer. Clin Nucl Med. 2008; 33(2):97–101

[34] Liu T, Cheng T, Xu W, Yan WL, Liu J, Yang HL. A meta-analysis of 18FDG-PET, MRI and bone scintigraphy for diagnosis of bone metastases in patients with breast cancer. Skeletal Radiol. 2011; 40(5):523–531

[35] Rong J, Wang S, Ding Q, Yun M, Zheng Z, Ye S. Comparison of 18 FDG PET-CT and bone scintigraphy for detection of bone metastases in breast cancer patients. A meta-analysis. Surg Oncol. 2013; 22(2):86–91

[36] Nakamoto Y, Cohade C, Tatsumi M, Hammoud D, Wahl RL. CT appearance of bone metastases detected with FDG PET as part of the same PET/CT examination. Radiology. 2005; 237 (2):627–634

[37] Taira AV, Herfkens RJ, Gambhir SS, Quon A. Detection of bone metastases: assessment of integrated FDG PET/CT imaging. Radiology. 2007; 243(1):204–211

[38] Nakai T, Okuyama C, Kubota T, et al. Pitfalls of FDG-PET for the diagnosis of osteoblastic bone metastases in patients with breast cancer. Eur J Nucl Med Mol Imaging. 2005; 32 (11):1253–1258

[39] Israel O, Goldberg A, Nachtigal A, et al. FDG-PET and CT patterns of bone metastases and their relationship to previously administered anti-cancer therapy. Eur J Nucl Med Mol Imaging. 2006; 33(11):1280–1284

[40] Fujimoto R, Higashi T, Nakamoto Y, et al. Diagnostic accuracy of bone metastases detection in cancer patients: comparison between bone scintigraphy and whole-body FDG-PET. Ann Nucl Med. 2006; 20(6):399–408

[41] Rohren EM, Provenzale JM, Barboriak DP, Coleman RE. Screening for cerebral metastases with FDG PET in patients undergoing whole-body staging of non-central nervous system malignancy. Radiology. 2003; 226(1):181–187

[42] Larcos G, Maisey MN. FDG-PET screening for cerebral metastases in patients with suspected malignancy. Nucl Med Commun. 1996; 17(3):197–198

[43] Boland GW, Dwamena BA, Jagtiani Sangwaiya M, et al. Characterization of adrenal masses by using FDG PET: a systematic review and meta-analysis of diagnostic test performance. Radiology. 2011; 259(1):117–126

[44] Gratz S, Kemke B, Kaiser W, Heinis J, Behr TM, Höffken H. Incidental non-secreting adrenal masses in cancer patients: intra-individual comparison of 18F-fluorodeoxyglucose positron emission tomography/computed tomography with computed tomography and shift magnetic resonance imaging. J Int Med Res. 2010; 38(2):633–644

[45] Perri M, Erba P, Volterrani D, et al. Adrenal masses in patients with cancer: PET/CT characterization with combined CT histogram and standardized uptake value PET analysis. AJR Am J Roentgenol. 2011; 197(1):209–216

[46] Park SY, Park BK, Kim CK. The value of adding (18)F-FDG PET/CT to adrenal protocol CT for characterizing adrenal metastasis (≥ 10 mm) in oncologic patients. AJR Am J Roentgenol. 2014; 202(2):W153–60

[47] Boland GW, Blake MA, Holalkere NS, Hahn PF. PET/CT for the characterization of adrenal masses in patients with cancer: qualitative versus quantitative accuracy in 150 consecutive patients. AJR Am J Roentgenol. 2009; 192(4):956–962

[48] Kunikowska J, Matyskiel R, Toutounchi S, Grabowska-Derlatka L, Koperski L, Królicki L. What parameters from 18F-FDG PET/CT are useful in evaluation of adrenal lesions? Eur J Nucl Med Mol Imaging. 2014; 41(12):2273–2280

[49] Kim JY, Kim SH, Lee HJ, et al. Utilisation of combined 18F-FDG PET/CT scan for differential diagnosis between benign and malignant adrenal enlargement. Br J Radiol. 2013; 86 (1028):20130190

[50] Watanabe H, Kanematsu M, Goshima S, et al. Adrenal-to-liver SUV ratio is the best parameter for differentiation of adrenal metastases from adenomas using 18F-FDG PET/CT. Ann Nucl Med. 2013; 27(7):648–653

[51] Jana S, Zhang T, Milstein DM, Isasi CR, Blaufox MD. FDG-PET and CT characterization of adrenal lesions in cancer patients. Eur J Nucl Med Mol Imaging. 2006; 33(1):29–35

[52] Evans PD, Miller CM, Marin D, et al. FDG-PET/CT characterization of adrenal nodules: diagnostic accuracy and interreader agreement using quantitative and qualitative methods. Acad Radiol. 2013; 20(8):923–929

[53] Metser U, Miller E, Lerman H, Lievshitz G, Avital S, Even-Sapir E. 18F-FDG PET/CT in the evaluation of adrenal masses. J Nucl Med. 2006; 47(1):32–37

[54] Votrubova J, Belohlavek O, Jaruskova M, et al. The role of FDG-PET/CT in the detection of recurrent colorectal cancer. Eur J Nucl Med Mol Imaging. 2006; 33(7):779–784

[55] Chong S, Lee KS, Kim HY, et al. Integrated PET-CT for the characterization of adrenal gland lesions in cancer patients: diagnostic efficacy and interpretation pitfalls. Radiographics. 2006; 26(6):1811–1824, discussion 1824–1826

12 Therapy Response

Sandip Basu and Eugene C. Lin

12.1 Introduction

This is a general overview of PET for therapy response. While information about the role of PET in specific tumors is found in the concerned chapters, we have summarized the major PET-based response evaluation criteria utilized in oncological settings and the considerations need to be made in routine assessment process.

12.2 General Principles

Therapy response imaging can be divided into two categories: interim (early prediction) and end of treatment (late prediction).

Interim PET. The goal of imaging is to predict response early during therapy. In this case, the cancer should be one in which viable alternative therapies are available if the first-line therapy is ineffective. If there is lack of response, the initial therapy can potentially be changed early during the course of therapy. If there is a good response, the initial therapy can potentially be modified to decrease potential toxicity (e.g., omission of bleomycin in the treatment of Hodgkin's disease). PET is particularly valuable in this setting, as response early during therapy often does not result in change on conventional imaging modalities. Currently, interim PET is primarily recommended in the context of clinical trials.

End of treatment. The goal of imaging is to evaluate response after completion of therapy and predict future outcome. PET is particularly valuable as conventional imaging techniques are often not able to differentiate tumor from scar tissue.

12.3 Pearls

1. Definition of response:
   a) There have been two published general criteria for defining response which are applicable to all tumors. One early proposed general criterion, evolved through a consensus meeting in February 1998, is the European Organization for Research and Treatment of Cancer (EORTC) PET Criteria published in 1999.[2] The Positron Emission Tomography Response Criteria in Solid Tumors (PERCIST)[3] was published in 2009;

the salient points and differences between EORTC and PERCIST are illustrated in ▶ Table 12.1.
   b) The EORTC and PERCIST criteria address the issue of whether changes in metabolic uptake are significant with regard to reproducibility, rather than the issue what changes in metabolic uptake constitute differences in outcome (histopathological response, or changes in disease-free or overall survival). For the latter question, the definition of response is specific to the particular tumor, specific therapy, and the timing of the study, and substantially greater changes in metabolic activity (e.g., 50–80%) are necessary. Published thresholds (amount of decrease in activity) to define response in this setting are usually specific to particular tumors, time intervals, and treatment methods. These are likely applicable only in those scenarios. If published thresholds are used, the method of standardized uptake value (SUV) determination used and the time intervals of imaging after therapy should be duplicated as closely as possible.

2. **Reproducibility.** Reproducibility of tumor uptake measurements is better if studies are performed in the same center on the same scanner. In single-center studies, the coefficient of variation in tumor FDG uptake in serial studies has been about 10 to 15%.[4] However, this is greater if different scanners are used for the baseline and follow-up scans. In multicenter trials, the variation in FDG uptake in serial studies has been 30 to 40%.[4,5]
   a) The mean difference in serial SUV measurements is around 10%.[6,7,8]
   b) For most lesions, changes in SUV greater than 20% are outside the 95% range for spontaneous fluctuation and can potentially be considered to reflect true changes in glucose metabolism.[8]
   c) However, the range of spontaneous fluctuation depends on the initial SUV. The higher the SUV, the less the range of fluctuation.[8]

3. **Non-SUV metrics**.[9] SUV measurements are feasible for the measurement of tumor response in the majority of cases, and are the easiest method to implement in a busy clinical practice.

Table 12.1 Salient differentiating points between the EORTC criteria and the PERCIST criteria

Characteristic	EORTC	PERCIST
Measurability of lesion at baseline	1. In baseline scan, ROI is drawn over the region in the tumor having greatest SUVmax. Also the entire tumor uptake is noted 2. Same ROI volume should be as far as possible and should be as close to the original tumor 3. Uptake should be noted in terms of SUVmax or SUVmean (unit: MBq/L) 4. Changes in the extent of tumor should be noted 5. Size of tumor should be measured wherever possible by anatomical imaging wherever possible (owing to lesser spatial resolution of PET)	1. Measurable target lesion is the single hottest lesion having the highest SUL within a ROI volume drawn having a greatest diameter of 1.2 cm. The SULpeak should be at least 1.5 times greater than SULmean + 2 SD (ROI in right lobe of liver should be 3 cm spherical ROI). If the liver is diseased then the SULpeak should be more than two times the SULmean over a 1-cm spherical ROI over the thoracic aorta extended over 2 cm in z-axis. 2. Maximal SULpeak is assessed. Preferable similar region of tumor is assessed, but it may not be always so. 3. Uptake measurements should be made peak and maximal single voxel tumor SUL. Other PET metrics like SULmean at 50 and 70% of SULpeak and total lesion glycolysis can be collected as exploratory data. 4. Maximum 5 lesions; typically the 5 hottest target lesions, and not more than 2 lesions per organ are considered
Normalization of uptake	All the scanners should be able to produce similar data. An empirical variation of 25% was found to be a useful cutoff point, but more studies are required to find out appropriate cutoffs of statistical significance	Normal SUL of the liver must be within 20% (or < 0.3 units of SUL) in between and baseline and post therapy scans. If liver is diseased, blood pool SUL must be within 20% (or < 0.3 units of SUL) in between and baseline and post therapy scans. Uptake time between the baseline study and posttherapy study must be 15 min within each other. Typically, these are at a mean of 60 min and should not be less than 50 min. Same scanner, similar injected dose, same acquisition protocol, same method of reconstruction should be used. Scanners should be properly calibrated and provide reproducible data
Objective response	CMR: Complete resolution of all the FDG avid lesions so that it is similar to the surrounding tissue PMR: Reduction of > 15% in SUV after first cycle of chemotherapy and > 25% after first cycle of chemotherapy. SMD: Increase in tumor SUV < 25% or decrease in tumor SUV < 15% and not more than 20% increase in extent of tumor. PMD: Increase in tumor SUV > 25% and increase in extent of tumor (20% increase in greatest dimension). Nonmeasurable lesions: CR disappearance of all lesions at 4 wk; PR decrease of at least 50% at 4 wk; PD is increase of at least 25% in existing lesions and NC is when PR or PD criteria is not met	CMR: Complete resolution of all the FDG avid lesions so that it is similar to liver or to blood pool. No new lesions are noted. Also percentage decline in SUL levels are recorded at specific time interval. PMR: Reduction of > 30% in SULpeak. Also absolute drop should be more than 0.8 units. Comparison should be preferable in the same lesion, but another lesion may be considered if it is the hottest lesion. ROI should preferably be in the same region. Also there should no increase in size of tumor (no PD as per RECIST). No new lesions should be seen. Also percentage decline in SUL levels is recorded at specific time interval SMD: no CMR, PMR, or PMD is seen PMD: increase of at least > 30% in SULpeak. Also absolute increase should be more than 0.8 units or appearance of new lesions or visible increase in extent of tumor uptake (75% in TLG with no decline in SUL) Except for visceral lesions, PMD should be followed up in 1 mo. Also percentage change in SUVpeak at what time intervals should also be noted. For this percentage change evaluation, the five hottest measurable lesions should be considered. Nonmeasurable lesions: CMR is complete disappearance of all lesions; PMD is unequivocal increase in nontarget lesions or appearance of new lesions; non-PMD is persistence of one or more nontarget lesions

Table 12.1 continued

Characteristic	EORTC	PERCIST
Overall response		1. Best response is measurable disease from treatment start to progression or recurrence 2. Non-PMD in measurable or no measurable target lesions will reduce CR in target lesion to overall PMR 3. Non-PMD in nontarget lesions will reduce PR in target lesions
Duration of response		1. Overall CMR: date from where CMR was achieved to date of recurrence 2. Overall response: date from where CMR or PMR was achieved to date of recurrence 3. SMD: from date of treatment to date at which PMD was noted

Abbreviations: CMR, complete metabolic response; EORTC, European Organization for Research and Treatment of Cancer; PERCIST, Positron Emission Tomography Response Criteria in Solid Tumors; PMR, partial metabolic response; PMD, progressive metabolic disease; ROI, region of interest; SMD, stable metabolic disease; SUV, standardized uptake value; TLG, total lesion glycosis.
Source: Adapted from Wahl et al.[3]

Patients with diabetes mellitus in particular may benefit from tracer kinetic approaches, as clearance and distribution of FDG may be altered. Recent PET-CT scanners provide advanced software packages, which provide readily available parameters such as metabolic tumor volume and metabolic index (max) and metabolic index (mean); some of these parameters are discussed in Chapter 6. Some other special softwares also provide partial volume-corrected SUV (pvcSUV), global metabolic burden, or whole body metabolic burden as additional parameters for PET quantification (▶ Fig. 12.1).

4. **Midtreatment versus posttreatment results**.[10] A given treatment dose of radiation or chemotherapy will typically kill the same fraction rather than the same number cells regardless of the size of the tumor. Thus, small tumors may still require multiple cycles of therapy to cure. This has implications for the interpretation of PET results in therapy response. As the resolution of PET is limited for small tumor volumes, PET can likely detect only the first few log units (90% reduction in tumor mass) of tumor cell killing. Thus, a tumor that is PET negative after therapy may still require multiple cycles of therapy to eliminate. Midtreatment and posttreatment PET results often have different implications.

    a) *Midtreatment.* Midtreatment PET scans provide information on the rate of tumor cell killing. A negative PET scan after a few cycles of therapy implies that the rate of tumor cell killing is sufficient to produce cure if the therapy is completed. While the negative PET scan could be seen with a few or many log units of tumor cell killing, even a few log units of response early in the therapy cycle implies a rapid rate of response. A positive PET scan implies that the rate of tumor cell killing may be inadequate to produce cure if the entire cycle is completed.

    b) *Posttreatment.* A positive PET scan after completion of therapy usually indicates a slow rate of tumor cell killing and a resistant cancer, as many cycles of therapy have not resulted in even a few log units of tumor cell killing. However, a negative posttreatment PET scan could have two possible implications. Due to limited resolution, a negative posttreatment PET scan cannot differentiate between a few log units and many log units of tumor cell killing (i.e., between minimal residual disease and complete response). Thus, a negative posttreatment PET scan typically has a lower predictive value than a negative midtreatment scan. High sensitivity is usually preferred to specificity in the posttherapy setting, as false-negative results are usually less desirable than false-positive results.

5. Variable response in different lesions in the same patient (▶ Fig. 12.2) indicates tumor heterogeneity, which may contribute to tumor treatment resistance.

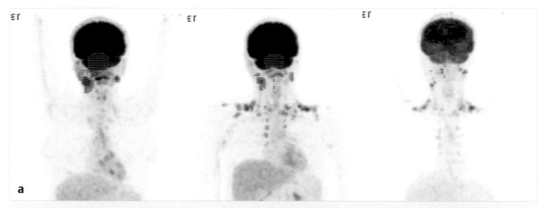

Fig. 12.1 **(a)** A 22 year-old male initially presenting with right-side neck swelling, which on FNAC (from right level II node) showed metastatic undifferentiated carcinoma likely arising from nasopharynx; CT nasopharynx showed mildly enhancing lesion in the right lateral wall and right half of roof of nasopharynx and biopsy from demonstrated undifferentiated carcinoma with staging as T3cN2M0. Baseline FDG-PET/CT (left column) showed metabolically active disease in the nasopharynx and bilateral cervical lymph node groups. The patient underwent two cycles of chemotherapy with paclitaxel, ifosfamide, and cisplatin. Postchemo PET-CT (midcolumn) showed persistence of lesions but decrease in the metabolic activity in them indicating partial response to therapy. He underwent further five cycles of chemotherapy with paclitaxel, ifosfamide, and cisplatin followed by 35 cycles of radiotherapy (70 Gy/35#/55 days). Follow-up FDG-PET/CT (right column) at 8 months of initial diagnosis showed complete metabolic response in the primary as well as in the lymph node groups. (*Continued*)

a) However, if there is a lack of response in one region and response in all other regions, a nonneoplastic etiology in the nonresponding region should be considered (▶ Fig. 12.3).

6. **Normal tissue response.** Increased inflammatory uptake in normal tissues postradiation positively correlates with tumor response. Normal tissue radiosensitivity may correlate with tumor radiosensitivity.[11]

7. **Increases versus decreases in SUV**. In general, a larger percentage change is needed to indicate a true metabolic change when the uptake increases, compared to decreasing uptake. For example, a decrease in SUV from 5 to 4 is a 20% change, and an increase in SUV from 4 to 5 is a 25% change, but the variability is the same in both cases. In an analysis of SUV repeatability in two multicenter trials,[4] decreases in uptake by more than 30% and increases of more than 40% were unlikely to represent measurement variability.

12.4 Pitfalls

See Chapter 4 for recommended minimum scan times after therapy. Chemotherapy and radiotherapy can cause false-positive and false-negative results.

1. **False-positive results**:
   a) False-positive results are usually seen early after therapy. A false-positive flare phenomenon has been described in responders to tamoxifen,[12] in patients undergoing chemotherapy for liver metastases in the first 2 weeks,[13] and in patients with glioblastoma treated with chemotherapy.[14] In some cases, this may be associated with an improved response to therapy.[12,14]
   b) However, flare phenomenon seen on other modalities such as bone scan may not result in a similar flare phenomenon on PET.[15]
   c) After radiation, uptake around the periphery of a tumor may be secondary to a fibrous pseudocapsule.[16]

2. **False-negative results.** False-negative results from presumed tumor "stunning" are usually seen for a much longer time frame than false-positive results.

3. **SUV measurement error.** There are numerous potential sources of error in SUV measurement discussed in Chapters 5 and 9. Some sources of measurement error specific to therapy response are as follows:
   a) Decreases in size of the tumor will artifactually decrease SUVs due to partial volume effects.

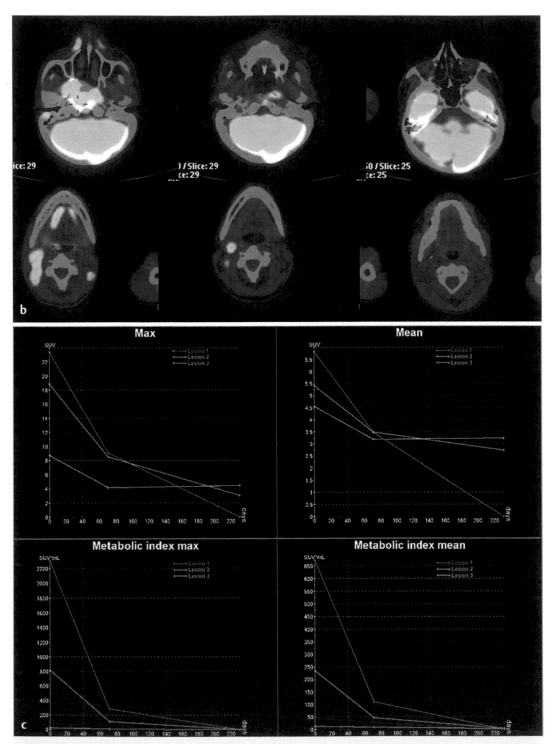

Fig. 12.1 (*continued*) **(b)** The graphical representation and **(c)** the tabular format of SUVmax, SUVmean, metabolic index (max), and metabolic index (mean) in the primary and two prominent cervical lymph node sites are demonstrated in the pretreatment and posttreatment PET-CT studies. (Reproduced with permission from Basu et al.[1])

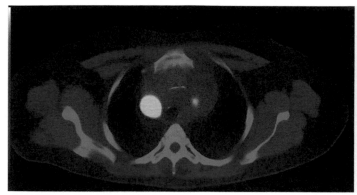

Fig. 12.2 Mixed tumor response. Axial PET/CT scan demonstrates extensive superior and anterior mediastinal adenopathy in a lymphoma patient posttherapy. Most of the nodes do not have increased FDG uptake, but two of the nodes have intense increased uptake. This finding often indicates increased tumor resistance to treatment.

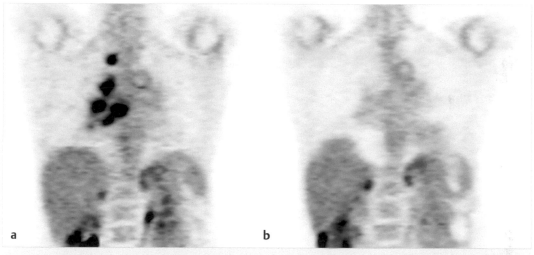

Fig. 12.3 False-positive uptake or mixed response? **(a)** Coronal PET scan demonstrates extensive right lung and mediastinal disease along with bilateral adrenal uptake in a patient with small cell lung cancer. The adrenal uptake was initially interpreted as adrenal metastasis. **(b)** Coronal PET scan after therapy demonstrates complete resolution of the lung and mediastinal uptake. The bilateral adrenal uptake is slightly increased. This lack of concordance in a single region suggests that the adrenal uptake is nonneoplastic. The uptake was secondary to adrenal hyperplasia.

b) Changes in the surrounding background activity between exams can affect the degree of "spill in" of background activity and thus the SUV.[16]

4. **Infection.** Infection is always a potential cause of false-positive PET results; however, it should be more strongly considered in patients who have received bone-marrow suppressing therapies.

5. **Lack of baseline PET study.** The lack of a baseline PET exam can result in both false-positive and false-negative results.

a) **False positives.** High levels of FDG uptake after therapy may not indicate therapy failure if the level of uptake prior to therapy was even greater. In this case, the response may have been partial.

b) **False negatives.** Minimal FDG uptake after therapy may not indicate therapy response if there was minimal uptake prior to therapy.

c) **Low pretherapy FDG uptake.** Lesions with low initial FDG uptake (SUV < 3 or tumor-to-background ratio < 5) may have a lower maximum detectable percentage change in SUV.[17,18] This may be secondary to a background of unmetabolized FDG included in SUV measurements.[17] This suggests that SUV measurements are less sensitive in detecting response in lesions with low initial FDG uptake. Measurements of the metabolic rate of FDG may be more helpful in lesions with low initial uptake.

6. **Cortical bone lesions**. Cortical bone lesions may be more difficult to assess for treatment response than marrow lesions. Cortical lesions often heal more slowly than marrow lesions and osseous remodeling can result in prolonged FDG uptake which limits assessment of residual malignancy.

7. **Hepatic and splenic lesions**. If hepatic and splenic involvement is demonstrated by initial staging, these lesions should usually be followed by contrast-enhanced CT or contrast-enhanced PET/CT. These lesions may be difficult to detect by PET and noncontrast PET/CT if they decrease in size after therapy.[19]

8. **Lung lesions.** SUV measurement variability in the lungs is higher, possibly due to respiratory motion.[4]

12.4.1 Disease-Specific PET Response Evaluation Criteria

Disease-specific PET response evaluation criteria have been developed in various malignancies, and noted among them is lymphoma. The lymphoma-specific response evaluation criteria include

a) Imaging Subcommittee of the International Harmonization Project in Lymphoma: IHP criteria—2007.[19]

b) Second, third, and fourth International Workshops on Positron Emission Tomography in Lymphoma held in 2010, 2011, and 2012 in Menton, France. The most recent one, known as Deauville's five-point scale criteria, published its report in 2014[20] and is recommended for clinical routine and clinical trials using FDG-PET/CT in the initial staging and assessment of treatment response in Hodgkin's lymphoma (HL) and FDG avid non-Hodgkin's lymphomas (NHL).

12.4.2 Salient Points in Deauville's Five-Point Score–Based Response Assessment

The two reference organs for assessment of FDG uptake are (1) mediastinum (blood pool) and (2) liver. The scale of FDG uptake ranges from 1 to 5, where 1 is best and 5 is the worst.

Each FDG avid lesion is scored as below:

1. No uptake.
2. Uptake ≤ mediastinum.
3. Uptake > mediastinum but ≤ liver.
4. Uptake moderately higher than liver.
5. Uptake markedly higher than liver and/or new lesions.
6. New areas of uptake unlikely to be related to lymphoma.

12.4.3 Definition of Response by Deauville's Criteria

• **Complete response (CR):** scores 1, 2, or 3 together with the absence of FDG avid bone marrow lesion(s) are interpreted as complete metabolic response (CR), irrespective of a persistent mass on CT

• **Partial response (PR):** Deauville score of 4 or 5, provided
  ○ uptake is decreased compared with baseline and
  ○ absence of structural progression development on CT

• **Stable disease (SD):** Deauville's score of 4 or 5 without significant change in FDG uptake from baseline.

• **Progressive disease (PD):** Deauville's score of 4 to 5 with increasing intensity compared to baseline or any interim scan and/or any new FDG avid focus consistent with malignant lymphoma.

References

[1] Basu S, Kumar R, Ranade R. Assessment of treatment response using PET. PET Clin. 2015; 10(1):9–26

[2] Young H, Baum R, Cremerius U, et al. European Organization for Research and Treatment of Cancer (EORTC) PET Study Group. Measurement of clinical and subclinical tumour response using [18F]-fluorodeoxyglucose and positron emission tomography: review and 1999 EORTC recommendations. Eur J Cancer. 1999; 35(13):1773–1782

[3] Wahl RL, Jacene H, Kasamon Y, Lodge MA. From RECIST to PERCIST: evolving considerations for PET response criteria in solid tumors. J Nucl Med. 2009; 50 Suppl 1:122S–150S

[4] Weber WA, Gatsonis CA, Mozley PD, et al. ACRIN 6678 Research Team, MK-0646–008 Research Team. Repeatability of 18F-FDG PET/CT in advanced non-small cell lung cancer: prospective assessment in 2 multicenter trials. J Nucl Med. 2015; 56(8):1137–1143

[5] Frings V, van Velden FH, Velasquez LM, et al. Repeatability of metabolically active tumor volume measurements with FDG PET/CT in advanced gastrointestinal malignancies: a multicenter study. Radiology. 2014; 273(2):539–548

[6] Minn H, Zasadny KR, Quint LE, Wahl RL. Lung cancer: reproducibility of quantitative measurements for evaluating 2-[F-18]-fluoro-2-deoxy-D-glucose uptake at PET. Radiology. 1995; 196(1):167–173

[7] Nakamoto Y, Zasadny KR, Minn H, Wahl RL. Reproducibility of common semi-quantitative parameters for evaluating lung

cancer glucose metabolism with positron emission tomography using 2-deoxy-2-[18F]fluoro-D-glucose. Mol Imaging Biol. 2002; 4(2):171–178

[8] Weber WA, Ziegler SI, Thödtmann R, Hanauske AR, Schwaiger M. Reproducibility of metabolic measurements in malignant tumors using FDG PET. J Nucl Med. 1999; 40(11):1771–1777

[9] Avril NE, Weber WA. Monitoring response to treatment in patients utilizing PET. Radiol Clin North Am. 2005; 43(1):189–204

[10] Kasamon YL, Jones RJ, Wahl RL. Integrating PET and PET/CT into the risk-adapted therapy of lymphoma. J Nucl Med. 2007; 48 Suppl 1:19S–27S

[11] Hicks RJ, Mac Manus MP, Matthews JP, et al. Early FDG-PET imaging after radical radiotherapy for non-small-cell lung cancer: inflammatory changes in normal tissues correlate with tumor response and do not confound therapeutic response evaluation. Int J Radiat Oncol Biol Phys. 2004; 60(2):412–418

[12] Mortimer JE, Dehdashti F, Siegel BA, Trinkaus K, Katzenellenbogen JA, Welch MJ. Metabolic flare: indicator of hormone responsiveness in advanced breast cancer. J Clin Oncol. 2001; 19(11):2797–2803

[13] Findlay M, Young H, Cunningham D, et al. Noninvasive monitoring of tumor metabolism using fluorodeoxyglucose and positron emission tomography in colorectal cancer liver metastases: correlation with tumor response to fluorouracil. J Clin Oncol. 1996; 14(3):700–708

[14] De Witte O, Hildebrand J, Luxen A, Goldman S. Acute effect of carmustine on glucose metabolism in brain and glioblastoma. Cancer. 1994; 74(10):2836–2842

[15] Shimizu N, Masuda H, Yamanaka H, Oriuchi N, Inoue T, Endo K. Fluorodeoxyglucose positron emission tomography scan of prostate cancer bone metastases with flare reaction after endocrine therapy. J Urol. 1999; 161(2):608–609

[16] Soret M, Bacharach SL, Buvat I. Partial-volume effect in PET tumor imaging. J Nucl Med. 2007; 48(6):932–945

[17] Doot RK, Dunnwald LK, Schubert EK, et al. Dynamic and static approaches to quantifying 18F-FDG uptake for measuring cancer response to therapy, including the effect of granulocyte CSF. J Nucl Med. 2007; 48(6):920–925

[18] McDermott GM, Welch A, Staff RT, et al. Monitoring primary breast cancer throughout chemotherapy using FDG-PET. Breast Cancer Res Treat. 2007; 102(1):75–84

[19] Juweid ME, Stroobants S, Hoekstra OS, et al. Imaging Subcommittee of International Harmonization Project in Lymphoma. Use of positron emission tomography for response assessment of lymphoma: consensus of the Imaging Subcommittee of International Harmonization Project in Lymphoma. J Clin Oncol. 2007; 25(5):571–578

[20] Meignan M, Barrington S, Itti E, Gallamini A, Haioun C, Polliack A. Report on the 4th International Workshop on Positron Emission Tomography in Lymphoma held in Menton, France, 3–5 October 2012. Leuk Lymphoma. 2014; 55(1):31–37

13 Brain Neoplasms

Eugene C. Lin

13.1 Primary Brain Tumors[1]

Although FDG PET imaging may not be indicated in the majority of newly diagnosed brain tumors, it is useful in specific situations. It should be noted that FDG PET is intrinsically limited for assessing brain tumors due to generally low tumor-to-background contrast. FDG uptake in low-grade tumors is often similar to white matter, while FDG uptake in high-grade tumors may be less than or similar to gray matter. Amino acid tracers, such as 11C-methyl-L-methioninine (MET), 18F-fluoro-ethyl-tyrosine (FET), and 18F-FDOPA generally have higher tumor-to-background contrast due to high uptake in neoplasms and low uptake in normal brain parenchyma.[2] However, this chapter will focus on FDG PET, which is mostly utilized in clinical practice. Possible clinical applications include

1. **Determining the best biopsy site for optimal grading of the tumor.** Despite the overall low degree of FDG uptake in low-grade gliomas, PET may be more useful for stereotactic biopsy target selection in low-grade gliomas (inhomogeneous gliomas without contrast enhancement) than in high-grade gliomas[3] as contrast enhancement can be used in the latter case.
2. **Metabolic grading of the tumor.** The degree of glucose metabolism correlates with prognosis and outcome in these patients (▶ Fig. 13.1). This is independent of other prognostic factors.[4] For example, in one study,[5] hypometabolic

low-grade gliomas were associated with a longer average survival compared to hypermetabolic low-grade gliomas. In one report,[6] the accuracy of FDG PET/CT for grading glioma was superior to that of MRI.
In a meta-analysis,[7] 18F-FET PET was much more accurate than FDG PET for the brain tumor diagnosis (distinguishing tumoral from nontumoral lesions), but both tracers performed similarly for glioma grading.

3. **Evaluating possible transformation of a low-grade glioma to a high-grade tumor.** Increased FDG uptake in a previously diagnosed low-grade lesion is suggestive of malignant transformation and associated with decreased survival.[8]

13.2 Pearls

1. **Factors affecting FDG uptake:**
   a) **Corticosteroids.** Corticosteroids decrease glucose metabolism in normal brain tissue, but do not affect metabolism within brain tumors. However, corticosteroid administration will limit evaluation of brain tumors, as overall image quality and anatomic detail are adversely affected.[9,10] Many of the effects of corticosteroids may be due to increased blood glucose levels.
   b) **Cushing's disease.** Patients with Cushing's disease have decreased brain glucose metabolism.

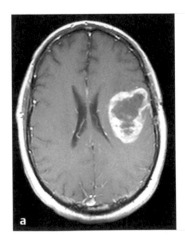
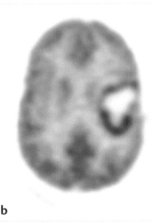

a

b

Fig. 13.1 High-grade glioma. **(a)** Axial MRI scan demonstrates peripheral enhancement of a left frontal high-grade glioma. **(b)** Axial PET scan demonstrates intense uptake greater than gray matter corresponding to the enhancement seen on MRI.

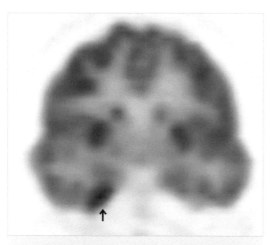

Fig. 13.2 Meningioma. Coronal PET scan demonstrates focal uptake (*arrow*) along the medial surface of the right temporal lobe corresponding to a meningioma.

c) **Sedatives and anticonvulsants:** Sedatives and anticonvulsants can also reduce glucose metabolism.

d) **Gray matter uptake of FDG.** Uptake of FDG is substantially reduced in any area of the brain which is adjacent to white matter edema seen on magnetic resonance imaging (MRI) or computed tomography (CT) images. This is probably a reversible process and should disappear with reduction in the degree of edema.[10] The decreased gray matter uptake secondary to edema may improve the contrast between the tumor and adjacent structures.

e) **Glucose level.** High blood glucose decreases FDG uptake in both the tumor and the cortex, but there is a greater decrease in cortical activity; thus, often a higher tumor-to-background ratio is noted in hyperglycemic states.

f) **Hyperglycemia.** While most patients should not be scanned in a hyperglycemic state, a high blood glucose may potentially be advantageous in the detection of tumors near or in the cortex.[11]

g) **Delayed imaging.** Delayed imaging (3–8 hours after injection) increases uptake in the tumor relative to normal brain. This is most helpful in tumors near the gray matter.[12]

2. **Standardized uptake value (SUV).** SUV may not be as useful in the brain, as it may not correlate well with regional glucose metabolism. Tumor to white matter or cortex ratios may be preferable.[13]

13.3 Pitfalls

1. **False negatives.** Small low-grade neoplasms are often undetectable on PET. A minority of high-grade tumors are also undetectable on PET.

2. **False positives:**
   a) Low-grade neoplasms such as pilocytic astrocytoma, pleomorphic xanthoastrocytoma, ganglioglioma, and oligodendroglioma can be hypermetabolic.[13,14]
   b) Benign lesions such as meningioma (▶ Fig. 13.2), pituitary adenoma (▶ Fig. 13.3), and histiocytosis X can be hypermetabolic.
      • There is a substantial range of uptake in meningiomas, with some lesions as high as normal gray matter, while others are hypometabolic. Glucose consumption in meningiomas may be related to tumor aggressiveness and probability of recurrence.[15]
   c) Seizures at the time of FDG administration can cause false-positive results due to activated cortex adjacent to the tumor site.
   d) A hypermetabolic flare phenomenon may be seen in glioblastoma treated with chemotherapy if PET is performed 24 hours after the first dose.[5] This may predict longer survival.

13.4 Tumor versus Radiation Necrosis

It is often difficult to differentiate tumor recurrence versus radiation necrosis on CT or MRI, as both entities demonstrate contrast enhancement. FDG PET is valuable in this situation (▶ Fig. 13.4, ▶ Fig. 13.5). This is the main indication for performing FDG PET imaging in patients with brain tumors.[16]

13.4.1 Accuracy/Comparison to Other Modalities

1. **FDG PET for recurrent glioma** (meta-analysis). Sensitivity 77%, specificity 78%[17]:
   a) MRI coregistration may increase sensitivity for tumor recurrence.[18] The sensitivity is 65% without MRI coregistration compared to 86% with coregistration.

2. **Magnetic resonance spectroscopy (MRS).** In a meta-analysis,[19] PET and MRS had comparable accuracy, but MRS had the highest pooled sensitivity and PET had the highest pooled specificity.

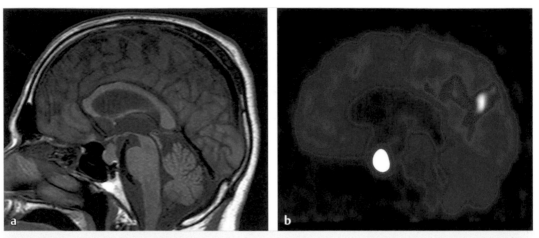

Fig. 13.3 Pituitary adenoma. **(a)** Sagittal T1-weighted MRI scan demonstrates a pituitary macroadenoma. **(b)** Sagittal PET scan demonstrates intense uptake in this adenoma.

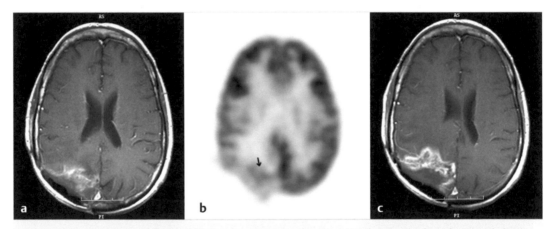

Fig. 13.4 Tumor recurrence. **(a)** Axial MRI scan demonstrates enhancement at the margin of a right parietal glioma resection site postradiation, equivocal for radiation necrosis vs. tumor. **(b)** Axial PET scan demonstrates increased uptake (*arrow*) in the area of enhancement seen on MRI, consistent with tumor recurrence. Note that it is important to differentiate this activity from normal gray matter activity decreased in intensity postradiation. There was no gray matter in this region by MRI correlation. **(c)** Follow-up axial MRI done several months after the PET scan demonstrates further increased enhancement in this region which now has the exact configuration as the uptake seen on PET.

3. **Thallium SPECT**. Compared to thallium SPECT, PET has higher specificity but lower sensitivity.[20] Thallium SPECT may be more valuable in the assessment of low-grade glioma recurrence.

13.5 Pearls

1. **Imaging correlation.** Correlation with MRI and CT scans is extremely helpful. Without such correlation, the findings from PET will often be misinterpreted.

2. **Postsurgical changes.** Postsurgical changes usually do not cause significant increased uptake and will not interfere with PET imaging for tumor recurrence.[14]

3. **Radiation effects:**
   a) In most cases, a hypometabolic area will be seen following radiation adjacent to and distant from the primary tumor. This finding could be secondary to edema.[16]
   b) Occasionally, there can be increased uptake in the tumor after radiation, likely related to migration of macrophages to the radiated

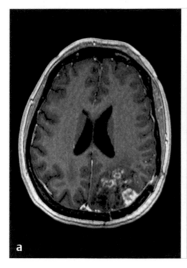 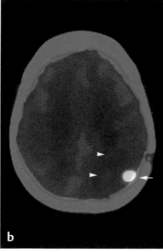

Fig. 13.5 Different levels of uptake in tumor recurrence. Three foci of enhancement in the left parietal lobe are seen on a contrast-enhanced MRI **(a)** in a patient status post resection of a left parietal glioma and radiation. **(b)** The two medial foci (*arrowheads*) demonstrate mild uptake greater than white matter on axial PET/CT. Using this level of uptake as a criterion for tumor recurrence would increase sensitivity but decrease specificity. The larger peripheral focus (*arrows*) demonstrates intense uptake greater than gray matter. Using this level of uptake as a criterion for tumor recurrence would decrease sensitivity but increase specificity.

site. This uptake is usually diffuse and moderate (between white and gray matter). In rare cases, the uptake is nodular and greater than or equal to gray matter, and cannot be differentiated from recurrent tumor.[14]

c) Intracavitary radioimmunotherapy can cause increased FDG accumulation (rim of increased uptake). The peripheral increased activity in this case is usually not secondary to tumor. However, if the activity is nodular, tumor recurrence is likely.[14]

4. Interpretation criteria:

a) ***Visual interpretation criteria***. The main criterion for diagnosing recurrence of tumor on PET is relatively increased uptake compared to the adjacent or contralateral white matter.

The ipsilateral white matter may be less suitable as a reference because[21]

- Tumor cells may infiltrate around a focal lesion causing diffuse increased white matter uptake ipsilaterally.

- Areas of encephalomalacia from prior surgery can cause apparent decreased white matter uptake. However, this will be apparent when PET and MRI images are compared.

Uptake greater than contralateral gray matter can also be used as a criterion for a positive study (▶ Fig. 13.5): this increases specificity but decreases sensitivity.[21] We do not advocate this as an optimal criterion, as the majority of recurrences will be false negative.

b) **SUV:**

- In one study,[22] a SUVmax cutoff of 5.7 had a 75% accuracy for detection of progression, and a normalized SUVmax (ratio of SUV in the lesion to the SUV in the contralateral normal white matter) cutoff of 1.9 had an accuracy of 83%. Glucose-corrected SUVmax > 4.3[23] has also been used to differentiate recurrent high-grade glioma from posttreatment change.

  Combining MRS (normalized choline/creatinine ratio) and PET results (normalized SUVmax) improves accuracy.[22]

5. Low-grade brain tumors are usually hypometabolic, and therefore it might be thought that differentiation of radiation necrosis versus tumor may pose a challenge in these patients. However, in most cases, recurrence is typically of the high-grade type and is hypermetabolic on PET. The degree of uptake does reflect the aggressiveness of the recurrent tumor.

6. Typically PET scan is ordered because enhancement is seen on MRI which is nondiagnostic for tumor versus radiation necrosis. It is important to determine the exact location of the area of enhancement seen on MRI on the PET scan, either by visual comparison or with coregistration of the two image sets.

a) Any area of increased activity on PET should correspond to an area of enhancement on MRI before it is interpreted as tumor activity. However, the area of PET uptake may be slightly larger than the area of MRI enhancement (▶ Fig. 13.4). Areas of increased uptake

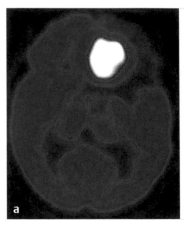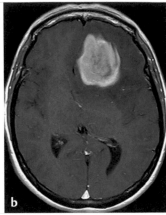

Fig. 13.6 CNS lymphoma. Axial PET **(a)** and contrast-enhanced MRI **(b)** in a patient with diffuse large B-cell lymphoma demonstrate intense uptake in an enhancing frontal lobe mass and decreased uptake in the surrounding edema. Both the intense uptake in the lesion and the decreased white matter uptake are helpful in differentiating CNS lymphoma from glioma.

definitely outside the enhancement area on MRI could represent other etiologies as a seizure focus in the cortex at the margin of the lesion.

13.6 Pitfalls

1. A seizure at the time of FDG administration can cause a false-positive result.
    a) Seizure foci are often seen in the cortex adjacent to the original tumor site.
2. If the recurrent tumor has a thin rim of tissue, PET may appear negative for tumor activity secondary to partial-volume effects.
3. Active small lesions near the cortex may be difficult to detect due to the high normal gray matter activity. Often, this does not pose a problem, as adjacent edema and/or prior radiation usually results in decreased normal gray matter activity and therefore improves lesion contrast. Fusion imaging with MRI is very helpful and should be employed to minimize errors related to such circumstances.
4. Avoiding imaging earlier than 3 to 4 months after radiation therapy may reduce false positives.[24]
5. Lesions involving the deep white matter and basal ganglia/thalamus can result in hypometabolism of the cortical gray matter secondary to disconnection; this has been described in primary central nervous system (CNS) lymphoma and gliomatosis cerebri.[25]
6. Accuracy is limited in lesions < 2 cm.[26]

13.7 Lymphoma

Potential uses of FDG PET in patients with known or suspected lymphoma include differentiation from glioma or toxoplasmosis. FDG PET can also be used to evaluate treatment response at an early stage, preceding changes on MRI. In addition, FDG uptake may have prognostic value in newly diagnosed primary CNS lymphoma.[25]

13.7.1 Lymphoma versus Glioma

Central nervous system lymphomas (▶ Fig. 13.6) have a significantly higher SUV than other enhancing brain lesions (e.g., gliomas and brain metastases). In addition, the FDG uptake in primary CNS lymphoma tends to be more homogeneous than the uptake in other brain tumors. In three studies,[27,28,29] SUVmax cutoffs of 12 and 15 differentiated primary CNS lymphoma from glioma or metastases. However, in one study,[30] the ratio of the SUV in the tumor to the normal contralateral cortex (cutoff 2.0) was more accurate than SUV in the primary tumor. The tumor to the ipsilateral white matter SUVmax ratio can also be helpful in lesions with markedly increased SUVmax. Since there may be a lesser degree of edema surrounding gliomas, this would result a higher metabolic activity in the white matter compared to lymphomas with more edema. A higher tumor to ipsilateral white matter SUVmax ratio (cutoff 4.65) may be helpful in differentiating lymphoma from gliomas with a high SUVmax.[31]

13.7.2 Lymphoma versus Toxoplasmosis

PET has been effective in differentiating lymphoma from toxoplasmosis in small series. Toxoplasmosis is hypometabolic, while lymphomas usually are hypermetabolic. PET may be superior to MRS in differentiating lymphoma from toxoplasmosis.[32]

13.8 Pitfalls

1. **Steroids.** Steroids have a cytotoxic effect in lymphoma, and reduce FDG uptake in the tumor.[25] This could potentially cause false-negative results.
2. **Primary CNS lymphoma.** Primary CNS lymphoma may demonstrate atypical radiological features such as disseminated or nonenhancing lesions. FDG PET/CT may be limited in these patients, as primary CNS lymphoma with atypical radiological findings may not demonstrate substantially increased FDG uptake.[25]
3. **Progressive multifocal leukoencephalopathy.** Progressive multifocal leukoencephalopathy can be hypermetabolic and cause a false-positive result.[33]

References

[1] Fullham MJ. Central Nervous System. Principles and Practice of Positron Emission Tomography. Philadelphia, PA: Lippincott Williams & Wilkins; 2002:276–297

[2] Galldiks N, Langen KJ, Pope WB. From the clinician's point of view - What is the status quo of positron emission tomography in patients with brain tumors? Neuro-oncol. 2015; 17 (11):1434–1444

[3] la Fougère C, Suchorska B, Bartenstein P, Kreth FW, Tonn JC. Molecular imaging of gliomas with PET: opportunities and limitations. Neuro-oncol. 2011; 13(8):806–819

[4] Colavolpe C, Metellus P, Mancini J, et al. Independent prognostic value of pre-treatment 18-FDG-PET in high-grade gliomas. J Neurooncol. 2012; 107(3):527–535

[5] De Witte O, Hildebrand J, Luxen A, Goldman S. Acute effect of carmustine on glucose metabolism in brain and glioblastoma. Cancer. 1994; 74(10):2836–2842

[6] Song PJ, Lu QY, Li MY, Li X, Shen F. Comparison of effects of 18F-FDG PET-CT and MRI in identifying and grading gliomas. J Biol Regul Homeost Agents. 2016; 30(3):833–838

[7] Dunet V, Pomoni A, Hottinger A, Nicod-Lalonde M, Prior JO. Performance of 18F-FET versus 18F-FDG-PET for the diagnosis and grading of brain tumors: systematic review and meta-analysis. Neuro-oncol. 2016; 18(3):426–434

[8] Wray R, Solnes L, Mena E, Meoded A, Subramaniam RM. (18) F-Flourodeoxy-glucose PET/computed tomography in brain tumors: value to patient management and survival outcomes. PET Clin. 2015; 10(3):423–430

[9] Fulham MJ, Brunetti A, Aloj L, Raman R, Dwyer AJ, Di Chiro G. Decreased cerebral glucose metabolism in patients with brain tumors: an effect of corticosteroids. J Neurosurg. 1995; 83(4):657–664

[10] Roelcke U, Blasberg RG, von Ammon K, et al. Dexamethasone treatment and plasma glucose levels: relevance for fluorine-18-fluorodeoxyglucose uptake measurements in gliomas. J Nucl Med. 1998; 39(5):879–884

[11] Ishizu K, Nishizawa S, Yonekura Y, et al. Effects of hyperglycemia on FDG uptake in human brain and glioma. J Nucl Med. 1994; 35(7):1104–1109

[12] Spence AM, Muzi M, Mankoff DA, et al. 18F-FDG PET of gliomas at delayed intervals: improved distinction between tumor and normal gray matter. J Nucl Med. 2004; 45(10): 1653–1659

[13] Bénard F, Romsa J, Hustinx R. Imaging gliomas with positron emission tomography and single-photon emission computed tomography. Semin Nucl Med. 2003; 33(2):148–162

[14] Wong TZ, van der Westhuizen GJ, Coleman RE. Positron emission tomography imaging of brain tumors. Neuroimaging Clin N Am. 2002; 12(4):615–626

[15] Cornelius JF, Langen KJ, Stoffels G, Hänggi D, Sabel M, Jakob Steiger H. Positron emission tomography imaging of meningioma in clinical practice: review of literature and future directions. Neurosurgery. 2012; 70(4):1033–1041, discussion 1042

[16] Hustinx R, Pourdehnad M, Kaschten B, Alavi A. PET imaging for differentiating recurrent brain tumor from radiation necrosis. Radiol Clin North Am. 2005; 43(1):35–47

[17] Nihashi T, Dahabreh IJ, Terasawa T. Diagnostic accuracy of PET for recurrent glioma diagnosis: a meta-analysis. AJNR Am J Neuroradiol. 2013; 34(5):944–950, S1–S11

[18] Chao ST, Suh JH, Raja S, Lee SY, Barnett G. The sensitivity and specificity of FDG PET in distinguishing recurrent brain tumor from radionecrosis in patients treated with stereotactic radiosurgery. Int J Cancer. 2001; 96(3):191–197

[19] Wang X, Hu X, Xie P, Li W, Li X, Ma L. Comparison of magnetic resonance spectroscopy and positron emission tomography in detection of tumor recurrence in posttreatment of glioma: a diagnostic meta-analysis. Asia Pac J Clin Oncol. 2015; 11(2): 97–105

[20] Alexiou GA, Tsiouris S, Kyritsis AP, Voulgaris S, Argyropoulou MI, Fotopoulos AD. Glioma recurrence versus radiation necrosis: accuracy of current imaging modalities. J Neurooncol. 2009; 95(1):1–11

[21] Ricci PE, Karis JP, Heiserman JE, Fram EK, Bice AN, Drayer BP. Differentiating recurrent tumor from radiation necrosis: time for re-evaluation of positron emission tomography? AJNR Am J Neuroradiol. 1998; 19(3):407–413

[22] Imani F, Boada FE, Lieberman FS, Davis DK, Mountz JM. Molecular and metabolic pattern classification for detection of brain glioma progression. Eur J Radiol. 2014; 83(2):e100–e105

[23] Nozawa A, Rivandi AH, Kanematsu M, et al. Glucose-corrected standardized uptake value in the differentiation of high-grade glioma versus post-treatment changes. Nucl Med Commun. 2015; 36(6):573–581

[24] Palumbo B. Brain tumour recurrence: brain single-photon emission computerized tomography, PET and proton magnetic resonance spectroscopy. Nucl Med Commun. 2008; 29 (8):730–735

[25] Kawai N, Miyake K, Yamamoto Y, Nishiyama Y, Tamiya T. 18F-FDG PET in the diagnosis and treatment of primary central nervous system lymphoma. BioMed Res Int. 2013; 2013: 247152

[26] Dankbaar JW, Snijders TJ, Robe PA, et al. The use of (18)F-FDG PET to differentiate progressive disease from treatment induced necrosis in high grade glioma. J Neurooncol. 2015; 125 (1):167–175

[27] Das K, Mittal BR, Vasistha RK, Singh P, Mathuriya SN. Role of (18)F-fluorodeoxyglucose positron emission tomography scan in differentiating enhancing brain tumors. Indian J Nucl Med. 2011; 26(4):171–176

[28] Kosaka N, Tsuchida T, Uematsu H, Kimura H, Okazawa H, Itoh H. 18F-FDG PET of common enhancing malignant brain tumors. AJR Am J Roentgenol. 2008; 190(6):W365–9

[29] Makino K, Hirai T, Nakamura H, et al. Does adding FDG-PET to MRI improve the differentiation between primary cerebral

lymphoma and glioblastoma? Observer performance study. Ann Nucl Med. 2011; 25(6):432–438

[30] Yamaguchi S, Hirata K, Kobayashi H, et al. The diagnostic role of (18)F-FDG PET for primary central nervous system lymphoma. Ann Nucl Med. 2014; 28(7):603–609

[31] Meric K, Killeen RP, Abi-Ghanem AS, et al. The use of 18F-FDG PET ratios in the differential diagnosis of common malignant brain tumors. Clin Imaging. 2015; 39(6):970–974

[32] Westwood TD, Hogan C, Julyan PJ, et al. Utility of FDG-PETCT and magnetic resonance spectroscopy in differentiating between cerebral lymphoma and non-malignant CNS lesions in HIV-infected patients. Eur J Radiol. 2013; 82(8):e374–e379

[33] Pierce MA, Johnson MD, Maciunas RJ, et al. Evaluating contrast-enhancing brain lesions in patients with AIDS by using positron emission tomography. Ann Intern Med. 1995; 123 (8):594–598

14 Head and Neck Cancer

Eugene C. Lin

14.1 Cervical Metastasis, Unknown Primary

1. PET can be useful for identifying the primary tumor in patients presenting with metastasis to cervical nodes if no primary site has been found by other tests (▶ Fig. 14.1, ▶ Fig. 14.2, ▶ Fig. 14.3). National Comprehensive Cancer Network (NCCN) guidelines[1] suggest that PET/CT scan (before random biopsies) should only be done if a needle biopsy reveals squamous cell carcinoma, adenocarcinoma, or anaplastic/undifferentiated cancer and no primary site has been found by other tests.
2. In addition, PET can identify unsuspected distant metastases and define regional disease in N2 patients.

14.2 Accuracy/Comparison to Other Modalities

1. **PET/CT for cervical nodal metastases of unknown primary site** (meta-analysis)[2]: Primary tumor detection rate of 30 to 44%, sensitivity of 97%, specificity of 68%.
   a) PET may have poor sensitivity in particular for occult tonsillar cancer.[3]
2. PET is more accurate than conventional imaging.[4]

14.2.1 Pearls/Pitfalls

1. The primary areas to search for primary tumors are the nasopharynx, base of tongue (▶ Fig. 14.1), tonsils (▶ Fig. 14.2), and pyriform sinuses (▶ Fig. 14.3).
2. **False-positive results**. False-positive results may arise from high metabolism in lymphatic tissue in Waldeyer's ring, salivary excretion, and swallowing movements. Physiological activity in these regions can both mimic and obscure a

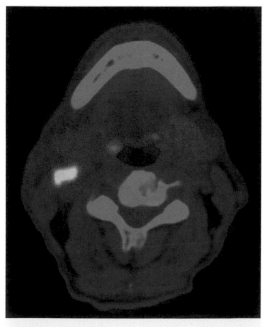

Fig. 14.1 Primary tumor localization: tongue base. Axial PET/CT in a patient with a malignant right neck node demonstrates uptake in the primary tumor in the right tongue base.

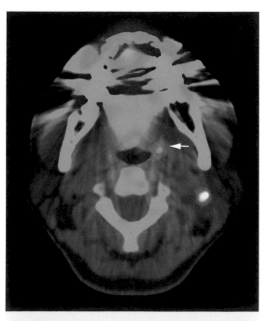

Fig. 14.2 Primary tumor localization: tonsil. Axial PET/CT in a patient with a malignant left neck node demonstrates uptake in the primary tumor in the left tonsil (*arrow*).

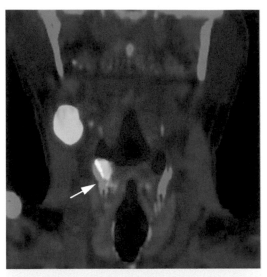

Fig. 14.3 Primary tumor localization: pyriform sinus. Coronal PET/CT in a patient with a malignant right neck node demonstrates uptake in the primary tumor in the right pyriform sinus (*arrow*).

primary tumor. The most common sites of false-positive results are in the tonsils (40%), the base of the tongue (20%), and the hypopharynx.[5,6]

a) The use of SUVmax ratios with the contralateral tonsil may be helpful in distinguishing tonsillar carcinoma from physiological uptake. In one report,[7] a cutoff SUVmax ratio of 1.48 was highly accurate in distinguishing tonsillar carcinoma from physiological uptake.

3. **False-negative results**. Primary tumors which are not identified by PET are generally superficial with a depth < 4 mm.[8]

4. **Timing of PET/CT**. Although some authors have suggested performing PET/CT after negative panendoscopy, random biopsies can result in false-positive PET/CT results. Performing PET/CT before endoscopy decreases the incidence of false-positive results.[6] The PET/CT results can then be used to direct biopsy.

a) If PET/CT is performed after biopsy, there is no clear "safe" time frame in which to perform the PET/CT. In one study,[9] numerous false-positive areas of FDG uptake were identified more than 5 weeks after biopsy.

14.3 Staging

NCCN guidelines[1] state that PET/CT may be considered in the workup of cancers of the nasopharynx, oral cavity, oropharynx, hypopharynx, larynx, and sinus. Evidence-based guidelines[10] recommend PET/CT in M and bilateral nodal staging of patients with head and neck squamous cell carcinoma where conventional imaging is equivocal or where treatment may significantly be modified. In particular, PET/CT is most helpful in patients with a moderate or high risk of distant metastatic disease (e.g., patients with nasopharyngeal carcinoma, stage III–IV diseases, or unexplained symptoms at earlier stages). PET/CT also has high accuracy in detecting synchronous second primary tumors. In addition, the degree of pretreatment FDG uptake also has prognostic significance. In a multicenter prospective trial,[11] the addition of PET to the pre-therapeutic conventional staging of patients with head and neck squamous cell carcinoma altered management in 13.7% of patients.

PET cannot replace CT or MRI for T staging. While clinically proven primary tumors are visualized by PET in the majority of cases, PET does not have the resolution to evaluate local spread. PET/CT is primarily valuable for nodal staging.

14.3.1 Nodal Staging

Although PET/CT is more accurate than CT or MRI for nodal metastases, it does not detect very small metastatic deposits (< 5 mm). Neck dissection in patients with a negative PET may be performed on pretest likelihood of metastatic disease (e.g., based on T-stage and histopathologic features). In patients with T4 disease, false-negative results are more likely and PET is less helpful. PET is more helpful in patients with T1 to T3 disease. The use of PET in this population can reduce the probability of occult neck metastases to less than 15%. In addition, false-positive results are not infrequent and are more common in the contralateral neck side, and in clinical N0 necks.[12,13] Pathologic confirmation should be considered for PET-positive nodes. PET/CT may have the most potential value where the probability of occult nodal metastases is higher (e.g., in patients with oral or oropharyngeal cancer). The sensitivity of PET in this setting is variable, ranging from 33 to 67%.[14,15,16]

14.3.2 Clinical N0 Neck

The use of PET/CT in staging patients with clinically N0 necks (negative neck palpation) is controversial. PET/CT is not recommended by some authors[5] in these patients. The goal of imaging would be to reduce the risk of occult metastases to below 15 to 20%, as patients with higher risk often undergo elective neck dissection or radiation treatment. For example, in one study,[17] PET/CT was more sensitive than CT or MRI for the nodal metastases, and a negative PET/CT reduced the probability of occult neck metastases in clinically N0 patients to 12%. In one meta-analysis,[18] the sensitivity of PET/CT was 79% overall but only 50% in clinical N0 patients (specificity was comparable). In another meta-analysis,[19] PET had a sensitivity of 48% and specificity of 86%. In the same meta-analysis,[19] a staging strategy of CT or MRI with sentinel node biopsy had the best performance in these patients. However, sentinel node biopsy may not be readily available for routine clinical use. As PET is insensitive compared to sentinel node biopsy, but specificity is high, one potential use of PET is to perform sentinel node biopsy if PET is negative and neck dissection if PET is positive. This may reduce the number of unnecessary neck dissections.[20]

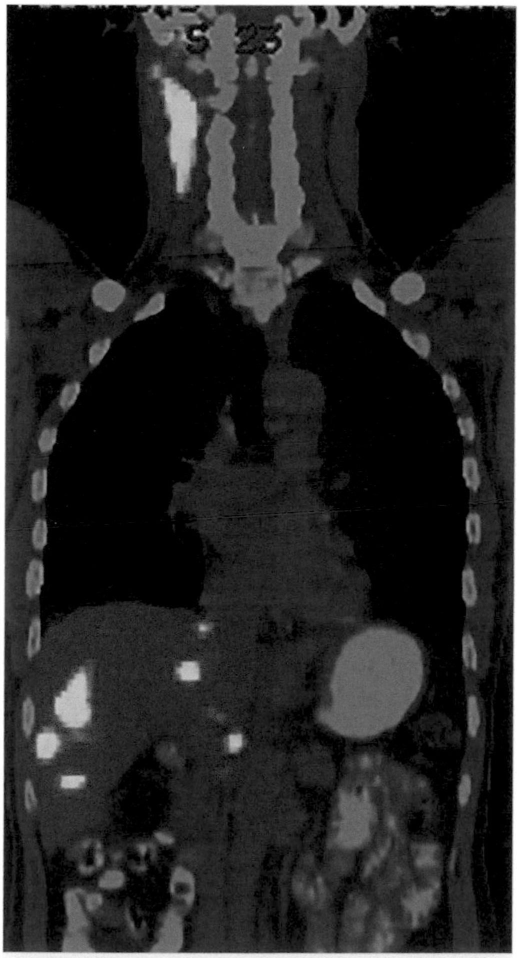

14.3.3 Detecting Distant Metastases

The most common sites of distant disease in head and neck cancer are the thorax, bones, and liver. PET can detect metastases in the mediastinum, bone marrow, and liver (▶ Fig. 14.4) but may be limited in the detection of small lung metastases. PET is particularly useful for detecting mediastinal disease in stage III and IV cancers.

14.3.4 Detection of Synchronous Lesions

The most common areas for second primary tumors are the lung (▶ Fig. 14.5) and aerodigestive tract (▶ Fig. 14.6).[21,22] The overall incidence of coincidental secondary primary tumors is 5 to 10%. PET has an accuracy of 80% for coincidental lung lesions. In one study,[23] PET/CT detected 84% of synchronous primaries, and therapy was changed in 80% of patients due to detection of synchronous primaries. In another study, PET/CT was superior to panendoscopy for the detection of

Fig. 14.4 Nasopharyngeal carcinoma with distant metastases. Coronal PET/CT in a patient with nasopharyngeal carcinoma demonstrates metastases to right cervical nodes and the liver.

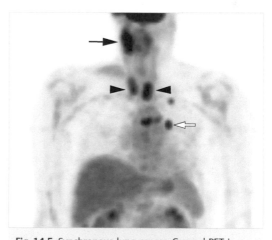

Fig. 14.5 Synchronous lung cancer. Coronal PET in a patient with a right parotid malignancy (*arrow*) demonstrates a synchronous left upper lobe lung cancer (*open arrow*) with mediastinal metastases and another nodule in the left apex. Uptake in the thyroid (*arrowheads*) is nonspecific but related to thyroiditis in this patient.

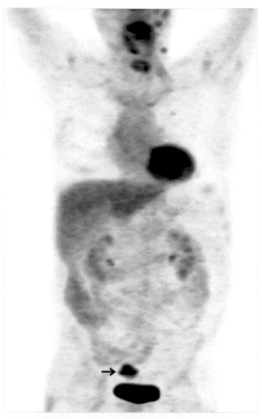

Fig. 14.6 Synchronous colon cancer. Coronal PET scan in a head and neck cancer patient with metastatic cervical nodes also demonstrates a synchronous sigmoid carcinoma (*arrow*).

synchronous primaries,[24] and the authors suggest that the extent of endoscopy can be reduced to the area of the primary tumor if PET/CT is negative.

14.3.5 Prognosis

Pretreatment tumor FDG uptake is an independent prognostic factor.[25] In a meta-analysis,[26] low FDG uptake before treatment is correlated with better disease-free survival, overall survival, and local control.

14.4 Accuracy/Comparison to Other Modalities

1. **Regional nodal metastases** (meta-analysis—per neck side analysis)[27]: Sensitivity of 84%, specificity of 84%.
2. **PET/CT for M staging** (meta-analysis)[28]: Sensitivity of 88%, specificity of 95%.

3. **PET/CT for bone metastases** (meta-analysis)[29]: Sensitivity of 89%, specificity of 99%.
   a) In comparative studies, PET and PET/CT are substantially more sensitive than bone scintigraphy (85 vs. 55%), but both modalities have comparable high specificity.[29]
4. **PET versus CT/MRI** (▶ Table 14.1)[21]:
   a) PET is more sensitive than CT and MRI and more specific than CT, MRI, and ultrasound.[21]

Table 14.1 Sensitivity and specificity of PET compared with other imaging modalities in the staging of head and neck cancer

	Sensitivity %	Specificity %
PET	87–90	80–93
CT/MRI	61–97	21–100

14.4.1 Pearls/Pitfalls

1. Knowledge of the common sites and incidence of cervical metastases for different primary tumors is helpful in the interpretation of PET scans.[30]
   a) Oral cavity tumors have high incidence of metastases despite being clinically node negative.
   b) Laryngeal tumors have a low incidence of metastases even in advanced stages of disease.
   c) Supraglottic larynx tumors often spread to nodes bilaterally (▶ Fig. 14.7).
   d) Nasopharyngeal tumors often spread to nodes bilaterally and to the posterior triangle (▶ Fig. 14.8).
2. The most common site of reactive lymphadenopathy is the jugulodigastric node. Reactive nodes are often enlarged and less intense than the primary and nodal metastases.[31]
3. **Scan volume.** It is helpful to include the abdomen and pelvis in the scan volume because of the possibility of coincidental tumors and distant metastases.
4. **Bone invasion.** In a meta-analysis,[32] PET/CT had a mean sensitivity of 83% and a mean specificity of 90% for the detection of mandibular invasion by head and neck cancers, compared to 96 and 66%, respectively, for SPECT. In patients with oral cancer, PET does not improve identification of bone infiltration compared to CT.[33]
5. **SUV.** The use of size-based SUV cutoffs may be helpful for nodal staging. In one study, SUV

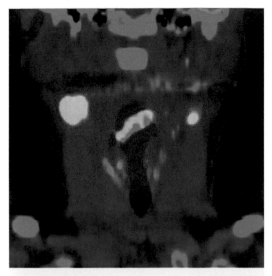

Fig. 14.7 Metastatic supraglottic cancer. Coronal PET/CT demonstrates a supraglottic cancer with metastases to bilateral neck nodes. Supraglottic cancers have a propensity for bilateral nodal metastases.

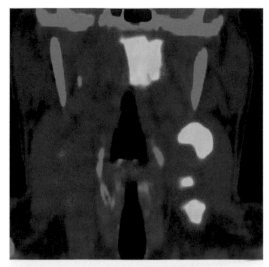

Fig. 14.8 Metastatic nasopharyngeal cancer. Coronal PET/CT demonstrates a large left nasopharyngeal cancer with metastases to bilateral neck nodes. Nasopharyngeal cancers have a propensity for bilateral nodal metastases.

cutoffs of 1.9, 2.5, and 3.0 for lymph nodes < 10 mm, 10 to 15 mm, and > 15 mm yielded a 79% sensitivity and 99% specificity for nodal staging.[34] The use of the ratio of nodal/liver SUVmax is helpful in correcting for interscanner variability. In one report,[35] a nodal/liver ratio of ≥ 0.90 yielded a sensitivity of 74% and specificity of 93%.

6. **Dedicated head and neck protocol.** The use of a dedicated head and neck PET protocol (longer acquisition, higher count study reconstructed with smaller pixels) improves detection of disease in small nodes. In one study, dedicated head and neck PET/CT was 7.4% more sensitive for detecting lymph nodes, all in the 5- to 10-mm range, although specificity was reduced.[36] However, SUVs with a dedicated protocol are significantly higher than with a standard protocol. Thus, SUVs from a dedicated PET study cannot be compared to those from a standard PET.

7. **Hardware artifacts.** Nonremovable metallic dental implants can generate artifacts adjacent to dental implants that mimic FDG uptake on attenuation-corrected images.[37] However, in one report,[38] if artifacts are reduced using an algorithm which corrects for overestimated and underestimated pixel values, quantification of PET images is not affected.

14.5 Recurrence

PET is very valuable for detecting recurrent disease, as CT and MRI are limited in the postoperative/posttherapy neck. NCCN guidelines[1] state that in patients with a clinically negative neck, a negative PET-CT is 90% reliable and further imaging is optional.

14.5.1 Accuracy

1. **PET and PET/CT for primary site residual/recurrent disease** (meta-analysis)[39]: sensitivity of 86%, specificity of 82%.

2. **PET and PET/CT for residual/recurrent neck disease** (meta-analysis)[39]: sensitivity of 72%, specificity of 88%.

3. **PET and PET/CT for distant metastases** (meta-analysis)[39]: sensitivity of 85%, specificity of 95%.

4. **PET/CT for residual/recurrent nasopharyngeal cancer after radiotherapy** (meta-analysis)[40]: sensitivity of 93%, specificity of 87%.

5. PET is sensitive and specific for disease at regional and distant sites. Specificity is lower in the head and neck region due to false-positive results from inflammation related to infection or other processes.[41] The primary value of PET is its high negative predictive value (NPV).[42]

6. Follow-up PET/CT studies are helpful in equivocal cases. If PET/CT results in the neck are equivocal, a repeat PET/CT in 4 to 6 weeks can identify those patients who can be safely observed without surgery.[43] Similarly, if PET is positive and biopsy is negative, a follow-up scan can be performed. Decreased activity on the follow-up scan indicates that the initial result was likely false positive due to an inflammatory process.[44]

14.6 Comparison with Other Modalities

1. **Other radionuclides.** PET is more sensitive than sestamibi, tetrofosmin, or thallium. Specificity is comparable. However, sestamibi or tetrofosmin combined with CT is comparable to PET (▶ Table 14.2).[45,46]

Table 14.2 Sensitivity and specificity of PET compared after radionuclides in the detection of recurrent disease

	Sensitivity %	Specificity %
PET	100	96
Tc-99 m sestamibi	73	96
Tc-99 m tetrofosmin	64	96

2. **MRI** (▶ Table 14.3)[47]

Table 14.3 Sensitivity and specificity of PET compared with MRI in the detection of recurrent disease

	Sensitivity %	Specificity %
PET	100	93
MRI	62	43

14.6.1 Pearls/Pitfalls

1. **SUV.** SUV cutoffs of 3.0 to 3.2 have been used to detect recurrence.[41,48] However, an increasing SUV on dual time point PET imaging is of greater value than a single SUV measurement. However, SUV cutoffs should be used with caution in this setting.
2. **Tumor stunning.** Both false-positive results secondary to inflammation and false-negative results secondary to tumor stunning are possible. NCCN guidelines[1] suggest that if PET-CT is used

for follow-up, the first scan should be performed at a minimum of 12 weeks after treatment. If possible, longer delays should be considered, as one study suggests that a delay in PET imaging for at least 4 months after radiation can be helpful in avoiding false-negative results from presumed tumor stunning.[49]

3. **Laryngeal uptake:** Laryngeal uptake of FDG can be noted normally, particularly in the posterior portion (see Chapter 7).
   a) It is better to use asymmetry of uptake rather than absolute uptake in the larynx as a criterion of abnormality.
   b) Anterior uptake is more suggestive of a malignant process than uptake in posterior structures.
   c) However, laryngeal uptake may be asymmetric due to postoperative changes or vocal cord paralysis.

4. **Postoperative.** PET/CT should be performed at least 4 to 6 weeks after surgery to minimize inflammatory uptake.[50] Besides the typical physiologic areas of uptake, abnormal patterns of uptake can be seen from postoperative distortion of normal anatomy or as a result of postsurgical or therapeutic inflammation. In one study,[51] typical postsurgical findings were inflammatory uptake of the tongue and oral cavity due to transoral resections, a shifted submandibular gland related to a myocutaneous flap, and uptake around voice prostheses. However, reconstruction hardware typically does not interfere with interpretability. Osteotomy sites do have slightly greater (25% on average) uptake but less than seen in tumor.[52] PET/CT can be used in free flap patients with acceptable levels of accuracy.

5. **Radiation effects.** Diffuse FDG uptake in the radiation field is usually secondary to postradiation inflammation. Increased laryngeal or oropharyngeal uptake can be noted for prolonged periods after chemoradiotherapy. Typically, this uptake is diffuse and of mild to moderate intensity. Focal, asymmetric uptake greater than surrounding tissues, particularly muscle, is suspicious for residual or recurrent disease as long as it does not fuse to anatomic structures.[53]

6. **Length of surveillance.** There are limited retrospective data on how long PET/CT should be used for surveillance. In one study, head and neck patients with a negative 3-month PET/CT had little benefit from subsequent PET/CT surveillance.[54] In another study,[55] PET/CT

surveillance beyond the first 24 months was thought to be of limited value as 95% of asymptomatic recurrences occurred within 24 months after chemoradiotherapy.

14.7 Therapy Response/ Prognosis[56]

Potential applications of PET in therapy response are as follows:

1. **Evaluation of residual disease following radiotherapy or chemoradiotherapy.** PET is useful in evaluating therapy response in preoperative induction chemoradiotherapy, chemoradiotherapy protocols which are aimed at organ preservation, and definitive radiotherapy.[21,22]

   In many patients with locally advanced head and neck squamous cell cancer, radiotherapy with or without chemotherapy regimens can be employed which attempt to preserve organ function (e.g., larynx and tongue). While a complete response may be achieved at the primary site, many of these patients will present with cervical nodal metastases. If a complete nodal response is achieved by clinical and CT evaluation, the isolated nodal failure rates are 5% or less. However, patients with a residual nodal abnormality on CT (> 1.0–1.5 cm) will typically undergo a neck dissection, although up to 70 to 80% of these cases will not have residual tumor. PET/CT can be helpful in restaging patients with residual CT abnormalities and selecting patients who do not require a neck dissection.

   PET/CT has a high NPV following radiotherapy or chemoradiotherapy in patients with node-positive cancers who achieve complete response at the primary site, regardless of the residual CT abnormality. In a prospective study,[43] node-positive patients with PET-negative lymph nodes after radiotherapy, with or without chemotherapy, were spared neck dissection, regardless of whether residual lymph nodes were present on CT or clinical exam. Long-term results of this study[57] demonstrated an NPV of 97% for PET at a median follow-up of 62 months. However, it should be noted that PET was helpful only when there was a residual CT abnormality, and a complete nodal response by CT also has a high NPV and PET did not add additional benefit.[43] In a prospective randomized controlled trial[58] of patients with squamous cell carcinoma and N2

or N3 disease, PET/CT surveillance was assessed 12 weeks after the completion of chemoradiotherapy. Neck dissection was performed only if PET/CT showed an incomplete or equivocal response. PET/CT-guided surveillance was noninferior to planned neck dissection. PET/CT surveillance resulted in approximately 80% of patients being spared neck dissection, and was more cost-effective. PET/CT was equally effective in HPV-positive and HPV-negative patients. As nodal disease may take longer to involute in HPV-positive patients, the authors suggest that patients with HPV-positive cancers, and enlarged nodes with no FDG uptake, can be considered for close follow-up with CT or PET/CT.

2. **Prognosis.** PET is helpful for both early and late prediction of outcome.
   a) **Primary tumor.** High SUV (> 10) in the primary tumor is correlated with poor prognosis.[59]
   b) **Nodes.** Nodal SUV does not predict prognosis.[60]
   c) **Interim PET.** Low levels of tumor metabolic activity after one cycle of chemotherapy or radiation predict complete remission and longer survival.
   End of treatment PET. High SUV after treatment predicts local recurrence and decreased survival.

14.8 Accuracy/Comparison to Other Modalities

1. PET and PET/CT for response assessment and surveillance (meta-analysis)[61]:
   a) Primary site: Sensitivity of 80%, specificity of 88%, positive predictive value (PPV) of 59%, NPV of 95%.
   b) Neck: Sensitivity of 73%, specificity of 88%, PPV of 52%, NPV of 95%.
2. Postradiotherapy (▶ Table 14.4)[62]

Table 14.4 Sensitivity and specificity of PET compared with other imaging modalities in the evaluation of therapy response

	Sensitivity %	Specificity %
PET/CT	77	93
CT	92	47

14.8.1 Pitfalls

1. PET has limitations in assessing response to postoperative adjuvant chemoradiotherapy.
   a) Postsurgical inflammatory reactions can cause false-positive results and therefore render subsequent response assessment inaccurate.
   b) Microscopic residual disease cannot be detected.
2. **Timing**. As in all settings, there should be a substantial time interval between radiotherapy and PET imaging. Typically false-negative results are more commonly seen if imaging is performed early after radiation. NCCN guidelines[1] suggest a minimum delay of 12 weeks after treatment. In a systematic review,[63] sensitivity was greater for scans performed 10 weeks or more after therapy. In a meta-analysis,[39] specificity was greater for scans performed more than 12 weeks after radiotherapy with or without chemotherapy. If postradiotherapy neck dissection is being considered, PET may be more valuable if it can be accurately performed earlier after therapy (within 12 weeks), as fibrosis can increase the technical difficulty and morbidity of delayed neck dissection.[64]
3. Visual grading criteria, such as the Deauville's criteria used for lymphoma,[65] or similar criteria[66,67] are also effective in therapy response assessment in patients with head and neck cancer.
4. **Osteoradionecrosis**. Osteoradionecrosis can cause false-positive results.[68] As mean and maximum SUVs can overlap between patients with osteoradionecrosis and tumor recurrence,[69] the CT findings may be more reliable. A solid or cystic mass is associated with tumor recurrence, while bony sclerosis is associated with osteoradionecrosis. Dual time point PET may also be helpful, as the SUV may decrease over time in osteoradionecrosis.[70]

14.8.2 Radiotherapy Planning

Potential applications of PET in radiotherapy planning are as follows[71]:
1. Coregistration of PET and treatment planning by CT.
2. Detection of additional/distant disease by PET.
3. Delineation of radiation therapy target volume. Gross tumor volume (GTV) assessment by PET is closer to the surgical specimen than CT or MRI, although all imaging modalities overestimate tumor extension. PET/CT has several potential advantages: reduction in size of the GTV, reduction of interobserver variability in GTV delineation, identifying parts of the GTV potentially requiring additional radiation dose, and identifying tumor extension missed by CT or MRI.[72] The GTV identified by PET is dependent on the segmentation method used (e.g., visual interpretation results in higher volumes than semiautomatic methods). However, all methods show a smaller tumor volume on PET/CT compared to only CT. Also, PET/CT often suggests tumor extension outside the CT-based tumor volume.[73]

14.9 Characterization of Head and Neck Tumors

1. **Parotid lesions**. PET cannot distinguish between benign and malignant parotid tumors (▶ Fig. 14.9, ▶ Fig. 14.10).[74] Warthin's tumors and pleomorphic adenomas can have FDG

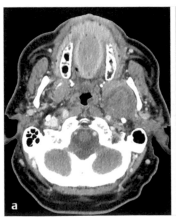
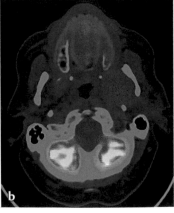

Fig. 14.9 Pleomorphic adenoma. **(a)** Axial CT and **(b)** PET/CT demonstrate a biopsy-proven pleomorphic adenoma in the deep lobe of the left parotid with mild FDG uptake.

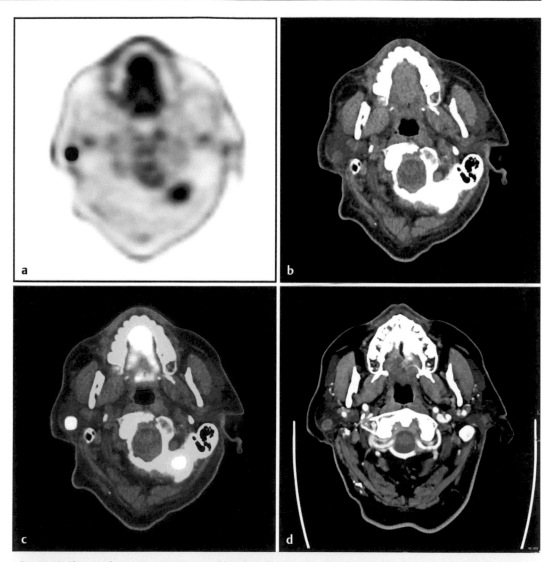

Fig. 14.10 Pleomorphic sarcoma. A 51-year-old male with biopsy-proven pleomorphic sarcoma of the right parotid gland. FDG PET/CT demonstrates an FDG-avid lesion in the right parotid gland **(a,c)**, corresponding to a 12 × 10 mm soft-tissue density on the CT image **(b)**, with moderate enhancement on contrast-enhanced CT **(d)**. (Courtesy of Gang Cheng, MD, Philadelphia, PA)

uptake. High-grade salivary gland tumors tend to have more uptake than lower grade tumors, but there is substantial overlap.[75] In addition, some malignant parotid lesions, such as adenoid cystic carcinoma, low-grade mucoepidermoid carcinoma, and necrotic squamous cell carcinoma can have minimal FDG uptake.[50] In a meta-analysis,[76] the pooled risk of malignancy of focal parotid incidental uptake was 9.6% in all detected lesions.

However, in patients with head and neck cancer/melanoma, lymphoma, or FDG-avid cervical lymph nodes, there are higher odds that the focal parotid uptake represents metastases.[77] PET and PET/CT may be superior to CT for staging patients with known salivary gland malignancies.[75,78,79]

2. **Cystic neck masses.** PET/CT may not be accurate in identifying malignancy in adults with cystic neck masses.[80]

14.10 PET/CT

PET/CT is of particular value in head and neck evaluations given the complex anatomy and relative lack of anatomic landmarks on PET.

1. The use of PET/CT compared to PET alone will decrease fraction of equivocal lesions by 53%, greatly improve lesion localization (▶ Fig. 9.1), slightly improve accuracy, and change management in 18% of cases.[21],[22]
2. Particular attention must be paid to the possibility of mislocalization on PET/CT studies due to movement of the head between the CT and PET studies (▶ Fig. 9.6; ▶ Fig. 9.7).
3. If PET/CT or fusion with CT or MRI is not available, potential anatomic landmarks that can be used to aid in localization include the tonsils, palate, tongue, floor of mouth, salivary glands, mandible, and cervical spine.

References

[1] Pfister DG, Spencer S, Brizel DM, et al. Head and neck cancers, version 1.2015. J Natl Compr Canc Netw. 2015; 13(7):847–855, quiz 856
[2] Zhu L, Wang N. 18F-fluorodeoxyglucose positron emission tomography-computed tomography as a diagnostic tool in patients with cervical nodal metastases of unknown primary site: a meta-analysis. Surg Oncol. 2013; 22(3):190–194
[3] Nabili V, Zaia B, Blackwell KE, Head CS, Grabski K, Sercarz JA. Positron emission tomography: poor sensitivity for occult tonsillar cancer. Am J Otolaryngol. 2007; 28(3):153–157
[4] Greven KM, Keyes JW, Jr, Williams DW, III, McGuirt WF, Joyce WT, III. Occult primary tumors of the head and neck: lack of benefit from positron emission tomography imaging with 2-[F-18]fluoro-2-deoxy-D-glucose. Cancer. 1999; 86(1):114–118
[5] Funk GF. A head and neck surgeon's perspective on best practices for the use of PET/CT scans for the diagnosis and treatment of head and neck cancers. Arch Otolaryngol Head Neck Surg. 2012; 138(8):748–752
[6] Johansen J, Petersen H, Godballe C, Loft A, Grau C. FDG-PET/CT for detection of the unknown primary head and neck tumor. Q J Nucl Med Mol Imaging. 2011; 55(5):500–508
[7] Davison JM, Ozonoff A, Imsande HM, Grillone GA, Subramaniam RM. Squamous cell carcinoma of the palatine tonsils: FDG standardized uptake value ratio as a biomarker to differentiate tonsillar carcinoma from physiologic uptake. Radiology. 2010; 255(2):578–585
[8] Hannah A, Scott AM, Tochon-Danguy H, et al. Evaluation of 18 F-fluorodeoxyglucose positron emission tomography and computed tomography with histopathologic correlation in the initial staging of head and neck cancer. Ann Surg. 2002; 236(2):208–217
[9] Wartski M, Le Stanc E, Gontier E, et al. In search of an unknown primary tumour presenting with cervical metastases: performance of hybrid FDG-PET-CT. Nucl Med Commun. 2007; 28(5):365–371
[10] Yoo J, Henderson S, Walker-Dilks C. Evidence-based guideline recommendations on the use of positron emission tomography imaging in head and neck cancer. Clin Oncol (R Coll Radiol). 2013; 25(4):e33–e66
[11] Lonneux M, Hamoir M, Reychler H, et al. Positron emission tomography with [18F]fluorodeoxyglucose improves staging and patient management in patients with head and neck squamous cell carcinoma: a multicenter prospective study. J Clin Oncol. 2010; 28(7):1190–1195
[12] Kastrinidis N, Kuhn FP, Hany TF, Ahmad N, Huber GF, Haerle SK. 18F-FDG-PET/CT for the assessment of the contralateral neck in patients with head and neck squamous cell carcinoma. Laryngoscope. 2013; 123(5):1210–1215
[13] Lee SH, Huh SH, Jin SM, Rho YS, Yoon DY, Park CH. Diagnostic value of only 18F-fluorodeocyglucose positron emission tomography/computed tomography-positive lymph nodes in head and neck squamous cell carcinoma. Otolaryngol Head Neck Surg. 2012; 147(4):692–698
[14] Ng SH, Yen TC, Chang JT, et al. Prospective study of [18F]fluorodeoxyglucose positron emission tomography and computed tomography and magnetic resonance imaging in oral cavity squamous cell carcinoma with palpably negative neck. J Clin Oncol. 2006; 24(27):4371–4376
[15] Schöder H, Carlson DL, Kraus DH, et al. 18F-FDG PET/CT for detecting nodal metastases in patients with oral cancer staged N0 by clinical examination and CT/MRI. J Nucl Med. 2006; 47(5):755–762
[16] Wensing BM, Vogel WV, Marres HA, et al. FDG-PET in the clinically negative neck in oral squamous cell carcinoma. Laryngoscope. 2006; 116(5):809–813
[17] Roh JL, Park JP, Kim JS, et al. 18F fluorodeoxyglucose PET/CT in head and neck squamous cell carcinoma with negative neck palpation findings: a prospective study. Radiology. 2014; 271(1):153–161
[18] Kyzas PA, Evangelou E, Denaxa-Kyza D, Ioannidis JP. 18F-fluorodeoxyglucose positron emission tomography to evaluate cervical node metastases in patients with head and neck squamous cell carcinoma: a meta-analysis. J Natl Cancer Inst. 2008; 100(10):712–720
[19] Liao LJ, Hsu WL, Wang CT, Lo WC, Lai MS. Analysis of sentinel node biopsy combined with other diagnostic tools in staging cN0 head and neck cancer: a diagnostic meta-analysis. Head Neck. 2016; 38(4):628–634
[20] Kovács AF, Döbert N, Gaa J, Menzel C, Bitter K. Positron emission tomography in combination with sentinel node biopsy reduces the rate of elective neck dissections in the treatment of oral and oropharyngeal cancer. J Clin Oncol. 2004; 22(19):3973–3980
[21] Schöder H, Yeung HW. Positron emission imaging of head and neck cancer, including thyroid carcinoma. Semin Nucl Med. 2004; 34(3):180–197
[22] Schöder H, Yeung HW, Gonen M, Kraus D, Larson SM. Head and neck cancer: clinical usefulness and accuracy of PET/CT image fusion. Radiology. 2004; 231(1):65–72
[23] Strobel K, Haerle SK, Stoeckli SJ, et al. Head and neck squamous cell carcinoma (HNSCC)–detection of synchronous primaries with (18)F-FDG-PET/CT. Eur J Nucl Med Mol Imaging. 2009; 36(6):919–927
[24] Haerle SK, Strobel K, Hany TF, Sidler D, Stoeckli SJ. (18)F-FDG-PET/CT versus panendoscopy for the detection of synchronous second primary tumors in patients with head and neck squamous cell carcinoma. Head Neck. 2010; 32(3):319–325
[25] Kim SY, Roh JL, Kim MR, et al. Use of 18F-FDG PET for primary treatment strategy in patients with squamous cell carcinoma of the oropharynx. J Nucl Med. 2007; 48(5):752–757
[26] Xie P, Li M, Zhao H, Sun X, Fu Z, Yu J. 18F-FDG PET or PET-CT to evaluate prognosis for head and neck cancer: a meta-analysis. J Cancer Res Clin Oncol. 2011; 137(7):1085–1093

[27] Yongkui L, Jian L, Wanghan, Jingui L. 18FDG-PET/CT for the detection of regional nodal metastasis in patients with primary head and neck cancer before treatment: a meta-analysis. Surg Oncol. 2013; 22(2):e11–e16

[28] Xu GZ, Zhu XD, Li MY. Accuracy of whole-body PET and PET-CT in initial M staging of head and neck cancer: a meta-analysis. Head Neck. 2011; 33(1):87–94

[29] Yi X, Fan M, Liu Y, Zhang H, Liu S. 18 FDG PET and PET-CT for the detection of bone metastases in patients with head and neck cancer. A meta-analysis. J Med Imaging Radiat Oncol. 2013; 57(6):674–679

[30] Lowe VJ, Stack BC, Jr. Esophageal cancer and head and neck cancer. Semin Roentgenol. 2002; 37(2):140–150

[31] Mak D, Corry J, Lau E, Rischin D, Hicks RJ. Role of FDG-PET/CT in staging and follow-up of head and neck squamous cell carcinoma. Q J Nucl Med Mol Imaging. 2011; 55(5):487–499

[32] Li C, Sheng S, Men Y, Sun H, Xia H, Li L. Emission computed tomography for the diagnosis of mandibular invasion by head and neck cancers: a systematic review and meta-analysis. J Oral Maxillofac Surg. 2015; 73(9):1875. e1–1875.e11

[33] Goerres GW, Schmid DT, Schuknecht B, Eyrich GK. Bone invasion in patients with oral cavity cancer: comparison of conventional CT with PET/CT and SPECT/CT. Radiology. 2005; 237(1):281–287

[34] Murakami R, Uozumi H, Hirai T, et al. Impact of FDG-PET/CT imaging on nodal staging for head-and-neck squamous cell carcinoma. Int J Radiat Oncol Biol Phys. 2007; 68(2):377–382

[35] Lim RS, Ramdave S, Beech P, et al. Utility of SUVmax on 18 F-FDG PET in detecting cervical nodal metastases. Cancer Imaging. 2016; 16(1):39

[36] Yamamoto Y, Wong TZ, Turkington TG, Hawk TC, Coleman RE. Head and neck cancer: dedicated FDG PET/CT protocol for detection–phantom and initial clinical studies. Radiology. 2007; 244(1):263–272

[37] Goerres GW, Schmid DT, Eyrich GK. Do hardware artefacts influence the performance of head and neck PET scans in patients with oral cavity squamous cell cancer? Dentomaxillofac Radiol. 2003; 32(6):365–371

[38] Nahmias C, Lemmens C, Faul D, et al. Does reducing CT artifacts from dental implants influence the PET interpretation in PET/CT studies of oral cancer and head and neck cancer? J Nucl Med. 2008; 49(7):1047–1052

[39] Cheung PK, Chin RY, Eslick GD. Detecting residual/recurrent head neck squamous cell carcinomas using PET or PET/CT: systematic review and meta-analysis. Otolaryngol Head Neck Surg. 2016; 154(3):421–432

[40] Zhou H, Shen G, Zhang W, Cai H, Zhou Y, Li L. 18F-FDG PET/CT for the diagnosis of residual or recurrent nasopharyngeal carcinoma after radiotherapy: a metaanalysis. J Nucl Med. 2016; 57(3):342–347

[41] Wong RJ, Lin DT, Schöder H, et al. Diagnostic and prognostic value of [(18)F]fluorodeoxyglucose positron emission tomography for recurrent head and neck squamous cell carcinoma. J Clin Oncol. 2002; 20(20):4199–4208

[42] Ryan WR, Fee WE, Jr, Le QT, Pinto HA. Positron-emission tomography for surveillance of head and neck cancer. Laryngoscope. 2005; 115(4):645–650

[43] Porceddu SV, Pryor DI, Burmeister E, et al. Results of a prospective study of positron emission tomography-directed management of residual nodal abnormalities in node-positive head and neck cancer after definitive radiotherapy with or without systemic therapy. Head Neck. 2011; 33(12):1675–1682

[44] Terhaard CH, Bongers V, van Rijk PP, Hordijk GJ. F-18-fluorodeoxy-glucose positron-emission tomography scanning in detection of local recurrence after radiotherapy for laryngeal/pharyngeal cancer. Head Neck. 2001; 23(11):933–941

[45] Kao CH, Shiau YC, Shen YY, Yen RF. Detection of recurrent or persistent nasopharyngeal carcinomas after radiotherapy with technetium-99 m methoxyisobutylisonitrile single photon emission computed tomography and computed tomography: comparison with 18-fluoro-2-deoxyglucose positron emission tomography. Cancer. 2002; 94(7):1981–1986

[46] Kao CH, Tsai SC, Wang JJ, Ho YJ, Yen RF, Ho ST. Comparing 18-fluoro-2-deoxyglucose positron emission tomography with a combination of technetium 99 m tetrofosmin single photon emission computed tomography and computed tomography to detect recurrent or persistent nasopharyngeal carcinomas after radiotherapy. Cancer. 2001; 92(2):434–439

[47] Yen RF, Hung RL, Pan MH, et al. 18-fluoro-2-deoxyglucose positron emission tomography in detecting residual/recurrent nasopharyngeal carcinomas and comparison with magnetic resonance imaging. Cancer. 2003; 98(2):283–287

[48] Yao M, Luo P, Hoffman HT, et al. Pathology and FDG PET correlation of residual lymph nodes in head and neck cancer after radiation treatment. Am J Clin Oncol. 2007; 30(3):264–270

[49] Keyes JW, Jr, Watson NE, Jr, Williams DW, III, Greven KM, McGuirt WF. FDG PET in head and neck cancer. AJR Am J Roentgenol. 1997; 169(6):1663–1669

[50] Purohit BS, Ailianou A, Dulguerov N, Becker CD, Ratib O, Becker M. FDG-PET/CT pitfalls in oncological head and neck imaging. Insights Imaging. 2014; 5(5):585–602

[51] Meerwein CM, Queiroz M, Kollias S, Hüllner M, Veit-Haibach P, Huber GF. Post-treatment surveillance of head and neck cancer: pitfalls in the interpretation of FDG PET-CT/MRI. Swiss Med Wkly. 2015; 145:w14116

[52] Oliver C, Muthukrishnan A, Mountz J, Deeb E, Johnson J, Deleyiannis F. Interpretability of PET/CT imaging in head and neck cancer patients following composite mandibular resection and osteocutaneous free flap reconstruction. Head Neck. 2008; 30(2):187–193

[53] Schöder H, Fury M, Lee N, Kraus D. PET monitoring of therapy response in head and neck squamous cell carcinoma. J Nucl Med. 2009; 50 Suppl 1:74S–88S

[54] Ho AS, Tsao GJ, Chen FW, et al. Impact of positron emission tomography/computed tomography surveillance at 12 and 24 months for detecting head and neck cancer recurrence. Cancer. 2013; 119(7):1349–1356

[55] Beswick DM, Gooding WE, Johnson JT, Branstetter BF, IV. Temporal patterns of head and neck squamous cell carcinoma recurrence with positron-emission tomography/computed tomography monitoring. Laryngoscope. 2012; 122(7): 1512–1517

[56] Kostakoglu L, Goldsmith SJ. PET in the assessment of therapy response in patients with carcinoma of the head and neck and of the esophagus. J Nucl Med. 2004; 45(1):56–68

[57] Sjövall J, Chua B, Pryor D, et al. Long-term results of positron emission tomography-directed management of the neck in node-positive head and neck cancer after organ preservation therapy. Oral Oncol. 2015; 51(3):260–266

[58] Mehanna H, Wong WL, McConkey CC, et al. PET-NECK Trial Management Group. PET-CT surveillance versus neck dissection in advanced head and neck cancer. N Engl J Med. 2016; 374(15):1444–1454

[59] Halfpenny W, Hain SF, Biassoni L, Maisey MN, Sherman JA, McGurk M. FDG-PET. A possible prognostic factor in head and neck cancer. Br J Cancer. 2002; 86(4):512–516

[60] Schwartz DL, Rajendran J, Yueh B, et al. FDG-PET prediction of head and neck squamous cell cancer outcomes. Arch Otolaryngol Head Neck Surg. 2004; 130(12):1361–1367

[61] Gupta T, Master Z, Kannan S, et al. Diagnostic performance of post-treatment FDG PET or FDG PET/CT imaging in head and neck cancer: a systematic review and meta-analysis. Eur J Nucl Med Mol Imaging. 2011; 38(11):2083–2095

[62] Andrade RS, Heron DE, Degirmenci B, et al. Posttreatment assessment of response using FDG-PET/CT for patients treated with definitive radiation therapy for head and neck cancers. Int J Radiat Oncol Biol Phys. 2006; 65(5):1315–1322

[63] Isles MG, McConkey C, Mehanna HM. A systematic review and meta-analysis of the role of positron emission tomography in the follow up of head and neck squamous cell carcinoma following radiotherapy or chemoradiotherapy. Clin Otolaryngol. 2008; 33(3):210–222

[64] Frank SJ, Chao KS, Schwartz DL, Weber RS, Apisarnthanarax S, Macapinlac HA. Technology insight: PET and PET/CT in head and neck tumor staging and radiation therapy planning. Nat Clin Pract Oncol. 2005; 2(10):526–533

[65] Sjövall J, Bitzén U, Kjellén E, Nilsson P, Wahlberg P, Brun E. Qualitative interpretation of PET scans using a Likert scale to assess neck node response to radiotherapy in head and neck cancer. Eur J Nucl Med Mol Imaging. 2016; 43(4):609–616

[66] Marcus C, Ciarallo A, Tahari AK, et al. Head and neck PET/CT: therapy response interpretation criteria (Hopkins Criteria)-interreader reliability, accuracy, and survival outcomes. J Nucl Med. 2014; 55(9):1411–1416

[67] Min M, Lin P, Lee M, et al. Prognostic value of 2-[(18)F] fluoro-2-deoxy-D-glucose positron emission tomography-computed tomography scan carried out during and after radiation therapy for head and neck cancer using visual therapy response interpretation criteria. Clin Oncol (R Coll Radiol). 2016; 28(6):393–401

[68] Liu SH, Chang JT, Ng SH, Chan SC, Yen TC. False positive fluorine-18 fluorodeoxy-D-glucose positron emission tomography finding caused by osteoradionecrosis in a nasopharyngeal carcinoma patient. Br J Radiol. 2004; 77(915): 257–260

[69] Alhilali L, Reynolds AR, Fakhran S. Osteoradionecrosis after radiation therapy for head and neck cancer: differentiation from recurrent disease with CT and PET/CT imaging. AJNR Am J Neuroradiol. 2014; 35(7):1405–1411

[70] Wang CH, Liang JA, Ding HJ, et al. Utility of TL-201 SPECT in clarifying false-positive FDG-PET findings due to osteoradionecrosis in head and neck cancer. Head Neck. 2010; 32(12):1648–1654

[71] Daisne JF, Duprez T, Weynand B, et al. Tumor volume in pharyngolaryngeal squamous cell carcinoma: comparison at CT, MR imaging, and FDG PET and validation with surgical specimen. Radiology. 2004; 233(1):93–100

[72] Troost EG, Schinagl DA, Bussink J, et al. Innovations in radiotherapy planning of head and neck cancers: role of PET. J Nucl Med. 2010; 51(1):66–76

[73] Schinagl DA, Vogel WV, Hoffmann AL, van Dalen JA, Oyen WJ, Kaanders JH. Comparison of five segmentation tools for 18F-fluoro-deoxy-glucose-positron emission tomography-based target volume definition in head and neck cancer. Int J Radiat Oncol Biol Phys. 2007; 69(4):1282–1289

[74] Rubello D, Nanni C, Castellucci P, et al. Does 18F-FDG PET/CT play a role in the differential diagnosis of parotid masses. Panminerva Med. 2005; 47(3):187–189

[75] Roh JL, Ryu CH, Choi SH, et al. Clinical utility of 18F-FDG PET for patients with salivary gland malignancies. J Nucl Med. 2007; 48(2):240–246

[76] Treglia G, Bertagna F, Sadeghi R, Muoio B, Giovanella L. Prevalence and risk of malignancy of focal incidental uptake detected by fluorine-18-fluorodeoxyglucose positron emission tomography in the parotid gland: a meta-analysis. Eur Arch Otorhinolaryngol. 2015; 272(12):3617–3626

[77] Mabray MC, Behr SC, Naeger DM, Flavell RR, Glastonbury CM. Predictors of pathologic outcome of focal FDG uptake in the parotid gland identified on whole-body FDG PET imaging. Clin Imaging. 2015; 39(6):1073–1079

[78] Jeong HS, Chung MK, Son YI, et al. Role of 18F-FDG PET/CT in management of high-grade salivary gland malignancies. J Nucl Med. 2007; 48(8):1237–1244

[79] Otsuka H, Graham MM, Kogame M, Nishitani H. The impact of FDG-PET in the management of patients with salivary gland malignancy. Ann Nucl Med. 2005; 19(8):691–694

[80] Ferris RL, Branstetter BF, Nayak JV. Diagnostic utility of positron emission tomography-computed tomography for predicting malignancy in cystic neck masses in adults. Laryngoscope. 2005; 115(11):1979–1982

15 Thyroid Cancer

Eugene C. Lin

15.1 Thyroid Nodules

Uptake in thyroid nodules can be seen as an incidental finding (▶ Fig. 15.1). The pooled prevalence of thyroid "incidentalomas" on FDG PET studies is between 2 and 3%.[1,2] The pooled risk of malignancy has been reported as approximately 1/3[1,2]; however, the risk was 20% in a meta-analysis confined to studies with definitive histological results.[3] Approximately 84% of malignant incidentalomas are papillary thyroid carcinoma.[1] In patients with an extrathyroidal malignancy, focal thyroid uptake represents metastatic disease in only 1% of cases.[3]

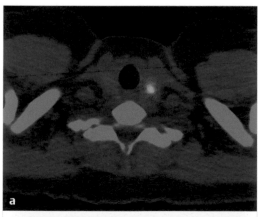

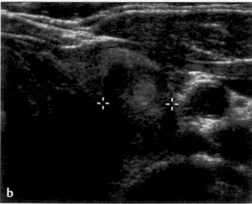

Fig. 15.1 Thyroid nodule. **(a)** Axial PET/CT demonstrates focal uptake in the left thyroid. **(b)** Ultrasound confirms the presence of a left thyroid nodule.

American Thyroid Association (ATA) guidelines[4] recommend fine needle aspiration (FNA) for sonographically confirmed thyroid nodules ≥ 1 cm with FDG uptake. FDG-positive nodules < 1 cm which do not meet FNA criteria can be monitored like high-risk thyroid nodules which do not meet FNA criteria.

1. **SUV).** Malignant thyroid nodules have a higher mean SUVmax than benign nodules. There have been numerous SUV cutoffs suggested for distinguishing benign from malignant thyroid nodules. These should be used with caution as published cutoffs vary greatly (from 2.0 to 8.5).[5] In one study,[6] SUVs were unable to distinguish benign from malignant nodules. A meta-analysis has suggested a SUV threshold of 3.3 or more.[7] However, given the variability in SUV measurement between institutions and the heterogeneity of the studies, focal uptake in the thyroid generally requires further workup as malignancy cannot be excluded based on SUV alone.

2. **Evaluation of nodules with nondiagnostic FNA results.** FDG PET/CT can be helpful in evaluating thyroid nodules with nondiagnostic fine needle aspiration biopsy (FNAB) results, potentially avoiding surgery. However, ATA guidelines[4] do not recommend routine use of PET/CT in this situation. The primary value of PET/CT in these cases is the high sensitivity and negative predictive value. In two meta-analyses,[8,9] the sensitivities were 89 and 95%, with specificities of 55 and 48%. A negative PET scan can accurately exclude thyroid cancer in patients with nodules > 15 mm and indeterminate FNAB results,[8] as all false-negative results are seen in tumors < 15 mm. Patients with a positive PET should be worked up further, but approximately 50% of these patients will have benign lesions. A cost-effectiveness analysis[10] indicates that full implementation of preoperative FDG PET/CT in indeterminate thyroid nodules is cost-effective and could prevent up to 47% of unnecessary surgeries. However, one multivariate analysis[11] found that adding FDG-PET findings to neck ultrasound provided no diagnostic benefit in patients with indeterminate FNAB.

    a) ***SUV cutoff.*** As a high negative predictive value is the primary value of PET/CT in this setting, a low SUVmax cutoff of 2.0 can used, which will have a high sensitivity (90%) with low specificity (42%).[9]

b) The sensitivity, accuracy, and negative predictive value of FDG PET/CT for cytologically indeterminate thyroid nodules is higher than that of neck ultrasound or 99mTc-MIBI scintigraphy.[12]

15.1.1 Pearls

1. Most malignant thyroid nodules > 1 cm will have FDG uptake.
2. Approximately one-third of benign thyroid nodules have FDG uptake.[13]
3. **Hürthle's cell and follicular neoplasms**. Hürthle's cell and follicular neoplasms can be preoperative diagnostic challenges, as they are considered indeterminate on FNA cytology.
   a) **Hürthle's cell adenomas**. Hürthle's cell adenomas often have substantial increased uptake, with a SUV > 5.[13,14] Hürthle's cell adenomas have significantly higher FDG uptake than follicular adenomas.[15]
   b) **Follicular neoplasms**. SUVs can overlap between follicular neoplasms and benign thyroid nodules.[16] However, in one report,[17] a SUVmax cutoff of 3.25 had an accuracy of 81% in discriminating between benign and malignant non-Hürthle's cell follicular neoplasms.
4. **Follicular variant papillary thyroid cancer.** Follicular variant papillary thyroid cancer typically has a low SUV (< 2).[18] This is consistent with the reclassification of encapsulated follicular variant papillary thyroid cancers as noninvasive follicular thyroid neoplasm with papillary-like nuclear features.[19]
5. **CT correlation.** Correlation with computed tomography (CT) images can be helpful in determining whether thyroid FDG uptake is benign or malignant. The following features suggest benign FDG uptake[20]:
   a) The FDG uptake corresponds to a very low attenuation lesion (< 25 Hounsfield units on CT).
   b) There is no nodule on CT which corresponds to the FDG uptake.
   c) The FDG uptake is diffuse.
6. **Incidental thyroid nodules on CT.** Incidental thyroid nodules may be noted on the CT portion of PET/CT studies. Some of these nodules can be safely ignored. One study indicates that the absence of FDG uptake in a thyroid nodule > 1 cm has a high negative predictive

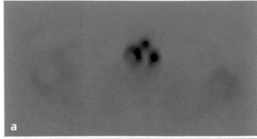

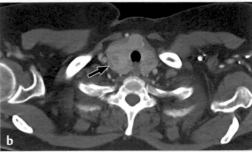

Fig. 15.2 Thyroid nodule without FDG uptake. **(a)** Axial PET demonstrates diffuse increased FDG uptake in the thyroid with lack of uptake corresponding to a right thyroid nodule (*arrow*) identified on an axial contrast-enhanced CT **(b)**. Given the size of this nodule and lack of FDG uptake, it is most likely benign.

value for malignancy,[13] while another study[8] indicates that the optimal threshold is 1.5 cm (▶ Fig. 15.2). However, PET will often miss carcinomas smaller than 1 cm in size.[14]

7. **Nodule size.** Size of thyroid nodules does not influence FDG uptake.[7,21]
8. **Change over time.** SUV in both benign and malignant thyroid nodules is typically stable over time.[21]
9. **Prognostic value.** When taking all other prognostic factors into account, the degree of uptake in differentiated thyroid cancer in nodules incidentally detected by PET/CT does not add further prognostic information.[22]

15.1.2 Pitfalls

1. **Thyroid nodule mimics.** Structures adjacent to the thyroid can mimic thyroid nodules. Before thyroid nodules are diagnosed by PET, anatomic correlation is necessary.
   a) **Nodes.** Medial neck lymph nodes can be adjacent to the thyroid (▶ Fig. 15.3).
   b) **Vocal cord.** Asymmetric vocal cord uptake secondary to vocal cord paralysis can mimic thyroid uptake (▶ Fig. 7.14).
   c) Parathyroid adenomas can have uptake.

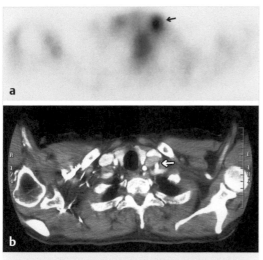

Fig. 15.3 Medial neck node mimicking a thyroid nodule. **(a)** Focal uptake in the left neck (*arrow*) on axial PET scan is suspicious for a thyroid nodule. **(b)** CT scan demonstrates a medial node (*arrow*) immediately lateral to the left thyroid lobe, corresponding to the area of FDG uptake. Conversely, a thyroid nodule can mimic a medial neck node.

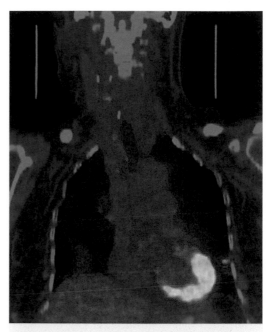

Fig. 15.4 Recurrent thyroid cancer. Coronal PET/CT scan demonstrates metastatic disease to right neck nodes, superior mediastinal nodes, and lungs.

2. **Diffuse uptake.** Diffuse uptake is highly likely to be benign (e.g., secondary to chronic thyroiditis), although it can obscure thyroid nodule uptake. However, the incidence of malignancy in diffuse uptake has been reported as 4.7%,[23] which is not significantly higher than the risk in patients with nodular goiters (5%) and may not require further workup.

3. **Diffuse plus focal and multifocal uptake**. The diffuse pattern of uptake should be separated from multifocal and diffuse plus focal uptake. The two latter patterns of uptake carry a risk of malignancy comparable to focal uptake, and should generally be worked up further.[23,24]

15.2 Initial Staging

PET/CT has little role in the routine preoperative staging of thyroid cancer. As there is no effective neoadjuvant therapy and all patients undergo surgical resection regardless of tumor stage, PET/CT would be unlikely to change management. However, as lymph node metastases do affect prognosis and prophylactic lateral neck node dissection is not typically performed, PET/CT could potentially be helpful in preoperative evaluation of the neck nodes.[24] In one report,[25] contrast-enhanced PET/ CT was more sensitive and accurate than neck CT for preoperative lymph node staging. ATA guidelines[4] suggest that PET/CT may be considered as a part of initial staging in poorly differentiated thyroid cancers and invasive Hürthle's cell carcinomas, particularly in patients with evidence of other disease on imaging or with elevated thyroglobulin.

15.3 Recurrent Thyroid Cancer

15.3.1 Differentiated Thyroid Cancer Patients with an Elevated Serum Thyroglobulin and Negative Radioiodine Scans

ATA guidelines[4] indicate that PET/CT (▶ Fig. 15.4) should be considered in high-risk differentiated thyroid cancer patients with an elevated serum thyroglobulin (generally > 10 ng/mL) and negative radioiodine scans. FDG PET/CT results lead to a change in management in 20 to 40% of patients who fall in this category.[26] In the national oncologic PET registry,[27] the use of PET for the detection of suspected recurrence resulted in a change in management in 33.2% of cases, with an imaging-adjusted impact (change from treatment to nontreatment, or nontreatment to treatment) of 17%. PET/CT is also effective in patients with negative radioiodine scan, undetectable thyroglobulin, and elevated antithyroglobulin antibody levels.[28]

In these patients, imaging of the neck and chest can be performed first to search for metastatic disease, typically with neck ultrasound and neck and chest CT. If anatomic imaging is negative for surgically curable disease, or the thyroglobulin is out of proportion to the identified surgically resectable disease, a PET/CT scan could be performed. If PET/CT is positive and biopsy confirms metastatic disease, resection can be performed. If PET/CT is negative, empiric radioiodine therapy or follow-up imaging in 6 to 12 months can be considered.[29] One advantage of performing PET prior to empiric radioiodine therapy is that PET-positive tumors generally do not concentrate radioiodine, and radioiodine therapy will be unlikely to alter the outcome in these patients. Therefore, empiric radioiodine therapy should primarily be considered in patients with no detectable FDG uptake.

If PET was not performed prior to empiric radioiodine therapy, and the whole body scan after therapy is negative, a PET scan should be considered, particularly in patients with unstimulated serum thyroglobulin levels > 10 to 20 ng/mL or with aggressive histologies.

15.3.2 Prognosis

ATA guidelines[4] indicate that PET/CT may be considered as a prognostic tool in patients with metastatic disease to identify lesions and patients at highest risk for rapid disease progression and disease-specific mortality. FDG uptake in patients with metastatic differentiated thyroid cancer is an independent prognostic factor for survival, and a negative predictive factor for response to radioiodine treatment. A large volume of metabolically active diseased sites and high SUVs (> 10) are strong negative predictors of survival.[30]

15.3.3 Accuracy/Comparison to Other Modalities

1. **PET/CT for differentiated thyroid cancer with negative radioiodine scan** (meta-analysis)[31]: Sensitivity of 93%, specificity of 81%, accuracy of 93%.
2. **PET and PET/CT for papillary thyroid cancer only without regard to radioiodine scan**

results (meta-analysis)[32]: Sensitivity of 77%, specificity of 85%.
A correlation between 1 and 131 negativity and PET sensitivity and specificity was not found in the above meta-analysis.
3. **PET for Hürthle's cell carcinoma:** Sensitivity of 96%, specificity of 95%.[33]
4. **Anatomic region:**
   a) PET is most valuable for the detection of cervical lymph node metastases.[34]
   b) *Bone metastases*. There is conflicting evidence regarding the value of FDG PET/CT for the detection of bone metastases relative to other modalities. One study suggests that FDG PET is comparable in sensitivity but superior in specificity and accuracy to bone scan,[35] while another study[36] suggests that FDG PET has superior sensitivity and specificity compared to bone scan. One report[37] suggests that the sensitivity of FDG PET/CT is significantly lower than that of bone scan (with SPECT) or 18F-flouride PET/CT, and another report[38] suggests that bone scan may identify metastases which are PET negative. Compared to 131-I SPECT/CT, FDG PET/CT was not significantly different on patient-based analysis, but 131-I SPECT/CT was superior on a lesion-based analysis.[36]
5. **FDG and other radionuclide studies: Papillary/Follicular cancer** (► Table 15.1)[39]

Table 15.1 Sensitivity and specificity of PET compared to other radionuclides in papillary/follicular cancer

	Sensitivity %	Specificity %
PET	75	90
Iodine-131	50	99
Sestamibi/thallium	53	92

a) *Relationship between FDG and radioiodine uptake*. There is usually an inverse relation between FDG and radioiodine uptake in thyroid metastases (flip flop phenomena). Poorly differentiated metastases have FDG uptake but no or minimal radioiodine uptake, and the reverse is true in well-differentiated metastatic lesions. A flip flop phenomena may be less common in younger patients. In one study[40] of patients with thyroid cancer and lung metastases, young patients had a greater likelihood of iodine uptake even when FDG accumulates in lung metastases.

Somatostatin receptor scintigraphy with Tc99m-depreotide is also able to detect disease in the setting of detectable thyroglobulin and negative radioiodine scan. There may also be a flip flop phenomenon between FDG and Tc-99 m depreotide; e.g., poorly differentiated lesions may have FDG uptake but no or minimal depreotide uptake.[41]

b) FDG-positive lesions are resistant to high-dose iodine-131 treatment.[42] Thyroglobulin levels are much more likely to normalize in PET-negative patients than in PET-positive patients after radioiodine therapy.[43]

FDG uptake correlates with thallium and sestamibi uptake.[44,45] However, FDG is preferred to thallium or sestamibi due to its superior resolution and higher sensitivity.

15.3.4 Pearls

1. **Histology.** PET is also useful in the Hürthle cell[33] and insular cell,[46] subtypes of follicular cancer.
2. **Thyroglobulin level.** The rate of PET scan positivity is low, ranging from < 10 to 30%, if thyroid-stimulating hormone (TSH)-stimulated thyroglobulin is < 10 ng/mL.[4] ATA guidelines recommend PET/CT only in patients with a stimulated thyroglobulin ≥ 10 ng/mL. However, this level could be lowered in patients with aggressive pathologic variants, and PET/CT could be useful in patients with undetectable thyroglobulin levels and persistent thyroglobulin antibodies. It should be noted that several studies[47,48,49,50] suggest that PET/CT may be valuable at thyroglobulin levels lower than 10 ng/mL. In addition, a few studies have shown a relationship between thyroglobulin doubling time (e.g., < 1 year) and FDG positivity,[51,52] suggesting that PET/CT may be valuable in patients with rapid thyroglobulin doubling time regardless of level.
3. **Thyroid hormone withdrawal/recombinant TSH.** While radioiodine imaging is most helpful when performed in patients with elevated TSH levels (thyroid hormone withdrawal or recombinant TSH administration), the value in FDG PET imaging is more controversial. There are several other factors to consider with FDG PET imaging:
   a) While thyroid carcinomas may increase their metabolic demand after TSH stimulation, the tumors which have FDG uptake are usually poorly differentiated and may be less dependent on TSH.
   b) A TSH-stimulated hypothyroid state can decrease metabolic organ activity, and may decrease metabolic activity in tumor cells. Using recombinant TSH has two advantages over thyroid hormone withdrawal: patients are spared from a prolonged hypothyroid state and the possible negative effects of hypothyroidism on tumor FDG uptake are avoided.

Conflicting studies indicate both increased and decreased sensitivity with an elevated TSH after thyroid hormone withdrawal.[39,44,53] The discrepant results may represent the conflicting effects of increased tumor metabolism from TSH stimulation and decreased metabolism from hypothyroidism.

In a meta-analysis,[54] PET scans under TSH stimulation versus thyroid hormone suppression showed statistically significant differences in the number of patients with PET true-positive lesions, detected lesions, and tumor-to-background ratios. Clinical management was altered in 9% of patients. ATA guidelines[4] state that the sensitivity of FDG PET may be slightly improved with TSH stimulation (with more potential benefit in patients with normal neck ultrasound and neck and chest CT), but the clinical benefit of identifying additional small foci is unclear.

There is currently no evidence that TSH stimulation improves the prognostic value of PET/CT in patients with thyroid cancer.

- *Thyroglobulin and TSH stimulation.* In patients with a thyroglobulin > 100 ng/mL, TSH stimulation is probably not necessary due the high sensitivity of PET in this subpopulation.[55]

15.3.5 Pitfalls

1. **Pulmonary metastases.** PET has poor sensitivity for pulmonary metastases from thyroid cancer < 1 cm. If pulmonary metastases are of clinical concern, a chest CT should be performed.
2. **Muscle/brown fat.** Neck muscle or brown fat uptake can be mistaken for cervical or mediastinal nodal disease (▶ Fig. 15.5, ▶ Fig. 15.6). Anatomic correlation is necessary to avoid such errors; this is particularly important in thyroid cancer where the prevalence of cervical node disease is high.
3. **Vocal cord.** Unilateral vocal cord activity can cause false-positive results (▶ Fig. 7.14).

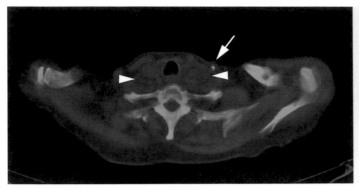

Fig. 15.5 Muscle uptake and nodal metastases. Axial PET/CT scan demonstrates increased uptake in a left neck node (*arrow*) secondary to metastatic thyroid cancer. Note the proximity of the node to muscle uptake (*arrowheads*).

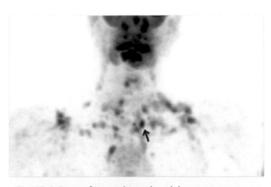

Fig. 15.6 Brown fat uptake and nodal metastases. Extensive brown fat uptake in the neck, supraclavicular regions, and superior mediastinum on a coronal PET scan severely limits evaluation in a patient with suspected metastatic thyroid cancer. A single superior mediastinal nodal metastasis (*arrow*) was present. This is slightly more intense than the brown fat uptake but otherwise similar in appearance. PET/CT was necessary to identify this node.

15.4 Medullary Thyroid Cancer

ATA guidelines[56] do not recommend FDG PET/CT to detect distant metastases preoperatively. In the postoperative setting, FDG PET/CT may be superior to conventional imaging modalities in detecting metastases.[57] FDG PET/CT has additional value in accurately identifying patients' progressive disease. Survival is significantly lower in FDG PET/CT-positive patients compared to those with negative results. However, the ATA guidelines suggest that due to the expense of PET/CT, selection criteria and a medico-economic evaluation are needed before routine clinical use.

Calcitonin level. Although there is some conflicting evidence, calcitonin level likely affects the sensitivity of FDG PET in medullary thyroid cancer. One study[46] suggests there is no correlation between calcitonin levels and lesion detection (the less differentiated lesions with FDG uptake may secrete less calcitonin). In contrast, another study[58] suggests that PET is most useful if the calcitonin level is > 1,000 pg/mL, and of limited use if the calcitonin level is < 500 pg/mL. A patient with a calcitonin level < 500 pg/mL is likely to have a negative FDG PET scan.[59] In a meta-analysis,[60] the detection rate was significantly increased (86%) in patients with serum calcitonin ≥ 1,000 pg/mL and calcitonin doubling times < 24 months.

15.4.1 Accuracy/Comparison to Other Modalities

1. **PET and PET/CT for recurrent or metastatic disease** (meta-analysis)[61]: Sensitivity of 68%, specificity of 69%.
2. **Comparison with CT**. The relative accuracy of PET and CT in medullary thyroid cancer has been variable in different studies, with some studies demonstrating higher accuracy for PET,[57] while other studies have suggested that CT has higher accuracy.[62,63]
3. **Anatomic location**. The performance of CT and FDG PET in medullary thyroid cancer depends on the location of the disease. In patients with medullary thyroid cancer, PET has the highest sensitivity in the neck and mediastinum, and is superior to CT in detecting neck, supraclavicular, and mediastinal nodal disease, while CT is superior for detecting liver and lung metastases.[59]

References

[1] Bertagna F, Treglia G, Piccardo A, Giubbini R. Diagnostic and clinical significance of F-18-FDG-PET/CT thyroid incidentalomas. J Clin Endocrinol Metab. 2012; 97(11):3866–3875

[2] Treglia G, Bertagna F, Sadeghi R, Verburg FA, Ceriani L, Giovanella L. Focal thyroid incidental uptake detected by 18F-fluorodeoxyglucose positron emission tomography. Meta-analysis on prevalence and malignancy risk. Nucl Med (Stuttg). 2013; 52(4):130–136

[3] Nayan S, Ramakrishna J, Gupta MK. The proportion of malignancy in incidental thyroid lesions on 18-FDG PET study: a systematic review and meta-analysis. Otolaryngol Head Neck Surg. 2014; 151(2):190–200

[4] Haugen BR, Alexander EK, Bible KC, et al. 2015 American Thyroid Association Management Guidelines for Adult Patients with Thyroid Nodules and Differentiated Thyroid Cancer: The American Thyroid Association Guidelines Task Force on Thyroid Nodules and Differentiated Thyroid Cancer. Thyroid. 2016; 26(1):1–133

[5] Bloom AD, Adler LP, Shuck JM. Determination of malignancy of thyroid nodules with positron emission tomography. Surgery. 1993; 114(4):728–734, discussion 734–735

[6] Bogsrud TV, Karantanis D, Nathan MA, et al. The value of quantifying 18F-FDG uptake in thyroid nodules found incidentally on whole-body PET-CT. Nucl Med Commun. 2007; 28(5):373–381

[7] Qu N, Zhang L, Lu ZW, Wei WJ, Zhang Y, Ji QH. Risk of malignancy in focal thyroid lesions identified by (18)F-fluorodeoxyglucose positron emission tomography or positron emission tomography/computed tomography: evidence from a large series of studies. Tumour Biol. 2014; 35(6):6139–6147

[8] Vriens D, de Wilt JH, van der Wilt GJ, Netea-Maier RT, Oyen WJ, de Geus-Oei LF. The role of [18F]-2-fluoro-2-deoxy-d-glucose-positron emission tomography in thyroid nodules with indeterminate fine-needle aspiration biopsy: systematic review and meta-analysis of the literature. Cancer. 2011; 117 (20):4582–4594

[9] Wang N, Zhai H, Lu Y. Is fluorine-18 fluorodeoxyglucose positron emission tomography useful for the thyroid nodules with indeterminate fine needle aspiration biopsy? A meta-analysis of the literature. J Otolaryngol Head Neck Surg. 2013; 42:38

[10] Vriens D, Adang EM, Netea-Maier RT, et al. Cost-effectiveness of FDG-PET/CT for cytologically indeterminate thyroid nodules: a decision analytic approach. J Clin Endocrinol Metab. 2014; 99(9):3263–3274

[11] Deandreis D, Al Ghuzlan A, Auperin A, et al. Is (18)F-fluorodeoxyglucose-PET/CT useful for the presurgical characterization of thyroid nodules with indeterminate fine needle aspiration cytology? Thyroid. 2012; 22(2):165–172

[12] Piccardo A, Puntoni M, Treglia G, et al. Thyroid nodules with indeterminate cytology: prospective comparison between 18F-FDG-PET/CT, multiparametric neck ultrasonography, 99mTc-MIBI scintigraphy and histology. Eur J Endocrinol. 2016; 174(5):693–703

[13] de Geus-Oei LF, Pieters GF, Bonenkamp JJ, et al. 18F-FDG PET reduces unnecessary hemithyroidectomies for thyroid nodules with inconclusive cytologic results. J Nucl Med. 2006; 47 (5):770–775

[14] Mitchell JC, Grant F, Evenson AR, Parker JA, Hasselgren PO, Parangi S. Preoperative evaluation of thyroid nodules with 18FDG-PET/CT. Surgery. 2005; 138(6):1166–1174, discussion 1174–1175

[15] Pathak KA, Klonisch T, Nason RW, Leslie WD. FDG-PET characteristics of Hürthle cell and follicular adenomas. Ann Nucl Med. 2016; 30(7):506–509

[16] Kim JM, Ryu JS, Kim TY, et al. 18F-fluorodeoxyglucose positron emission tomography does not predict malignancy in thyroid nodules cytologically diagnosed as follicular neoplasm. J Clin Endocrinol Metab. 2007; 92(5): 1630–1634

[17] Pathak KA, Goertzen AL, Nason RW, Klonisch T, Leslie WD. A prospective cohort study to assess the role of FDG-PET in differentiating benign and malignant follicular neoplasms. Ann Med Surg (Lond). 2016; 12:27–31

[18] Kim BS, Ryu HS, Kang KH. The value of preoperative PET-CT in papillary thyroid cancer. J Int Med Res. 2013; 41(2):445–456

[19] Nikiforov YE, Seethala RR, Tallini G, et al. Nomenclature revision for encapsulated follicular variant of papillary thyroid carcinoma: a paradigm shift to reduce overtreatment of indolent tumors. JAMA Oncol. 2016; 2(8):1023–1029

[20] Choi JY, Lee KS, Kim HJ, et al. Focal thyroid lesions incidentally identified by integrated 18F-FDG PET/CT: clinical significance and improved characterization. J Nucl Med. 2006; 47 (4):609–615

[21] Boeckmann J, Bartel T, Siegel E, Bodenner D, Stack BC, Jr. Can the pathology of a thyroid nodule be determined by positron emission tomography uptake? Otolaryngol Head Neck Surg. 2012; 146(6):906–912

[22] Piccardo A, Puntoni M, Bertagna F, et al. 18F-FDG uptake as a prognostic variable in primary differentiated thyroid cancer incidentally detected by PET/CT: a multicentre study. Eur J Nucl Med Mol Imaging. 2014; 41(8):1482–1491

[23] Kang BJ, O JH, Baik JH, Jung SL, Park YH, Chung SK. Incidental thyroid uptake on F-18 FDG PET/CT: correlation with ultrasonography and pathology. Ann Nucl Med. 2009; 23(8):729–737

[24] Lang BH, Law TT. The role of 18F-fluorodeoxyglucose positron emission tomography in thyroid neoplasms. Oncologist. 2011; 16(4):458–466

[25] Chong A, Ha JM, Han YH, et al. Preoperative lymph node staging by FDG PET/CT with contrast enhancement for thyroid cancer: a multicenter study and comparison with neck CT. Clin Exp Otorhinolaryngol. 2017; 10(1):121–128

[26] Abraham T, Schöder H. Thyroid cancer–indications and opportunities for positron emission tomography/computed tomography imaging. Semin Nucl Med. 2011; 41(2):121–138

[27] Hillner BE, Siegel BA, Shields AF, et al. Relationship between cancer type and impact of PET and PET/CT on intended management: findings of the national oncologic PET registry. J Nucl Med. 2008; 49(12):1928–1935

[28] Ozkan E, Soydal C, Araz M, Aras G, Ibis E. The additive clinical value of 18F-FDG PET/CT in defining the recurrence of disease in patients with differentiated thyroid cancer who have isolated increased antithyroglobulin antibody levels. Clin Nucl Med. 2012; 37(8):755–758

[29] Lal G, Fairchild T, Howe JR, Weigel RJ, Sugg SL, Menda Y. PET-CT scans in recurrent or persistent differentiated thyroid cancer: is there added utility beyond conventional imaging? Surgery. 2010; 148(6):1082–1089, discussion 1089–1090

[30] Wang W, Larson SM, Tuttle RM, et al. Resistance of [18f]-fluorodeoxyglucose-avid metastatic thyroid cancer lesions to treatment with high-dose radioactive iodine. Thyroid. 2001; 11(12):1169–1175

[31] Caetano R, Bastos CR, de Oliveira IA, et al. Accuracy of positron emission tomography and positron emission tomography-CT in the detection of differentiated thyroid cancer recurrence with negative (131) I whole-body scan results: a meta-analysis. Head Neck. 2016; 38(2):316–327

[32] Miller ME, Chen Q, Elashoff D, Abemayor E, St John M. Positron emission tomography and positron emission tomography-CT

evaluation for recurrent papillary thyroid carcinoma: meta-analysis and literature review. Head Neck. 2011; 33(4):562–565

[33] Pryma DA, Schöder H, Gönen M, Robbins RJ, Larson SM, Yeung HW. Diagnostic accuracy and prognostic value of 18F-FDG PET in Hürthle cell thyroid cancer patients. J Nucl Med. 2006; 47(8):1260–1266

[34] Chung JK, So Y, Lee JS, et al. Value of FDG PET in papillary thyroid carcinoma with negative 131I whole-body scan. J Nucl Med. 1999; 40(6):986–992

[35] Ito S, Kato K, Ikeda M, et al. Comparison of 18F-FDG PET and bone scintigraphy in detection of bone metastases of thyroid cancer. J Nucl Med. 2007; 48(6):889–895

[36] Qiu ZL, Xue YL, Song HJ, Luo QY. Comparison of the diagnostic and prognostic values of 99mTc-MDP-planar bone scintigraphy, 131I-SPECT/CT and 18F-FDG-PET/CT for the detection of bone metastases from differentiated thyroid cancer. Nucl Med Commun. 2012; 33(12):1232–1242

[37] Ota N, Kato K, Iwano S, et al. Comparison of 18F-fluoride PET/CT, 18F-FDG PET/CT and bone scintigraphy (planar and SPECT) in detection of bone metastases of differentiated thyroid cancer: a pilot study. Br J Radiol. 2014; 87(1034): 20130444

[38] Phan HT, Jager PL, Plukker JT, Wolffenbuttel BH, Dierckx RA, Links TP. Detection of bone metastases in thyroid cancer patients: bone scintigraphy or 18F-FDG PET? Nucl Med Commun. 2007; 28(8):597–602

[39] Grünwald F, Biersack HJ. FDG PET in thyroid cancer: thyroxine or not? J Nucl Med. 2000; 41(12):1996–1998

[40] Isoda T, BaBa S, Maruoka Y, et al. Impact of patient age on the iodine/FDG "flip-flop" phenomenon in lung metastasis from thyroid cancer. Ann Nucl Med. 2016; 30(8):518–524

[41] Rodrigues M, Li S, Gabriel M, Heute D, Greifeneder M, Virgolini I. 99mTc-depreotide scintigraphy versus 18F-FDG-PET in the diagnosis of radioiodine-negative thyroid cancer. J Clin Endocrinol Metab. 2006; 91(10):3997–4000

[42] Wang W, Larson SM, Fazzari M, et al. Prognostic value of [18F]fluorodeoxyglucose positron emission tomographic scanning in patients with thyroid cancer. J Clin Endocrinol Metab. 2000; 85(3):1107–1113

[43] Salvatore B, Paone G, Klain M, et al. Fluorodeoxyglucose PET/CT in patients with differentiated thyroid cancer and elevated thyroglobulin after total thyroidectomy and (131)I ablation. Q J Nucl Med Mol Imaging. 2008; 52(1):2–8

[44] Grünwald F, Kälicke T, Feine U, et al. Fluorine-18 fluorodeoxyglucose positron emission tomography in thyroid cancer: results of a multicentre study. Eur J Nucl Med. 1999; 26(12): 1547–1552

[45] Shiga T, Tsukamoto E, Nakada K, et al. Comparison of (18)F-FDG, (131)I-Na, and (201)Tl in diagnosis of recurrent or metastatic thyroid carcinoma. J Nucl Med. 2001; 42(3):414–419

[46] Diehl M, Graichen S, Menzel C, Lindhorst E, Grünwald F. F-18 FDG PET in insular thyroid cancer. Clin Nucl Med. 2003; 28 (9):728–731

[47] Giovanella L, Ceriani L, De Palma D, Suriano S, Castellani M, Verburg FA. Relationship between serum thyroglobulin and 18FDG-PET/CT in 131I-negative differentiated thyroid carcinomas. Head Neck. 2012; 34(5):626–631

[48] Na SJ, Yoo IeR, O JH, et al. Diagnostic accuracy of (18)F-fluorodeoxyglucose positron emission tomography/computed tomography in differentiated thyroid cancer patients with elevated thyroglobulin and negative (131)I whole body scan: evaluation by thyroglobulin level. Ann Nucl Med. 2012; 26 (1):26–34

[49] Rosenbaum-Krumme SJ, Görges R, Bockisch A, Binse I. 18F-FDG PET/CT changes therapy management in high-risk DTC after first radioiodine therapy. Eur J Nucl Med Mol Imaging. 2012; 39(9):1373–1380

[50] Vera P, Kuhn-Lansoy C, Edet-Sanson A, et al. Does recombinant human thyrotropin-stimulated positron emission tomography with [18F]fluoro-2-deoxy-D-glucose improve detection of recurrence of well-differentiated thyroid carcinoma in patients with low serum thyroglobulin? Thyroid. 2010; 20(1):15–23

[51] Giovanella L, Trimboli P, Verburg FA, et al. Thyroglobulin levels and thyroglobulin doubling time independently predict a positive 18F-FDG PET/CT scan in patients with biochemical recurrence of differentiated thyroid carcinoma. Eur J Nucl Med Mol Imaging. 2013; 40(6):874–880

[52] Kelders A, Kennes LN, Krohn T, Behrendt FF, Mottaghy FM, Verburg FA. Relationship between positive thyroglobulin doubling time and 18F-FDG PET/CT-positive, 131I-negative lesions. Nucl Med Commun. 2014; 35(2):176–181

[53] van Tol KM, Jager PL, Piers DA, et al. Better yield of (18)fluorodeoxyglucose-positron emission tomography in patients with metastatic differentiated thyroid carcinoma during thyrotropin stimulation. Thyroid. 2002; 12(5):381–387

[54] Ma C, Xie J, Lou Y, Gao Y, Zuo S, Wang X. The role of TSH for 18F-FDG-PET in the diagnosis of recurrence and metastases of differentiated thyroid carcinoma with elevated thyroglobulin and negative scan: a meta-analysis. Eur J Endocrinol. 2010; 163(2):177–183

[55] Stokkel MP, Duchateau CS, Dragoiescu C. The value of FDG-PET in the follow-up of differentiated thyroid cancer: a review of the literature. Q J Nucl Med Mol Imaging. 2006; 50 (1):78–87

[56] Wells SA, Jr, Asa SL, Dralle H, et al. American Thyroid Association Guidelines Task Force on Medullary Thyroid Carcinoma. Revised American Thyroid Association guidelines for the management of medullary thyroid carcinoma. Thyroid. 2015; 25 (6):567–610

[57] Diehl M, Risse JH, Brandt-Mainz K, et al. Fluorine-18 fluorodeoxyglucose positron emission tomography in medullary thyroid cancer: results of a multicentre study. Eur J Nucl Med. 2001; 28(11):1671–1676

[58] Ong SC, Schöder H, Patel SG, et al. Diagnostic accuracy of 18F-FDG PET in restaging patients with medullary thyroid carcinoma and elevated calcitonin levels. J Nucl Med. 2007; 48(4): 501–507

[59] Wong KK, Laird AM, Moubayed A, et al. How has the management of medullary thyroid carcinoma changed with the advent of 18F-FDG and non-18F-FDG PET radiopharmaceuticals. Nucl Med Commun. 2012; 33(7):679–688

[60] Treglia G, Cocciolillo F, Di Nardo F, et al. Detection rate of recurrent medullary thyroid carcinoma using fluorine-18 dihydroxyphenylalanine positron emission tomography: a meta-analysis. Acad Radiol. 2012; 19(10):1290–1299

[61] Cheng X, Bao L, Xu Z, Li D, Wang J, Li Y. 18F-FDG-PET and 18F-FDG-PET/CT in the detection of recurrent or metastatic medullary thyroid carcinoma: a systematic review and meta-analysis. J Med Imaging Radiat Oncol. 2012; 56(2):136–142

[62] Giraudet AL, Vanel D, Leboulleux S, et al. Imaging medullary thyroid carcinoma with persistent elevated calcitonin levels. J Clin Endocrinol Metab. 2007; 92(11):4185–4190

[63] Gotthardt M, Battmann A, Höffken H, et al. 18F-FDG PET, somatostatin receptor scintigraphy, and CT in metastatic medullary thyroid carcinoma: a clinical study and an analysis of the literature. Nucl Med Commun. 2004; 25(5):439–443

16 Thoracic Neoplasms

Eugene C. Lin

16.1 Solitary Pulmonary Nodule

PET is a well-established modality for evaluating indeterminate solitary pulmonary nodules. American College of Chest Physicians (ACCP) guidelines[1] recommend PET for characterization of solid, indeterminate nodules > 8 mm in diameter with a low to intermediate pretest probability of malignancy (5–65%). British Thoracic Society guidelines recommend PET in pulmonary nodules if the initial risk of malignancy is > 10%.[2]

A 2012 systematic review concluded that PET is cost-effective in the management of solitary pulmonary nodules.[3] PET is most cost-effective when used in nodules with a pretest probability of malignancy between 12 and 69%.[4] In particular, PET may be most cost-effective when clinical pretest probability and CT results are discordant (e.g., when pretest probability is low and CT characteristics are indeterminate).[1] However, PET may not be cost-effective in areas where the specificity is lower (e.g., if tuberculosis is endemic).[5]

1. If the pretest probability of malignancy is very low, observation alone is considered acceptable in most circumstances.
2. If the pretest probability is high, biopsy should be considered instead. With a pretest probability of 80%, the probability of malignancy is still 14% with a negative PET.
   a) Although PET does not reliably exclude malignancy in patients with high pretest probability, continued surveillance is another option, as patients with non-hypermetabolic malignant tumors may have a favorable prognosis even when surgical treatment is delayed by a period of observation.[1,6,7]

16.1.1 Accuracy

1. **PET** (meta-analysis)[8]: Sensitivity of 95%, specificity of 82%.
2. **PET/CT:** Sensitivity of 97%, specificity of 85%.[9]
   a) By incorporating the CT findings into the PET/CT interpretation (e.g., a highly suspicious nodule on CT would be interpreted as positive even if PET is negative), the sensitivity of CT and specificity of PET are synergistic. This approach results in a higher accuracy compared to PET alone,[9] and may be particularly helpful for nodules < 1 cm.
3. A negative PET scan indicates that a nodule is highly likely to be benign, but follow-up is still necessary as a small number of nodules will be malignant and have low FDG uptake.
   a) It is important to take the pretest probability of malignancy into account with a negative PET scan result.
4. A positive result indicates that the nodule is most likely malignant.
   a) Although false-positive results are noted with PET, PET has higher specificity than competing modalities.
5. A negative PET result is usually more accurate than a positive result, as false-negative findings are less common than false-positive lesions for malignancy.

16.1.2 Comparison with Other Modalities

British Thoracic Society guidelines do not recommend performing either dynamic contrast-enhanced CT or SPECT if PET/CT is available.[2]

1. **Dynamic contrast-enhanced CT:** Sensitivity of 98%, specificity of 58%.[10]
   a) In two studies comparing PET and contrast-enhanced CT, PET had a slightly lower sensitivity and much higher specificity in one[11] and a greater sensitivity and comparable specificity in another.[12] Overall, PET is more accurate than contrast-enhanced CT for pulmonary nodule evaluation. CT should primarily be used in nodules less than 1 cm, if PET is not available, or in low-risk patients.
   b) PET scan can be useful after a positive dynamic contrast CT exam if biopsy is not desirable. Over half of false-positive lesions on contrast CT can be shown to be true negative on PET.[13]
2. **Technetium-99 m Depreotide (somatostatin analog) SPECT.** PET is more sensitive than technetium-99 m depreotide, and specificity is comparable.[14,15]

3. An additional benefit of PET over other modalities is that if a PET is performed to evaluate a solitary pulmonary nodule and is positive for malignancy, PET is also the most accurate modality for staging.

16.1.3 Pearls

1. **Interpretation.**[16] A nodule is positive for malignancy if
   a) Standardized uptake value (SUV) is > 2.5.
   b) Visual analysis. Intensity is greater than that of the mediastinum (▶ Fig. 16.1).
      • Visual and SUV analyses are comparable in accuracy.
      • Visual analysis can be done with an ordinal scale.[2] This is particularly helpful if PET/CT is used in conjunction with prediction tools.
      • Absent—Uptake indiscernible from background lung tissue.

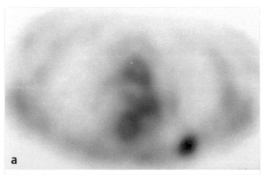

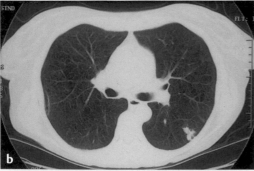

Fig. 16.1 Peripheral lung nodule. (a) Axial PET scan demonstrates focal uptake in the peripheral left thorax. PET often has difficulty localizing peripheral lesions and it cannot be determined whether this is in the lung or chest wall. (b) Axial CT scan at the same level demonstrates an irregular lung nodule corresponding to the FDG uptake. The degree of FDG uptake in this nodule is consistent with malignancy.

• Faint—Uptake less than or equal to mediastinal blood pool.
• Moderate—Uptake greater than mediastinal blood pool.
• Intense—Uptake marked greater than mediastinal blood pool.
   c) Lower thresholds (SUV > 2.0 and intensity equal or greater than mediastinum) have also been used successfully.[9]
   d) *Small nodules.* Use caution when evaluating small nodules. For nodules smaller than 1 cm, SUV values will be substantially lower due to partial volume effects. Visual analysis threshold should also be lowered.
      • If a nodule less than 1 cm demonstrates any FDG uptake, it should be considered potentially malignant.[17]

2. **What size pulmonary nodule should be evaluated?**
   a) Detection of malignancy in nodules as small as 5 mm[7] has been reported. As a practical consideration, PET is best used in nodules greater than 1 cm in size, although 8 mm is reasonable if nodule is in the upper lungs.
      • However, there is limited evidence for the accuracy of PET in nodules ≤ 1 cm.[18]
   b) Small nodules in the upper and anterior lungs are more optimal sites for assessment by PET than other sites because
      • There is less respiratory motion in the upper lungs.
      • Significant scatter from the liver in the lower lungs obscures small lesions.
      • There is normally slightly increased activity in the posterior and lower lungs, related to atelectasis, particularly if the PET is acquired primarily in expiration, which may decrease the contrast between the lesion and the adjacent tissues and therefore limit detectability. Respiratory misregistration artifact (seen on PET/CT but not on PET) can artifactually decrease uptake in lung nodules near the hemidiaphragms.
   c) PET could be considered in nodules < 1 cm in intermediate-risk patients if negative nodules are closely observed.[19,20,21]

3. **Scan time.** Scanning should begin approximately 50 minutes after FDG injection to best separate malignant from benign lesions.[22]

4. **Dual point imaging.** Dual point imaging (e.g., imaging at 1 and 3 hours and using a threshold of 10% SUV increase for malignancy) has been suggested as an aid to nodule characterization

with PET.[23] Malignant lesions should show increased uptake on delayed images, while benign inflammatory lesions are stable or less active on the second scan. However, two meta-analyses[24,25] did not find a difference in accuracy between dual time point and single time point PET.

a) This technique may be particularly helpful for equivocal lesions with SUVs around 2.5.

b) Benign lesions (in particular granulomas) can sometimes demonstrate increasing uptake, but this is typically less than that seen in malignancies. However, uptake in malignant lesions should not decrease.[26]

5. **Histology:**

a) ***Carcinoids versus hamartomas.*** In one report,[27] the SUVmax in pulmonary carcinoids (mean: 3.9) was higher than in hamartomas (mean: 1.9). However, more aggressive atypical carcinoids could not be distinguished from typical carcinoids by FDG uptake.

b) ***Squamous cell carcinoma versus adenocarcinoma and large cell carcinoma***. Squamous cell carcinomas have greater FDG uptake than adenocarcinomas or large cell carcinomas.[28]

6. **Round atelectasis.** Round atelectasis usually does not have FDG uptake (▶ Fig. 16.2). PET can be used to differentiate atypical round atelectasis from malignant tumors.[29]

16.1.4 Pitfalls

1. **False positives.** Active granulomatous/inflammatory process (TB, fungal infection, rheumatoid nodule, sarcoid, lipoid pneumonia, talc granulomata, inflammatory pseudotumor, organizing pneumonia), benign tumors (sclerosing hemangioma, leiomyoma).[30]

a) PET should be used with caution in areas with a high incidence of tuberculosis, as it has a high false-positive rate in this setting.[31]

b) In some cases, the infectious/inflammatory processes are associated with FDG-avid mediastinal lymph nodes which mimic nodal metastases. For example, in one report,[32] at least one positive mediastinal node was detected in 76% of patients with FDG-avid organizing pneumonia.

2. **False negatives.** Lepidic-predominant adenocarcinomas (minimally invasive or in situ) (▶ Fig. 16.3), mucinous adenocarcinoma,

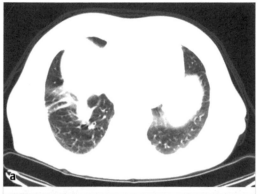
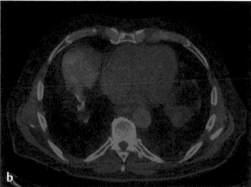

Fig. 16.2 Round atelectasis. **(a)** Axial CT scan demonstrates round atelectasis in the right lung base. **(b)** Corresponding PET/CT scan does not demonstrate uptake in the area of round atelectasis.

carcinoid, mucoepidermoid carcinoma,[30] small lesions.

a) Most false-negative malignant pulmonary nodules on PET imaging are differentiated adenocarcinoma.[33]

b) The sensitivity of PET for the multifocal form of bronchioalveolar carcinoma is substantially higher than for the solitary form.[3]

c) The average SUV in a pulmonary carcinoid tumor is 3.0.[35]

d) The false-negative rate may be higher if PET is used to evaluate nodules detected during screening chest CT, as these nodules, if malignant, tend to be small and/or low grade.[36]

3. **Subsolid nodules.** In general, PET is not indicated to evaluate purely subsolid nodules or part-solid nodules with a solid component that is 8 mm or less.[1] However, ACCP guidelines do recommend PET for the evaluation of part-solid nodules only if the solid component is > 8 mm.

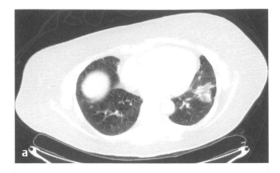

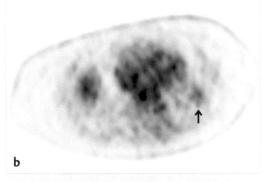

Fig. 16.3 Bronchoalveolar carcinoma. **(a)** Axial CT scan demonstrates ground-glass opacity in the left lower lobe secondary to bronchoalveolar carcinoma. **(b)** Axial PET scan demonstrates mild FDG uptake (*arrow*) in this lesion.

a) As subsolid nodules, if malignant, are often secondary to lepidic predominant adenocarcinoma, a paradoxical pattern has been noted in which higher SUV can be noted in inflammatory subsolid nodules compared to malignant nodules.[37,38] For example, using a higher SUV as an indicator of malignancy for nonsolid nodules, the sensitivity was 10% and specificity was 20% in one report.[39] Thus, evaluation of subsolid nodules may be more accurate using a low SUV as an indicator of malignancy (e.g., in one study,[38] a SUV cutoff above 1.5 was successfully used to diagnose benign nodules with nonsolid components).

b) Increased FDG avidity in clinical stage IA lung adenocarcinoma is correlated with increased aggressiveness and poorer prognosis.[40,41] Although false-negative PET results are more common in patients with subsolid nodules, low FDG avidity does indicate a favorable prognosis following surgical resection. However, it is unclear whether low FDG avidity is correlated with favorable prognosis

if surgical resection is delayed by a period of observation.

4. **Lack of CT correlate.** A focus of FDG uptake in the lung should not be considered to represent a nodule if there is no CT correlate, as the latter can detect almost any nodule in the lung. This may not be true if a CT performed during respiration (as part of a PET/CT) is used for correlation as small lung nodules may not be detected. If there is no corresponding CT lesion, consider the following possibilities:

   a) *Misregistration on PET/CT* (see Chapter 8). If the study is a PET/CT, the PET uptake and lung nodule may be misregistered and appear to be in different sites from each other. In addition, a liver dome lesion could appear to be in the lung base due to misregistration (▶ Fig. 9.10).

   b) *Injected clot.* Injection of radioactive clot (following blood draw) in the syringe can result in pulmonary hot spots without a CT correlate (▶ Fig. 7.25). A similar phenomenon is seen on pulmonary perfusion images during ventilation perfusion scans.

5. **Lesions with FDG uptake and SUV < 2.5.** There is some evidence that lesions with SUV < 2.5 should be further stratified by level of visual uptake. In one study,[33] lesions with faint or no visible uptake had a very low probability of malignancy, while lesions that were visually evident had a probability of malignancy of 60%, even if SUV was < 2.5. A SUV cutoff of 1.6 was proposed by the author of this study. Another study suggests using a SUV cutoff of 2.0 for nodules < 1 cm.[42]

   In practice, the author recommends reporting discordant visual and SUV findings (e.g., visual uptake greater than mediastinum but SUV < 2.5) as suspicious for malignancy. This is particularly true for small nodules where SUV may be artifactually low due to partial volume effects. If a nodule is not small (> 2 cm) and there is uptake less than the mediastinum and SUV < 2.5, the author reports this as probably benign. Small nodules (between 1 and 2 cm) with definite uptake less than mediastinum and SUV < 2.5 are the most problematic. If the SUV is > 1.6 for these nodules, or the uptake is equal to the mediastinal blood pool, the author reports these nodules as indeterminate and at least recommends very close follow-up. The author also gives greater weight to the CT characteristics in these nodules.

6. **Lung base nodules.** PET/CT should be used with caution in nodules near the hemidiaphragms. Due to photopenic respiratory misregistration artifact (see Chapter 9), SUVs can be artifactually decreased in these nodules.

7. **Screening detected lung nodules**. There have been several studies assessing the utility of PET-CT in the context of lung cancer screening studies, where patients have a higher risk of malignancy than the general population. In general, the sensitivity is lower (69–90%) and specificity higher (82–93%) for PET/CT in a screening population compared to the general population.[2] Thus, a positive scan typically warrants invasive diagnostic tests, while negative scans have a lower exclusion value for malignancy.

16.2 Pulmonary Metastasis versus Benign Nodule

PET can be used to evaluate an indeterminate pulmonary lesion(s) in a patient with a known primary tumor. Minimal data exist for this application of PET. Please note that in this setting, a metastasis cannot be distinguished from other causes of uptake including bronchogenic carcinoma.

16.2.1 Accuracy

Using a cutoff SUV of 2.5 or lesion-to-background ratio of 3.0, PET can distinguish pulmonary metastasis from benign nodule with an accuracy of 91%.[43]

16.3 Non-Small Cell Lung Cancer: Staging

PET is a standard modality for staging non-small cell lung cancer (NSCLC). The addition of PET to the conventional workup will prevent unnecessary surgery in one out of five patients,[44] and results in changing stage from that determined by conventional modalities in over half of patients.[45]

1. However, the primary value of PET/CT in many cases will be in identifying distant metastases rather than in mediastinal staging, as, with the possible exception of a negative PET study in peripheral T1ab N0 patients, patients will require invasive confirmation regardless of whether the PET is positive or negative for mediastinal nodal metastases. A Cochrane review[46] examining the accuracy of PET/CT in differentiating N0 and N1 from N2 and N3 disease indicated that PET/CT alone was not sufficiently accurate to make a decision about whether to offer surgery. The Cochrane authors suggest that PET/CT could be used in deciding whether the next step is biopsy or surgical resection (if PET/CT is negative and nodes are small). National Comprehensive Cancer Network (NCCN) and European Society of Thoracic Surgery (ESTS) guidelines[47,48] suggest peripheral T1ab N0 patients with negative PET studies can forgo invasive mediastinal staging.

2. Compared to conventional staging, PET correctly identifies about 20% more patients with N2, N3, or distant metastases.[49]

3. However, there is a significant rate of incorrect upstaging, which has ranged from 5 to 42% in randomized controlled trials.[49] Therefore, suspected PET finding should be confirmed if possible.

4. PET has little value in staging pure ground-glass adenocarcinomas. As the incidence of nodal metastasis and distant metastasis is low, no true positives were seen in several reports.[50,51]

5. **Mediastinal staging**[20]:
   a) PET is most useful in patients without enlarged mediastinal nodes on CT and no clinical evidence of systemic metastases. In one analysis,[52] considering effectiveness only (and not cost), the optimal strategy was to perform PET, transbronchial needle aspiration (TBNA), endobronchial ultrasound (EBUS), and endoscopic ultrasound (EUS) if the initial CT is negative. If TBNA or PET is positive, mediastinoscopy is performed only if EBUS and EUS are negative. If TBNA or PET is negative, mediastinoscopy is performed only if EBUS and EUS give contradictory results.
   b) In patients with enlarged mediastinal nodes, PET is usually less valuable as a negative PET may not preclude mediastinoscopy due to possible false-negative results.
   c) PET has a limited role in clinical stage I (peripheral) tumors, as the incidence of mediastinal metastases is low.

6. **Distant staging**[20]:
   a) PET is most useful in patients with a positive clinical evaluation suggesting systemic metastasis (clinical stage IV), or radiographic evidence of mediastinal lymph node enlargement (clinical stage III).
      • In these situations, PET should be performed in conjunction with a head CT or MRI.

b) PET may also be useful to detect distant metastases in patients with clinical stage II tumors (particularly central tumors or adenocarcinoma).

c) PET has a limited role in clinical stage I (peripheral) tumors as the incidence of unsuspected distant metastases is low.

16.3.1 Accuracy/Comparison to Other Modalities

1. **PET/CT for mediastinal staging** (meta-analysis)[46]:
   a) Sensitivity of 77%, specificity of 90% (visual analysis).
   b) Sensitivity of 81%, specificity of 79% (SUV threshold of 2.5):
      - PET/CT has superior accuracy than that of CT, PET alone, or visual correlation of CT and PET for tumor and nodal staging.
      - *Tumor stage*. PET/CT is superior to PET for T staging. The CT component allows for determination of tumor size and extension in adjacent soft tissues. PET/CT is ideally suited for assessing chest wall and mediastinal invasion (▶ Fig. 16.4). The advantages of PET/CT compared to PET are probably greater for T staging than nodal staging.[53]
      - *Nodal stage*. PET/CT increases confidence in diagnosing nodal disease, and decreases equivocal results substantially.
         - PET/CT has superior sensitivity to PET alone for left hilar, subaortic, and right paratracheal nodes and higher accuracy for subcarinal and interlobar nodes.[54]

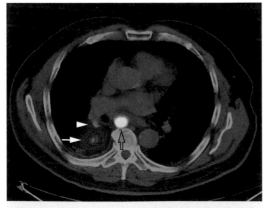

Fig. 16.4 Mediastinal and hilar metastases. Axial PET/CT scan demonstrates a right lower lobe carcinoma (*arrow*) with right hilar (*arrowhead*) and subcarinal (*open arrow*) nodal metastases.

2. **PET versus CT for mediastinal staging** (▶ Table 16.1).[49]

Table 16.1 Sensitivity and specificity of PET versus CT in the mediastinal staging of non-small cell lung cancer

	Sensitivity %	Specificity %
PET	80	88
CT	55	81

a) PET is superior to CT for N0, N2, and N3 disease but not N1 disease.[55]

b) PET has a lower frequency of false-positive findings in the upper mediastinal nodes.

c) PET has a lower frequency of false-negative findings in adenocarcinoma and false-positive findings in squamous cell carcinoma.

3. **PET/CT for distant staging** (meta-analysis)[56]: sensitivity of 93%, specificity of 96%.
   a) PET will detect unsuspected distant metastases in approximately 10% of patients.[45]

4. **Bone marrow metastases**:
   a) PET/CT (meta-analysis)[57]: Sensitivity of 92%, specificity of 98%.
   b) PET/CT has higher sensitivity and specificity than PET, MRI, or bone scan, while PET is superior to MRI or bone scan.[57] Compared to bone scintigraphy, PET is equal or greater in sensitivity and more specific for the diagnosis of bone marrow metastases from lung carcinoma (▶ Fig. 16.5).
   PET is more valuable for detecting bone marrow metastases in lung carcinoma than in other primary neoplasms since the bone lesions are often lytic with this malignancy.

5. **Adrenal metastases** (▶ Fig. 16.6)**: PET:** Sensitivity of 100%, specificity of 80%.

6. **Brain metastases**:
   a) *PET:* Sensitivity 60%
   b) Cannot substitute for CT or MRI.

7. **Malignant versus benign pleural disease.** PET can be used to differentiate malignant from benign pleural disease. It can evaluate both effusions (▶ Fig. 16.7) and pleural thickening. In patients with indeterminate pleural abnormalities on contrast-enhanced CT, PET/CT has better diagnostic performance than the CT.[58]
   a) *Accuracy.* In a meta-analysis,[59] PET and PET/CT had a sensitivity of 95 and specificity of 82%, for distinguishing benign from malignant pleural lesions overall. In a meta-analysis[60] focused on pleural abnormalities in patients with primarily lung cancer, PET

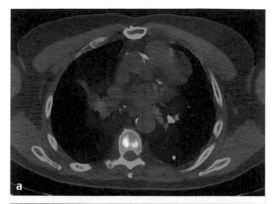

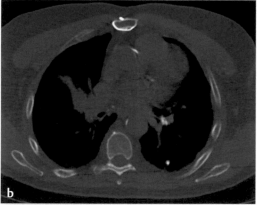

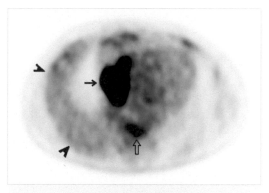

Fig. 16.7 Malignant effusion. Axial PET scan demonstrates uptake in a malignant right effusion (*arrowheads*) in a patient with a large central right lung carcinoma (*arrow*). A bone metastasis is also noted (*open arrow*).

Fig. 16.5 Bone metastasis. Axial PET/CT (**a**) demonstrates a right lung cancer metastatic to a vertebral body. The metastasis is not visible on CT (**b**).

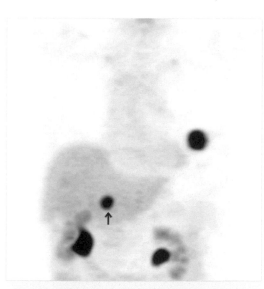

Fig. 16.6 Adrenal metastasis. Coronal PET scan demonstrates a left lung cancer metastatic to the right adrenal (*arrow*).

and PET/CT had a sensitivity of 86% and specificity of 80% for assessing pleural abnormalities.

b) **Degree of uptake.** Intense uptake is highly predictive of malignancy; however, moderate uptake should be interpreted with caution since it also can be seen in infection and other inflammatory disorders. Visual grading (e.g., pleural activity higher than mediastinal background activity)[58] is comparable in accuracy to SUV cutoffs.

- A SUV cutoff of 2.2 and 2.8[58] has an accuracy of 82% for distinguishing between benign and malignant pleural processes.[61] Pleural metastases from thoracic primaries tend to have more uptake than metastases from extrathoracic primaries.

c) Correlation with anatomic imaging is necessary to discover false-positive results due to peripheral but nonpleural (e.g., rib) uptake (▶ Fig. 7.46).

16.3.2 Pearls

1. **Do positive PET scans in the mediastinum require mediastinoscopy?** Positive results on PET scan should be confirmed by mediastinoscopy or lymph node sampling, before excluding surgery as an option. The false-positive rate of PET in the mediastinum is 13 to

22%.[20] However, PET is useful in guiding more invasive methods of mediastinal node sampling.

2. Confirmation can be avoided only if the pretest probability of metastasis is very high (> 85–90%), e.g., if there is diffuse mediastinal infiltration on CT. In patients with discrete, measurable mediastinal nodal enlargement, or in patients without nodal enlargement but a central tumor or suspected N1 disease (which raises probability of N2, 3 nodal involvement), invasive confirmation is needed regardless of the results of PET/CT.

3. **Do negative PET scans in the mediastinum obviate the need for invasive staging?** Invasive can potentially be avoided before thoracotomy if PET is negative, but only in cases where the pretest probability of nodal metastases is low. The false-negative rate of PET in the mediastinum is 5 to 8% compared to an average false-negative rate for mediastinoscopy of 9%.[20] However, mediastinoscopy can detect microscopic disease which will be missed on PET.

   NCCN guidelines[48] suggest that mediastinoscopy is appropriate in central T1ab, T2, and T3 lesions if PET/CT is negative. ESTS guidelines[62] suggest that invasive staging should be performed in patients with cN1, central tumors, or tumors > 3 cm (mainly, adenocarcinoma with high FDG uptake). A European Society of Medical Oncology consensus conference[63] suggests invasive staging for the same reasons as the ESTS guidelines, but also includes CT-enlarged lymph nodes (short axis > 1 cm).

   A minimally invasive strategy combining PET, endobronchial ultrasound needle aspiration, and endoscopic ultrasound needle aspiration can be used to exclude mediastinal nodal metastases. In one report,[64] the combined negative predictive value of these modalities was 93%.

   One situation where a negative PET could preclude mediastinoscopy is in patients with a peripheral clinical T1a (≤ 2 cm) lesion with normal-sized lymph nodes and a negative PET. In this situation, approximately 4% of patients will have unsuspected mediastinal disease.[49] ACCP guidelines[1] suggest that invasive preoperative evaluation is not necessary in this scenario (however, ACCP guidelines also do not recommend PET in peripheral clinical T1a tumors to begin with). ESTS guidelines[62] recommend that further mediastinal staging

can be omitted in patients with peripheral tumors < 3 cm (T1ab) with nonenlarged, PET-negative nodes.

Mediastinoscopy is usually indicated if the pretest probability of mediastinal nodal involvement is high (e.g., central tumor, adenocarcinoma, hilar involvement). The negative predictive value of PET is much lower in the presence of PET-positive N1 nodes and/or a centrally located primary tumor.[65] Patients with the following tumor characteristics may benefit from invasive staging.[66,67,68] However, there is no standard approach to quantify the probability of pathologic N2 disease based on these factors. In a multivariate prediction model,[69] only N1 disease by PET/CT was associated with pathologic N2 disease.

a) Staged as N1 with PET/CT.

b) Adenocarcinoma. In a meta-analysis, there was a higher risk of mediastinal nodal disease (risk ratio: 2.72) compared to other tumor histologies.[70]

c) Upper lobe (particularly right upper lobe) or central tumors.

d) Tumors with SUV ≥ 10. In a meta-analysis,[70] high FDG uptake in the primary lesion was associated with a greater risk of occult nodal metastases.

e) Lymph nodes > 15 mm in short axis on CT. If an enlarged lymph node is seen on CT and PET is negative, ACCP guidelines[49] suggest invasive staging of the mediastinum. However, if lymph node enlargement is substantial, it may be less likely that PET is false negative. Tumor burdens large enough to cause large degrees of nodal enlargement commonly demonstrate high FDG uptake. The sensitivity of PET/CT is higher in nodes > 1 cm, but specificity and accuracy are lower.[71]

f) Tumor size > 3 cm. In a meta-analysis, the negative predictive value of PET/CT for mediastinal metastases was 94% for tumors ≤ 3 cm and 89% for tumors > 3 cm.[70]

4. **Pattern of uptake.** Understanding the standard pattern of lymphatic spread of lung lesions by location is helpful in avoiding false-positive results. For example, left upper lobe malignancies will usually first metastasize to the aortopulmonary window nodes. The first level of nodal drainage is usually the most intense if multiple nodes are involved (▶ Fig. 11.13). This can help distinguish metastatic disease from benign causes of

adenopathy, such as sarcoidosis, in which the nodes usually appear with similar intensity (▶ Fig. 11.14).

5. Patients with other pulmonary pathologies (e.g., interstitial pneumonitis, tuberculosis) are more likely to have false-positive results, even if the disease is inactive.

6. **SUVs and visual analysis:**
   a) *SUV cutoff*. SUV cutoffs of 2.5 to 5.3 have been used to distinguish between benign and malignant adenopathy.[72,73] When evaluating specific SUV cutoffs, there is a tradeoff between optimal accuracy (which will require higher SUV cutoffs) and the clinical role of PET/CT, which is to potentially preclude mediastinoscopy in negative cases (requiring a lower SUV cutoff to minimize false-negative results). One study[74] suggests using a SUV of 2.5, as the resulting high negative predictive value of 96% may allow the omission of mediastinoscopy in PET-negative cases. However, the highest diagnostic accuracy was achieved with a SUV of 4.5 in this study.
   b) It is not clear whether using SUVs is superior to visual interpretation (using uptake greater than mediastinum as positive); in one study, there was no difference,[73] while in another, use of visual criteria resulted in overdiagnosis.[75]
   c) In equivocal, mildly positive, nodes, the use of ratios may be helpful. For example, threshold ratios of 0.20 to 0.30 (ratio of SUV node/SUV tumor) have been accurate in predicting nodal malignancy,[76,77,78] as well as a threshold ratio of 3.0 for SUV node/SUV tumor size.[78]

7. **Lymph node density**. Lymph node density can be helpful in the evaluation of lymph nodes with intermediate degrees of FDG uptake ($2.0 < SUVmax \leq 4.0$). Malignant lymph nodes will typically be higher in density than benign lymph nodes, although very high densities can be seen in benign nodes. In one report,[79] 71% of malignant lymph nodes had median Hounsfield units (HU) between 25 and 45. By using additional density criteria (median HU: 25–45) in lymph nodes with intermediate FDG uptake, the sensitivity improved from 70 to 88%. Other reports have used cutoff values of 7.5 and 20 HU[80,81] to distinguish between benign and malignant lymph nodes. A 20 HU cutoff may be useful specifically to exclude a benign etiology,

as in one report[80] > 99% of benign lymph nodes were below the 20 HU cutoff.

8. **Dexamethasone suppression**. Dexamethasone suppression has the potential to reduce false-positive findings secondary to inflammation. In one report,[82] patients with NSCLC were studied without dexamethasone and with 8 mg of oral dexamethasone administered 24 hours prior to PET/CT. The glucose levels were not elevated by this dose, and visual uptake and SUV in true-positive nodes was not affected. In false-positive nodes, the visual uptake was decreased and there was a mean decrease in SUVmax of 20%. Twenty-one percent of false-positive nodes were true negative after dexamethasone administration.

16.3.3 Pitfalls

1. The accuracy of PET/CT is reduced in countries where tuberculosis is endemic (▶ Fig. 16.8). In a meta-analysis,[83] studies from tuberculosis endemic countries showed lower sensitivity on a node-basis and lower specificity on a patient-basis.

2. Mild bilateral hilar nodal uptake from inflammatory etiologies is often seen in the lung cancer population as well as patients without any known underlying disease. However, this should be interpreted with caution in tuberculosis endemic countries, as metastatic lymph nodes can be hidden in a "benign" pattern of bilateral mediastinal and hilar nodal uptake.[83]

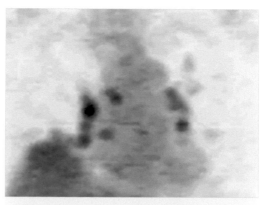

Fig. 16.8 Pulmonary tuberculosis. MIP PET in a patient with pulmonary tuberculosis demonstrates FDG uptake in bilateral hilar and mediastinal nodes and the left lung.

3. False-positive mediastinal and hilar nodes often have histologic findings of follicular hyperplasia, anthracotic pigmentation, and macrophage infiltration.[84]

4. Inaccurate mediastinal nodal staging is more often seen in patients with rheumatoid arthritis, diabetes, tuberculosis, and pneumonia.[85]

5. The highest rate of inaccuracy is nodal station 4 (lower paratracheal) followed by station 7 (inferior mediastinal) and station 9 (pulmonary ligament).[85]

6. **Adrenal hyperplasia.** Adrenal hyperplasia may have increased uptake. In patients with carcinoid or small cell tumors, adrenal hyperplasia can mimic bilateral adrenal metastases (▶ Fig. 7.38).

7. **Talc pleurodesis.** Prior talc pleurodesis can cause increased pleural uptake, likely secondary to inflammation (▶ Fig. 16.9). Within 5 months of talc pleurodesis, both increased FDG uptake and increased pleural thickness are noted. After 5 months, pleural thickness stabilizes, which FDG uptake persists or increases further.[86] Calcification forms slowly. Correlation with CT can be helpful in distinguishing malignant pleural disease from changes from talc pleurodesis. If a calcified pleural lesion shows

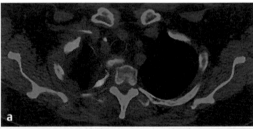
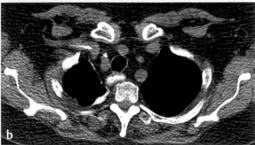

Fig. 16.9 Talc pleurodesis. **(a)** Axial PET/CT in a patient with a history of mesothelioma and talc pleurodesis demonstrates mild increased uptake corresponding to an area of increased pleural density on the corresponding axial CT **(b)**. This uptake is secondary to the prior talc pleurodesis.

FDG uptake, this is most likely inflammatory. Mild interval increases in pleural FDG uptake in calcified pleural lesions are also likely inflammatory. However, an increase in both FDG uptake and thickness in a noncalcified pleural lesion, or new FDG uptake in a noncalcified lesion, are suspicious for malignancy.

8. Pleural dissemination without an effusion from peripheral lung adenocarcinomas often presents as small pleural nodules and uneven pleural thickening. This is often beyond the resolution of PET, and in a patient with peripheral lung adenocarcinoma these findings on the CT portion of a PET/CT exam should be reported as suspicious for pleural dissemination even in the absence of FDG uptake.[87]

9. As false-positive results can result in incorrect M1 staging, metastatic disease identified by PET requires additional confirmation, particularly if there is a single site.[88]

16.3.4 NSCLC: Prognosis/Therapy Response

PET has several potential applications for therapy response and prognosis in NSCLC: prognosis of newly diagnosed tumors, restaging after neoadjuvant therapy, early assessment of therapy response, and restaging after therapy completion.[89,90,91] For restaging, PET is primarily useful in stage III disease and stage IV disease with solitary metastasis. In these cases, PET should ideally be performed 2 to 3 months after therapy. PET may not be helpful in restaging patients with stage I and II diseases.[92]

1. **Prognosis.** PET may be a useful tool for identifying patients at a high risk of recurrence; this may help guide therapy in resected stage I and II NSCLC.[93] In a meta-analysis,[94] high values of SUVmax, metabolic tumor volume, and total lesion glycolysis predicted a higher risk of recurrence or death in patients with surgical NSCLC. In a meta-analysis,[95] 11 of 13 studies found that a high primary tumor SUV was a poor prognostic factor for survival, with a hazard risk of 2.27. In contrast to the primary tumor, the prognostic ability of regional nodal SUV is less certain.[96] PET also provides prognostic information for tumors which tend to have less FDG uptake, such as bronchioalveolar carcinoma and stage I adenocarcinomas. For these tumors, even

relatively low levels of FDG uptake (SUV ≥ 2.5 in bronchioalveolar carcinoma and 3.3 in stage I adenocarcinoma) are associated with poor prognosis.[97,98]

In recurrent lung cancer, the SUV in the recurrent tumor is also an independent prognostic factor in survival.[99]

In addition, the primary tumor FDG uptake has been studied as a prognostic factor in patients receiving radiotherapy, both before and after treatment. In a meta-analysis,[100] both the pretherapy and posttherapy primary tumor SUV predicted survival and local control. PET may also have prognostic value after neoadjuvant therapy for stage III NSCLC.[101]

2. **Interim PET.** Patients with inoperable disease treated with systemic chemotherapy have overall response rates of 40%, but many patients experience significant treatment-related toxicity. Early prediction of tumor response can potentially spare some patients the additional cost and toxicity of ineffective treatment, as well as allow for other potentially more effective treatments. Multiple studies have suggested that PET may be able to predict tumor response and patient outcome as early as after one course of chemotherapy, as well as predict the response to newer targeted agents such as epidermal growth factor receptor tyrosine kinase inhibitors.[102] In one study,[103] PET studies performed at 1 and 3 weeks after the initiation of chemotherapy predicted survival. However, as issues such as timing of imaging and thresholds to define response are not established, further studies are necessary before PET can be used for this purpose in a clinical setting.

3. **End-of-treatment PET.** PET may have a potential role in restaging and response prediction after induction therapy for locally advanced disease (▶ Fig. 16.10). Therapeutic options for stage III patients include definitive chemo-radiotherapy, and neoadjuvant therapy (either chemotherapy alone or chemo-radiotherapy), followed by surgical resection. In patients receiving neoadjuvant therapy before planned surgical resection, assessment of clearance of tumor from mediastinal lymph nodes is very important. Survival is substantially higher in patients with mediastinal clearance and complete resection of disease, and surgical resection is often avoided if there is residual tumor in the mediastinal nodes after induction therapy. Parameters that can be assessed include residual tumor viability, persistent mediastinal disease, and distant disease.

In general, PET is less accurate for assessing the mediastinum after induction therapy than in untreated patients. PET/CT has superior sensitivity to PET for this application without compromising the specificity.[104] Histologic confirmation is still necessary in most cases, but PET may be useful in guiding mediastinoscopy or endoscopic procedures, or in detecting extrathoracic metastatic disease.

In the neoadjuvant setting, PET is more accurate in predicting the T component than the N status.[47] PET is sensitive but nonspecific for the detection of residual disease in the primary tumor.[105] PET is specific but has limited sensitivity for restaging of mediastinal nodes.[105] After neoadjuvant chemotherapy, PET is more accurate than CT in detecting residual tumor, except in N1 nodes where PET and CT are comparable.

The data on restaging with PET (primarily in stage IIIA–N2 disease) after neoadjuvant therapy are conflicting. While PET or PET/CT may be more accurate in assessing response than CT[106] or repeat mediastinoscopy,[107] the published accuracy ranges from 50 to 95%.[19,108] In a meta-analysis of the value of PET in predicting pathological tumor response of NSCLC to neoadjuvant therapy,[25] the sensitivity and specificity were 83 and 84%, respectively, and the predictive value of PET was superior to that of CT. In a

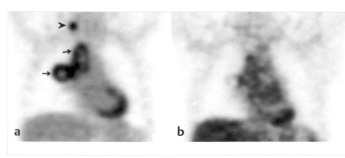

Fig. 16.10 Therapy follow-up for lung cancer. **(a)** Coronal PET scan demonstrates uptake in necrotic right hilar and mediastinal nodes (*arrows*) and a right supraclavicular node (*arrowhead*). **(b)** Posttherapy coronal PET scan demonstrates that the supraclavicular activity has resolved and the hilar and mediastinal activity has decreased.

systematic review[109] of restaging after induction therapy for stage IIIa lung cancer, a complete response at all sites carries a false-negative rate of 50% for CT and 30% for PET, while mediastinal node involvement had a false-negative rate of 25% and false-positive rate of 33% for PET. Of the studies which report N2 data for PET restaging after induction chemotherapy only, the false-positive rates were 25 to 40% and false-negative rates were 23 to 36%.[110] One study[110] of patients undergoing induction chemotherapy for stage IIIA/pN2 disease did not find that postinduction PET avidity for N2 nodes was associated with pathological persistent disease, disease-free survival, or overall survival.

PET has also been used to predict survival after definitive chemoradiation therapy for locally advanced disease. In the largest prospective study,[111] higher posttreatment tumor SUV (peak or max) was associated with worse survival in stage III NSCLC. Although a clear cutoff value useful for routine clinical use could be identified, there were no long-term survivors with a posttreatment SUV (peak) > 7. In a secondary analysis of the same study,[112] high residual metabolic activity in regional lymph nodes on posttreatment PET was associated with worse local-regional control.

16.3.5 Pearls/Pitfalls

1. PET is particularly useful when posttreatment scarring and pleural thickening limit the role of CT for assessing disease.
2. Radiation pneumonitis has a characteristic linear border and diffuse intense uptake (▶ Fig. 7.26). Uptake on PET can be seen before radiographic findings. Tumor recurrence has more focal uptake and can usually be differentiated from radiation pneumonitis. However, radiation pneumonitis can occasionally have heterogeneous uptake in the early stages, and thus PET imaging should be delayed for 3 to 6 months after radiotherapy if possible.[113]

16.4 NSCLC: Recurrence[89,114]

PET is useful in the evaluation of local recurrence following treatment.
1. Residual thoracic abnormalities on CT are common as a result of treatment. PET can differentiate between local recurrence and posttreatment changes. In a meta-analysis,[115] PET/CT had a better diagnostic accuracy than

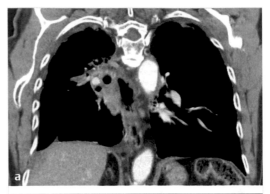

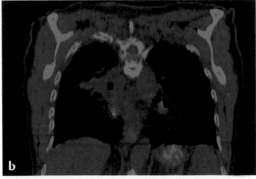

Fig. 16.11 Recurrent lung cancer. **(a)** Coronal contrast-enhanced CT in a patient with lung cancer status post radiotherapy demonstrates extensive soft tissue in the right hilar region. Tumor cannot be differentiated from fibrosis in this case. **(b)** Coronal PET/CT at the same level demonstrates two small foci of tumor in the hilar soft tissue.

conventional imaging for the detection of lung cancer recurrence (▶ Fig. 16.11). The sensitivity and specificity of PET/CT was 90 and 90%, respectively, compared to 78 and 80% for conventional imaging.
2. PET/CT has comparable sensitivity to PET for recurrence, but has substantially higher specificity.[116]
3. The SUV in the recurrent tumor is an independent survival factor.[99]

16.5 Radiation Therapy Planning

PET/CT is potentially valuable in radiation therapy (RT) planning, primarily in better defining the RT field or gross tumor volume (GTV), resulting in significant changes in RT delivery. For RT delivery to the primary tumor, the primary advantage has been in patients with atelectasis, defining the tumor boundary differently and allowing for sparing of lung tissue. The other major change in RT delivery is a change in nodal status (e.g., including CT-negative but PET-positive nodes in the RT field, and excluding CT-positive but PET-negative nodes). Other potential applications are allowing dose heterogeneity in one target by determining biological differences within the tumor, assessing the tumor during and after chemoradiotherapy, and response-modulated radiotherapy based on changing the target volumes during the course of treatment.[117] In a multicenter trial,[118] the GTV was smaller for PET/CT-derived volumes compared to CT-derived volumes, and nodal contours were altered for 51% of patients. Changes in the target volume of over 20% and stage alteration of 20 to 50% have been observed when PET has been incorporated in target volume delineation.[119]

16.6 Radiofrequency Ablation

PET/CT has been used for response assessment, and the detection and prediction of local recurrence after radiofrequency ablation (RFA) of lung tumors. In one report,[120] PET/CT detected a higher number of early treatment failures than chest CT, without false-negative findings. This led to changes in treatment strategy in 26%. In particular, PET/CT can detect malignant lesions inside the ablation zone which do not alter morphology or contrast enhancement patterns. However, one limitation of PET/CT is the relatively poor specificity. In a multicenter prospective study,[121] the sensitivity and specificity were 91 and 63%, respectively, for PET/CT performed at 3 months after RFA. In particular, specificity was low for lesions close to the pleura.

16.6.1 Timing

There has been some variability in published reports regarding the optimal timing for PET/CT after RFA, but suggestions range from 3 to 6 months.[120,121,122,123] Earlier PET/CT imaging after RFA is not necessary and less accurate than imaging at 3 to 6 months.[122,123]

16.6.2 Interpretation

Inflammation at the periphery of the necrotic zone is noted as early as 2 to 3 days after RFA.[124] On PET/CT exams, this results in a ring of peripheral activity around a central photopenic area. There is variability in the literature regarding the time course of the ring of peripheral activity. It has been suggested that the uptake should reach back-ground mediastinal blood pool by 2 months[125]; however, one report[126] indicates that the ring may persist at 6 months but will resolve by 12 months. In this same report, the peripheral ring was replaced by a central increase in activity at 6 and 12 months, which was hypothesized to be due to the outer reactive lung being drawn into the center of the ablated lesion. However, this delayed central increased activity has not been identified in other reports or after liver RFA.

Postablation FDG uptake has been categorized into favorable and unfavorable patterns.[127] Favorable uptake patterns suggesting nonrecurrence are diffuse, heterogeneous, rim, and rim + focal (the focus not corresponding to the original tumor nodule). Unfavorable uptake patterns suggesting recurrence are focal, and rim + focal (the focus corresponding to the original tumor nodule). A high postablation SUV and progressive increase in FDG uptake during follow-up also predict local recurrence.

Inflammatory FDG uptake can occur in both the RFA needle path and in mediastinal nodes.[120] This can occur early (24 hours) or late (3 months) after the procedure.

16.7 Small Cell Lung Cancer

Compared to conventional imaging, PET or PET/CT can result in a change in stage in 10 to 17% of patients.[128,129,130] In a systematic review of imaging for the pretreatment staging of small cell lung cancer,[131] FDG PET/CT was more sensitive than CT or bone scintigraphy for detecting osseous metastases, and more sensitive for detecting any distant metastases. In a meta-analysis,[132] the sensitivity and specificity of PET and PET/CT for the detection of extensive disease in small-cell lung cancer was 97 and 98%, respectively.

16.8 Mesothelioma

PET/CT is helpful in diagnosing and staging pleural mesothelioma. NCCN guidelines[48] suggest that PET-CT has a role in pretreatment evaluation only in patients being considered for surgery. The primary role of PET/CT staging is to identify disease outside the affected hemithorax and in precluding surgery in patients with extrathoracic disease.

In a best evidence review,[133] PET/CT had a combined sensitivity and specificity of 88 and 93%, respectively; however, sensitivity was substantially lower for stage N2 (37%) and T4 disease (67%). PET/CT was more accurate than PET, and PET was more accurate than CT or MRI. Compared to PET/CT, CT

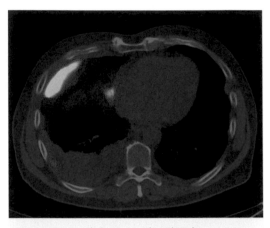

Fig. 16.12 Mesothelioma. Axial PET/CT demonstrates medial and lateral pleural uptake in a patient with mesothelioma.

has a lower specificity for stage II (77 vs. 100%) and stage III (75 vs. 100%) disease. In addition, PET/CT has lower interobserver variability than CT.[134] However, PET/CT may understage patients, as it does not accurately identify advanced tumor stage (T4) or mediastinal nodal disease (N2).[135]

In addition, PET/CT may be helpful in predicting disease recurrence and survival. In patients with resectable disease, the metabolic response after neoadjuvant chemotherapy is an independent prognostic factor for survival.[136] PET/CT also predicts survival in patients undergoing palliative chemotherapy.[137]

1. PET may have limited sensitivity for determining the extent of the local tumor (► Fig. 16.12) (subtle transdiaphragmatic extension is particularly hard to detect) and mediastinal nodal metastases.
2. A high level of uptake in the primary tumor is associated with the presence of N2 disease and with poor survival.
3. SUV > 10 is associated with poor survival.[138]
4. Localized fibrous tumor of the pleura (benign mesothelioma) typically has low (< 2.5 SUV) uptake.[139]
5. Most benign pleural processes have a SUV < 2.2.[54]
6. Prior talc pleurodesis does not alter the accuracy of PET/CT staging of mesothelioma.[135]

References

[1] Gould MK, Donington J, Lynch WR, et al. Evaluation of individuals with pulmonary nodules: when is it lung cancer? Diagnosis and management of lung cancer, 3rd ed: American College of Chest Physicians evidence-based clinical practice guidelines. Chest. 2013; 143(5) Suppl:e93S–e120S

[2] Callister ME, Baldwin DR, Akram AR, et al. British Thoracic Society Pulmonary Nodule Guideline Development Group, British Thoracic Society Standards of Care Committee. British Thoracic Society guidelines for the investigation and management of pulmonary nodules. Thorax. 2015; 70 Suppl 2: ii1–ii54

[3] Cao JQ, Rodrigues GB, Louie AV, Zaric GS. Systematic review of the cost-effectiveness of positron-emission tomography in staging of non–small-cell lung cancer and management of solitary pulmonary nodules. Clin Lung Cancer. 2012; 13(3): 161–170

[4] Gambhir SS, Shepherd JE, Shah BD, et al. Analytical decision model for the cost-effective management of solitary pulmonary nodules. J Clin Oncol. 1998; 16(6):2113–2125

[5] Deppen SA, Davis WT, Green EA, et al. Cost-effectiveness of initial diagnostic strategies for pulmonary nodules presenting to thoracic surgeons. Ann Thorac Surg. 2014; 98(4): 1214–1222

[6] Cheran SK, Nielsen ND, Patz EF, Jr. False-negative findings for primary lung tumors on FDG positron emission tomography: staging and prognostic implications. AJR Am J Roentgenol. 2004; 182(5):1129–1132

[7] Marom EM, Sarvis S, Herndon JE, II, Patz EF, Jr. T1 lung cancers: sensitivity of diagnosis with fluorodeoxyglucose PET. Radiology. 2002; 223(2):453–459

[8] Cronin P, Dwamena BA, Kelly AM, Carlos RC. Solitary pulmonary nodules: meta-analytic comparison of cross-sectional imaging modalities for diagnosis of malignancy. Radiology. 2008; 246(3):772–782

[9] Kim SK, Allen-Auerbach M, Goldin J, et al. Accuracy of PET/CT in characterization of solitary pulmonary lesions. J Nucl Med. 2007; 48(2):214–220

[10] Swensen SJ, Viggiano RW, Midthun DE, et al. Lung nodule enhancement at CT: multicenter study. Radiology. 2000; 214(1):73–80

[11] Christensen JA, Nathan MA, Mullan BP, Hartman TE, Swensen SJ, Lowe VJ. Characterization of the solitary pulmonary nodule: 18F-FDG PET versus nodule-enhancement CT. AJR Am J Roentgenol. 2006; 187(5):1361–1367

[12] Yi CA, Lee KS, Kim BT, et al. Tissue characterization of solitary pulmonary nodule: comparative study between helical dynamic CT and integrated PET/CT. J Nucl Med. 2006; 47(3): 443–450

[13] Rohren EM, Lowe VJ. Update in PET imaging of nonsmall cell lung cancer. Semin Nucl Med. 2004; 34(2):134–153

[14] Blum J, Handmaker H, Lister-James J, Rinne N. A multicenter trial with a somatostatin analog (99m)Tc depreotide in the evaluation of solitary pulmonary nodules. Chest. 2000; 117 (5):1232–1238

[15] Ferran N, Ricart Y, Lopez M, et al. Characterization of radiologically indeterminate lung lesions: 99mTc-depreotide SPECT versus 18F-FDG PET. Nucl Med Commun. 2006; 27 (6):507–514

[16] Lowe VJ, Fletcher JW, Gobar L, et al. Prospective investigation of positron emission tomography in lung nodules. J Clin Oncol. 1998; 16(3):1075–1084

[17] Hagge RJ, Coleman RE. Positron emission tomography: lung cancer. Semin Roentgenol. 2002; 37(2):110–117

[18] Herder GJ, Golding RP, Hoekstra OS, et al. The performance of (18)F-fluorodeoxyglucose positron emission tomography in small solitary pulmonary nodules. Eur J Nucl Med Mol Imaging. 2004; 31(9):1231–1236

[19] Detterbeck FC, Vansteenkiste JF, Morris DE, Dooms CA, Khandani AH, Socinski MA. Seeking a home for a PET, part

3: Emerging applications of positron emission tomography imaging in the management of patients with lung cancer. Chest. 2004; 126(5):1656–1666

[20] Detterbeck FC, Falen S, Rivera MP, Halle JS, Socinski MA. Seeking a home for a PET, part 2: Defining the appropriate place for positron emission tomography imaging in the staging of patients with suspected lung cancer. Chest. 2004; 125 (6):2300–2308

[21] Detterbeck FC, Falen S, Rivera MP, Halle JS, Socinski MA. Seeking a home for a PET, part 1: Defining the appropriate place for positron emission tomography imaging in the diagnosis of pulmonary nodules or masses. Chest. 2004; 125 (6):2294–2299

[22] Lowe VJ, DeLong DM, Hoffman JM, Coleman RE. Optimum scanning protocol for FDG-PET evaluation of pulmonary malignancy. J Nucl Med. 1995; 36(5):883–887

[23] Demura Y, Tsuchida T, Ishizaki T, et al. 18F-FDG accumulation with PET for differentiation between benign and malignant lesions in the thorax. J Nucl Med. 2003; 44(4):540–548

[24] Barger RL, Jr, Nandalur KR. Diagnostic performance of dual-time 18F-FDG PET in the diagnosis of pulmonary nodules: a meta-analysis. Acad Radiol. 2012; 19(2):153–158

[25] Zhang L, Wang Y, Lei J, Tian J, Zhai Y. Dual time point 18FDG-PET/CT versus single time point 18FDG-PET/CT for the differential diagnosis of pulmonary nodules: a meta-analysis. Acta Radiol. 2013; 54(7):770–777

[26] Núñez R, Kalapparambath A, Varela J. Improvement in sensitivity with delayed imaging of pulmonary lesions with FDG-PET. Rev Esp Med Nucl. 2007; 26(4):196–207

[27] Uhlén N, Grundberg O, Jacobsson H, et al. 18F-FDG PET/CT diagnosis of bronchopulmonary carcinoids versus pulmonary hamartomas. Clin Nucl Med. 2016; 41(4):263–267

[28] de Geus-Oei LF, van Krieken JH, Aliredjo RP, et al. Biological correlates of FDG uptake in non-small cell lung cancer. Lung Cancer. 2007; 55(1):79–87

[29] McAdams HP, Erasmus JJ, Patz EF, Goodman PC, Coleman RE. Evaluation of patients with round atelectasis using 2-[18F]-fluoro-2-deoxy-D-glucose PET. J Comput Assist Tomogr. 1998; 22(4):601–604

[30] Shim SS, Lee KS, Kim BT, Choi JY, Chung MJ, Lee EJ. Focal parenchymal lung lesions showing a potential of false-positive and false-negative interpretations on integrated PET/CT. AJR Am J Roentgenol. 2006; 186(3):639–648

[31] Li Y, Su M, Li F, Kuang A, Tian R. The value of 18F-FDG-PET/CT in the differential diagnosis of solitary pulmonary nodules in areas with a high incidence of tuberculosis. Ann Nucl Med. 2011; 25(10):804–811

[32] Erdoğan Y, Özyürek BA, Özmen Ö, et al. The evaluation of FDG PET/CT scan findings in patients with organizing pneumonia mimicking lung cancer. Mol Imaging Radionucl Ther. 2015; 24(2):60–65

[33] Hashimoto Y, Tsujikawa T, Kondo C, et al. Accuracy of PET for diagnosis of solid pulmonary lesions with 18F-FDG uptake below the standardized uptake value of 2.5. J Nucl Med. 2006; 47(3):426–431

[34] Heyneman LE, Patz EF. PET imaging in patients with bronchioloalveolar cell carcinoma. Lung Cancer. 2002; 38(3):261–266

[35] Krüger S, Buck AK, Blumstein NM, et al. Use of integrated FDG PET/CT imaging in pulmonary carcinoid tumours. J Intern Med. 2006; 260(6):545–550

[36] Lindell RM, Hartman TE, Swensen SJ, et al. Lung cancer screening experience: a retrospective review of PET in 22 non-small cell lung carcinomas detected on screening chest CT in a high-risk population. AJR Am J Roentgenol. 2005; 185(1):126–131

[37] Chun EJ, Lee HJ, Kang WJ, et al. Differentiation between malignancy and inflammation in pulmonary ground-glass nodules: The feasibility of integrated (18)F-FDG PET/CT. Lung Cancer. 2009; 65(2):180–186

[38] Tsushima Y, Tateishi U, Uno H, et al. Diagnostic performance of PET/CT in differentiation of malignant and benign nonsolid solitary pulmonary nodules. Ann Nucl Med. 2008; 22 (7):571–577

[39] Nomori H, Watanabe K, Ohtsuka T, Naruke T, Suemasu K, Uno K. Evaluation of F-18 fluorodeoxyglucose (FDG) PET scanning for pulmonary nodules less than 3 cm in diameter, with special reference to the CT images. Lung Cancer. 2004; 45(1):19–27

[40] Tsutani Y, Miyata Y, Nakayama H, et al. Solid tumor size on high-resolution computed tomography and maximum standardized uptake on positron emission tomography for new clinical T descriptors with T1 lung adenocarcinoma. Ann Oncol. 2013; 24(9):2376–2381

[41] Uehara H, Tsutani Y, Okumura S, et al. Prognostic role of positron emission tomography and high-resolution computed tomography in clinical stage IA lung adenocarcinoma. Ann Thorac Surg. 2013; 96(6):1958–1965

[42] Veronesi G, Bellomi M, Veronesi U, et al. Role of positron emission tomography scanning in the management of lung nodules detected at baseline computed tomography screening. Ann Thorac Surg. 2007; 84(3):959–965, discussion 965–966

[43] Hsu WH, Hsu NY, Shen YY, Yen RF, Kao CH. Differentiating solitary pulmonary metastases in patients with extrapulmonary neoplasmas using FDG-PET. Cancer Invest. 2003; 21 (1):47–52

[44] van Tinteren H, Hoekstra OS, Smit EF, et al. Effectiveness of positron emission tomography in the preoperative assessment of patients with suspected non-small-cell lung cancer: the PLUS multicentre randomised trial. Lancet. 2002; 359 (9315):1388–1393

[45] Pieterman RM, van Putten JW, Meuzelaar JJ, et al. Preoperative staging of non-small-cell lung cancer with positron-emission tomography. N Engl J Med. 2000; 343(4):254–261

[46] Schmidt-Hansen M, Baldwin DR, Zamora J. FDG-PET/CT imaging for mediastinal staging in patients with potentially resectable non-small cell lung cancer. JAMA. 2015; 313(14):1465–1466

[47] De Leyn P, Dooms C, Kuzdzal J, et al. Preoperative mediastinal lymph node staging for non-small cell lung cancer: 2014 update of the 2007 ESTS guidelines. Transl Lung Cancer Res. 2014; 3(4):225–233

[48] Ettinger DS, Wood DE, Akerley W, et al. NCCN guidelines insights: non-small cell lung cancer, version 4.2016. J Natl Compr Canc Netw. 2016; 14(3):255–264

[49] Silvestri GA, Gonzalez AV, Jantz MA, et al. Methods for staging non-small cell lung cancer: Diagnosis and management of lung cancer, 3rd ed: American College of Chest Physicians evidence-based clinical practice guidelines. Chest. 2013; 143(5) Suppl:e211S–e250S

[50] Cho H, Lee HY, Kim J, et al. Pure ground glass nodular adenocarcinomas: Are preoperative positron emission tomography/computed tomography and brain magnetic resonance imaging useful or necessary? J Thorac Cardiovasc Surg. 2015; 150(3):514–520

[51] Kim TJ, Park CM, Goo JM, Lee KW. Is there a role for FDG PET in the management of lung cancer manifesting predominantly as ground-glass opacity? AJR Am J Roentgenol. 2012; 198(1):83–88

[52] Luque M, Díez FJ, Disdier C. Optimal sequence of tests for the mediastinal staging of non-small cell lung cancer. BMC Med Inform Decis Mak. 2016; 16:9

[53] Czernin J, Allen-Auerbach M, Schelbert HR. Improvements in cancer staging with PET/CT: literature-based evidence as of September 2006. J Nucl Med. 2007; 48 Suppl 1:78S–88S

[54] Cerfolio RJ, Ojha B, Bryant AS, Raghuveer V, Mountz JM, Bartolucci AA. The accuracy of integrated PET-CT compared with dedicated PET alone for the staging of patients with nonsmall cell lung cancer. Ann Thorac Surg. 2004; 78(3): 1017–1023, discussion 1017–1023

[55] Ebihara A, Nomori H, Watanabe K, et al. Characteristics of advantages of positron emission tomography over computed tomography for N-staging in lung cancer patients. Jpn J Clin Oncol. 2006; 36(11):694–698

[56] Li J, Xu W, Kong F, Sun X, Zuo X. Meta-analysis: accuracy of 18FDG PET-CT for distant metastasis staging in lung cancer patients. Surg Oncol. 2013; 22(3):151–155

[57] Qu X, Huang X, Yan W, Wu L, Dai K. A meta-analysis of 18FDG-PET-CT, 18FDG-PET, MRI and bone scintigraphy for diagnosis of bone metastases in patients with lung cancer. Eur J Radiol. 2012; 81(5):1007–1015

[58] Jung MY, Chong A, Seon HJ, et al. Indeterminate pleural metastasis on contrast-enhanced chest CT in non-small cell lung cancer: improved differential diagnosis with (18)F-FDG PET/CT. Ann Nucl Med. 2012; 26(4):327–336

[59] Treglia G, Sadeghi R, Annunziata S, et al. Diagnostic accuracy of 18F-FDG-PET and PET/CT in the differential diagnosis between malignant and benign pleural lesions: a systematic review and meta-analysis. Acad Radiol. 2014; 21(1):11–20

[60] Treglia G, Sadeghi R, Annunziata S, et al. Diagnostic performance of fluorine-18-fluorodeoxyglucose positron emission tomography in the assessment of pleural abnormalities in cancer patients: a systematic review and a meta-analysis. Lung Cancer. 2014; 83(1):1–7

[61] Duysinx BC, Larock MP, Nguyen D, et al. 18F-FDG PET imaging in assessing exudative pleural effusions. Nucl Med Commun. 2006; 27(12):971–976

[62] De Leyn P, Dooms C, Kuzdzal J, et al. Revised ESTS guidelines for preoperative mediastinal lymph node staging for non-small-cell lung cancer. Eur J Cardiothorac Surg. 2014; 45(5): 787–798

[63] Eberhardt WE, De Ruysscher D, Weder W, et al. Panel Members. 2nd ESMO consensus conference in lung cancer: locally advanced stage III non-small-cell lung cancer. Ann Oncol. 2015; 26(8):1573–1588

[64] Hauer J, Szlubowski A, Żanowska K, et al. Minimally invasive strategy for mediastinal staging of patients with lung cancer. Pol Arch Med Wewn. 2015; 125(12):910–913

[65] Verhagen AF, Bootsma GP, Tjan-Heijnen VC, et al. FDG-PET in staging lung cancer: how does it change the algorithm? Lung Cancer. 2004; 44(2):175–181

[66] Cerfolio RJ, Bryant AS, Eloubeidi MA. Routine mediastinoscopy and esophageal ultrasound fine-needle aspiration in patients with non-small cell lung cancer who are clinically N2 negative: a prospective study. Chest. 2006; 130(6):1791–1795

[67] de Langen AJ, Raijmakers P, Riphagen I, Paul MA, Hoekstra OS. The size of mediastinal lymph nodes and its relation with metastatic involvement: a meta-analysis. Eur J Cardiothorac Surg. 2006; 29(1):26–29

[68] Murgu SD. Diagnosing and staging lung cancer involving the mediastinum. Chest. 2015; 147(5):1401–1412

[69] Farjah F, Lou F, Sima C, Rusch VW, Rizk NP. A prediction model for pathologic N2 disease in lung cancer patients with a negative mediastinum by positron emission tomography. J Thorac Oncol. 2013; 8(9):1170–1180

[70] Wang J, Welch K, Wang L, Kong FM. Negative predictive value of positron emission tomography and computed tomography for stage T1–2N0 non-small-cell lung cancer: a meta-analysis. Clin Lung Cancer. 2012; 13(2):81–89

[71] Al-Sarraf N, Gately K, Lucey J, Wilson L, McGovern E, Young V. Lymph node staging by means of positron emission tomography is less accurate in non-small cell lung cancer patients with enlarged lymph nodes: analysis of 1,145 lymph nodes. Lung Cancer. 2008; 60(1):62–68

[72] Bryant AS, Cerfolio RJ, Klemm KM, Ojha B. Maximum standard uptake value of mediastinal lymph nodes on integrated FDG-PET-CT predicts pathology in patients with non-small cell lung cancer. Ann Thorac Surg. 2006; 82(2):417–422, discussion 422–423

[73] Vansteenkiste JF, Stroobants SG, De Leyn PR, et al. Lymph node staging in non-small-cell lung cancer with FDG-PET scan: a prospective study on 690 lymph node stations from 68 patients. J Clin Oncol. 1998; 16(6):2142–2149

[74] Hellwig D, Graeter TP, Ukena D, et al. 18F-FDG PET for mediastinal staging of lung cancer: which SUV threshold makes sense? J Nucl Med. 2007; 48(11):1761–1766

[75] Hara M, Shiraki N, Itoh M, et al. A problem in diagnosing N3 disease using FDG-PET in patients with lung cancer–high false positive rate with visual assessment. Ann Nucl Med. 2004; 18(6):483–488

[76] Koksal D, Demirag F, Bayiz H, et al. The correlation of SUV-max with pathological characteristics of primary tumor and the value of Tumor/ Lymph node SUVmax ratio for predicting metastasis to lymph nodes in resected NSCLC patients. J Cardiothorac Surg. 2013; 8:63

[77] Mattes MD, Moshchinsky AB, Ahsanuddin S, et al. Ratio of lymph node to primary tumor SUV on PET/CT accurately predicts nodal malignancy in non-small-cell lung cancer. Clin Lung Cancer. 2015; 16(6):e253–e258

[78] Moloney F, Ryan D, McCarthy L, et al. Increasing the accuracy of 18F-FDG PET/CT interpretation of "mildly positive" mediastinal nodes in the staging of non-small cell lung cancer. Eur J Radiol. 2014; 83(5):843–847

[79] Lee JW, Kim EY, Kim DJ, et al. The diagnostic ability of 18F-FDG PET/CT for mediastinal lymph node staging using 18F-FDG uptake and volumetric CT histogram analysis in non-small cell lung cancer. Eur Radiol. 2016; 26(12):4515–4523

[80] Flechsig P, Frank P, Kratochwil C, et al. Radiomic analysis using density threshold for FDG-PET/CT-based N-staging in lung cancer patients. Mol Imaging Biol. 2017; 19(2):315–322

[81] Giesel FL, Schneider F, Kratochwil C, et al. Correlation between SUVmax and CT radiomic analysis using lymph node density in PET/CT-based lymph node staging. J Nucl Med. 2017; 58(2):282–287

[82] Nakajo M, Nakajo M, Nakayama H, et al. Dexamethasone suppression FDG PET/CT for differentiating between true- and false-positive pulmonary and mediastinal lymph node metastases in non-small cell lung cancer: a pilot study of FDG PET/CT after oral administration of dexamethasone. Radiology. 2016; 279(1):246–253

[83] Pak K, Park S, Cheon GJ, et al. Update on nodal staging in non-small cell lung cancer with integrated positron emission tomography/computed tomography: a meta-analysis. Ann Nucl Med. 2015; 29(5):409–419

[84] Shim SS, Lee KS, Kim BT, et al. Non-small cell lung cancer: prospective comparison of integrated FDG PET/CT and CT alone for preoperative staging. Radiology. 2005; 236(3): 1011–1019

[85] Al-Sarraf N, Aziz R, Doddakula K, et al. Factors causing inaccurate staging of mediastinal nodal involvement in non-small cell lung cancer patients staged by positron emission tomography. Interact Cardiovasc Thorac Surg. 2007; 6(3): 350–353

[86] Nguyen NC, Tran I, Hueser CN, Oliver D, Farghaly HR, Osman MM. F-18 FDG PET/CT characterization of talc pleurodesis-induced pleural changes over time: a retrospective study. Clin Nucl Med. 2009; 34(12):886–890

[87] Shim SS, Lee KS, Kim BT, et al. Integrated PET/CT and the dry pleural dissemination of peripheral adenocarcinoma of the lung: diagnostic implications. J Comput Assist Tomogr. 2006; 30(1):70–76

[88] Reed CE, Harpole DH, Posther KE, et al. American College of Surgeons Oncology Group Z0050 trial. Results of the American College of Surgeons Oncology Group Z0050 trial: the utility of positron emission tomography in staging potentially operable non-small cell lung cancer. J Thorac Cardiovasc Surg. 2003; 126(6):1943–1951

[89] Vansteenkiste JF, Stroobants SG. Positron emission tomography in the management of non-small cell lung cancer. Hematol Oncol Clin North Am. 2004; 18(1):269–288

[90] Kostakoglu L, Goldsmith SJ. 18F-FDG PET evaluation of the response to therapy for lymphoma and for breast, lung, and colorectal carcinoma. J Nucl Med. 2003; 44(2):224–239

[91] Bunyaviroch T, Coleman RE. PET evaluation of lung cancer. J Nucl Med. 2006; 47(3):451–469

[92] Podoloff DA, Advani RH, Allred C, et al. NCCN task force report: positron emission tomography (PET)/computed tomography (CT) scanning in cancer. J Natl Compr Canc Netw. 2007; 5 Suppl 1:S1–S22, quiz S23–S2

[93] Pillot G, Siegel BA, Govindan R. Prognostic value of fluorodeoxyglucose positron emission tomography in non-small cell lung cancer: a review. J Thorac Oncol. 2006; 1(2):152–159

[94] Liu J, Dong M, Sun X, Li W, Xing L, Yu J. Prognostic value of 18F-FDG PET/CT in surgical non-small cell lung cancer: a meta-analysis. PLoS One. 2016; 11(1):e0146195

[95] Berghmans T, Dusart M, Paesmans M, et al. European Lung Cancer Working Party for the IASLC Lung Cancer Staging Project. Primary tumor standardized uptake value (SUV-max) measured on fluorodeoxyglucose positron emission tomography (FDG-PET) is of prognostic value for survival in non-small cell lung cancer (NSCLC): a systematic review and meta-analysis (MA) by the European Lung Cancer Working Party for the IASLC Lung Cancer Staging Project. J Thorac Oncol. 2008; 3(1):6–12

[96] de Geus-Oei LF, van der Heijden HF, Corstens FH, Oyen WJ. Predictive and prognostic value of FDG-PET in nonsmall-cell lung cancer: a systematic review. Cancer. 2007; 110(8):1654–1664

[97] Ohtsuka T, Nomori H, Watanabe K, et al. Prognostic significance of [(18)F]fluorodeoxyglucose uptake on positron emission tomography in patients with pathologic stage I lung adenocarcinoma. Cancer. 2006; 107(10):2468–2473

[98] Raz DJ, Odisho AY, Franc BL, Jablons DM. Tumor fluoro-2-deoxy-D-glucose avidity on positron emission tomographic scan predicts mortality in patients with early-stage pure and mixed bronchioloalveolar carcinoma. J Thorac Cardiovasc Surg. 2006; 132(5):1189–1195

[99] Hellwig D, Gröschel A, Graeter TP, et al. Diagnostic performance and prognostic impact of FDG-PET in suspected recurrence of surgically treated non-small cell lung cancer. Eur J Nucl Med Mol Imaging. 2006; 33(1):13–21

[100] Na F, Wang J, Li C, Deng L, Xue J, Lu Y. Primary tumor standardized uptake value measured on F18-Fluorodeoxyglucose positron emission tomography is of prediction value for survival and local control in non-small-cell lung cancer receiving radiotherapy: meta-analysis. J Thorac Oncol. 2014; 9(6):834–842

[101] Dooms C, Vansteenkiste J. Positron emission tomography in nonsmall cell lung cancer. Curr Opin Pulm Med. 2007; 13(4):256–260

[102] Skoura E, Datseris IE, Platis I, Oikonomopoulos G, Syrigos KN. Role of positron emission tomography in the early prediction of response to chemotherapy in patients with non-small-cell lung cancer. Clin Lung Cancer. 2012; 13(3):181–187

[103] Nahmias C, Hanna WT, Wahl LM, Long MJ, Hubner KF, Townsend DW. Time course of early response to chemotherapy in non-small cell lung cancer patients with 18F-FDG PET/CT. J Nucl Med. 2007; 48(5):744–751

[104] Vansteenkiste J, Dooms C. Positron emission tomography in nonsmall cell lung cancer. Curr Opin Oncol. 2007; 19(2):78–83

[105] Ryu JS, Choi NC, Fischman AJ, Lynch TJ, Mathisen DJ. FDG-PET in staging and restaging non-small cell lung cancer after neoadjuvant chemoradiotherapy: correlation with histopathology. Lung Cancer. 2002; 35(2):179–187

[106] Cerfolio RJ, Bryant AS, Ojha B. Restaging patients with N2 (stage IIIa) non-small cell lung cancer after neoadjuvant chemoradiotherapy: a prospective study. J Thorac Cardiovasc Surg. 2006; 131(6):1229–1235

[107] De Leyn P, Stroobants S, De Wever W, et al. Prospective comparative study of integrated positron emission tomography-computed tomography scan compared with remediastinoscopy in the assessment of residual mediastinal lymph node disease after induction chemotherapy for mediastinoscopy-proven stage IIIA-N2 Non-small-cell lung cancer: a Leuven Lung Cancer Group Study. J Clin Oncol. 2006; 24(21):3333–3339

[108] Knoepp UW, Ravenel JG. CT and PET imaging in non-small cell lung cancer. Crit Rev Oncol Hematol. 2006; 58(1):15–30

[109] de Cabanyes Candela S, Detterbeck FC. A systematic review of restaging after induction therapy for stage IIIa lung cancer: prediction of pathologic stage. J Thorac Oncol. 2010; 5(3):389–398

[110] Ripley RT, Suzuki K, Tan KS, et al. Postinduction positron emission tomography assessment of N2 nodes is not associated with ypN2 disease or overall survival in stage IIIA non-small cell lung cancer. J Thorac Cardiovasc Surg. 2016; 151(4):969–977, 979.e1–979.e3

[111] Machtay M, Duan F, Siegel BA, et al. Prediction of survival by [18F]fluorodeoxyglucose positron emission tomography in patients with locally advanced non-small-cell lung cancer undergoing definitive chemoradiation therapy: results of the ACRIN 6668/RTOG 0235 trial. J Clin Oncol. 2013; 31(30):3823–3830

[112] Markovina S, Duan F, Snyder BS, Siegel BA, Machtay M, Bradley JD. Regional lymph node uptake of [(18)F]fluorodeoxyglucose after definitive chemoradiation therapy predicts local-regional failure of locally advanced non-small cell lung cancer: results of ACRIN 6668/RTOG 0235. Int J Radiat Oncol Biol Phys. 2015; 93(3):597–605

[113] Bruzzi JF, Munden RF. PET/CT imaging of lung cancer. J Thorac Imaging. 2006; 21(2):123–136

[114] Vansteenkiste J, Fischer BM, Dooms C, Mortensen J. Positron-emission tomography in prognostic and therapeutic assessment of lung cancer: systematic review. Lancet Oncol. 2004; 5(9):531–540

[115] He YQ, Gong HL, Deng YF, Li WM. Diagnostic efficacy of PET and PET/CT for recurrent lung cancer: a meta-analysis. Acta Radiol. 2014; 55(3):309–317

[116] Keidar Z, Haim N, Guralnik L, et al. PET/CT using 18F-FDG in suspected lung cancer recurrence: diagnostic value and impact on patient management. J Nucl Med. 2004; 45(10):1640–1646

[117] Berberoğlu K. Use of positron emission tomography/computed tomography in radiation treatment planning for lung cancer. Mol Imaging Radionucl Ther. 2016; 25(2):50–62

[118] Bradley J, Bae K, Choi N, et al. A phase II comparative study of gross tumor volume definition with or without PET/CT fusion in dosimetric planning for non-small-cell lung cancer (NSCLC): primary analysis of Radiation Therapy Oncology Group (RTOG) 0515. Int J Radiat Oncol Biol Phys. 2012; 82 (1):435–41.e1

[119] Chi A, Nguyen NP. The utility of positron emission tomography in the treatment planning of image-guided radiotherapy for non-small cell lung cancer. Front Oncol. 2014; 4:273

[120] Deandreis D, Leboulleux S, Dromain C, et al. Role of FDG PET/CT and chest CT in the follow-up of lung lesions treated with radiofrequency ablation. Radiology. 2011; 258(1):270–276

[121] Bonichon F, Palussière J, Godbert Y, et al. Diagnostic accuracy of 18F-FDG PET/CT for assessing response to radiofrequency ablation treatment in lung metastases: a multicentre prospective study. Eur J Nucl Med Mol Imaging. 2013; 40(12):1817–1827

[122] Higuchi M, Honjo H, Shigihara T, Shishido F, Suzuki H, Gotoh M. A phase II study of radiofrequency ablation therapy for thoracic malignancies with evaluation by FDG-PET. J Cancer Res Clin Oncol. 2014; 140(11):1957–1963

[123] Yoo DC, Dupuy DE, Hillman SL, et al. Radiofrequency ablation of medically inoperable stage IA non-small cell lung cancer: are early posttreatment PET findings predictive of treatment outcome? AJR Am J Roentgenol. 2011; 197(2): 334–340

[124] Purandare NC, Rangarajan V, Shah SA, et al. Therapeutic response to radiofrequency ablation of neoplastic lesions: FDG PET/CT findings. Radiographics. 2011; 31(1):201–213

[125] Abtin FG, Eradat J, Gutierrez AJ, Lee C, Fishbein MC, Suh RD. Radiofrequency ablation of lung tumors: imaging features of the postablation zone. Radiographics. 2012; 32(4):947–969

[126] Sharma A, Lanuti M, He W, Palmer EL, Shepard JA, Digumarthy SR. Increase in fluorodeoxyglucose positron emission tomography activity following complete radiofrequency ablation of lung tumors. J Comput Assist Tomogr. 2013; 37(1):9–14

[127] Singnurkar A, Solomon SB, Gönen M, Larson SM, Schöder H. 18F-FDG PET/CT for the prediction and detection of local recurrence after radiofrequency ablation of malignant lung lesions. J Nucl Med. 2010; 51(12):1833–1840

[128] Brink I, Schumacher T, Mix M, et al. Impact of [18F]FDG-PET on the primary staging of small-cell lung cancer. Eur J Nucl Med Mol Imaging. 2004; 31(12):1614–1620

[129] Fischer BM, Mortensen J, Langer SW, et al. A prospective study of PET/CT in initial staging of small-cell lung cancer: comparison with CT, bone scintigraphy and bone marrow analysis. Ann Oncol. 2007; 18(2):338–345

[130] Bradley JD, Dehdashti F, Mintun MA, Govindan R, Trinkaus K, Siegel BA. Positron emission tomography in limited-stage small-cell lung cancer: a prospective study. J Clin Oncol. 2004; 22(16):3248–3254

[131] Mitchell MD, Aggarwal C, Tsou AY, Torigian DA, Treadwell JR. Imaging for the pretreatment staging of small cell lung cancer: a systematic review. Acad Radiol. 2016; 23(8):1047–1056

[132] Lu YY, Chen JH, Liang JA, Chu S, Lin WY, Kao CH. 18F-FDG PET or PET/CT for detecting extensive disease in small-cell lung cancer: a systematic review and meta-analysis. Nucl Med Commun. 2014; 35(7):697–703

[133] Zahid I, Sharif S, Routledge T, Scarci M. What is the best way to diagnose and stage malignant pleural mesothelioma? Interact Cardiovasc Thorac Surg. 2011; 12(2):254–259

[134] Frauenfelder T, Kestenholz P, Hunziker R, et al. Use of computed tomography and positron emission tomography/computed tomography for staging of local extent in patients with malignant pleural mesothelioma. J Comput Assist Tomogr. 2015; 39(2):160–165

[135] Pilling J, Dartnell JA, Lang-Lazdunski L. Integrated positron emission tomography-computed tomography does not accurately stage intrathoracic disease of patients undergoing trimodality therapy for malignant pleural mesothelioma. Thorac Cardiovasc Surg. 2010; 58(4):215–219

[136] Tsutani Y, Takuwa T, Miyata Y, et al. Prognostic significance of metabolic response by positron emission tomography after neoadjuvant chemotherapy for resectable malignant pleural mesothelioma. Ann Oncol. 2013; 24(4):1005–1010

[137] Sharif S, Zahid I, Routledge T, Scarci M. Does positron emission tomography offer prognostic information in malignant pleural mesothelioma? Interact Cardiovasc Thorac Surg. 2011; 12(5):806–811

[138] Flores RM, Akhurst T, Gonen M, et al. Positron emission tomography predicts survival in malignant pleural mesothelioma. J Thorac Cardiovasc Surg. 2006; 132(4):763–768

[139] Cortes J, Rodriguez J, Garcia-Velloso MJ, et al. [(18)F]-FDG PET and localized fibrous mesothelioma. Lung. 2003; 181 (1):49–54

17 Breast Cancer

Eugene C. Lin

17.1 Breast Masses

Positron emission tomography (PET) with 18F-fluorodeoxyglucose (FDG) is relatively sensitive for detecting breast lesions which are larger than 1 cm, but insensitive for low-grade lesions and lesions less than 1 cm. PET is not currently used in screening or diagnosing primary breast cancer. PET may be more cost-effective and accurate with dedicated breast imaging PET machines. High-resolution positron emission mammography (PEM) is an approved device to perform PET imaging of the breast under gentle compression. Advantages of PEM are higher spatial resolution, shorter imaging time, and reduced soft-tissue attenuation. PEM may be of value to define extent of disease for surgical planning, detect multifocal or bilateral disease, and monitor response to therapy.

Breast lesions are sometimes detected as incidental findings on PET studies performed for other indications and should be reported when discovered. In a study of 4,038 female patients undergoing FDG PET/CT for reasons other than breast cancer,[1] unexpected foci of breast uptake were identified in 0.82% of patients.

17.1.1 Accuracy

1. **Positron Emission MammographyPEM** (meta-analysis).[2] Sensitivity of 85%, specificity of 79%.
   a) *Ductal carcinoma in-situ*. In one report,[3] PEM was able to identify ductal carcinoma in-situ in 10 of 11 cases.
   b) *PEM versus PET*. In one study,[4] PEM had an index lesion depiction sensitivity of 93% which was significantly better than whole body PET (68%).
2. **Tumor size.** Sensitivity is highly dependent on tumor size[5] and grade.[6]
   a) Detection rate for T1a and b tumors (< 1 cm) is low, and tumors < 0.5 cm (T1a) will likely not be detected.
   b) Sensitivity increases substantially for T2 lesions (2–5 cm) and T3 lesions (> 5 cm).

17.1.2 Comparison to Other Modalities

1. **99mTc-Sestamibi**:
   a) The sensitivity of PET and sestamibi for breast lesions is comparable.[7]
   b) Tumors usually have higher uptake relative to normal tissue on PET than on sestamibi.

17.1.3 Contrast-Enhanced Breast MRI

1. PET is less sensitive but more specific than MRI for characterizing and detecting breast lesions.[8]
2. MRI has superior sensitivity for lesions < 1 cm and lobular carcinoma.
3. In a study of presurgical planning for the ipsilateral breast,[9] PEM and MRI had comparable breast level sensitivity, although MRI had greater lesion level sensitivity. PEM had greater specificity at the breast and lesion levels. As PEM was more specific, it was less likely to prompt unnecessary biopsies. However, MRI was more sensitive for additional malignant lesions (lesion level sensitivity) and more accurate in assessing disease extent and need for mastectomy. The combination of PEM and MRI increased cancer detection compared to MRI alone, although even the combined modalities did not fully depict disease extent, particularly in cases with extensive intraductal component, or multifocal or multicentric disease. In another study,[10] PEM was substantially less sensitive than MRI in identifying contralateral malignancies in women with newly diagnosed breast cancer.

Pearls

1. **Standardized uptake value (SUV).** SUVmax of 2.0 or tumor-to-background ratio of 2.5 is potential cutoff between benign and malignant.[11,12,13] SUVmax > 1.9 has been employed for PEM.[14] In a multivariate regression analysis,[15] the SUV did not differentiate benign from malignant incidental breast lesions; only the BI-RADS category (on ultrasound and mammography) did so.
   a) However, as there is no definitive SUV cutoff for benignity, any focal abnormal uptake of FDG should undergo further workup.
   b) In general, breast cancer has lower metabolic activity than most other malignancies.
2. **Incidental breast uptake.** Focal FDG uptake in the breast is sometimes seen incidentally and is associated with a high likelihood of

malignancy.[16] In a meta-analysis,[17] the pooled risk of malignancy in incidental FDG avid breast lesions was 48%. Initial workup of incidentally detected breast abnormality on PET should include the standard examinations in such settings: physical exam and mammography. Contrast-enhanced breast MRI may be particularly helpful after negative initial workup due to its high sensitivity for breast lesions. Ultrasound may also be helpful in selected circumstances.

3. **Delayed/dual time point imaging.** Delayed imaging increases tumor visualization by PET.[18] Tumors will accumulate FDG over time while normal breast tissue will reveal decreased or unchanged FDG uptake. Dual time point imaging improves the sensitivity and accuracy of PET for primary breast cancer, particularly for noninvasive, small invasive, and invasive lobular and mixed carcinomas.[19]

4. **Dense breasts.** Dense breasts have more FDG uptake, but the uptake in dense breasts is not substantial and therefore will not interfere with detectability of breast lesions. Even in dense breasts, the maximum SUV in normal tissue is usually relatively low (< 1).[20] In one analysis,[4] the performance characteristics of PEM were not affected by patient menopausal/hormonal status or breast density.

5. **Degree of FDG uptake.** A higher SUVmax has been reported to be associated with larger tumor size, higher histological grade, higher stage, axillary nodal metastases, a high Ki-67 index, estrogen receptor (ER) negativity, progesterone receptor (PR) negativity, and human epidermal growth factor 2 (HER2) positivity.[21]

   a) Triple negative breast cancers (ER and PR negative, lacking HER2 overexpression) are typically highly FDG avid.[22] Inflammatory breast cancers also typically have high FDG uptake.

   b) Luminal breast cancers (hormone receptor positive, HER2 negative) typically have low metabolic activity.

Pitfalls

1. **False negatives.** Small lesions, invasive lobular carcinoma (ILC; ▶ Fig. 17.1), tubular carcinoma, carcinoma in situ, ER-positive tumors.

2. **False positives**[23,24]:

   a) *Inflammatory.* Abscess, soft-tissue inflammation, fat necrosis, tuberculosis, sarcoidosis, silicone granuloma.

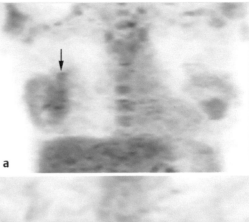

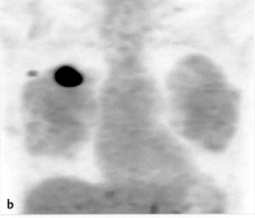

Fig. 17.1 Histology and FDG uptake in breast neoplasms. **(a)** MIP PET demonstrates mild FDG uptake in an invasive lobular carcinoma in the right breast (*arrow*). **(b)** MIP PET demonstrates intense FDG uptake in an invasive ductal carcinoma in the right breast.

   b) *Traumatic.* Postbiopsy, hematoma, seroma (▶ Fig. 17.2; often has a ring-like pattern of uptake).

   c) *Benign neoplasms.* Ductal adenoma, dysplastic tissue, intraductal papilloma, fibrocystic disease and inspissated cysts, and fibroadenomas (rare, the majority of fibroadenomas do not have significant uptake).[5]

17.2 Staging

National Comprehensive Cancer Network (NCCN) guidelines[25] recommend against the use of PET/CT in early-stage (stage I–IIB) breast cancer patients. In this patient population, there is a low prior probability of detectable metastatic disease and a high rate of false-positive scans. NCCN guidelines

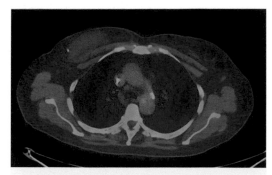

Fig. 17.2 Breast seroma. Axial PET/CT scan demonstrates peripheral uptake around a right breast seroma.

state that PET/CT is optional (category 2B—appropriate based on lower-level evidence) in stage IIIA (T3, N1, MO), invasive stage III, stage IV, and inflammatory breast cancer. The guidelines suggest that PET/CT is most helpful when standard imaging results are equivocal or suspicious, but there is also a potential role in the detection of regional nodal involvement and distant metastatic disease in locally advanced breast cancer.

European Society of Medical Oncology guidelines[26] state that PET/CT can replace traditional imaging for staging in high-risk patients who are candidates for neoadjuvant chemotherapy (NAC), and patients with locally advanced and/or inflammatory disease with a high risk of metastatic disease. However, PET/CT is not recommended for staging local/regional disease due to limited specificity compared to sentinel lymph node biopsy (SLNB) and axillary node dissection.

However, some authors have suggested that a staging PET/CT may be warranted in patients with stage IIB disease, particularly younger patients where patient age is a factor in tumor aggressiveness. In a retrospective study,[27] PET/CT revealed distant metastases in 17% of asymptomatic stage IIB breast cancer patients younger than 40 years. In another retrospective study[28] of patients with stage IIb triple-negative breast cancer, PET/CT revealed distant metastases in 15% of patients, and stage IIb patients upstaged to stage 4 by PET/CT had significantly shorter survival. In a prospective study of patients with clinical stage II and III breast cancers,[29] PET/CT had substantial yield and prognostic value in patients with clinical stage IIB or higher breast cancer. PET/CT revealed distant metastases in 2.3% of stage IIA patients, and 10.7% of stage IIB patients.

Tumor histology is another potential factor to consider when deciding whether to perform a staging PET/CT. ILC demonstrates lower SUVs than invasive ductal carcinoma (IDC). In one report,[30] the relative risk of identifying unsuspected FDG-avid distant metastases in patients with stage III IDC was 2.8 times that in patients with stage III ILC. In particular, all IDC patients upstaged with PET/CT had FDG avid metastases, while only 70% of ILC patients upstaged with PET/CT had FDG avid metastases (the remaining patients were upstaged by CT findings).

PET is relatively insensitive for axillary nodal metastasis, but has a high specificity. While PET cannot replace sentinel node biopsy, a positive PET scan suggests that axillary nodal dissection could be performed instead of sentinel node biopsy.[31,32] In one study,[33] selective sentinel node biopsy and axillary node dissection based on PET/CT results in substantially reduced unnecessary sentinel node biopsies.

PET is superior to CT for the detection of mediastinal and internal mammary nodal metastases.[34] PET is also relatively sensitive in detecting distant metastases. PET is most valuable in staging in specific circumstances[35,36]:

1. The primary tumor is T3 or T4.
2. Stage 4 disease.
3. Neoadjuvant therapy is planned without axillary dissection or sentinel node sampling.
4. Equivocal findings are seen on CT, ultrasound, or MR,
5. The primary lesion is medial or superior, which indicates a higher risk for internal mammary metastases or supraclavicular metastases. Patients with inner quadrant breast tumors are six times more likely to have isolated extra-axillary metastases identified by PET.[37]

17.2.1 Accuracy/Comparison to Other Modalities

In a comparison of PET/CT to conventional imaging in staging patients with locally advanced or inflammatory breast cancer,[38] PET/CT outperformed conventional imaging for bone metastases, liver metastases, and distant lymph nodes, whereas CT was more sensitive for lung metastases.

1. **Multifocal disease (PET).** Sensitivity of 92%, specificity of 90%.
   a) PET is superior to conventional imaging (mammography and ultrasound combined).
   b) However, contrast-enhanced MRI is more sensitive than PET (▶ Fig. 17.3).[8,39]

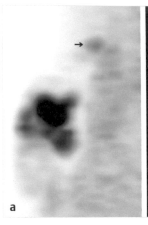
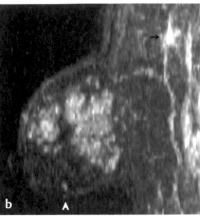

Fig. 17.3 Multifocal breast cancer on PET and MRI. **(a)** Sagittal PET scan demonstrates a multifocal breast cancer. Uptake in an axillary node (*arrow*) is also seen. **(b)** Sagittal contrast-enhanced MRI scan in the same patient demonstrates the enhancing lesions corresponding to the areas of increased uptake on PET. Enhancement in the axillary node that had FDG uptake (*arrow*) is also seen. However, the MRI identified a small tumor in the inferior breast (*arrowhead*) not seen on PET.

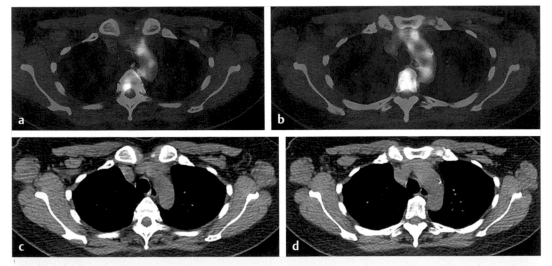

Fig. 17.4 Rotter's node metastases from breast cancer. **(a,b)** Axial PET/CT in a patient with breast cancer demonstrates interpectoral (Rotter's) node metastases. These are considered to be level II nodes. **(c,d)** The corresponding CT demonstrates nonenlarged nodes corresponding to the FDG uptake.

2. **Axillary nodes:**
   a) PET has a lower sensitivity and specificity than SLNB and cannot substitute for axillary nodal dissection in most patients.
   b) PET/CT (meta-analysis)[40]: Sensitivity of 56%, specificity of 96%.
3. **Extra-axillary nodes.** As PET/CT has limited sensitivity in axillary staging, the primary value in nodal evaluation is in the detection of nodes outside of axillary level I and II nodes (▶ Fig. 17.4) which would typically be surgically cleared. In particular, PET/CT can accurately detect N3 metastases (indicating stage IIIC) in the internal mammary, supraclavicular, and level III (superior to the pectoralis minor but infraclavicular) nodes. Detection of extra-axillary nodes missed by conventional imaging can lead to changes in the extent of surgical clearance or radiation fields.[41] PET is more accurate than CT for the diagnosis of internal mammary (▶ Fig. 17.5) and mediastinal nodal metastases (▶ Fig. 17.6).[34,42]

PET versus CT in the diagnosis of extra-axillary nodes (▶ Table 17.1)

4. **Distant metastases.** PET has a sensitivity of 84 to 93% and a specificity of 55 to 86% for the detection of distant metastases.[34] In patients with locally advanced breast cancer, the

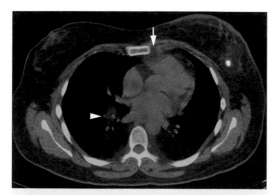

Fig. 17.5 Metastatic breast cancer. Axial PET/CT demonstrates a primary left breast cancer with internal mammary node (*arrow*) and lung (*arrowhead*) metastases. Paravertebral brown fat uptake is also noted.

Table 17.1 Sensitivity and specificity of PET versus CT in the diagnosis of internal mammary and mediastinal metastases

	Sensitivity %	Specificity %
PET	85	90
CT	54	85

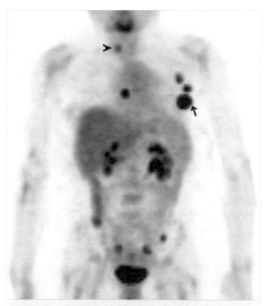

Fig. 17.6 Metastatic disease from breast cancer. Coronal PET scan demonstrates increased uptake in a left breast cancer (*arrow*). Metastases are present to left axillary lymph nodes, the mediastinum, and the left iliac bone. Uptake is present in an incidentally noted right thyroid nodule (*arrowhead*).

addition of PET to the workup for staging will result in detection of distant metastases not detected by conventional imaging in 8% of cases.[43] **PET/CT versus conventional imaging in the diagnosis of distant metastases** (meta-analysis; ▶ Table 17.2).[44]

Table 17.2 Sensitivity and specificity of PET/CT versus conventional imaging in the diagnosis of distant metastases

	Sensitivity %	Specificity %
PET/CT	97	95
Conventional imaging	56	91

5. **Bone marrow metastases:**

   Although FDG PET/CT is limited in the detection of sclerotic metastases, PET/CT has a high accuracy in the detection of bone metastases in breast cancer patients (▶ Fig. 17.7). In addition, there is a high concordance between the results of PET/CT and bone scintigraphy (BS) in patients with breast cancer.[45] While some authors[46] state that BS is not necessary if PET/CT is performed, other authors[47,48] conclude that BS should be performed in addition to PET/CT given the limitation for sclerotic metastases. In

an early meta-analysis,[49] it was inconclusive whether FDG PET or bone scan was superior, but FDG PET had a higher specificity. In another meta-analysis,[50] FDG PET had a lower sensitivity and higher specificity than BS on a per lesion basis, but per patient basis there was no difference in sensitivity. In a meta-analysis[51] of PET/CT specifically, FDG PET/CT had a higher sensitivity and accuracy than BS. While PET may have poor sensitivity for sclerotic bone metastases, these are detectable on CT, and NCCN guidelines[25] suggest that BS may not be necessary if both PET and CT components of a staging PET/CT identify bone metastases.

a) PET/CT versus bone scintigraphy in the diagnosis of bone metastases from breast cancer (meta-analysis; ▶ Table 17.3).[51]

Table 17.3 Sensitivity and specificity of PET/CT versus bone scintigraphy in the diagnosis of bone metastases from breast cancer

	Sensitivity %	Specificity %
PET/CT	93	99
BS	81	96

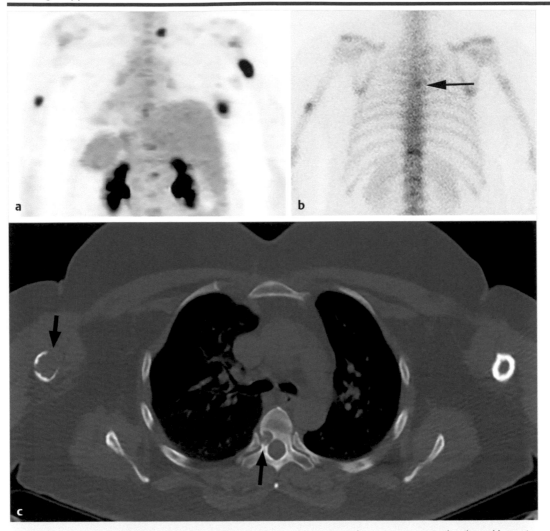

Fig. 17.7 Bone metastases from breast cancer. **(a)** MIP PET scan demonstrates bone metastases in the ribs and humeri. **(b)** The rib metastases are not identified on a bone scan and the humeral metastases are less well visualized. **(c)** An axial CT demonstrates both right humerus and spine metastases (*arrows*) at the same level. The spine metastasis is not visualized on the PET scan but is faintly visualized on the bone scan (**b**, *arrow*).

b) Lytic and blastic metastases. FDG PET is superior to bone scan for detecting osteolytic metastases, but is inferior for visualizing osteoblastic metastases, with a sensitivity of 56 to 74% for blastic metastases.[52,53] PET is more sensitive than bone scan for mixed lytic and sclerotic metastases and substantially more sensitive for invisible (not detected on CT) metastases.[54] However, many blastic metastases missed on PET could potentially be detected on the CT portion of a PET/CT study.

c) Patients with more aggressive tumors may benefit more from PET given the high likelihood of osteolytic bone metastases with these malignancies.

d) Histology. The histologic subtype of breast cancer affects the appearance of untreated osseous metastases on PET/CT. In one study,[55] patients with ILC had bone metastases which were more likely sclerotic with a lower SUV than metastases in patients with IDC. Less than half of sclerotic metastases in patients with ILC were FDG avid. This suggests that breast cancer histology should play a role in the interpretation of non-FDG avid sclerotic lesions, which are more suspicious for metastases in patients with ILC.

Pearls

Axillary staging

1. A SUV cutoff of > 2.3 has a sensitivity of 60% and specificity of 100% for axillary nodal metastasis.[28]
2. Multiple foci of axillary uptake are specific but insensitive.
3. PET is more sensitive for detecting lesions in patients with T2 or T3 disease (> 2 cm).
4. Sensitivity increased as the degree of FDG uptake in primary tumor increases and the axillary tumor load increases.[56]
5. Sensitivity increases with large primary tumors, but specificity is the highest for the small lesions.[57]
6. PET has little role in axillary staging for patients with palpable nodes, as these patients will undergo axillary lymph node dissection (ALND) after pathologic confirmation of nodal metastasis. PET has a high sensitivity and low specificity in this group of patients.[58]
7. A negative PET scan should not preclude ALND.
8. A positive PET scan is helpful as the false-positive rate in the axilla in breast cancer is relatively low, and identification of multiple foci of uptake further increases specificity.
9. Similarly, identifying multiple foci of axillary uptake could potentially obviate ALND in patients receiving NAC.
10. Patients with a positive axillary PET scan could potentially forego sentinel node biopsy and proceed to ALND.[59]

Pitfalls

Sternal metastases and internal mammary nodal metastases can be confused on PET due to their possible close proximity. These metastases should be easily differentiated with PET/CT.

17.3 Tumor Recurrence

PET is accurate in detecting both locoregional and distant tumor recurrence, and is useful both in asymptomatic patients with elevated tumor markers and patients with clinical suspicion for recurrence and negative tumor markers. PET can be used to evaluate suspected recurrence, or to identify multifocal or distant disease in locoregional recurrence. Between 16 and 30% of patients with a locoregional recurrence have distant metastases identified by PET.[62] PET is most helpful when aggressive local therapy is planned as the detection of additional disease often alters management.

17.3.1 Accuracy/Comparison to Other Modalities

In a meta-analysis,[63] PET/CT was more sensitive than CT, but the increase in specificity was not significant. PET/CT has an approximately 10% increase in diagnostic accuracy compared to PET alone.[37] Limited data that PET/CT and MRI are comparable in sensitivity and specificity.

17.3.2 PET/CT Versus CT for the Diagnosis of Breast Cancer Recurrence

See meta-analysis in ▶ Table 17.4.

Table 17.4 Sensitivity and specificity of PET/CT versus CT for the diagnosis of breast cancer recurrence

	Sensitivity %	Specificity %
PET/CT	95	89
CT	80	77

Pearls/Pitfalls

1. **Locoregional recurrence**:
   a) PET is valuable in differentiating locoregional recurrence from postoperative changes. CT/MRI is often limited in this capacity.
      - Areas where PET is particularly useful are the chest wall (▶ Fig. 17.8) and brachial plexus (▶ Fig. 17.9) region.
      - However anatomic imaging is often still necessary to depict relationships to adjacent structures (e.g., neurovascular invasion).
   b) PET is useful in evaluating the axillary, supraclavicular, mediastinal, and internal mammary nodes.
      - However, if the patient has had an ALND, sensitivity for axillary lymph node metastases is decreased.[64]
2. **Distant recurrence**:
   a) PET detects more lymph node metastases than conventional imaging.
   b) PET should be employed in conjunction with bone scan to detect bone metastases.
3. **Elevated tumor markers**:
   a) In a meta-analysis,[65] the sensitivity and specificity of PET in breast cancer recurrence detection in the presence of elevated tumor

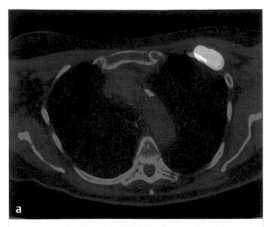

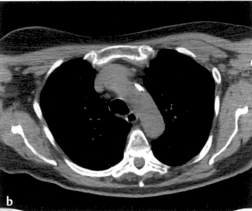

Fig. 17.8 Chest wall metastases. **(a)** Axial PET/CT scan in a patient with breast cancer demonstrates a left chest wall metastasis. This is difficult to visualize on the corresponding CT **(b)**.

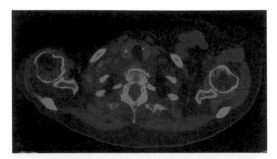

Fig. 17.9 Brachial plexus disease. Axial PET/CT scan in a patient with breast cancer demonstrates uptake secondary to recurrence in the right brachial plexus region.

17.4 Therapy Response/ Prognosis

PET/CT can be used for early response assessment in patients receiving NAC.[68,69] As only 13 to 26% of patients receiving NAC will achieve a pathological complete response,[70] PET/CT could potentially be valuable in early prediction of final pathological response, allowing nonresponders to be switched to an alternate therapy earlier. For example, platinum-based chemotherapy could potentially be added in poorly responding triple-negative breast cancer patients. While PET/CT overall has a moderate sensitivity and specificity for differentiating responders from nonresponders, specific thresholds (amount of decrease in SUV) used vary substantially between studies.[70] Currently, it is recommended that early response assessment by PET/CT in breast cancer patients receiving NAC should be done primarily in the context of clinical trials.[71]

PET/CT can also be used for early response assessment in patients with metastatic disease, and also for response assessment after completion of therapy.

1. PET is useful to evaluate response during induction therapy for advanced disease and during preoperative chemoradiotherapy (▶ Fig. 17.10). In one study, PET altered therapy most frequently in patients with suspected or proven locoregional recurrence under consideration for aggressive therapy, and in patients with known metastases being evaluated for therapy response.[72]
2. **Prognosis.** SUV ≥ 3.0 in the primary breast tumor is usually associated with poor survival.
3. **Interim PET.** Change in FDG uptake after one to three courses of chemotherapy[73,74] predicts

markers were 88 and 69%, respectively, with a pooled accuracy of 83%.
b) PET should be considered in patients with equivocal conventional imaging results and asymptomatically elevated tumor markers. In one report,[66] PET/CT had a higher sensitivity and accuracy than standard workup in asymptomatic patients presenting with rising CA 15–3 and/or CEA serum levels, with the diagnosis of recurrence leading to treatment modification in 54% of patients.
c) The likelihood of detecting recurrence is higher if CA 15–3 blood level is > 60 U/mL.[67]
d) False-negative results are noted in patients with invasive lobular cancer and elevated CA 15–3.

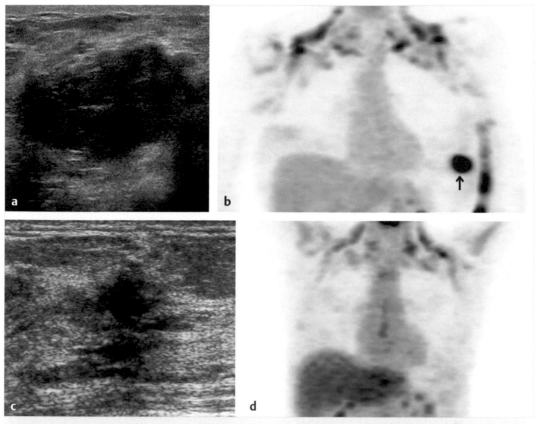

Fig. 17.10 Breast cancer: response to neoadjuvant therapy. Ultrasound **(a)** demonstrates a large left breast cancer with intense uptake (*arrow*) on a coronal PET scan **(b)**. After neoadjuvant therapy, the mass is much smaller on ultrasound **(c)** and not visualized on PET **(d)**.

pathological response and survival in locally advanced and metastatic breast tumors.

a) A SUV decrease of more than 55% below baseline may distinguish responders from nonresponders with an accuracy of 88% after the first cycle of chemotherapy.[75]

b) However, patients with decreased uptake may still have microscopic residual disease.

c) An additional PET scan after additional cycles of chemotherapy may be helpful to confirm initial results.

4. **Posttherapy response**. After therapy, PET is more accurate than conventional imaging for predicting outcome.[76]

a) However, the sensitivity for lymph node disease after completion of therapy is low, and a negative PET scan has a very low predictive value for complete response.[69] This is particularly true for axillary nodal disease.

b) PET may be particularly helpful for assessment of treatment response in bone-dominant breast cancer.[77]

17.4.1 Accuracy/Comparison to Other Modalities

PET/CT Versus MRI for Assessing Pathological Complete Response to NAC

See meta-analysis in ▶ Table 17.5.[78]

Table 17.5 Sensitivity and specificity of PET/CT versus MRI for assessing pathological complete response to NAC

	Sensitivity %	Specificity %
PET/CT	86	72
MRI	65	88

However, the timing of imaging for NAC response assessment has a substantial influence on diagnostic accuracy. In a meta-analysis,[79] the accuracy of MRI was superior to PET/CT after completion of therapy, but PET/CT outperformed MRI for intratherapy assessment.

17.4.2 Pearls/Pitfalls

1. **Timing.** In a meta-analysis,[80] the accuracy of PET/CT performed to predict neoadjuvant response was superior if performed early (after the first or second cycle of therapy) than later.

2. **SUV.** In a meta-analysis,[80] a SUV reduction rate of 55 to 65% was best correlated with pathology. However, it should be noted that optimal cutoffs for early prediction of pathological complete response and survival vary with the type of chemotherapy.[81] In addition, it is currently unclear whether measuring absolute SUVs or relative change in SUVs better identifies nonresponders.[82]

3. **Receptor expression.** The accuracy of PET/CT in monitoring treatment response depends on receptor expression. Specifically, changes in FDG uptake are correlated with response to NAC in HER2 tumors (including ER + and triple-negative tumors),[83,84] but not HER2 + tumors.

4. **MRI.** PET and MRI are complementary in monitoring response. PET predicts lack of response more accurately than MRI. When PET predicts response, MRI is able to define the extent of residual disease accurately.[85] However, PEM may potentially be superior to PET for monitoring therapy response.

5. **Tumors with low FDG uptake.** Low tumor metabolic activity may be an indicator of chemotherapeutic resistance. In a multicenter trial,[86] none of the patients with a baseline SUV less than 3.0 achieved a complete histopathological response to chemotherapy. These tumors were better differentiated and often steroid-receptor positive. PET also is less effective in predicting response in tumors with low FDG uptake. In one study, PET could predict response only in tumors with a tumor-to-background ratio greater than 5.[87]

6. **Metabolic flare.** In patients treated with tamoxifen, responders can demonstrate increased activity initially from metabolic flare. This may be secondary to the initial agonist effects of tamoxifen before antagonist effects are dominant. The flare reaction implies that ERs are functional, and is an early predictor of tumor sensitivity to endocrine therapy.[88] This is typically seen at 7 to 10 days after therapy, but the time course could be variable. The flare phenomenon can be seen with 18F bone PET scanning, but is not typically seen with FDG PET during most chemotherapeutic regimens. However, a flare response has been described during the treatment of breast cancer with second-line chemotherapy and bevacizumab,[89] which has also been described with the use of bevacizumab in lung cancer.[90]

7. **Antiaromatase therapy.** Patients on antiaromatase therapy will show an opposite effect from metabolic flare. Antiaromatase therapy lowers estradiol levels and reduces the tumor agonist effect. Therefore, responding patients will show an early drop in tumor FDG uptake after antiaromatase induction.[88]

References

[1] Litmanovich D, Gourevich K, Israel O, Gallimidi Z. Unexpected foci of 18F-FDG uptake in the breast detected by PET/CT: incidence and clinical significance. Eur J Nucl Med Mol Imaging. 2009; 36(10):1558–1564

[2] Caldarella C, Treglia G, Giordano A. Diagnostic performance of dedicated positron emission mammography using fluorine-18-fluorodeoxyglucose in women with suspicious breast lesions: a meta-analysis. Clin Breast Cancer. 2014; 14 (4):241–248

[3] Berg WA, Weinberg IN, Narayanan D, et al. Positron Emission Mammography Working Group. High-resolution fluorodeoxyglucose positron emission tomography with compression ("positron emission mammography") is highly accurate in depicting primary breast cancer. Breast J. 2006; 12(4):309–323

[4] Schilling K, Narayanan D, Kalinyak JE, et al. Positron emission mammography in breast cancer presurgical planning: comparisons with magnetic resonance imaging. Eur J Nucl Med Mol Imaging. 2011; 38(1):23–36

[5] Avril N, Rosé CA, Schelling M, et al. Breast imaging with positron emission tomography and fluorine-18 fluorodeoxyglucose: use and limitations. J Clin Oncol. 2000; 18(20):3495–3502

[6] Kumar R, Chauhan A, Zhuang H, Chandra P, Schnall M, Alavi A. Clinicopathologic factors associated with false negative FDG-PET in primary breast cancer. Breast Cancer Res Treat. 2006; 98(3):267–274

[7] Yutani K, Shiba E, Kusuoka H, et al. Comparison of FDG-PET with MIBI-SPECT in the detection of breast cancer and axillary lymph node metastasis. J Comput Assist Tomogr. 2000; 24(2):274–280

[8] Heinisch M, Gallowitsch HJ, Mikosch P, et al. Comparison of FDG-PET and dynamic contrast-enhanced MRI in the evaluation of suggestive breast lesions. Breast. 2003; 12(1):17–22

[9] Berg WA, Madsen KS, Schilling K, et al. Breast cancer: comparative effectiveness of positron emission mammography and MR imaging in presurgical planning for the ipsilateral breast. Radiology. 2011; 258(1):59–72

[10] Berg WA, Madsen KS, Schilling K, et al. Comparative effectiveness of positron emission mammography and MRI in the contralateral breast of women with newly diagnosed breast cancer. AJR Am J Roentgenol. 2012; 198(1):219–232

[11] Dehdashti F, Mortimer JE, Siegel BA, et al. Positron tomographic assessment of estrogen receptors in breast cancer: comparison with FDG-PET and in vitro receptor assays. J Nucl Med. 1995; 36(10):1766–1774

[12] Dehdashti F, Siegel BA. Evaluation of breast and gynecologic cancers by positron emission tomography. Semin Roentgenol. 2002; 37(2):151–168

[13] Levine EA, Freimanis RI, Perrier ND, et al. Positron emission mammography: initial clinical results. Ann Surg Oncol. 2003; 10(1):86–91

[14] Müller FH, Farahati J, Müller AG, Gillman E, Hentschel M. Positron emission mammography in the diagnosis of breast cancer. Is maximum PEM uptake value a valuable threshold for malignant breast cancer detection? Nucl Med (Stuttg). 2016; 55(1):15–20

[15] Shin KM, Kim HJ, Jung SJ, et al. Incidental breast lesions identified by (18)F-FDG PET/CT: which clinical variables differentiate between benign and malignant breast lesions? J Breast Cancer. 2015; 18(1):73–79

[16] Korn RL, Yost AM, May CC, et al. Unexpected focal hypermetabolic activity in the breast: significance in patients undergoing 18F-FDG PET/CT. AJR Am J Roentgenol. 2006; 187(1):81–85

[17] Bertagna F, Treglia G, Orlando E, et al. Prevalence and clinical significance of incidental F18-FDG breast uptake: a systematic review and meta-analysis. Jpn J Radiol. 2014; 32(2):59–68

[18] Boerner AR, Weckesser M, Herzog H, et al. Optimal scan time for fluorine-18 fluorodeoxyglucose positron emission tomography in breast cancer. Eur J Nucl Med. 1999; 26(3):226–230

[19] Mavi A, Urhan M, Yu JQ, et al. Dual time point 18F-FDG PET imaging detects breast cancer with high sensitivity and correlates well with histologic subtypes. J Nucl Med. 2006; 47(9):1440–1446

[20] Vranjesevic D, Schiepers C, Silverman DH, et al. Relationship between 18F-FDG uptake and breast density in women with normal breast tissue. J Nucl Med. 2003; 44(8):1238–1242

[21] Kitajima K, Miyoshi Y. Present and future role of FDG-PET/CT imaging in the management of breast cancer. Jpn J Radiol. 2016; 34(3):167–180

[22] Groheux D, Cochet A, Humbert O, Alberini JL, Hindié E, Mankoff D. 18F-FDG PET/CT for staging and restaging of breast cancer. J Nucl Med. 2016; 57 Suppl 1:17S–26S

[23] Adejolu M, Huo L, Rohren E, Santiago L, Yang WT. False-positive lesions mimicking breast cancer on FDG PET and PET/CT. AJR Am J Roentgenol. 2012; 198(3):W304–14

[24] Dong A, Wang Y, Lu J, Zuo C. Spectrum of the breast lesions with increased 18F-FDG uptake on PET/CT. Clin Nucl Med. 2016; 41(7):543–557

[25] Gradishar WJ, Anderson BO, Balassanian R, et al. Invasive breast cancer version 1.2016, NCCN Clinical Practice Guidelines in Oncology. J Natl Compr Canc Netw. 2016; 14(3):324–354

[26] Senkus E, Kyriakides S, Ohno S, et al. ESMO Guidelines Committee. Primary breast cancer: ESMO Clinical Practice Guidelines for diagnosis, treatment and follow-up. Ann Oncol. 2015; 26 Suppl 5:v8–v30

[27] Riedl CC, Slobod E, Jochelson M, et al. Retrospective analysis of 18F-FDG PET/CT for staging asymptomatic breast cancer patients younger than 40 years. J Nucl Med. 2014; 55(10):1578–1583

[28] Ulaner GA, Castillo R, Goldman DA, et al. (18)F-FDG-PET/CT for systemic staging of newly diagnosed triple-negative breast cancer. Eur J Nucl Med Mol Imaging. 2016; 43(11):1937–1944

[29] Groheux D, Hindié E, Delord M, et al. Prognostic impact of (18)FDG-PET-CT findings in clinical stage III and IIB breast cancer. J Natl Cancer Inst. 2012; 104(24):1879–1887

[30] Hogan MP, Goldman DA, Dashevsky B, et al. Comparison of 18F-FDG PET/CT for systemic staging of newly diagnosed invasive lobular carcinoma versus invasive ductal carcinoma. J Nucl Med. 2015; 56(11):1674–1680

[31] Kumar R, Zhuang H, Schnall M, et al. FDG PET positive lymph nodes are highly predictive of metastasis in breast cancer. Nucl Med Commun. 2006; 27(3):231–236

[32] Veronesi U, De Cicco C, Galimberti VE, et al. A comparative study on the value of FDG-PET and sentinel node biopsy to identify occult axillary metastases. Ann Oncol. 2007; 18(3):473–478

[33] Kim J, Lee J, Chang E, et al. Selective sentinel node plus additional non-sentinel node biopsy based on an FDG-PET/CT scan in early breast cancer patients: single institutional experience. World J Surg. 2009; 33(5):943–949

[34] Quon A, Gambhir SS. FDG-PET and beyond: molecular breast cancer imaging. J Clin Oncol. 2005; 23(8):1664–1673

[35] Wahl RL. Current status of PET in breast cancer imaging, staging, and therapy. Semin Roentgenol. 2001; 36(3):250–260

[36] Wahl RL. PET Imaging in Breast Cancer. In: Valk PE, Bailey DL, Townsend DW, et al., eds. Positron Emission Tomography: Basic Science and Clinical Practice. London, UK: Springer-Verlag; 2003:595–610

[37] Tran A, Pio BS, Khatibi B, Czernin J, Phelps ME, Silverman DH. 18F-FDG PET for staging breast cancer in patients with inner-quadrant versus outer-quadrant tumors: comparison with long-term clinical outcome. J Nucl Med. 2005; 46(9):1455–1459

[38] Groheux D, Giacchetti S, Delord M, et al. 18F-FDG PET/CT in staging patients with locally advanced or inflammatory breast cancer: comparison to conventional staging. J Nucl Med. 2013; 54(1):5–11

[39] Rieber A, Schirrmeister H, Gabelmann A, et al. Pre-operative staging of invasive breast cancer with MR mammography and/or PET: boon or bunk? Br J Radiol. 2002; 75(898):789–798

[40] Cooper KL, Harnan S, Meng Y, et al. Positron emission tomography (PET) for assessment of axillary lymph node status in early breast cancer: a systematic review and meta-analysis. Eur J Surg Oncol. 2011; 37(3):187–198

[41] Aukema TS, Straver ME, Peeters MJ, et al. Detection of extra-axillary lymph node involvement with FDG PET/CT in patients with stage II-III breast cancer. Eur J Cancer. 2010; 46(18):3205–3210

[42] Eubank WB, Mankoff DA, Takasugi J, et al. 18fluorodeoxyglucose positron emission tomography to detect mediastinal or internal mammary metastases in breast cancer. J Clin Oncol. 2001; 19(15):3516–3523

[43] van der Hoeven JJ, Krak NC, Hoekstra OS, et al. 18F-2-fluoro-2-deoxy-d-glucose positron emission tomography in staging of locally advanced breast cancer. J Clin Oncol. 2004; 22(7):1253–1259

[44] Hong S, Li J, Wang S. 18FDG PET-CT for diagnosis of distant metastases in breast cancer patients. A meta-analysis. Surg Oncol. 2013; 22(2):139–143

[45] Morris PG, Lynch C, Feeney JN, et al. Integrated positron emission tomography/computed tomography may render bone scintigraphy unnecessary to investigate suspected metastatic breast cancer. J Clin Oncol. 2010; 28(19):3154–3159

[46] Caglar M, Kupik O, Karabulut E, Høilund-Carlsen PF. Detection of bone metastases in breast cancer patients in the PET/CT era: do we still need the bone scan? Rev Esp Med Nucl Imagen Mol. 2016; 35(1):3–11

[47] Escalona S, Blasco JA, Reza MM, Andradas E, Gómez N. A systematic review of FDG-PET in breast cancer. Med Oncol. 2010; 27(1):114–129

[48] Sahin E, Zincirkeser S, Akcan AB, Elboga U. Is (99m)Tc-MDP whole body bone scintigraphy adjuvant to (18)F-FDG-PET for the detection of skeletal metastases? J BUON. 2014; 19(1): 291–296

[49] Shie P, Cardarelli R, Brandon D, Erdman W, Abdulrahim N. Meta-analysis: comparison of F-18 fluorodeoxyglucose-positron emission tomography and bone scintigraphy in the detection of bone metastases in patients with breast cancer. Clin Nucl Med. 2008; 33(2):97–101

[50] Liu T, Cheng T, Xu W, Yan WL, Liu J, Yang HL. A meta-analysis of 18FDG-PET, MRI and bone scintigraphy for diagnosis of bone metastases in patients with breast cancer. Skeletal Radiol. 2011; 40(5):523–531

[51] Rong J, Wang S, Ding Q, Yun M, Zheng Z, Ye S. Comparison of 18 FDG PET-CT and bone scintigraphy for detection of bone metastases in breast cancer patients. A meta-analysis. Surg Oncol. 2013; 22(2):86–91

[52] Abe K, Sasaki M, Kuwabara Y, et al. Comparison of 18FDG-PET with 99mTc-HMDP scintigraphy for the detection of bone metastases in patients with breast cancer. Ann Nucl Med. 2005; 19(7):573–579

[53] Nakai T, Okuyama C, Kubota T, et al. Pitfalls of FDG-PET for the diagnosis of osteoblastic bone metastases in patients with breast cancer. Eur J Nucl Med Mol Imaging. 2005; 32 (11):1253–1258

[54] Chung A, Liou D, Karlan S, et al. Preoperative FDG-PET for axillary metastases in patients with breast cancer. Arch Surg. 2006; 141(8):783–788, discussion 788–789

[55] Dashevsky BZ, Goldman DA, Parsons M, et al. Appearance of untreated bone metastases from breast cancer on FDG PET/CT: importance of histologic subtype. Eur J Nucl Med Mol Imaging. 2015; 42(11):1666–1673

[56] van der Hoeven JJ, Hoekstra OS, Comans EF, et al. Determinants of diagnostic performance of [F-18]fluorodeoxyglucose positron emission tomography for axillary staging in breast cancer. Ann Surg. 2002; 236(5):619–624

[57] Ohta M, Tokuda Y, Suzuki Y, et al. Whole body PET for the evaluation of bony metastases in patients with breast cancer: comparison with 99Tcm-MDP bone scintigraphy. Nucl Med Commun. 2001; 22(8):875–879

[58] Greco M, Crippa F, Agresti R, et al. Axillary lymph node staging in breast cancer by 2-fluoro-2-deoxy-D-glucose-positron emission tomography: clinical evaluation and alternative management. J Natl Cancer Inst. 2001; 93(8):630–635

[59] Lovrics PJ, Chen V, Coates G, et al. A prospective evaluation of positron emission tomography scanning, sentinel lymph node biopsy, and standard axillary dissection for axillary staging in patients with early stage breast cancer. Ann Surg Oncol. 2004; 11(9):846–853

[60] Eubank WB, Mankoff DA, Vesselle HJ, et al. Detection of locoregional and distant recurrences in breast cancer patients by using FDG PET. Radiographics. 2002; 22(1):5–17

[61] Siggelkow W, Rath W, Buell U, Zimny M. FDG PET and tumour markers in the diagnosis of recurrent and metastatic breast cancer. Eur J Nucl Med Mol Imaging. 2004; 31 Suppl 1:S118–S124

[62] Tafra L. Positron emission tomography (PET) and mammography (PEM) for breast cancer: importance to surgeons. Ann Surg Oncol. 2007; 14(1):3–13

[63] Pennant M, Takwoingi Y, Pennant L, et al. A systematic review of positron emission tomography (PET) and positron emission tomography/computed tomography (PET/CT) for the diagnosis of breast cancer recurrence. Health Technol Assess. 2010; 14(50):1–103

[64] Czernin J, Allen-Auerbach M, Schelbert HR. Improvements in cancer staging with PET/CT: literature-based evidence as of September 2006. J Nucl Med. 2007; 48 Suppl 1:78S–88S

[65] Evangelista L, Cervino AR, Ghiotto C, Al-Nahhas A, Rubello D, Muzzio PC. Tumor marker-guided PET in breast cancer patients-a recipe for a perfect wedding: a systematic literature review and meta-analysis. Clin Nucl Med. 2012; 37(5):467–474

[66] Champion L, Brain E, Giraudet AL, et al. Breast cancer recurrence diagnosis suspected on tumor marker rising: value of whole-body 18FDG-PET/CT imaging and impact on patient management. Cancer. 2011; 117(8):1621–1629

[67] Aide N, Huchet V, Switsers O, et al. Influence of CA 15–3 blood level and doubling time on diagnostic performances of 18F-FDG PET in breast cancer patients with occult recurrence. Nucl Med Commun. 2007; 28(4):267–272

[68] Kostakoglu L, Goldsmith SJ. 18F-FDG PET evaluation of the response to therapy for lymphoma and for breast, lung, and colorectal carcinoma. J Nucl Med. 2003; 44(2):224–239

[69] Krak NC, Hoekstra OS, Lammertsma AA. Measuring response to chemotherapy in locally advanced breast cancer: methodological considerations. Eur J Nucl Med Mol Imaging. 2004; 31 Suppl 1:S103–S111

[70] Groheux D, Espié M, Giacchetti S, Hindié E. Performance of FDG PET/CT in the clinical management of breast cancer. Radiology. 2013; 266(2):388–405

[71] Avril N, Sassen S, Roylance R. Response to therapy in breast cancer. J Nucl Med. 2009; 50 Suppl 1:55S–63S

[72] Eubank WB, Mankoff D, Bhattacharya M, et al. Impact of FDG PET on defining the extent of disease and on the treatment of patients with recurrent or metastatic breast cancer. AJR Am J Roentgenol. 2004; 183(2):479–486

[73] Couturier O, Jerusalem G, N'Guyen JM, Hustinx R. Sequential positron emission tomography using [18F]fluorodeoxyglucose for monitoring response to chemotherapy in metastatic breast cancer. Clin Cancer Res. 2006; 12(21):6437–6443

[74] Rousseau C, Devillers A, Sagan C, et al. Monitoring of early response to neoadjuvant chemotherapy in stage II and III breast cancer by [18F]fluorodeoxyglucose positron emission tomography. J Clin Oncol. 2006; 24(34):5366–5372

[75] Schelling M, Avril N, Nährig J, et al. Positron emission tomography using [(18)F]Fluorodeoxyglucose for monitoring primary chemotherapy in breast cancer. J Clin Oncol. 2000; 18 (8):1689–1695

[76] Vranjesevic D, Filmont JE, Meta J, et al. Whole-body (18)F-FDG PET and conventional imaging for predicting outcome in previously treated breast cancer patients. J Nucl Med. 2002; 43(3):325–329

[77] Stafford SE, Gralow JR, Schubert EK, et al. Use of serial FDG PET to measure the response of bone-dominant breast cancer to therapy. Acad Radiol. 2002; 9(8):913–921

[78] Liu Q, Wang C, Li P, Liu J, Huang G, Song S. The role of (18)F-FDG PET/CT and MRI in assessing pathological complete response to neoadjuvant chemotherapy in patients with breast cancer: a systematic review and meta-analysis. BioMed Res Int. 2016; 2016:3746232

[79] Sheikhbahaei S, Trahan TJ, Xiao J, et al. FDG-PET/CT and MRI for evaluation of pathologic response to neoadjuvant chemotherapy in patients with breast cancer: a meta-analysis of diagnostic accuracy studies. Oncologist. 2016; 21(8):931–939

[80] Wang Y, Zhang C, Liu J, Huang G. Is 18F-FDG PET accurate to predict neoadjuvant therapy response in breast cancer? A meta-analysis. Breast Cancer Res Treat. 2012; 131(2):357–369

[81] Groheux D, Biard L, Giacchetti S, et al. 18F-FDG PET/CT for the early evaluation of response to neoadjuvant treatment in

triple-negative breast cancer: influence of the chemotherapy regimen. J Nucl Med. 2016; 57(4):536–543

[82] Avril S, Muzic RF, Jr, Plecha D, Traughber BJ, Vinayak S, Avril N. 18F-FDG PET/CT for monitoring of treatment response in breast cancer. J Nucl Med. 2016; 57 Suppl 1:34S–39S

[83] Cheng J, Wang Y, Mo M, et al. 18F-fluorodeoxyglucose (FDG) PET/CT after two cycles of neoadjuvant therapy may predict response in HER2-negative, but not in HER2-positive breast cancer. Oncotarget. 2015; 6(30):29388–29395

[84] Koolen BB, Pengel KE, Wesseling J, et al. FDG PET/CT during neoadjuvant chemotherapy may predict response in ER-positive/HER2-negative and triple negative, but not in HER2-positive breast cancer. Breast. 2013; 22(5):691–697

[85] Chen X, Moore MO, Lehman CD, et al. Combined use of MRI and PET to monitor response and assess residual disease for locally advanced breast cancer treated with neoadjuvant chemotherapy. Acad Radiol. 2004; 11(10):1115–1124

[86] Schwarz-Dose J, Untch M, Tiling R, et al. Monitoring primary systemic therapy of large and locally advanced breast cancer by using sequential positron emission tomography imaging with [18F]fluorodeoxyglucose. J Clin Oncol. 2009; 27(4):535–541

[87] McDermott GM, Welch A, Staff RT, et al. Monitoring primary breast cancer throughout chemotherapy using FDG-PET. Breast Cancer Res Treat. 2007; 102(1):75–84

[88] Humbert O, Cochet A, Coudert B, et al. Role of positron emission tomography for the monitoring of response to therapy in breast cancer. Oncologist. 2015; 20(2):94–104

[89] Balasubramanian Harisankar CN, Preethi R, John J. Metabolic flare phenomenon on 18 fluoride-fluorodeoxy glucose positron emission tomography-computed tomography scans in a patient with bilateral breast cancer treated with second-line chemotherapy and bevacizumab. Indian J Nucl Med. 2015; 30 (2):145–147

[90] Krupitskaya Y, Eslamy HK, Nguyen DD, Kumar A, Wakelee HA. Osteoblastic bone flare on F18-FDG PET in non-small cell lung cancer (NSCLC) patients receiving bevacizumab in addition to standard chemotherapy. J Thorac Oncol. 2009; 4(3): 429–431

18 Gastric, Esophageal, and Gastrointestinal Stromal Tumors

Eugene C. Lin

18.1 Gastric Cancer

National Comprehensive Cancer Network (NCCN) guidelines[1] suggest that positron emission tomography/computed tomography (PET/CT) is reasonable for staging patients without known M1 disease, except in patients with T1 disease.

1. Potential uses of PET in patients with gastric cancer are staging, detecting recurrence, determining prognosis, and evaluating therapy response.
2. **Prognosis:**
   a) Survival rate in patients with high 18F-fluorodeoxyglucose (FDG) uptake in the primary tumor is significantly lower than in patients with low FDG uptake.[2] However, as mucinous and signet ring cell carcinomas typically have low FDG uptake, low FDG uptake does not necessarily mean a better prognosis. The number of FDG avid lymph nodes is also a prognostic factor.[3]
   b) A negative PET scan after surgical treatment with curative intent is associated with significantly longer survival.[2]
3. **Therapy response (early prediction).** PET performed 14 days after initiation of chemotherapy predicts response to therapy.[4]

18.1.1 Accuracy/Comparison to Other Modalities

1. **PET.** Sensitivity of 71%, specificity of 74%[5] (advanced, metastatic, or recurrent gastric cancer).
2. **Primary tumor.** PET does not have a role in the detection of primary gastric cancer. In general, gastric cancer is less well detected than esophageal cancer, as sensitivity for early gastric cancer (sensitivity of 23–63%)[6] as well as signet-ring cell and mucinous histology is low. Published rates of sensitivities have ranged from 21 to 100% with specificities ranging from 78 to 100%.[7]
   a) A greater degree of FDG uptake is associated with greater depth of invasion, size of tumor, and lymph node metastases.[2]
   b) Signet-ring cell and mucinous carcinomas have low FDG uptake.[8,9]

3. **Nodal metastases** (meta-analysis; ▶ Table 18.1)[6]:

Table 18.1 Sensitivity and specificity of PET versus CT in the detection of nodal metastases in gastric cancer

	Sensitivity %	Specificity %	Accuracy %
PET	40	98	60
CT	77	78	66

a) The sensitivity of PET (▶ Fig. 18.1) ranges from 22 to 60%, which is inferior to the sensitivity of CT which ranges from 52 to 77%. In particular, CT is more sensitive for N1 nodes. However, the specificity of PET (62–100%) is higher than that of CT (62–94%).[7]
b) **Intestinal and diffuse-type adenocarcinoma**. The accuracy of lymph node staging depends on whether the tumor is intestinal or diffuse-type adenocarcinoma. In one report,[10] FDG uptake was superior to shortest lymph node diameter for the detection of metastases for intestinal-type adenocarcinoma, but the FDG uptake was less accurate for diffuse-type adenocarcinoma. In another report,[11] PET/CT improved the detection of extraregional lymph node metastases and distant metastases compared to CT alone in patients with intestinal/mixed-type tumors. However,

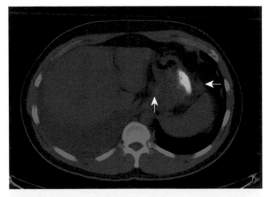

Fig. 18.1 Gastric cancer. Axial PET/CT scan demonstrates uptake in a primary gastric cancer with two local nodal metastases (*arrows*).

the sensitivity of lymph node assessment for diffuse-type cancers after neoadjuvant therapy was low.

4. **Body region**[8]:

   a) Accuracy for the primary lesion and for metastases to the liver (▶ Fig. 18.2), lymph nodes, and lung is high.

   Accuracy for pleural and peritoneal disease and bone marrow metastases is low.

   Accuracy for small perigastric nodes can also be low if obscured by uptake in the primary tumor.

5. **Distant metastases**. In a meta-analysis,[6] the overall accuracy of PET for M staging was 88% compared to 81% for CT.

   a) *Hepatic metastases* (systematic review; ▶ Table 18.2).[12]

Table 18.2 Sensitivity and specificity of PET versus CT in the detection of hepatic metastases in gastric cancer

	Sensitivity %	Specificity %
PET	70	96
CT	74	99

   b) *Peritoneal metastases* (systematic review; ▶ Table 18.3).[12]

Table 18.3 Sensitivity and specificity of PET versus CT in the detection of peritoneal metastases in gastric cancer

	Sensitivity %	Specificity %
PET	28	97
CT	33	99

   c) *Bone metastases* (▶ Table 18.4).[13]

   • However, 15% of solitary bone metastases in the same study were positive on PET

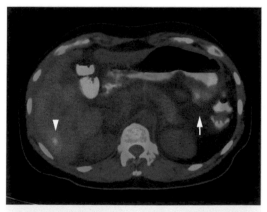

Fig. 18.2 Metastatic gastric cancer. Axial PET/CT scan demonstrates uptake in a gastric cancer (*arrow*) which has metastasized to the liver (*arrowhead*).

Table 18.4 Sensitivity and specificity of PET versus bone scan in the detection of bone metastases in gastric cancer

	Sensitivity %	Specificity %
PET	93.5	25
Bone scan	93.5	37.5

only, and PET was superior to bone scan for the detection of synchronous metastases.

6. **Recurrent gastric cancer.** In a meta-analysis,[14] the sensitivity and specificity of PET for recurrent gastric cancer were 78 and 82%, respectively. A meta-analysis of PET/CT[15] yielded a sensitivity of 86% and specificity of 88%. A meta-analysis[16] of both PET and PET/CT for the detection of gastric cancer recurrence yielded a sensitivity of 85% and specificity of 78% on a per-patient basis.

In addition, PET/CT has demonstrated good diagnostic accuracy in postoperative surveillance of asymptomatic gastric cancer patients.[17,18] However, the FDG avidity of the primary tumor affects the performance of PET/CT for detecting gastric cancer recurrence. In one report,[19] the sensitivity for recurrence was 81% in patients with FDG avid primary tumors, and 52% in patients with nonavid tumors. However, specificity was high (97%) and did not differ between the two groups.

18.1.2 Pearls/Pitfalls

1. **Histology.** Signet ring cell and mucinous carcinomas have low FDG uptake.

2. **Morphology.** The amount of uptake in the primary tumor may not correlate with histopathology.

   a) Poorly differentiated tumors may appear to have less uptake due to diffuse infiltration in the gastric wall.

   b) Well-differentiated tumors may appear to have more uptake due to mass formation.

3. **Other pathologies.** Increased gastric FDG uptake can be secondary to etiologies other than gastric cancer.

   a) Diffuse increased uptake can be secondary to gastritis or lymphoma.

   b) Focal increased uptake can be secondary to lymphoma (▶ Fig. 18.3). Gastric lymphoma tends to present with diffuse or segmental FDG uptake, while gastric carcinoma typically presents with local tracer uptake. In addition, gastric lymphoma typically has a higher SUVmax, and ratio of SUVmax to

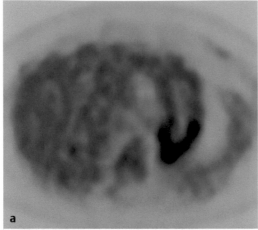

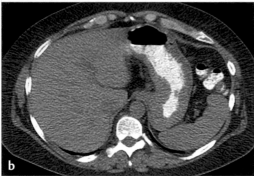

Fig. 18.3 Gastric lymphoma. **(a)** Axial PET demonstrates segmental increased uptake in the fundus (SUVmax 8.5) corresponding to wall thickening on CT **(b)** in a patient with mucosa-associated lymphoid tissue lymphoma. The segmental pattern of uptake and the high FDG uptake relative to the wall thickness suggest lymphoma rather than carcinoma.

maximum wall thickness, compared to gastric carcinoma.[20] A high ratio of SUVmax to maximum wall thickness is the most helpful finding in discriminating gastric lymphoma from carcinoma.

4. **Perigastric nodes**. Uptake in perigastric nodes is often not distinguishable from uptake in the immediately adjacent tumor, or adjacent physiologic gastric wall activity. However, this may have limited clinical significance, as these nodes are typically part of the standard dissection in patients with advanced gastric cancer.

5. **Gastric remnant**. Physiologic FDG uptake in a gastric remnant may be difficult to differentiate from recurrent tumor. Ingestion of water may

be helpful. Gastric FDG uptake secondary to malignancy will persist after water ingestion.

18.2 Esophageal Cancer

18.2.1 Primary Esophageal Tumor

PET has a limited role in evaluating primary esophageal tumors.

1. **Detection**
   a) PET can detect primary tumors with depth of invasion of T1b or greater, but Tis and T1a tumors are not detectable.[21]
   b) The overall detection rate of PET for primary esophageal carcinoma is 80%. However, this depends on the T stage. The detection rate for T3 and T4 tumors is close to 100%, but the detection rate for T1 tumors is 43%.[22]
   c) PET cannot assess the degree of tumor penetration into the esophageal wall and cannot determine T stage. However, PET is increasingly likely to identify the tumor with increasing depth of invasion.

2. **Level of uptake**[23]
   a) The amount of uptake correlates positively with depth of tumor invasion, presence of lymph node metastases, and lymphatic invasion.
   b) Adenocarcinomas and squamous cell carcinomas overall have similar degrees of FDG uptake, although adenocarcinomas, particularly at or near the gastroesophageal junction, often have lower uptake secondary to diffuse growth pattern and/or mucinous histopathology.[24,25,26]
   c) While high pretreatment SUV is correlated with diminished survival, it is unclear whether it is an independent prognostic marker (e.g., it could just be a marker of advanced stage). While most studies have shown that pretreatment FDG uptake is a predictor for survival in univariate analysis,[27] the two largest prospective studies did not demonstrate the independent prognostic value of baseline SUV.[28,29]
   d) Interestingly, two studies[30,31] have reported that patients with high primary tumor uptake had a better response to neoadjuvant chemoradiation. This suggests that a high baseline SUV may not predict survival if preoperative chemoradiation is given, as patients with high tumor uptake might have a better response to neoadjuvant chemoradiation.

3. **Pitfalls**
   a) Mild focal uptake at the gastroesophageal junction could be secondary to esophagitis, or could be a normal variant (▶ Fig. 7.30). SUV cutoffs of ≥ 3.5[32] and > 4 at the gastroesophageal junction have been suggested as raising concern for malignancy.[33]
   b) Hiatal hernias can cause large areas of uptake at the gastroesophageal junction.
   c) Benign strictures can have substantial FDG uptake after dilatation. Increased uptake can also be identified after endoscopic biopsy.
   d) Esophageal leiomyomas can have FDG uptake.[33,34]
   e) ***Respiratory misregistration.*** Respiratory misregistration artifact on PET/CT (which is greatest in the peridiaphragmatic region) may result in erroneous SUV measurements of distal esophageal tumors.[33,35]

18.3 Staging

NCCN guidelines[1] indicate that PET/CT is appropriate if there is no evidence of M1 disease.

1. The combination of PET and endoscopic ultrasound (EUS) can be the most cost-effective method of staging esophageal cancer.[33,36]
2. The primary value of PET is in[37]
   a) Detecting distant metastases (▶ Fig. 18.4, ▶ Fig. 18.5).
   b) Improving the specificity of lymph node staging.
3. However, PET may not be routinely useful in patients with early-stage esophageal cancer (T ≤ 2), as these patients have a low incidence of lymphatic metastases.[38]
4. In a multicenter prospective study,[39] PET/CT led to clinically important changes in stage in 24% of patients; 22% were upstaged, and 2% were downstaged. The overall incremental benefit in staging accuracy of PET compared to CT is 14%.[22] PET will identify unsuspected distant metastatic disease in 5 to 8%[40] of patients without evidence of metastases after conventional workup. In nine studies, PET evaluation changed the pretherapeutic stage compared to conventional staging in 5 to 27% of patients, (22% across all the studies).[41]
5. **Prognosis.** Greater tumor length on PET and increased number of PET-positive lymph nodes predict low survival rate.[42]

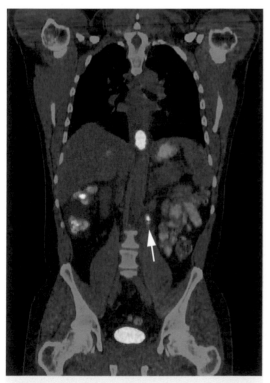

Fig. 18.4 Metastatic esophageal cancer. Coronal PET/CT in a patient with distal esophageal cancer demonstrates liver and retroperitoneal node (*arrow*) metastases.

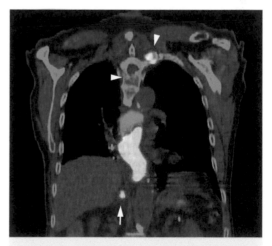

Fig. 18.5 Metastatic esophageal cancer. Coronal PET/CT in a patient with esophageal carcinoma demonstrates intense uptake in the primary tumor and adrenal (*arrow*) and bone (*arrowheads*) metastases.

18.3.1 Accuracy/Comparison to Other Modalities

1. **Nodal staging with PET/CT** (meta-analysis).[43] Sensitivity of 62%, specificity of 96%.
   a) **Locoregional nodes.**[38] PET is insensitive for locoregional disease and cannot replace CT/EUS for locoregional staging, but a positive result is more specific than CT/EUS for nodal disease (▶ Fig. 18.6). A large percentage of false-negative nodal groups on PET are in the immediate vicinity of the primary tumor.[22] EUS will detect more pathologic periesophageal and celiac axis nodes than PET or CT (▶ Table 18.5).[44]

Table 18.5 Sensitivity and specificity of PET versus CT versus EUS in the detection of nodal metastases

	Sensitivity %	Specificity %
PET	57	85
CT	50	83
EUS	80	70

   b) **Distant nodes** (▶ Table 18.6).[38]

Table 18.6 Sensitivity and specificity of PET versus CT and EUS in the detection of distant nodes

	Sensitivity %	Specificity %
PET	77	90
CT/EUS	46	69

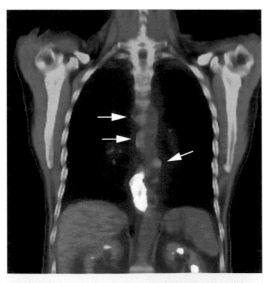

Fig. 18.6 Esophageal cancer with locoregional nodal metastases. Coronal PET/CT scan demonstrates multiple metastases to locoregional paraesophageal nodes (*arrows*) from a distal esophageal cancer. While endoscopic ultrasound would usually be more sensitive for the detection of these nodes, a positive PET study is more specific for metastatic disease.

2. **Distant metastases** (meta-analysis; ▶ Table 18.7).[45]

Table 18.7 Sensitivity and specificity of PET versus CT in the detection of distant metastases

	Sensitivity %	Specificity %
PET	71	93
CT	52	91

3. **Bone metastases.** PET may be more accurate than bone scintigraphy for bone metastases (▶ Table 18.8; ▶ Table 18.9).[46]

Table 18.8 Sensitivity and specificity of PET versus bone scan in the detection of bone metastases

	Sensitivity %	Specificity %
PET	92	94
Bone scan	77	84

Table 18.9 Sensitivity and specificity of PET versus EUS in the detection of bone metastases

	Sensitivity %	Specificity %
PET	42–100	27–100
EUS	20–100	36–100

4. **Anatomic region.** PET has the highest accuracy in the neck, upper thoracic, and abdominal regions but low sensitivity in the mid- and lower thoracic regions.[23]

18.3.2 Pearls/Pitfalls

1. Hilar uptake must be interpreted with caution, as it is the most common area of false-positive nodal uptake, particularly in smokers and in geographic locations where granulomatous disease is endemic.[47,48]
2. Small intracapsular locoregional metastases have a high false-negative rate.[49]
3. Uptake in the primary tumor may obscure the abnormal nodes adjacent to it.
4. PET/CT is least sensitive in the assessment of lymph nodes adjacent to the mid and lower thoracic esophagus.
5. **Gastrohepatic versus celiac nodes.** Resectable gastrohepatic lymph nodes should be distinguished from nonregional celiac nodes which are typically nonresectable. This may be difficult as lower gastrohepatic nodes may appear close to the celiac axis.[35]

6. **Synchronous neoplasms.** PET will detect unexpected synchronous primary neoplasms in 5.5% of patients with esophageal cancer.[50] Sites of pathologic uptake should be confirmed by other methods before being ascribed to metastases.

7. **Low uptake in primary tumor.** If the primary lesion in esophageal squamous cell cancer has low uptake (< 5 SUV in one report),[51] PET/CT has a low sensitivity for detecting lymph node metastases.

8. Mid and lower esophageal SCC tends to metastasize to the right paratracheal/supraclavicular nodes.[52]

18.4 Recurrence

PET is accurate for the detection of recurrent esophageal cancer (▶ Fig. 18.7), but it is not clearly superior to conventional imaging. In patients with recurrence SUV and disease, status on PET/CT predicts survival.[53]

18.4.1 Accuracy

Diagnosis of recurrent esophageal cancer with PET and PET/CT after initial treatment with curative intent (meta-analysis).[54] Sensitivity of 96%, specificity of 78%.

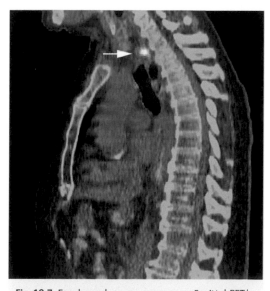

Fig. 18.7 Esophageal cancer recurrence. Sagittal PET/CT in an esophageal cancer patient status post esophagectomy and gastric pull-through demonstrates recurrence at the proximal anastomosis (*arrow*).

18.4.2 Pitfalls

There is a low false-negative rate when PET/CT is used to evaluate for recurrence. However, histopathological confirmation of suspected PET-positive lesions is required, as there is a considerable false-positive rate.[54] PET is not accurate for the diagnosis of perianastomotic recurrence, as inflammation often causes false-positive results. At local sites, the specificity of PET/CT is only 50%, although sensitivity is high.[53]

18.5 Therapy Response[55]

NCCN guidelines[1] recommend that PET/CT should be considered for the assessment of response to preoperative or definitive chemoradiotherapy before surgery or the initiation of postoperative treatment. However, PET/CT is not recommended for the selection of patients to surgery following preoperative chemoradiotherapy.

Neoadjuvant therapy. In patients with advanced stages (T3–4) of esophageal cancer, the prognosis is poor with esophagectomy alone. Neoadjuvant radiochemotherapy or chemotherapy can result in downstaging, higher resectability in subsequent surgery, and eradication of occult disease. Neoadjuvant therapy improves the survival of patients with advanced esophageal carcinoma by about 10% in 5 years, but this benefit is seen only in patients with a major histopathological response. Patients who show minor or no response would only be exposed to the toxicity of the therapy. Thus, it would be beneficial to identify nonresponders early in the course of neoadjuvant therapy, as these patients could potentially discontinue therapy and proceed to surgery.[56,57]

The primary value of PET/CT in neoadjuvant therapy is its negative predictive value—a PET/CT scan without a substantial change in SUV predicts a worse prognosis. In a systematic review,[58] the median negative predictive value of PET was 86.5%, using a SUV reduction of at least 35% as a threshold criterion. There is conflicting data on whether pretherapeutic SUV is associated with response and prognosis.[59]

Interim PET. The MUNICON trial[60] evaluated the ability to tailor treatment based on the chemoresponsiveness of esophageal cancers as assessed by PET. This trial was one of the first to evaluate the feasibility of a PET-guided treatment algorithm based on early metabolic response. A change in SUV greater than 35% at 2 weeks after the start of neoadjuvant chemotherapy was used to predict response. Metabolic responders continued neoadjuvant therapy and had a favorable outcome. Metabolic nonresponders discontinued chemotherapy and proceeded to surgery. Metabolic nonresponders had a poor prognosis, but discontinuing the chemotherapy in nonresponders did not compromise the prognosis, and reduced costs, time, and potential side effects. However, adding neoadjuvant radiation therapy for metabolic nonresponders did not lead to an improvement in the poor prognosis.[61]

It should be noted that early response evaluation has only been successfully evaluated in patients receiving chemotherapy without radiation. In some studies of patients being treated with chemotherapy plus radiation therapy, metabolic response did not predict tumor response.[62] This may be due to factors such as radiation-induced inflammation, and possible different mechanisms of cell death from radiotherapy compared to chemotherapy.[63]

End of treatment PET. Some studies have suggested that surgery can be omitted in patients who have achieved a pathological complete response after neoadjuvant therapy. However, overall, PET/CT offers a better prediction on long-term outcomes (survival) than on histopathological response.[64] In particular, reliable PET criteria have not been established to identify pathologic complete response. There are two general methods to predict complete pathologic response: interpreting a posttherapeutic FDG-negative tumor as a pathologic complete response and retrospectively identifying cutoff values. The percentage of residual tumor in FDG-negative tumors ranges from 17.8 to 70.6%.[41] In a study confined to patients with

esophageal adenocarcinoma,[30] a change in SUV of < 45% had a positive predictive value of 92% for incomplete pathologic response, but only a 38% positive predictive value for complete pathologic response. Other studies have found accuracies of around 75% using retrospective cutoffs.[41] In one study, two-thirds of patients with a post-chemoradiotherapy SUV < 2.5 had tumor in the surgical specimen, and two-thirds of patients had positive lymph nodes at surgery not detected by PET. Therefore, surgical resection is still indicated regardless of the posttherapy SUV in the primary tumor.

Interval metastases. There is conflicting evidence as to the effectiveness of PET in detecting interval metastases (which may preclude surgical resection) after neoadjuvant therapy for esophageal carcinoma (▶ Fig. 18.8). In several studies,[41] PET/CT detected interval metastases in 8% of patients. In another study, PET was not sensitive for interval metastases.[65]

18.5.1 Accuracy/Comparison to Other Modalities

1. **PET** (meta-analysis).[66] Sensitivity of 70%, specificity of 70%.
   a) **PET during neoadjuvant therapy** (meta-analysis).[67] Sensitivity of 85%, specificity of 59%.
   b) **PET after neoadjuvant therapy** (meta-analysis).[67] Sensitivity of 67%, specificity of 69%.
      • However, some analyses[68,69] have found no difference in accuracy of early PET and PET after completion of therapy.

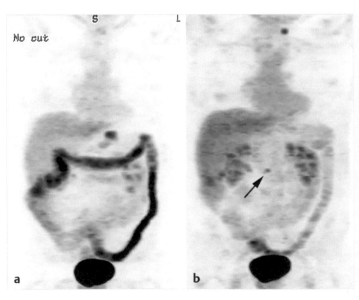

Fig. 18.8 Interval metastases. (a) MIP PET demonstrates increased uptake in a gastroesophageal junction cancer. (b) After neoadjuvant chemoradiotherapy, the uptake in the primary tumor is greatly decreased, but there are new interval metastases in left supraclavicular and retroperitoneal (*arrow*) nodes.

2. **CT and EUS.** The accuracy rates of PET and EUS are similar, but EUS is sometimes not feasible after chemotherapy and radiation. The accuracy of CT is significantly lower than that of PET and EUS.[70]

3. **PET versus EUS** (meta-analysis).[68]

4. **SUV.** A wide range of cutoff values (30–80%) for SUV reduction have been reported as discriminating between responders and nonresponders.[71] Both absolute SUVs and relative changes in SUV have been used for prognosis. In a meta-analysis,[69] relative changes in uptake was the better prognosticator. A posttherapy SUV of ≥ 4 is the better predictor of poor outcome and short survival than EUS mass size or CT wall thickness.[72]

5. The overall accuracy for predicting tumor response does not differ between adenocarcinoma and squamous cell carcinoma.[73]

18.5.2 Pitfalls

1. **Esophagitis.** After neoadjuvant radiotherapy, radiation esophagitis can interfere with optimal assessment of response to treatment.[74] Unlike the lung, the esophagus may react early to radiation and elevations in activity can be seen during the course of radiotherapy.[75] The delay in imaging after therapy necessary to avoid uptake from radiation esophagitis is not well established. Delays of 2 to 12 weeks after radiotherapy have been proposed.[76] Another possible approach is to image very early (< 2 weeks) after radiotherapy, before the development of esophagitis.[35]

2. **Esophageal ulceration.** Chemoradiotherapy-induced esophageal ulceration can result in false-positive findings of residual malignancy. Endoscopy is very helpful in increasing accuracy in these cases. If ulceration is absent at endoscopy, a SUV ≥ 4 is highly predictive of residual disease.[77]

18.6 Radiation Therapy Planning

Accurate delineation of the gross tumor volume (GTV) is necessary for successful radiotherapy of esophageal cancer. Potentially, PET could improve the accuracy of the delineation process. While incorporation of FDG PET/CT may improve assessment of GTV in various tumors, such as non-small cell lung cancer, the evidence is more limited in esophageal cancer. Although some studies suggest that PET/CT can accurately assess esophageal tumor length,[78] a systematic review[79] concluded that further validation is necessary before standard implementation of PET/CT in the tumor delineation process. In addition, sensitivity of PET/CT for locoregional nodes, which should be included in the radiation field, is variable.

18.7 Gastrointestinal Stromal Tumors

CT is the standard imaging modality for primary gastrointestinal stromal tumor (GIST). PET/CT is primarily valuable in assessing early response to imatinib mesylate (▶ Fig. 18.9) or in cases where CT or MRI results are equivocal.[80] However, PET is less sensitive than CT prior to treatment. Approximately 20% of lesions detected by CT have no FDG uptake (▶ Fig. 18.10).[81] In particular, PET is less sensitive for liver metastases.[82] PET may be more useful than CT for predicting response to therapy, but CT detects more lesions.[83]

In addition, PET may be helpful in predicting the malignant potential of GIST prior to surgery.[84] In one report,[85] a SUV > 3.0 was associated with a high malignant potential; in another report,[86] the SUV cutoff was > 5.

Standard morphologic criteria based on changes in tumor size are not optimal in the early assessment of treatment response in GIST patients. Treatment with imatinib induces changes such as decreased vascularity, hemorrhage, necrosis, and

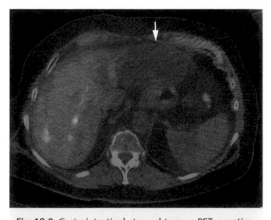

Fig. 18.9 Gastrointestinal stromal tumor: PET negative. Axial PET/CT demonstrates a large GIST tumor (*arrow*) without substantial FDG uptake.

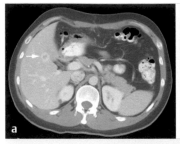 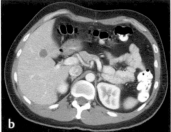 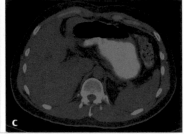

Fig. 18.10 Gastrointestinal stromal tumor: therapy response. **(a)** Axial CT demonstrates an enhancing liver metastasis (*arrow*) from a GIST. **(b)** After imatinib mesylate treatment, the metastasis is now completely hypodense and appears slightly larger. GIST metastases are difficult to follow by CT as they change primarily in density rather than size after treatment, and may actually increase in size early after treatment. PET/CT **(c)** done after therapy demonstrates lack of uptake in the liver metastasis.

cystic or mucoid degeneration which are consistent with therapeutic activity but are not necessarily associated with a change in tumor volume. In patients with FDG avid GISTs, decreases in FDG uptake precede changes in tumor size during imatinib treatment. The median time for tumor shrinkage on CT is 3 to 4 months, but may be 6 to 12 months or longer.[87] In general, the imaging changes during response to cytostatic agents like imatinib differ from the response to cytotoxic agents. In particular, other imaging findings in addition to change in size are relevant (such as decreased tumor density), and lesion size may even increase during response (e.g., from myxoid degeneration, necrosis, or hemorrhage). The Choi criteria for CT evaluation of GIST tumor response incorporate decreases in tumor density as well as size. Change in tumor size (particularly of hepatic metastases) on CT is often not apparent until late in therapy. Instead, tumors will decrease in attenuation on CT studies.[88]

PET may be helpful in evaluating equivocal metastatic lesions.[88] Pseudoprogression can be caused by an increase in lesion size secondary to myxoid degeneration or intratumoral hemorrhage. Intratumoral hemorrhage can increase tumor density and mask a treatment response.

Reduction in SUV 1 week after treatment predicts progression-free survival.[89] Early response evaluation with PET/CT may be useful in patients with marginally resectable GISTs, or those at greater surgical risk, when a timely decision whether or not to perform surgery is needed.

Early monitoring of therapeutic response may also be needed after adjusting the imatinib dose.

A subset of GIST patients have primary resistance and do not respond to imatinib and demonstrate disease progression in the first 6 months. With PET/CT, a drop in SUV to less than 2.5 or a 25% drop from baseline is seen in most responding GISTs in the first month of treatment.[90] Patients who do not demonstrate this decline likely have primary resistance, and may benefit from alternative treatment regiments. Secondary resistance manifests as disease progression in patients who have an initial good response for at least 6 months.

18.7.1 Accuracy

PET for prediction of response to treatment (meta-analysis). Sensitivity of 90%, specificity of 62%.[91]

18.7.2 Pearls

1. PET criteria to define a good response include a decrease in SUV < 70% and a decrease to an absolute SUV < 2.5.[92]
2. Tumors may become larger within the first 6 months of treatment (possibly secondary to hemorrhage, edema, or myxoid degeneration) despite regression clinically and on PET.
3. Lesions without FDG uptake (approximately 20%) could be followed by CT with evaluation of change in attenuation.
4. Recurrence after partial response to imatinib appears as a focal area of FDG uptake within a larger mass. This correlates with an enhancing nodule on CT.[93]

18.7.3 Pitfalls

In patients with imatinib refractory GISTs, termination of imatinib therapy may result in a "flare" phenomenon in which increased FDG uptake is seen within days of stopping treatment. This implies that tumor cell populations responsive to imatinib are still present, along with tumor cells which are resistant to imatinib. Potentially, these patients could remain on imatinib therapy in combination with another targeted drug directed at the resistant clones.[94]

References

[1] Ajani JA, D'Amico TA, Almhanna K, et al. Gastric cancer, version 3.2016, NCCN Clinical Practice Guidelines in Oncology. J Natl Compr Canc Netw. 2016; 14(10):1286–1312

[2] Mochiki E, Kuwano H, Katoh H, Asao T, Oriuchi N, Endo K. Evaluation of 18F-2-deoxy-2-fluoro-D-glucose positron emission tomography for gastric cancer. World J Surg. 2004; 28(3):247–253

[3] Wang X, Wei Y, Xue Y, Lu P, Yu L, Shen B. Predictive role of the number of 18F-FDG-positive lymph nodes detected by PET/CT for pre-treatment evaluation of locally advanced gastric cancer. PLoS One. 2016; 11(12):e0166836

[4] Ott K, Fink U, Becker K, et al. Prediction of response to preoperative chemotherapy in gastric carcinoma by metabolic imaging: results of a prospective trial. J Clin Oncol. 2003; 21 (24):4604–4610

[5] Yoshioka T, Yamaguchi K, Kubota K, et al. Evaluation of 18F-FDG PET in patients with advanced, metastatic, or recurrent gastric cancer. J Nucl Med. 2003; 44(5):690–699

[6] Seevaratnam R, Cardoso R, McGregor C, et al. How useful is preoperative imaging for tumor, node, metastasis (TNM) staging of gastric cancer? A meta-analysis. Gastric Cancer. 2012; 15 Suppl 1:S3–S18

[7] Smyth EC, Shah MA. Role of 18F 2-fluoro-2-deoxyglucose positron emission tomography in upper gastrointestinal malignancies. World J Gastroenterol. 2011; 17(46):5059–5074

[8] Chen J, Cheong JH, Yun MJ, et al. Improvement in preoperative staging of gastric adenocarcinoma with positron emission tomography. Cancer. 2005; 103(11):2383–2390

[9] Stahl A, Ott K, Weber WA, et al. FDG PET imaging of locally advanced gastric carcinomas: correlation with endoscopic and histopathological findings. Eur J Nucl Med Mol Imaging. 2003; 30(2):288–295

[10] Okumura Y, Aikou S, Onoyama H, et al. Evaluation of 18F-FDG uptake for detecting lymph node metastasis of gastric cancer: a prospective pilot study for one-to-one comparison of radiation dose and pathological findings. World J Surg Oncol. 2015; 13:327

[11] Lehmann K, Eshmuminov D, Bauerfeind P, et al. 18FDG-PET-CT improves specificity of preoperative lymph-node staging in patients with intestinal but not diffuse-type esophagogastric adenocarcinoma. Eur J Surg Oncol. 2017; 43(1):196–202

[12] Wang Z, Chen JQ. Imaging in assessing hepatic and peritoneal metastases of gastric cancer: a systematic review. BMC Gastroenterol. 2011; 11:19

[13] Ma DW, Kim JH, Jeon TJ, et al. 18F-fluorodeoxyglucose positron emission tomography-computed tomography for the evaluation of bone metastasis in patients with gastric cancer. Dig Liver Dis. 2013; 45(9):769–775

[14] Wu LM, Hu JN, Hua J, Gu HY, Zhu J, Xu JR. 18 F-fluorodeoxyglucose positron emission tomography to evaluate recurrent gastric cancer: a systematic review and meta-analysis. J Gastroenterol Hepatol. 2012; 27(3):472–480

[15] Zou H, Zhao Y. 18FDG PET-CT for detecting gastric cancer recurrence after surgical resection: a meta-analysis. Surg Oncol. 2013; 22(3):162–166

[16] Li P, Liu Q, Wang C, et al. Fluorine-18-fluorodeoxyglucose positron emission tomography to evaluate recurrent gastric cancer after surgical resection: a systematic review and meta-analysis. Ann Nucl Med. 2016; 30(3):179–187

[17] Lee DY, Lee CH, Seo MJ, Lee SH, Ryu JS, Lee JJ. Performance of (18)F-FDG PET/CT as a postoperative surveillance imaging modality for asymptomatic advanced gastric cancer patients. Ann Nucl Med. 2014; 28(8):789–795

[18] Lee JW, Lee SM, Son MW, Lee MS. Diagnostic performance of FDG PET/CT for surveillance in asymptomatic gastric cancer patients after curative surgical resection. Eur J Nucl Med Mol Imaging. 2016; 43(5):881–888

[19] Kim SJ, Cho YS, Moon SH, et al. Primary tumor 18F-FDG avidity affects the performance of 18F-FDG PET/CT for detecting gastric cancer recurrence. J Nucl Med. 2016; 57(4):544–550

[20] Li XF, Fu Q, Dong YW, et al. (18)F-fluorodeoxyglucose positron emission tomography/computed tomography comparison of gastric lymphoma and gastric carcinoma. World J Gastroenterol. 2016; 22(34):7787–7796

[21] Himeno S, Yasuda S, Shimada H, Tajima T, Makuuchi H. Evaluation of esophageal cancer by positron emission tomography. Jpn J Clin Oncol. 2002; 32(9):340–346

[22] Kato H, Miyazaki T, Nakajima M, et al. The incremental effect of positron emission tomography on diagnostic accuracy in the initial staging of esophageal carcinoma. Cancer. 2005; 103(1):148–156

[23] Kato H, Kuwano H, Nakajima M, et al. Comparison between positron emission tomography and computed tomography in the use of the assessment of esophageal carcinoma. Cancer. 2002; 94(4):921–928

[24] Dam HQ, Manzone TM, Sagar VV. Evolving role of (18)F-fluorodeoxyglucose positron emission tomography in the management of esophageal carcinoma. Surg Oncol Clin N Am. 2006; 15(4):733–749

[25] Esteves FP, Schuster DM, Halkar RK. Gastrointestinal tract malignancies and positron emission tomography: an overview. Semin Nucl Med. 2006; 36(2):169–181

[26] Piessen G, Petyt G, Duhamel A, Mirabel X, Huglo D, Mariette C. Ineffectiveness of 18F-fluorodeoxyglucose positron emission tomography in the evaluation of tumor response after completion of neoadjuvant chemoradiation in esophageal cancer. Ann Surg. 2013; 258(1):66–76

[27] Omloo JM, van Heijl M, Hoekstra OS, van Berge Henegouwen MI, van Lanschot JJ, Sloof GW. FDG-PET parameters as prognostic factor in esophageal cancer patients: a review. Ann Surg Oncol. 2011; 18(12):3338–3352

[28] Chatterton BE, Ho Shon I, Baldey A, et al. Positron emission tomography changes management and prognostic stratification in patients with oesophageal cancer: results of a multicentre prospective study. Eur J Nucl Med Mol Imaging. 2009; 36(3):354–361

[29] Omloo JM, Sloof GW, Boellaard R, et al. Importance of fluorodeoxyglucose-positron emission tomography (FDG-PET) and endoscopic ultrasonography parameters in predicting survival following surgery for esophageal cancer. Endoscopy. 2008; 40(6):464–471

[30] Kukar M, Alnaji RM, Jabi F, et al. Role of repeat 18F-fluorodeoxyglucose positron emission tomography examination in predicting pathologic response following neoadjuvant chemoradiotherapy for esophageal adenocarcinoma. JAMA Surg. 2015; 150(6):555–562

[31] Rizk NP, Tang L, Adusumilli PS, et al. Predictive value of initial PET-SUVmax in patients with locally advanced esophageal and gastroesophageal junction adenocarcinoma. J Thorac Oncol. 2009; 4(7):875–879

[32] Stagg J, Farukhi I, Lazaga F, et al. Significance of 18F-fluoro-deoxyglucose uptake at the gastroesophageal junction: comparison of PET to esophagogastroduodenoscopy. Dig Dis Sci. 2015; 60(5):1335–1342

[33] Salaun PY, Grewal RK, Dodamane I, Yeung HW, Larson SM, Strauss HW. An analysis of the 18F-FDG uptake pattern in the stomach. J Nucl Med. 2005; 46(1):48–51

[34] Meirelles GS, Ravizzini G, Yeung HW, Akhurst T. Esophageal leiomyoma: a rare cause of false-positive FDG scans. Clin Nucl Med. 2006; 31(6):342–344

[35] Bruzzi JF, Munden RF, Truong MT, et al. PET/CT of esophageal cancer: its role in clinical management. Radiographics. 2007; 27(6):1635–1652

[36] Wallace MB, Nietert PJ, Earle C, et al. An analysis of multiple staging management strategies for carcinoma of the esophagus: computed tomography, endoscopic ultrasound, positron emission tomography, and thoracoscopy/laparoscopy. Ann Thorac Surg. 2002; 74(4):1026–1032

[37] Flamen P, Lerut A, Van Cutsem E, et al. Utility of positron emission tomography for the staging of patients with potentially operable esophageal carcinoma. J Clin Oncol. 2000; 18 (18):3202–3210

[38] Lerut T, Flamen P, Ectors N, et al. Histopathologic validation of lymph node staging with FDG-PET scan in cancer of the esophagus and gastroesophageal junction: a prospective study based on primary surgery with extensive lymphadenectomy. Ann Surg. 2000; 232(6):743–752

[39] You JJ, Wong RK, Darling G, Gulenchyn K, Urbain JL, Evans WK. Clinical utility of 18F-fluorodeoxyglucose positron emission tomography/computed tomography in the staging of patients with potentially resectable esophageal cancer. J Thorac Oncol. 2013; 8(12):1563–1569

[40] Meyers BF, Downey RJ, Decker PA, et al. American College of Surgeons Oncology Group Z0060. The utility of positron emission tomography in staging of potentially operable carcinoma of the thoracic esophagus: results of the American College of Surgeons Oncology Group Z0060 trial. J Thorac Cardiovasc Surg. 2007; 133(3):738–745

[41] Schmidt T, Lordick F, Herrmann K, Ott K. Value of functional imaging by PET in esophageal cancer. J Natl Compr Canc Netw. 2015; 13(2):239–247

[42] Choi JY, Jang HJ, Shim YM, et al. 18F-FDG PET in patients with esophageal squamous cell carcinoma undergoing curative surgery: prognostic implications. J Nucl Med. 2004; 45(11):1843–1850

[43] Shi W, Wang W, Wang J, Cheng H, Huo X. Meta-analysis of 18FDG PET-CT for nodal staging in patients with esophageal cancer. Surg Oncol. 2013; 22(2):112–116

[44] Konski A, Doss M, Milestone B, et al. The integration of 18-fluoro-deoxy-glucose positron emission tomography and endoscopic ultrasound in the treatment-planning process for esophageal carcinoma. Int J Radiat Oncol Biol Phys. 2005; 61 (4):1123–1128

[45] van Vliet EP, Heijenbrok-Kal MH, Hunink MG, Kuipers EJ, Siersema PD. Staging investigations for oesophageal cancer: a meta-analysis. Br J Cancer. 2008; 98(3):547–557

[46] Kato H, Miyazaki T, Nakajima M, et al. Comparison between whole-body positron emission tomography and bone scintigraphy in evaluating bony metastases of esophageal carcinomas. Anticancer Res. 2005; 25 6C:4439–4444

[47] Yoon YC, Lee KS, Shim YM, Kim BT, Kim K, Kim TS. Metastasis to regional lymph nodes in patients with esophageal squamous cell carcinoma: CT versus FDG PET for presurgical detection prospective study. Radiology. 2003; 227(3):764–770

[48] Yuan S, Yu Y, Chao KS, et al. Additional value of PET/CT over PET in assessment of locoregional lymph nodes in thoracic esophageal squamous cell cancer. J Nucl Med. 2006; 47(8):1255–1259

[49] Luketich JD, Friedman DM, Weigel TL, et al. Evaluation of distant metastases in esophageal cancer: 100 consecutive positron emission tomography scans. Ann Thorac Surg. 1999; 68 (4):1133–1136, discussion 1136–1137

[50] van Westreenen HL, Westerterp M, Jager PL, et al. Synchronous primary neoplasms detected on 18F-FDG PET in staging of patients with esophageal cancer. J Nucl Med. 2005; 46(8):1321–1325

[51] Manabe O, Hattori N, Hirata K, et al. Diagnostic accuracy of lymph node metastasis depends on metabolic activity of the primary lesion in thoracic squamous esophageal cancer. J Nucl Med. 2013; 54(5):670–676

[52] Liu CJ, Cheng JC, Lee JM, Cheng MF, Tzen KY, Yen RF. Patterns of nodal metastases on 18F-FDG PET/CT in patients with esophageal squamous cell carcinoma are useful to guide treatment planning of radiotherapy. Clin Nucl Med. 2015; 40 (5):384–389

[53] Guo H, Zhu H, Xi Y, et al. Diagnostic and prognostic value of 18F-FDG PET/CT for patients with suspected recurrence from squamous cell carcinoma of the esophagus. J Nucl Med. 2007; 48(8):1251–1258

[54] Goense L, van Rossum PS, Reitsma JB, et al. Diagnostic performance of 18F-FDG PET and PET/CT for the detection of recurrent esophageal cancer after treatment with curative intent: a systematic review and meta-analysis. J Nucl Med. 2015; 56(7):995–1002

[55] Kostakoglu L, Goldsmith SJ. PET in the assessment of therapy response in patients with carcinoma of the head and neck and of the esophagus. J Nucl Med. 2004; 45(1):56–68

[56] Bollschweiler E, Hölscher AH, Schmidt M, Warnecke-Eberz U. Neoadjuvant treatment for advanced esophageal cancer: response assessment before surgery and how to predict response to chemoradiation before starting treatment. Chin J Cancer Res. 2015; 27(3):221–230

[57] Tao CJ, Lin G, Xu YP, Mao WM. Predicting the response of neoadjuvant therapy for patients with esophageal carcinoma: an in-depth literature review. J Cancer. 2015; 6(11):1179–1186

[58] Schröer-Günther M, Scheibler F, Wolff R, Westwood M, Baumert B, Lange S. The role of PET and PET-CT scanning in assessing response to neoadjuvant therapy in esophageal carcinoma. Dtsch Arztebl Int. 2015; 112(33–34):545–552

[59] Ott K, Weber W, Siewert JR. The importance of PET in the diagnosis and response evaluation of esophageal cancer. Dis Esophagus. 2006; 19(6):433–442

[60] Lordick F, Ott K, Krause BJ, et al. PET to assess early metabolic response and to guide treatment of adenocarcinoma of the oesophagogastric junction: the MUNICON phase II trial. Lancet Oncol. 2007; 8(9):797–805

[61] zum Büschenfelde CM, Herrmann K, Schuster T, et al. (18)F-FDG PET-guided salvage neoadjuvant radiochemotherapy of adenocarcinoma of the esophagogastric junction: the MUNICON II trial. J Nucl Med. 2011; 52(8):1189–1196

[62] Klaeser B, Nitzsche E, Schuller JC, et al. Limited predictive value of FDG-PET for response assessment in the preoperative treatment of esophageal cancer: results of a prospective multi-center trial (SAKK 75/02). Onkologie. 2009; 32(12):724–730

[63] Lordick F. The role of PET in predicting response to chemotherapy in oesophago-gastric cancer. Acta Gastroenterol Belg. 2011; 74(4):530–535

[64] Schollaert P, Crott R, Bertrand C, D'Hondt L, Borght TV, Krug B. A systematic review of the predictive value of (18)FDG-PET in esophageal and esophagogastric junction cancer after

neoadjuvant chemoradiation on the survival outcome stratification. J Gastrointest Surg. 2014; 18(5):894–905

[65] Downey RJ, Akhurst T, Ilson D, et al. Whole body 18FDG-PET and the response of esophageal cancer to induction therapy: results of a prospective trial. J Clin Oncol. 2003; 21(3):428–432

[66] Chen YM, Pan XF, Tong LJ, Shi YP, Chen T. Can 18F-fluorodeoxyglucose positron emission tomography predict responses to neoadjuvant therapy in oesophageal cancer patients? A meta-analysis. Nucl Med Commun. 2011; 32(11):1005–1010

[67] Cong L, Wang S, Gao T, Hu L. The predictive value of 18F-FDG PET for pathological response of primary tumor in patients with esophageal cancer during or after neoadjuvant chemoradiotherapy: a meta-analysis. Jpn J Clin Oncol. 2016; 46(12):1118–1126

[68] Ngamruengphong S, Sharma VK, Nguyen B, Das A. Assessment of response to neoadjuvant therapy in esophageal cancer: an updated systematic review of diagnostic accuracy of endoscopic ultrasonography and fluorodeoxyglucose positron emission tomography. Dis Esophagus. 2010; 23(3):216–231

[69] Zhu W, Xing L, Yue J, et al. Prognostic significance of SUV on PET/CT in patients with localised oesophagogastric junction cancer receiving neoadjuvant chemotherapy/chemoradiation: a systematic review and meta-analysis. Br J Radiol. 2012; 85(1017):e694–e701

[70] Westerterp M, van Westreenen HL, Reitsma JB, et al. Esophageal cancer: CT, endoscopic US, and FDG PET for assessment of response to neoadjuvant therapy–systematic review. Radiology. 2005; 236(3):841–851

[71] Sloof GW. Response monitoring of neoadjuvant therapy using CT, EUS, and FDG-PET. Best Pract Res Clin Gastroenterol. 2006; 20(5):941–957

[72] Swisher SG, Maish M, Erasmus JJ, et al. Utility of PET, CT, and EUS to identify pathologic responders in esophageal cancer. Ann Thorac Surg. 2004; 78(4):1152–1160, discussion 1152–1160

[73] Kwee RM. Prediction of tumor response to neoadjuvant therapy in patients with esophageal cancer with use of 18F FDG PET: a systematic review. Radiology. 2010; 254(3):707–717

[74] Gillham CM, Lucey JA, Keogan M, et al. (18)FDG uptake during induction chemoradiation for oesophageal cancer fails to predict histomorphological tumour response. Br J Cancer. 2006; 95(9):1174–1179

[75] Kong FM, Frey KA, Quint LE, et al. A pilot study of [18F]fluorodeoxyglucose positron emission tomography scans during and after radiation-based therapy in patients with non small-cell lung cancer. J Clin Oncol. 2007; 25(21):3116–3123

[76] Wieder HA, Brücher BL, Zimmermann F, et al. Time course of tumor metabolic activity during chemoradiotherapy of esophageal squamous cell carcinoma and response to treatment. J Clin Oncol. 2004; 22(5):900–908

[77] Erasmus JJ, Munden RF, Truong MT, et al. Preoperative chemo-radiation-induced ulceration in patients with esophageal cancer: a confounding factor in tumor response assessment in integrated computed tomographic-positron emission tomographic imaging. J Thorac Oncol. 2006; 1(5):478–486

[78] Rollins KE, Lucas E, Tewari N, James E, Hughes S, Catton JA. PET-CT offers accurate assessment of tumour length in oesophageal malignancy. Eur J Radiol. 2015; 84(2):195–200

[79] Muijs CT, Beukema JC, Pruim J, et al. A systematic review on the role of FDG-PET/CT in tumour delineation and radiotherapy planning in patients with esophageal cancer. Radiother Oncol. 2010; 97(2):165–171

[80] Kalkmann J, Zeile M, Antoch G, et al. German GIST Imaging Working Group. Consensus report on the radiological management of patients with gastrointestinal stromal tumours (GIST): recommendations of the German GIST Imaging Working Group. Cancer Imaging. 2012; 12:126–135

[81] Choi H, Charnsangavej C, de Castro Faria S, et al. CT evaluation of the response of gastrointestinal stromal tumors after imatinib mesylate treatment: a quantitative analysis correlated with FDG PET findings. AJR Am J Roentgenol. 2004; 183(6):1619–1628

[82] Goldstein D, Tan BS, Rossleigh M, Haindl W, Walker B, Dixon J. Gastrointestinal stromal tumours: correlation of F-FDG gamma camera-based coincidence positron emission tomography with CT for the assessment of treatment response–an AGITG study. Oncology. 2005; 69(4):326–332

[83] Goerres GW, Stupp R, Barghouth G, et al. The value of PET, CT and in-line PET/CT in patients with gastrointestinal stromal tumours: long-term outcome of treatment with imatinib mesylate. Eur J Nucl Med Mol Imaging. 2005; 32(2):153–162

[84] Kamiyama Y, Aihara R, Nakabayashi T, et al. 18F-fluorodeoxyglucose positron emission tomography: useful technique for predicting malignant potential of gastrointestinal stromal tumors. World J Surg. 2005; 29(11):1429–1435

[85] Yoshikawa K, Shimada M, Kurita N, et al. Efficacy of PET-CT for predicting the malignant potential of gastrointestinal stromal tumors. Surg Today. 2013; 43(10):1162–1167

[86] Tokumoto N, Tanabe K, Misumi T, Fujikuni N, Suzuki T, Ohdan H. The usefulness of preoperative 18FDG positron-emission tomography and computed tomography for predicting the malignant potential of gastrointestinal stromal tumors. Dig Surg. 2014; 31(2):79–86

[87] Boonsirikamchai P, Podoloff DA, Choi H. Imaging of gastrointestinal stromal tumors and assessment of benefit from systemic therapy. Hematol Oncol Clin North Am. 2009; 23(1):35–48, vii

[88] Blay JY, Bonvalot S, Casali P, et al. GIST Consensus Meeting Panelists. Consensus meeting for the management of gastrointestinal stromal tumors. Report of the GIST Consensus Conference of 20–21 March 2004, under the auspices of ESMO. Ann Oncol. 2005; 16(4):566–578

[89] Schuetze SM. Utility of positron emission tomography in sarcomas. Curr Opin Oncol. 2006; 18(4):369–373

[90] Tirumani SH, Jagannathan JP, Hornick JL, Ramaiya NH. Resistance to treatment in gastrointestinal stromal tumours: what radiologists should know. Clin Radiol. 2013; 68(8):e429–e437

[91] Hassanzadeh-Rad A, Yousefifard M, Katal S, et al. The value of (18) F-fluorodeoxyglucose positron emission tomography for prediction of treatment response in gastrointestinal stromal tumors: a systematic review and meta-analysis. J Gastroenterol Hepatol. 2016; 31(5):929–935

[92] Choi H, Charnsangavej C, Faria SC, et al. Correlation of computed tomography and positron emission tomography in patients with metastatic gastrointestinal stromal tumor treated at a single institution with imatinib mesylate: proposal of new computed tomography response criteria. J Clin Oncol. 2007; 25(13):1753–1759

[93] Shankar S, vanSonnenberg E, Desai J, Dipiro PJ, Van Den Abbeele A, Demetri GD. Gastrointestinal stromal tumor: new nodule-within-a-mass pattern of recurrence after partial response to imatinib mesylate. Radiology. 2005; 235(3):892–898

[94] Van den Abbeele AD. The lessons of GIST–PET and PET/CT: a new paradigm for imaging. Oncologist. 2008; 13 Suppl 2:8–13

19 Lymphoma

Eugene C. Lin

19.1 Staging

1. Positron emission tomography/computed tomography (PET/CT) is a standard modality for staging both Hodgkin's disease (HD) (▶ Fig. 19.1) and non-Hodgkin's lymphoma (NHL) (▶ Fig. 19.2, ▶ Fig. 19.3, ▶ Fig. 19.4). The Lugano classification[1] recommends PET/CT for routine staging of 18F-fluorodeoxyglucose (FDG)-avid nodal lymphomas (essentially all histologies except chronic lymphocytic leukemia/small lymphocytic lymphoma, lymphoplasmacytic lymphoma/Waldenström's macroglobulinemia, mycosis fungoides, and marginal zone NHLs).

2. **HD.** National Comprehensive Cancer Network (NCCN) guidelines[2] recommend baseline PET/CT as an essential test in HD. In HD, PET/CT can be of value in any stage, but it is most useful in stage I and II diseases where a change in stage will alter disease management. The use of PET/CT at diagnosis upstages 13 to 24% more patients than CT, with a small percentage downstaged. Patient management is changed in 7 to 15% of cases, when patients are upstaged from early-stage to advanced-stage disease.[3,4,5,6] The staging study can also serve as a baseline for comparison with posttherapy studies.

3. **NHL.** NCCN guidelines[7] recommend baseline PET/CT as an essential test in diffuse large B-cell (DLBCL) lymphoma and AIDS-related B-cell lymphoma and as a useful test in selected cases of many other NHL subtypes. In NHL, PET/CT can be of value in any stage, but it is most useful in staging aggressive disease. Clinical stage is modified in 15 to 20% of patients, and treatment is changed in 8%.[7] Upstaging occurs more often than downstaging.[8] Management change after upstaging is most common in follicular lymphoma with limited disease on CT.[8] In a meta-analysis,[9] the pooled summary proportion of patients with follicular lymphoma upstaged by PET compared to CT was 18.7%, but in one report,[10] the impact of PET in patients with follicular lymphoma was highest in patients with limited stage, with PET upstaging 62% of patients with limited disease. Staging PET/CT is also necessary as a baseline test if PET/CT is to be used to monitor response to treatment.

19.1.1 Accuracy

1. **PET: Sensitivity of 90%, specificity of 91%.**[11]
   a) HD: Sensitivity of 93%, specificity of 88%.
   b) NHL: Sensitivity of 87%, specificity of 94%.
2. **PET/CT:** Improved staging accuracy by 9%.[12]
3. **Histological subtype.** PET/CT has variable sensitivity depending on histological subtype of lymphoma.[13] In general, PET/CT has high sensitivity in the three major classes of this malignancy in clinical practice—diffuse large B cell and follicular lymphomas, and HD.

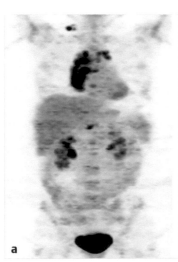
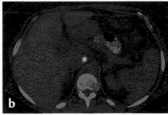
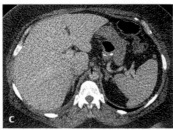

Fig. 19.1 Hodgkin's disease staging. **(a)** MIP PET demonstrates increased uptake in right neck and mediastinal nodes, and a single upper abdominal node. **(b)** Axial PET/CT demonstrates increased uptake in a small gastrohepatic ligament node. **(c)** Axial CT demonstrates a subcentimeter node (*arrow*) which would not be identified as abnormal by CT size criteria.

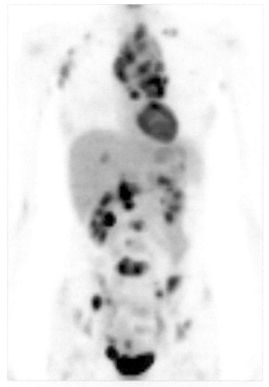

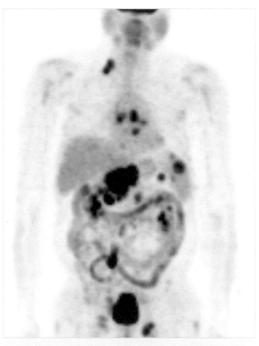

Fig. 19.2 Extensive lymphoma. Coronal PET scan in an NHL patient demonstrates uptake in mediastinal, supraclavicular, axillary, and retroperitoneal nodes, liver, and bone marrow (pelvis and lumbar spine).

Fig. 19.3 Extensive lymphoma. Coronal PET scan in an NHL patient demonstrates uptake in mediastinal, supraclavicular, abdominal, pelvic, and groin nodes and the spleen.

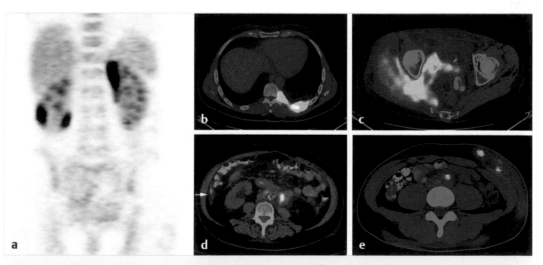

Fig. 19.4 Lymphoma: spectrum of disease. PET and PET/CT scans in different patients with NHL demonstrate disease involving the perirenal space (a), pleura (b), muscle (c), and peritoneum (arrow) (d), subcutaneous fat and retroperitoneal nodes (e). (Continued)

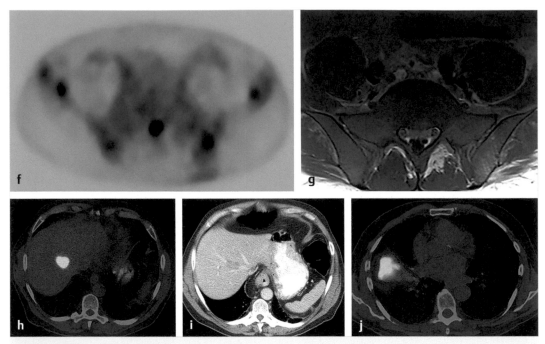

Fig. 19.4 (*continued*) PET and PET/CT scans in different patients with NHL demonstrate disease involving the bone and spinal canal (**f,g**), liver (**h,i**), and lung (**j**).

a) *HD.* The different histological subtypes of HD all have substantial FDG uptake, although the difference in degree of uptake is significant among the subtypes. Mixed cellularity has the most uptake, followed by nodular sclerosis and nodular lymphocytic predominant type.[14] However, the FDG uptake in the least FDG-avid subtype (lymphocytic predominance) is still very high.

b) **NHL.** Most indolent lymphomas have low FDG avidity; however, the sensitivity in follicular lymphoma is high.[15] The higher grade lymphomas are in general more FDG avid, but sensitivity in peripheral T-cell lymphoma is moderate.[13] Patients with NHL and SUV > 10 have a high likelihood of aggressive disease.[16]
DLBCL, follicular, Burkitt, and mantle cell lymphomas routinely have high FDG avidity.[17] DLBCL usually has the highest degree of FDG avidity.
Marginal zone lymphomas (MZLs), chronic lymphocytic leukemia/small lymphocytic lymphomas, and lymphoblastic lymphomas typically have limited FDG avidity.

FDG avidity is variable in the NHLs of T-cell origin. The aggressive nodal subtypes including peripheral T-cell and anaplastic large cell lymphoma typically have higher degrees of FDG avidity.

• *Follicular lymphoma.* PET/CT is accurate in both indolent and aggressive nodal follicular lymphoma.[18] Low-grade follicular lymphomas of the gastrointestinal tract usually have substantial FDG uptake,[19] but the degree of uptake is still less than that in high-grade NHL. However, sensitivity for bone marrow involvement in follicular lymphoma may be limited.[20]

• *MZL.* PET/CT has good sensitivity for nodal MZL but has poor sensitivity for extranodal MZL (in particular, splenic MZL).[21,22]

• *Mucosa-associated lymphoid tissue (MALT) lymphoma.* PET/CT has variable sensitivity for extranodal MZL of MALT type (MALT lymphoma). The sensitivity in patients with advanced disease is much higher than that in early-stage disease.[23] The sensitivity of PET/CT in typical MALT lymphomas is low, but MALT lymphomas with plasmacytic features usually have substantial FDG uptake.[24] MALT lymphomas of the gastrointestinal tract typically have low FDG uptake.[19]

Peripheral T-cell lymphoma. PET/CT has high sensitivity at nodal and noncutaneous nodal sites, but poor sensitivity at cutaneous sites[25] and for bone marrow involvement.[26] FDG uptake in cutaneous T-cell lymphoma is much more likely in stage IV disease.[27]

4. **Anatomic region.** PET/CT is more sensitive in the thorax than in the abdomen/pelvis.[28]

5. **Bone marrow involvement.** PET/CT can potentially replace bone marrow biopsy (BMB) in newly diagnosed HD and DLBCL. PET/CT and BMB have similar high specificity and positive predictive value (PPV), but PET/CT has significantly better sensitivity, negative predictive value (NPV), and accuracy.[29] PET/CT is able to detect sites of bone marrow involvement not sampled with iliac crest biopsy. The sensitivity is higher in HD and high-grade NHL, particularly DLBCL.

The Lugano classification[30] indicates that if PET/CT is performed in HD, a BMB is not necessary. A BMB is only needed for DLBCL if PET is negative and identifying a discordant histology is relevant in patient management. PET/CT can miss low-volume involvement (typically < 20% of the marrow) or coexistent low-grade lymphoma in DLBCL. However, in several studies, no patients with DLBCL staged by PET/CT were changed to advanced stage based on BMB alone, similar to HD. In addition, neither low-volume disease nor indolent NHL in the marrow have been shown to affect outcome.[31] Information from staging PET and BMB can be combined to optimize outcome prediction in patients with DLBCL. In one report,[32] only the combination of a positive PET and marrow biopsy conferred a poor prognosis compared to patients with no marrow involvement. Patients with only a positive PET or a positive marrow biopsy did not have a worse outcome. This suggests that DLBCL patients with normal marrow on staging PET will not gain additional prognostic information from a marrow biopsy, but a marrow biopsy may provide prognostic information if the marrow is abnormal on staging PET. A BMB remains the standard test for staging lymphomas other than HD and DLBCL.

a) *PET/CT for HD*: Sensitivity of 97%, specificity of 100%.[33]

b) *PET/CT for DLBCL*: Sensitivity of 89%, specificity of 100%.[34]

c) *PET and PET/CT for aggressive NHL*: Sensitivity of 74%, specificity of 84%.[35]

d) *PET and PET/CT for indolent NHL*: Sensitivity of 46%, specificity of 93%.[35]

6. **Splenic disease.** PET/CT is 97% accurate for the diagnosis of splenic involvement in HD.[36] The degree of splenic uptake in NHL depends on the subtype, with DLBCL having the highest uptake.[37]

a) Possible methods to the diagnosis of abnormal splenic uptake include uptake greater than that of the liver[36] or SUV > 4.[37] However, splenic uptake with DLBCL involvement often has a SUV > 20.

b) PET/CT is more accurate for detecting focal splenic involvement than gallium or CT.

19.1.2 Comparison to Other Modalities

1. **PET versus CT.** PET and CT have comparable specificity, but PET is approximately 15% more sensitive.[28]

a) The primary advantage of PET over CT is in nodal detection in the thorax and periphery; in the abdomen and pelvis, PET and CT provide comparable results.[38,39]

b) PET and CT are concordant in staging 80 to 90% of patients with DLBCL and follicular lymphoma. In contrast, PET and CT are less likely to be concordant in staging HD (60–80%).[40] In both cases, PET discordance usually results in upstaging. However, the higher rate of discordance in HD suggests that both PET and CT need to be performed in staging HD.

2. **PET/CT versus CT.** PET/CT (with low-dose nonenhanced CT) is more sensitive and specific than contrast-enhanced CT for both nodal and extranodal disease.

a) PET/CT is particularly valuable compared to CT in the exclusion of disease.
   • A common problem with CT is false-positive results from lung opacities interpreted as lymphoma; these can be accurately diagnosed by PET.

b) *Nodal disease* (▸ Table 19.1).

Table 19.1 Sensitivity and specificity of PET/CT versus CT in the detection of nodal disease

	Sensitivity %	Specificity %
PET/CT	94	100
CT	88	86

c) **Extranodal disease** (▶ Table 19.2).

Table 19.2 Sensitivity and specificity of PET/CT versus CT in the detection of extranodal disease

	Sensitivity %	Specificity %
PET/CT	88	100
CT	50	90

3. **PET versus gallium**. PET is superior to gallium for both initial staging and follow-up of lymphoma.[41]

19.1.3 Pearls/Pitfalls

1. **Thymus.** It is important to recognize thymic hyperplasia as a distinct entity in patients with anterior mediastinal uptake. Thymic hyperplasia (▶ Fig. 7.20; ▶ Fig. 7.21) is a common reaction following chemotherapy and as such is an expected phenomenon.
2. **Diffuse bone marrow activity.** Diffuse bone marrow uptake can be noted in a variety of nonneoplastic etiologies including myeloid hyperplasia post–granulocyte colony-stimulating factor (G-CSF) therapy (▶ Fig. 7.37). Diffuse marrow uptake should generally not be interpreted as lymphomatous involvement, but it can obscure lymphomatous bone marrow infiltration.
3. **Focal bone marrow activity.** Always consider a history of prior BMB as a cause of focal uptake in the posterior ilium. The most common pattern of bone marrow involvement in HD is multifocal, with at least one focus in the pelvis or vertebrae, and no corresponding CT lesions.[42]
4. **Spleen:**
   a) Splenic uptake post G-CSF therapy can mimic splenic involvement (▶ Fig. 7.37).
   b) The spleen is a common site for false-positive findings from infectious/inflammatory etiologies.
5. **Low-grade lymphomas.** Certain low-grade lymphomas such as small-cell lymphocytic lymphoma typically do not have substantial FDG uptake and may not be detected with high sensitivity by PET. In these cases, a positive scan often demonstrates hazy mild uptake.

19.2 Therapy Response

The predictive value of PET depends on the type of disease before therapy. HD, particularly in its early stages, usually has a higher response rate than NHL, and thus will have a lower pretest probability of residual disease following therapy. Thus, a negative PET in early stages of HD is predictive of a complete response, but a positive PET has fairly high false-positive rates. The opposite is true of advanced stage HD and NHL which has a higher pretest probability of residual disease following therapy. In these cases, a negative PET does not exclude minimal residual disease, but a positive PET is predictive of treatment failure.

While the bulk of the tumor in NHL is composed of malignant cells, the bulk of the tumor in HD is a benign inflammatory infiltrate. FDG uptake in HD may originate from this inflammatory component as well as the malignant cells.[43] In addition, patients with HD often receive radiation which may also result in inflammatory changes. Along with the lower pretest probability of residual disease in HD, these factors may account for the lower PPV of PET in HD compared to NHL. However, the PPV of PET in HD is still substantially higher than that of CT.

19.3 Hodgkin's Disease

Interim PET/CT: The prognostic value of interim PET/CT is clearly established for advanced disease, and is superior to traditional risk stratification based on clinical and laboratory evaluations.[6] However, it is currently unclear whether interim PET results can be used to safely change therapy, as it is not certain that alternative therapies will have a result that is better or even as good. NCCN guidelines[2] indicate that guiding therapy based on the results of interim PET/CT is investigational and not recommended outside the context of clinical trials.

The majority of studies have evaluated interim PET after two cycles of therapy. However, the prognostic value of interim PET may be comparable after four cycles.[44]

1. **Stage IA–IIA (favorable disease).** The role of interim PET in limited-stage HD is less clear than in advanced stage HD, as relapses occur in only 20 to 30% of patients with limited stage HD who are interim PET positive.[1] As most patients with limited-stage disease can be cured, the potential value of PET/CT would primarily lie in reducing treatment toxicity (e.g., elimination of radiation and abbreviation of therapy cycles in patients with a good early PET response). Although initial studies did not demonstrate a

prognostic significance for interim PET in stage I–II favorable diseases, more recent studies have suggested that interim PET based on the Deauville criteria is a good prognostic indicator in this setting.[45,46] PET/CT has a lower PPV in earlier stage disease[47] compared to more advanced stages, due to the inherently better prognosis and efficacy of combined chemoradiotherapy. While the PPVs are already lower in limited-stage HD, the presence of a bulky mass further lowers PPV. Overall, there is a high NPV and a moderate and variable PPV for interim PET/CT in this setting.[48]

The role of PET-adapted therapy in early-stage HD is under active investigation. It is still uncertain whether PET/CT can be used to select patients with early-stage HD who can be treated without radiation. In a randomized controlled trial,[49] patients with newly diagnosed stage IA or IIA HD received three cycles of chemotherapy with doxorubicin, bleomycin, vinblastine, and dacarbazine (ABVD) and underwent PET scanning. Patients with negative PET findings were randomly assigned to receive involved-field radiotherapy or no further treatment. Patient with positive PET findings received a fourth cycle of ABVD and radiotherapy. Although this study did not show noninferiority of the strategy of no further treatment with regard to progression-free survival, patients with negative PET findings had a very good prognosis with or without radiotherapy, suggesting that radiotherapy might be avoided in patients with a negative PET. In a meta-analysis,[47,50] progression-free survival was decreased in the PET-adapted treatment arm (without radiotherapy) in early-stage HL patients. However, although radiotherapy after initial chemotherapy may marginally improve the progression-free survival rate, the downside is irradiating all patients with negative PET findings, most of who have already been cured.

2. **Stage I–II (unfavorable disease) and stages III–IV.** The general aim of PET response-adapted therapy in this population is deescalate therapy for those patients with a good early PET response, or escalate therapy in poor PET responders, depending on initial treatment regimen. For example, a more intense initial treatment regimen (escalated bleomycin, etoposide, doxorubicin, cyclophosphamide, vincristine, procarbazine, prednisone (BEACOPP) could be continued with positive PET results, or deescalated with negative PET

results. Advanced stage HD patients treated with ABVD with negative interim PET have had 2-year progression-free survival rates of approximately 95% in retrospective series[47]; however, in several prospective series, the progression-free survival was approximately 85%.[51] Patients with positive PET scans have had progression-free survival rates of 0 to 53%, with poorer outcomes in advanced disease.[52] However, although the prognostic value of interim PET in advanced stage HD is clearly established, further trials are necessary before PET can be used to safely deescalate or escalate therapy.

In a randomized controlled trial,[51] patients with newly diagnosed advanced classic HD received two cycles of ABVD, with baseline and interim PET/CT. Patients with negative interim PET findings were randomly assigned to continue ABVD or omit bleomycin. Patients with positive PET findings received BEACOPP. Although the results fell just short of the specified noninferiority margin, the omission of bleomycin from ABVD after negative interim PET findings resulted in a lower incidence of pulmonary toxicity without significantly lower efficacy. Escalation of therapy in patients with a positive interim PET/CT resulted in a 3-year progression-free survival of 67.5%, similar to another trial of escalated therapy in interim PET/CT-positive patients where the 2-year progression-free survival was 64%.[53] Although the precise effect of escalation is uncertain due to lack of randomized comparisons, these survival rates are substantially superior to retrospective series without escalation.

Final response assessment.[6] British guidelines[54] recommend end-of-treatment PET/CT for all patients who have not achieved an interim PET-negative remission, as this may affect radiotherapy planning, biopsy considerations, and follow-up strategy. NCCN guidelines[2] recommend PET/CT for the evaluation of residual masses at the end of treatment (▶ Fig. 19.5).

Revised response criteria[55] for lymphoma include metabolic complete response, which allows for residual masses as long as they are not FDG avid. Due to the high NPV, radiotherapy could potentially be omitted in advanced stage patients with a residual mass but a negative end-of-treatment PET/CT.[47,56] British guidelines[54] indicate that patients treated with escalated BEACOPP who achieve an end-of-treatment PET-negative remission do not need consolidation radiotherapy to

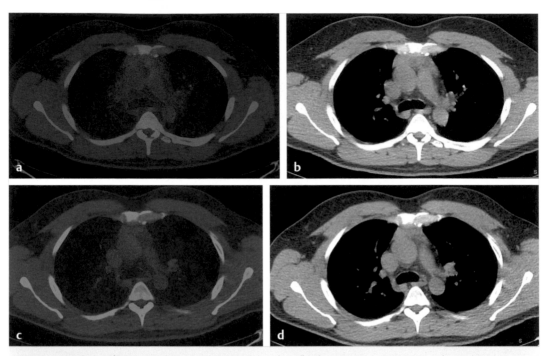

Fig. 19.5 Lymphoma therapy response. Axial PET/CT (**a**) and CT (**b**) demonstrate an anterior mediastinal mass in a patient with Hodgkin's disease posttherapy. This has uptake greater than the liver and should be interpreted as residual disease. After further therapy (**c**), the degree of FDG uptake is equal to the mediastinum and the mass is smaller on CT (**d**). This can be interpreted as a complete metabolic response.

residual tissue. In patients treated with ABVD, it is unclear whether radiotherapy can be safely omitted if there is residual PET-negative tissue of > 1.5 cm on CT.

While some reports suggest improved outcomes when a complete metabolic response is accompanied by a complete radiological response, other reports suggest that outcomes are not affected by the presence of a residual mass.[8] In a meta-analysis,[57] the disease relapse rate in HD patients with a PET-negative residual mass after first-line therapy was 6.8%, and there was no definite worse outcome than a metabolic complete response without a residual mass.

19.4 Diffuse Large B-Cell Lymphoma

Interim PET. Currently, there is less evidence for the value of interim PET in diffuse large-B cell lymphoma than in HD. For example, a European Society for Medical Oncology consensus conference[58]

indicated the results of interim PET may be applied in individual patients with early or advanced HD. However, the routine clinical use of interim PET was not recommended in patients with DLBCL due to the lack of therapeutic consequences. In a systematic review,[59] two studies reported interim PET to have independent prognostic value in predicting treatment failure in addition to the International Prognostic Index (IPI), while three studies did not. In one report,[60] a single interim PET scan could not differentiate chemoresistant lymphoma from complete response, as more than half of interim PET-positive patients became PET negative by the end of therapy and most slow responders had durable remissions. In a prospective study,[61] patients with any stage of DLBCL were treated with R-CHOP (rituximab, cyclophosphamide, doxorubicin, vincristine, and prednisone) with baseline, interim, and end-of-treatment PET/CT. Although 2-year event-free survival was significantly shorter for PET-positive compared to PET-negative patients (48 vs. 74%), overall survival did not differ. The NPV of interim PET/CT for 2-year event-free survival was 73% and the PPV was 59%, which was inferior to prognostic value of interim PET/CT in HD. The PPV of interim PET has been much more variable than the NPV, ranging from 18 to 74%, compared to a NPV of 73 to 86%. It has been suggested that this may be secondary to improved outcomes with rituximab, or more false-positive results with immunotherapy. End-of-treatment PET is likely a better predictor.[8]

Although interim PET/CT may have some prognostic value in DLBCL (less than in HD), studies which have examined change or escalation in therapy on the basis of interim PET/CT have not shown any benefit.[31]

Final response assessment. In R-CHOP-treated patients, progression-free survival ranges from 24 to 35% in patients with positive end-of-treatment PET.[31] In a meta-analysis[62] of R-CHOP-treated patients, the disease relapse rate in patients with a complete remission on end-of-treatment PET was 7 to 20% with a weighted summary proportion of 13.7%. However, patients who are at high risk by standard prognostic indices (such as the NCCN-IPI) may still be at high risk of relapse irrespective of a complete metabolic response.[31]

19.5 Follicular Lymphoma

Numerous studies have demonstrated that end-of-treatment PET/CT is predictive of progression-free survival, independent of the follicular lymphoma IPI, and is superior to CT assessment for this purpose. Interim PET is also predictive, but less so than end-of-treatment PET.[31]

19.5.1 Accuracy/Comparison to Other Modalities

1. **Interim PET in HD** (meta-analysis)[9]: Sensitivity of 71%, specificity of 90%.
2. **Interim PET/CT in DLBCL treated with R-CHOP** (meta-analysis)[63]: Sensitivity of 52%, specificity of 68%.
3. **Final response assessment in HD:** NPV of 94 to 100%, PPV of 91 to 92%.[52]
4. **Final response assessment in aggressive NHL:** NPV of 90 to 100%, PPV of 50 to 82%.[52]
5. **CT**. CT has a low PPV, as it is usually not possible to distinguish between viable tumor and necrosis or fibrosis in patients with residual masses identified on CT. The NPV of CT is similar to PET, but the PPV is substantially higher, resulting in a higher accuracy of PET (85%) compared to CT (40%).[64]

6. **Bone scintigraphy**. PET has fewer false-positive results than bone scintigraphy. In particular, PET can often accurately evaluate response in bone lesions when bone scintigraphy is false positive.

19.5.2 Pearls

1. End-of-therapy evaluation should not be omitted with negative interim PET, as negative interim PET can convert to positive in around 4% of patients.[65]
2. Interim PET should be performed at least 2, and preferably 3, weeks after the initiation of therapy, or 4 to 5 days before the start of the subsequent treatment cycle.[48]
3. In the Lugano classification,[30] a complete metabolic response with a persistent mass is considered a complete remission.
4. The Deauville criteria can be adapted for the role of interim PET. For example, if therapy escalation is being considered, a high cutoff such as liver uptake can be used to increase PPV and avoid overtreatment. If therapy de-escalation is being considered, a lower cutoff such as mediastinal blood pool can be used to increase NPV and minimize the risk of undertreatment. Most patients with uptake higher than mediastinum, but less than or equal to the liver (score of 3), have a good prognosis at the end of therapy of HD, DLBCL, and follicular lymphoma.[30] However, there are some settings in which a score of 3 could be considered an inadequate response to avoid undertreatment. For example, a more cautious approach might be preferred in response-adapted trails with possible treatment de-escalation.
5. British guidelines[54] state that while an end-of-treatment Deauville score of 4 or 5 likely represents an inadequate response, biopsy is recommended to exclude false-positive uptake, as a positive result is less reliable because false positives can occur from infection/inflammation and reactive changes after treatment.
6. In the Deauville classification, the terms moderately (score 4) and marked (score 5) were not initially defined, but it has been suggested that score 4 be applied to uptake > SUVmax in a large region of normal liver, and score 5 to uptake two to three times > SUVmax.[8]

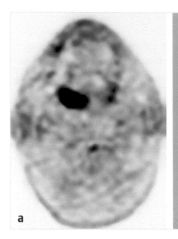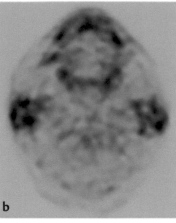

Fig. 19.6 Metabolic complete response. **(a)** Axial PET scan in a patient with diffuse large B-cell lymphoma demonstrates increased uptake in the right tonsil. **(b)** A follow-up axial PET scan after therapy demonstrates decreased and symmetric tonsillar uptake. Although the Deauville criteria cannot be applied as physiological tonsillar uptake may be greater than mediastinal or liver uptake, a metabolic complete response can be inferred if the uptake is no greater than the surrounding normal tissues.

7. The Deauville criteria may not be applicable if physiological uptake (e.g., in Waldeyer's ring) or high uptake secondary to marrow or splenic activation results in uptake greater than mediastinum or liver. In these cases, a complete metabolic response can be inferred if the uptake at sites of initial involvement is no greater than surrounding normal tissues.[8]

8. Some caution should be exercised when using liver activity to aid in interpretation as several studies demonstrate that liver SUVmean and SUVmax can change during chemotherapy.[66,67,68] In particular, the liver SUV can increase between the baseline and subsequent studies. In contrast, the mediastinal blood pool activity remains stable during chemotherapy.

9. Although the Deauville criteria are valid for assessing the prognostic value in interim PET/CT in DLBCL, a 66% change in SUVmax cutoff had better prognostic value and interobserver reproducibility in one report.[69]

10. **Baseline pretreatment scan:**

    a) If the disease seen on the pretreatment PET scan is not active, FDG PET should not be used for therapy monitoring. False-negative results will increase if baseline PET scans are not obtained on a routine basis.

    b) Acquiring baseline scans will also decrease false-positive results. As relapses typically occur in the region of previous disease seen on the baseline study, abnormalities on follow-up PET scans outside areas of previous disease should be interpreted with caution (e.g., inflammatory etiologies should be considered).

    c) Baseline scans are helpful but not mandatory in patients with subtypes of lymphomas which are routinely FDG avid, such as HD and diffuse B-cell lymphoma. Baseline scans are mandatory in patients with subtypes of lymphoma with variable FDG avidity, such as MALT lymphomas.[55]

11. **Immunomodulatory agents.** Patients treated with immunomodulatory agents, such as immune checkpoint inhibitors, may have atypical responses to therapy (▶ Fig. 19.6). For example, treatment with the monoclonal antibody rituximab as part of the R-CHOP regimen in DLBCL can cause an inflammatory "flare" response and false-positive findings on interim PET/CT studies.[70] A refinement of the Lugano classification lymphoma response criteria for these patients has been proposed,[1] with the introduction of the term "indeterminate response" to identify lesions with potential atypical response until confirmed as flare/pseudoprogression or true progressive disease by biopsy or subsequent imaging. For FDG PET/CT, an indeterminate response is an increase in FDG uptake of one or lesions with a concomitant increase in lesion size or number. These patients are not considered to have progressive disease unless there is evidence of progressive disease by an increase in lesions size or development of new lesions. If a patient initially classified as having an indeterminate response is later identified as having true progressive disease, the initial designation of indeterminate response is changed to progressive disease.

12. **False-positive findings:**
    a) In younger patients, rebound thymic hyperplasia is a potential source of false-positive results.
    b) Posttreatment uptake outside the sites of initial disease may present false-positive findings.
    c) Infectious etiologies should always be considered in immunocompromised patients.
13. **Postradiotherapy.** In general, PET imaging early after radiotherapy is not recommended. However, if patients are scanned early after radiotherapy for lymphoma, typical findings are mild and nonfocal uptake in the radiation field, which is usually distinguishable from sites with malignancy.[71]

19.6 Pretransplantation

High-dose chemotherapy and autologous stem cell transplantation (HDT and ASCT) are employed in patients who relapse from NHL or HD after conventional chemotherapy. However, patients must remain chemosensitive. Numerous studies have shown that PET/CT has prognostic value in patients with relapsed or refractory HD or DLBCL after salvage chemotherapy and before HCT and ASCT, and is superior to CT for this purpose.[8] In one report, patients who achieved a Deauville response of 1 to 3 after salvage chemotherapy had a 3-year progression-free and overall survival of 77 and 86%, respectively, compared to 49 and 54% for patients achieving Deauville 4. No other pre-HDT/ASCT risk factor significantly impacted survival. The risk of treatment failure is further increased if the PET is still positive after ASCT.[72]

However, not all patients with a positive PET after salvage chemotherapy will relapse, and often there are few therapeutic options besides HCT and ASCT. Thus, a positive PET scan after salvage chemotherapy should not exclude patients from transplantation, but modified approaches including HCT and ASCT or experimental therapies might be considered. Serial PET scans prior to transplantation may predict outcome better than a single scan.[73]

19.6.1 Pearls

1. Superior PPVs are obtained if PET is performed just prior to transplantation compared to early during salvage therapy.[27] After salvage therapy, resistant clones will become apparent when disease sites with sensitive histologies are destroyed.
2. The prognostic value of PET is higher prior to transplantation than after transplantation, because glucose metabolism may be transiently decreased after intense therapy.
3. Patients with negative PET studies prior to ASCT can be managed without post-ASCT PET imaging.[72]

19.6.2 Accuracy

Predicting treatment failure in refractory/relapsed aggressive NHL (meta-analysis): Sensitivity of 68%, specificity of 72%.[74]

19.7 Relapse

Limited data suggest that PET may be useful in the detection of subclinical relapse in both HD and NHL.

References

[1] Cheson BD, Kostakoglu L. FDG-PET for early response assessment in lymphomas; Part 1-Hodgkin lymphoma. Oncology (Williston Park). 2017; 31(1):45–49
[2] Hoppe RT, Advani RH, Ai WZ, et al. NCCN Hodgkin Lymphoma. Hodgkin lymphoma. J Natl Compr Canc Netw. 2011; 9 (9):1020–1058
[3] Cerci JJ, Trindade E, Buccheri V, et al. Consistency of FDG-PET accuracy and cost-effectiveness in initial staging of patients with Hodgkin lymphoma across jurisdictions. Clin Lymphoma Myeloma Leuk. 2011; 11(4):314–320
[4] Hutchings M, Loft A, Hansen M, et al. Position emission tomography with or without computed tomography in the primary staging of Hodgkin's lymphoma. Haematologica. 2006; 91(4):482–489
[5] Rigacci L, Vitolo U, Nassi L, et al. Intergruppo Italiano Linfomi. Positron emission tomography in the staging of patients with Hodgkin's lymphoma. A prospective multicentric study by the Intergruppo Italiano Linfomi. Ann Hematol. 2007; 86(12): 897–903
[6] Townsend W, Linch D. Hodgkin's lymphoma in adults. Lancet. 2012; 380(9844):836–847
[7] Zelenetz AD, Abramson JS, Advani RH, et al. NCCN Clinical Practice Guidelines in Oncology: non-Hodgkin's lymphomas. J Natl Compr Canc Netw. 2010; 8(3):288–334
[8] Barrington SF, Mikhaeel NG, Kostakoglu L, et al. Role of imaging in the staging and response assessment of lymphoma: consensus of the International Conference on Malignant Lymphomas Imaging Working Group. J Clin Oncol. 2014; 32 (27):3048–3058
[9] Adams HJ, Nievelstein RA, Kwee TC. Systematic review on the additional value of 18F-fluoro-2-deoxy-D-glucose positron emission tomography in staging follicular lymphoma. J Comput Assist Tomogr. 2017; 41(1):98–103
[10] Luminari S, Biasoli I, Arcaini L, et al. The use of FDG-PET in the initial staging of 142 patients with follicular lymphoma: a retrospective study from the FOLL05 randomized trial of the

Fondazione Italiana Linfomi. Ann Oncol. 2013; 24(8):2108–2112

[11] Isasi CR, Lu P, Blaufox MD. A metaanalysis of 18F-2-deoxy-2-fluoro-D-glucose positron emission tomography in the staging and restaging of patients with lymphoma. Cancer. 2005; 104(5):1066–1074

[12] Allen-Auerbach M, Quon A, Weber WA, et al. Comparison between 2-deoxy-2-[18F]fluoro-D-glucose positron emission tomography and positron emission tomography/computed tomography hardware fusion for staging of patients with lymphoma. Mol Imaging Biol. 2004; 6(6):411–416

[13] Elstrom R, Guan L, Baker G, et al. Utility of FDG-PET scanning in lymphoma by WHO classification. Blood. 2003; 101(10):3875–3876

[14] Hutchings M, Loft A, Hansen M, Ralfkiaer E, Specht L. Different histopathological subtypes of Hodgkin lymphoma show significantly different levels of FDG uptake. Hematol Oncol. 2006; 24(3):146–150

[15] Karam M, Novak L, Cyriac J, Ali A, Nazeer T, Nugent F. Role of fluorine-18 fluoro-deoxyglucose positron emission tomography scan in the evaluation and follow-up of patients with low-grade lymphomas. Cancer. 2006; 107(1):175–183

[16] Schöder H, Noy A, Gönen M, et al. Intensity of 18fluorodeoxyglucose uptake in positron emission tomography distinguishes between indolent and aggressive non-Hodgkin's lymphoma. J Clin Oncol. 2005; 23(21):4643–4651

[17] Kostakoglu L, Cheson BD. State-of-the-art research on "lymphomas: role of molecular imaging for staging, prognostic evaluation, and treatment response". Front Oncol. 2013; 3:212

[18] Wöhrer S, Jaeger U, Kletter K, et al. 18F-fluoro-deoxy-glucose positron emission tomography (18F-FDG-PET) visualizes follicular lymphoma irrespective of grading. Ann Oncol. 2006; 17(5):780–784

[19] Phongkitkarun S, Varavithya V, Kazama T, et al. Lymphomatous involvement of gastrointestinal tract: evaluation by positron emission tomography with (18)F-fluorodeoxyglucose. World J Gastroenterol. 2005; 11(46):7284–7289

[20] Fuster D, Chiang S, Andreadis C, et al. Can [18F]fluorodeoxyglucose positron emission tomography imaging complement biopsy results from the iliac crest for the detection of bone marrow involvement in patients with malignant lymphoma? Nucl Med Commun. 2006; 27(1):11–15

[21] Hoffmann M, Kletter K, Becherer A, Jäger U, Chott A, Raderer M. 18F-fluorodeoxyglucose positron emission tomography (18F-FDG-PET) for staging and follow-up of marginal zone B-cell lymphoma. Oncology. 2003; 64(4):336–340

[22] Tsukamoto N, Kojima M, Hasegawa M, et al. The usefulness of (18)F-fluorodeoxyglucose positron emission tomography ((18)F-FDG-PET) and a comparison of (18)F-FDG-pet with (67)gallium scintigraphy in the evaluation of lymphoma: relation to histologic subtypes based on the World Health Organization classification. Cancer. 2007; 110(3):652–659

[23] Perry C, Herishanu Y, Metzer U, et al. Diagnostic accuracy of PET/CT in patients with extranodal marginal zone MALT lymphoma. Eur J Haematol. 2007; 79(3):205–209

[24] Hoffmann M, Wöhrer S, Becherer A, et al. 18F-Fluoro-deoxyglucose positron emission tomography in lymphoma of mucosa-associated lymphoid tissue: histology makes the difference. Ann Oncol. 2006; 17(12):1761–1765

[25] Bishu S, Quigley JM, Bishu SR, et al. Predictive value and diagnostic accuracy of F-18-fluoro-deoxy-glucose positron emission tomography treated grade 1 and 2 follicular lymphoma. Leuk Lymphoma. 2007; 48(8):1548–1555

[26] Kako S, Izutsu K, Ota Y, et al. FDG-PET in T-cell and NK-cell neoplasms. Ann Oncol. 2007; 18(10):1685–1690

[27] Kirby AM, Mikhaeel NG. The role of FDG PET in the management of lymphoma: what is the evidence base? Nucl Med Commun. 2007; 28(5):335–354

[28] Schiepers C, Filmont JE, Czernin J. PET for staging of Hodgkin's disease and non-Hodgkin's lymphoma. Eur J Nucl Med Mol Imaging. 2003; 30 Suppl 1:S82–S88

[29] Berthet L, Cochet A, Kanoun S, et al. In newly diagnosed diffuse large B-cell lymphoma, determination of bone marrow involvement with 18F-FDG PET/CT provides better diagnostic performance and prognostic stratification than does biopsy. J Nucl Med. 2013; 54(8):1244–1250

[30] Harries N, Loeppky JA, Shaheen S, et al. MESF Project. A stair-climbing test for measuring mechanical efficiency of ambulation in adults with chronic stroke. Disabil Rehabil. 2015; 37(11):1004–1008

[31] Barrington SF, Mikhaeel NG. PET scans for staging and restaging in diffuse large B-cell and follicular lymphomas. Curr Hematol Malig Rep. 2016; 11(3):185–195

[32] Cerci JJ, Györke T, Fanti S, et al. IAEA Lymphoma Study Group. Combined PET and biopsy evidence of marrow involvement improves prognostic prediction in diffuse large B-cell lymphoma. J Nucl Med. 2014; 55(10):1591–1597

[33] Adams HJ, Kwee TC, de Keizer B, et al. Systematic review and meta-analysis on the diagnostic performance of FDG-PET/CT in detecting bone marrow involvement in newly diagnosed Hodgkin lymphoma: is bone marrow biopsy still necessary? Ann Oncol. 2014; 25(5):921–927

[34] Adams HJ, Kwee TC, de Keizer B, Fijnheer R, de Klerk JM, Nievelstein RA. FDG PET/CT for the detection of bone marrow involvement in diffuse large B-cell lymphoma: systematic review and meta-analysis. Eur J Nucl Med Mol Imaging. 2014; 41(3):565–574

[35] Chen YK, Yeh CL, Tsui CC, Liang JA, Chen JH, Kao CH. F-18 FDG PET for evaluation of bone marrow involvement in non-Hodgkin lymphoma: a meta-analysis. Clin Nucl Med. 2011; 36(7):553–559

[36] Rini JN, Manalili EY, Hoffman MA, et al. F-18 FDG versus Ga-67 for detecting splenic involvement in Hodgkin's disease. Clin Nucl Med. 2002; 27(8):572–577

[37] Rutherford SC, Andemariam B, Philips SM, et al. FDG-PET in prediction of splenectomy findings in patients with known or suspected lymphoma. Leuk Lymphoma. 2008; 49(4):719–726

[38] Jerusalem G, Beguin Y, Najjar F, et al. Positron emission tomography (PET) with 18F-fluorodeoxyglucose (18F-FDG) for the staging of low-grade non-Hodgkin's lymphoma (NHL). Ann Oncol. 2001; 12(6):825–830

[39] Buchmann I, Reinhardt M, Elsner K, et al. 2-(fluorine-18)fluoro-2-deoxy-D-glucose positron emission tomography in the detection and staging of malignant lymphoma. A bicenter trial. Cancer. 2001; 91(5):889–899

[40] Seam P, Juweid ME, Cheson BD. The role of FDG-PET scans in patients with lymphoma. Blood. 2007; 110(10):3507–3516

[41] Jhanwar YS, Straus DJ. The role of PET in lymphoma. J Nucl Med. 2006; 47(8):1326–1334

[42] Weiler-Sagie M, Kagna O, Dann EJ, Ben-Barak A, Israel O. Characterizing bone marrow involvement in Hodgkin's lymphoma by FDG-PET/CT. Eur J Nucl Med Mol Imaging. 2014; 41(6):1133–1140

[43] Kasamon YL, Jones RJ, Wahl RL. Integrating PET and PET/CT into the risk-adapted therapy of lymphoma. J Nucl Med. 2007; 48 Suppl 1:19S–27S

[44] Hutchings M, Loft A, Hansen M, et al. FDG-PET after two cycles of chemotherapy predicts treatment failure and progression-free survival in Hodgkin lymphoma. Blood. 2006; 107(1):52–59

[45] Kostakoglu L, Schöder H, Johnson JL, et al. Cancer Leukemia Group B. Interim [(18)F]fluorodeoxyglucose positron emission tomography imaging in stage I-II non-bulky Hodgkin lymphoma: would using combined positron emission tomography and computed tomography criteria better predict response than each test alone? Leuk Lymphoma. 2012; 53(11): 2143-2150

[46] Zinzani PL, Rigacci L, Stefoni V, et al. Early interim 18F-FDG PET in Hodgkin's lymphoma: evaluation on 304 patients. Eur J Nucl Med Mol Imaging. 2012; 39(1):4-12

[47] Hutchings M. FDG-PET response-adapted therapy: is 18F-fluorodeoxyglucose positron emission tomography a safe predictor for a change of therapy? Hematol Oncol Clin North Am. 2014; 28(1):87-103

[48] Kostakoglu L, Gallamini A. Interim 18F-FDG PET in Hodgkin lymphoma: would PET-adapted clinical trials lead to a paradigm shift? J Nucl Med. 2013; 54(7):1082-1093

[49] Radford J, Illidge T, Counsell N, et al. Results of a trial of PET-directed therapy for early-stage Hodgkin's lymphoma. N Engl J Med. 2015; 372(17):1598-1607

[50] Sickinger MT, von Tresckow B, Kobe C, Borchmann P, Engert A, Skoetz N. PET-adapted omission of radiotherapy in early stage Hodgkin lymphoma-a systematic review and meta-analysis. Crit Rev Oncol Hematol. 2016; 101:86-92

[51] Johnson P, Federico M, Kirkwood A, et al. Adapted treatment guided by interim PET-CT scan in advanced Hodgkin's lymphoma. N Engl J Med. 2016; 374(25):2419-2429

[52] Barrington SF, Mikhaeel NG. When should FDG-PET be used in the modern management of lymphoma? Br J Haematol. 2014; 164(3):315-328

[53] Press OW, Li H, Schöder H, et al. US Intergroup Trial of Response-adapted therapy for stage III to IV Hodgkin lymphoma using early interim fluorodeoxyglucose-positron emission tomography imaging: Southwest Oncology Group S0816. J Clin Oncol. 2016; 34(17):2020-2027

[54] Follows GA, Ardeshna KM, Barrington SF, et al. British Committee for Standards in Haematology. Guidelines for the first line management of classical Hodgkin lymphoma. Br J Haematol. 2014; 166(1):34-49

[55] Juweid ME, Stroobants S, Hoekstra OS, et al. Imaging Subcommittee of International Harmonization Project in Lymphoma. Use of positron emission tomography for response assessment of lymphoma: consensus of the Imaging Subcommittee of International Harmonization Project in Lymphoma. J Clin Oncol. 2007; 25(5):571-578

[56] Kobe C, Dietlein M, Franklin J, et al. Positron emission tomography has a high negative predictive value for progression or early relapse for patients with residual disease after first-line chemotherapy in advanced-stage Hodgkin lymphoma. Blood. 2008; 112(10):3989-3994

[57] Adams HJ, Nievelstein RA, Kwee TC. Outcome of Hodgkin lymphoma patients with a posttreatment 18F-fluoro-2-deoxy-D-glucose positron emission tomography (FDG-PET)-negative residual mass: systematic review and meta-analysis. Pediatr Hematol Oncol. 2015; 32(8):515-524

[58] Ladetto M, Buske C, Hutchings M, et al. ESMO Lymphoma Consensus Conference Panel Members. ESMO consensus conference on malignant lymphoma: general perspectives and recommendations for prognostic tools in mature B-cell lymphomas and chronic lymphocytic leukaemia. Ann Oncol. 2016; 27(12):2149-2160

[59] Adams HJ, Kwee TC. Prognostic value of interim FDG-PET in R-CHOP-treated diffuse large B-cell lymphoma: systematic review and meta-analysis. Crit Rev Oncol Hematol. 2016; 106:55-63

[60] Carr R, Fanti S, Paez D, et al. IAEA Lymphoma Study Group. Prospective international cohort study demonstrates inability of interim PET to predict treatment failure in diffuse large B-cell lymphoma. J Nucl Med. 2014; 55(12):1936-1944

[61] Mamot C, Klingbiel D, Hitz F, et al. Final results of a prospective evaluation of the predictive value of interim positron emission tomography in patients with diffuse large B-cell lymphoma treated with R-CHOP-14 (SAKK 38/07). J Clin Oncol. 2015; 33(23):2523-2529

[62] Adams HJ, Nievelstein RA, Kwee TC. Prognostic value of complete remission status at end-of-treatment FDG-PET in R-CHOP-treated diffuse large B-cell lymphoma: systematic review and meta-analysis. Br J Haematol. 2015; 170(2):185-191

[63] Sun N, Zhao J, Qiao W, Wang T. Predictive value of interim PET/CT in DLBCL treated with R-CHOP: meta-analysis. BioMed Res Int. 2015; 2015:648572

[64] Juweid ME. Utility of positron emission tomography (PET) scanning in managing patients with Hodgkin lymphoma. Hematology (Am Soc Hematol Educ Program). 2006; 259-265-510-511

[65] Dann EJ. PET/CT adapted therapy in Hodgkin disease: current state of the art and future directions. Curr Oncol Rep. 2012; 14(5):403-410

[66] Boktor RR, Walker G, Stacey R, Gledhill S, Pitman AG. Reference range for intrapatient variability in blood-pool and liver SUV for 18F-FDG PET. J Nucl Med. 2013; 54(5):677-682

[67] Ceriani L, Suriano S, Ruberto T, Zucca E, Giovanella L. 18F-FDG uptake changes in liver and mediastinum during chemotherapy in patients with diffuse large B-cell lymphoma. Clin Nucl Med. 2012; 37(10):949-952

[68] Chiaravalloti A, Danieli R, Abbatiello P, et al. Factors affecting intrapatient liver and mediastinal blood pool 18F-FDG standardized uptake value changes during ABVD chemotherapy in Hodgkin's lymphoma. Eur J Nucl Med Mol Imaging. 2014; 41 (6):1123-1132

[69] Itti E, Meignan M, Berriolo-Riedinger A, et al. An international confirmatory study of the prognostic value of early PET/CT in diffuse large B-cell lymphoma: comparison between Deauville criteria and ΔSUVmax. Eur J Nucl Med Mol Imaging. 2013; 40(9):1312-1320

[70] Johnson SA, Kumar A, Matasar MJ, Schöder H, Rademaker J. Imaging for staging and response assessment in lymphoma. Radiology. 2015; 276(2):323-338

[71] Castellucci P, Zinzani P, Nanni C, et al. 18F-FDG PET early after radiotherapy in lymphoma patients. Cancer Biother Radiopharm. 2004; 19(5):606-612

[72] Filmont JE, Gisselbrecht C, Cuenca X, et al. The impact of pre- and post-transplantation positron emission tomography using 18-fluorodeoxyglucose on poor-prognosis lymphoma patients undergoing autologous stem cell transplantation. Cancer. 2007; 110(6):1361-1369

[73] Schot BW, Pruim J, van Imhoff GW, Sluiter WJ, Vaalburg W, Vellenga E. The role of serial pre-transplantation positron emission tomography in predicting progressive disease in relapsed lymphoma. Haematologica. 2006; 91(4):490-495

[74] Adams HJ, Kwee TC. Pretransplant FDG-PET in aggressive non-Hodgkin lymphoma: systematic review and meta-analysis. Eur J Haematol. 2017; 98(4):337-347

20 Melanoma

Eugene C. Lin

20.1 Initial Staging/Recurrence

Positron emission tomography (PET) is most useful in staging high-risk disease at diagnosis and evaluation for recurrent disease if surgery is planned. It has a potential role in assessing response and surveillance for recurrence, but the exact value of PET in these settings is not well defined.

20.2 Initial Staging

1. PET is a useful modality for regional and distant staging of high-risk melanoma at initial diagnosis (▶ Fig. 20.1, ▶ Fig. 20.2, ▶ Fig. 20.3, ▶ Fig. 20.4).[1,2]
2. The value of PET for initial staging depends on the disease stage:
   a) PET is most valuable in stage III disease with regional lymph node metastases. Detection of distant disease will likely influence prognosis and management. PET/CT has changed management in patients with stage III disease in 10 to 49% of cases,[3] most likely by upstaging: 22 to 27% of patients are upstaged by PET.[4,5] In one analysis,[5] adding PET to the workup in stage III patients results in true positive upstaging in 27% of patients with an increase in cost of 7.2%.
   b) PET has minimal, if any, role in stage I and II disease. In these stages, the prevalence of nodal disease is small, and sentinel node biopsy has a much higher negative predictive value than PET. In a meta-analysis[6] of patients with stage I and II diseases, the sensitivity ranged from 0 to 67% and the specificity ranged from 77 to 100%. The sensitivity of PET for regional lymph node metastases in melanoma is only 17% relative to sentinel lymphadenectomy.[7]

   PET may have potential value in patients with a higher pretest likelihood of distant metastases: for example, in melanomas located in the trunk and upper arms, a Breslow thickness > 4 mm, ulceration, bleeding, lymphadenopathy, or high mitotic

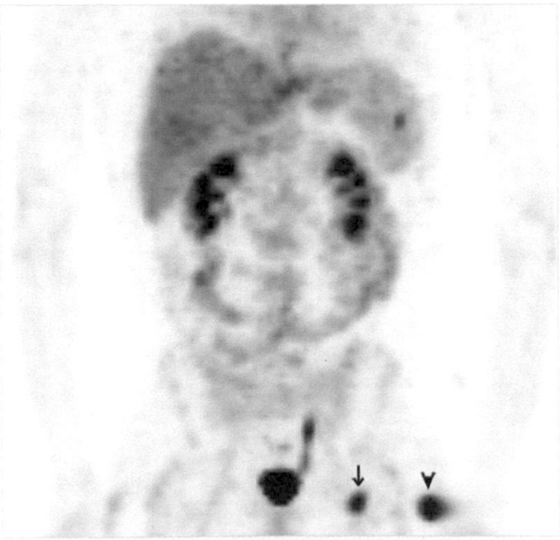

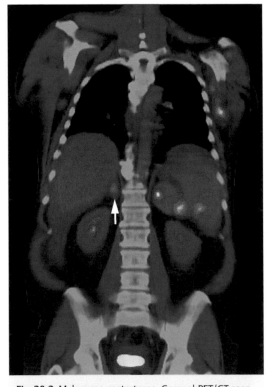

Fig. 20.1 Primary melanoma and metastases. Coronal PET scan demonstrates uptake in a primary left thigh melanoma (*arrowhead*), a left groin nodal metastasis (*arrow*), and a splenic metastasis.

Fig. 20.2 Melanoma metastases. Coronal PET/CT scan demonstrates melanoma metastases to the right adrenal (*arrow*), spleen, and axillary nodes.

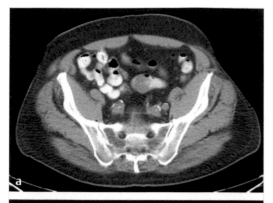

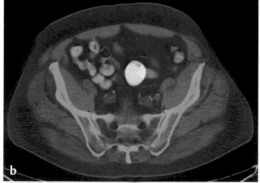

Fig. 20.3 Bowel metastasis. Axial CT (**a**) and PET/CT (**b**) demonstrate a bowel metastasis from melanoma. There is intense uptake in this metastatic lesion which is much more easily identified by PET than CT.

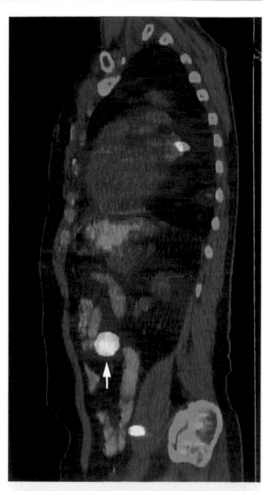

Fig. 20.4 Metastatic melanoma. Sagittal PET/CT image demonstrates metastases to the hilum, lung base, psoas muscle, and a mesenteric node (*arrow*).

rate.[7,8] However, note that in stage I and II disease, possible distant disease identified by PET has a high false-positive rate.[9]

PET may occasionally be of value in stage IV disease. In patients with potentially surgically remediable disease (solitary or limited distant metastases), PET is helpful in the detection of additional disease, which may obviate plans for surgery. PET is usually not helpful if metastases are multiple, as demonstration of additional metastases usually will not alter management. However, PET could be useful in this situation to determine response if experimental therapies employed.

3. PET is more useful in identifying distant disease than regional metastases given the established role of sentinel node imaging and biopsy. PET, or any other gross imaging technique, cannot replace sentinel node biopsy because these techniques will not detect micrometastases.[10]

a) However, if used in intermediate- and high-risk lesions, a positive PET study can guide biopsy of appropriate regional nodes.[11]

b) A sentinel node biopsy must be performed if PET is negative as micrometastases can be missed.

c) In general, there is a distinct and appropriate role for both PET and sentinel node biopsy and either or both should be employed accordingly.

4. **Isolated limb infusion**. Isolated limb infusion is often used to treat patients with in-transit melanoma (stage IIIB/C). In a prospective multicenter trial,[12] PET/CT identified only 59% of patients with a complete response, while 41% with a complete response had residual metabolic activity. However, PET/CT was still

useful in identifying a subgroup of patients with worse regional progression-free survival. The 3-year disease-free rate was 62% in patients with a complete response by both clinical/pathological exam and PET/CT, and 29% in patients with a complete response and residual PET/CT activity. In addition, PET/CT was an excellent method of surveillance in stage IIIB/IIIC patients after isolated limb infusion, as it could identify surgically resectable recurrent disease.

5. **Noncutaneous melanoma.** There is limited data on the use of PET in noncutaneous melanoma. Although a few studies have found that PET/CT is accurate in the diagnosis of metastases from uveal melanoma,[13,14] one study indicates that liver metastases in patients with uveal melanoma are substantially less FDG avid than metastases from cutaneous melanoma.[15] MRI is superior to PET/CT in the diagnosis of liver metastases from uveal melanoma.[16,17]

20.3 Recurrent Disease

For the follow-up of patients with stage IIB–IV melanoma,[1,2] National Comprehensive Cancer Network (NCCN) guidelines[18] state that imaging (including PET/CT) should be considered every 3 to 12 months to screen for recurrence or metastatic disease, but routine imaging to screen asymptomatic patients is not recommended after 3 to 5 years.

1. PET is a standard modality in the evaluation of recurrent melanoma. It is useful for:
   a) Diagnosis of recurrent or metastatic disease.
   b) Pretreatment staging of recurrent disease.
2. The primary indication for PET in recurrence is when surgery is planned.
   a) Detection of additional sites of disease will avoid unnecessary surgery.
   b) Equivocal findings on conventional imaging can be characterized.

20.4 Prognosis

High SUV in lymph node metastases is an independent negative prognostic factor for disease-free survival.[19] However, there is no impact on overall survival.

20.5 Accuracy/Comparison to Other Modalities

1. **Systemic metastases in stage III cutaneous melanoma** (meta-analysis)[20]: Sensitivity of 89% and specificity of 89%.

2. **Asymptomatic patients at high risk of relapse (PET and PET/CT)**[21]: Sensitivity of 96% and specificity of 92%.
3. **Comparison to other modalities**. In a meta-analysis[22] comparing PET/CT, PET, CT, and ultrasonography, PET/CT had the highest sensitivity, specificity, and diagnostic odds ratio for both staging and surveillance of distant metastases.
4. **Body region:**
   a) PET is more sensitive than CT for skin lesions, lymph node, soft tissue, liver, bone marrow, and bowel metastases (▶ Fig. 20.3).[23,24] However, MRI is more sensitive than PET for liver metastases.[25]
   b) CT is more sensitive for lung, brain metastases.

20.6 Pearls/Pitfalls

1. In melanoma, PET is limited in the brain, lungs, and liver. If there is concern for brain and lung metastases, PET must be supplemented with CT or MRI of the brain and chest CT (▶ Fig. 20.5). Lung metastases in melanoma are often very small and undetectable by PET. Although PET has limited sensitivity for lung metastases, it is still useful for assessment of the lungs. The higher specificity (92 vs. 70%)[24] of PET versus CT is useful to evaluate indeterminate lung lesions seen on CT. Liver MRI is substantially more sensitive than PET for liver metastases from melanoma.[25]
2. **Melanin content**. Melanin content does not influence lesion detectability by PET.[25]
3. **Peripheral lesions**. Skin or subcutaneous lesions may be missed on non–attenuation-corrected images due to the high skin activity on these images. However, it is also possible that peripheral subcutaneous lesions could also be better seen on non–attenuation-corrected images due to lack of attenuation relative to central structures.
4. Given that melanoma has the potential to metastasize to a wider range of anatomic sites than most neoplasms, false-positive results are often more of an issue in this cancer than in others. The full range of normal/benign variants and artifacts in PET imaging can cause false-positive findings. Because of this, close clinical and radiographic correlation is necessary to avoid such errors. Confirmation of assumed disease sites should be obtained if possible for optimal management.

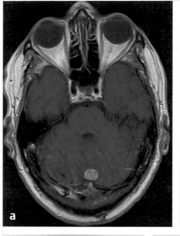
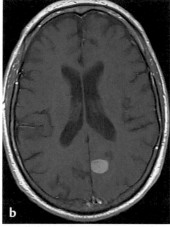
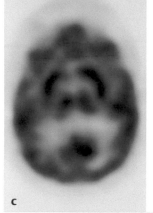
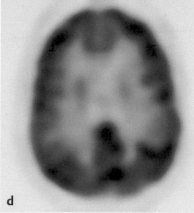

Fig. 20.5 Melanoma brain metastases. Axial contrast-enhanced MRI demonstrates enhancing metastases in the cerebellum **(a)** and occipital lobe **(b)** in a patient with melanoma. These metastases are difficult to identify prospectively on corresponding axial PET images through the cerebellum **(c)** and occipital lobe **(d)** due to intense gray matter activity.

5. **Interpretation**. The diagnostic accuracy of PET/CT in melanoma may be improved by using a high threshold approach to interpretation (i.e., subtle findings are interpreted as negative).[26] In particular, false positives are more prevalent in patients with suspected local recurrence only, suggesting a higher interpretation threshold could be used in this group.[3]

6. **Scan volume**. One study[27] suggests that scanning the lower extremities and skull in melanoma patients is of low yield. It has been suggested that "true" whole body PET/CT should only be performed if the melanoma arises in the lower extremities.[28]

7. **Immune modulation therapy.** Immunomodulation uses monoclonal antibodies to inhibit immune tolerance toward tumor cells by targeting regulators of T-lymphocyte activation. Ipilimumab is a monoclonal antibody which has been approved for first- and second-line treatment of unresectable or advanced melanoma. As immunomodulation potentiates T-lymphocytes, it can produce a variety of immune-related reactions which lead to false-positive FDG uptake (▶ Fig. 20.6). These include colitis, dermatitis, hypophysitis, arthritis, thyroiditis, and pancreatitis.[29,30] Some authors[29] suggest that mild nodal FDG uptake after immune modulation therapy is more likely due to inflammation, and recommend a follow-up PET/CT in 1 to 3 months.

8. **Tumor markers**. PET/CT has higher diagnostic accuracy and prognostic power than serum protein S100B or melanoma inhibitory activity in the follow-up of patients with melanoma.[31,32]

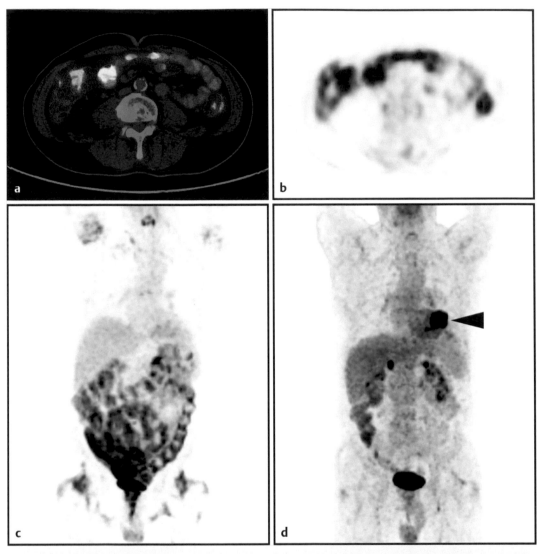

Fig. 20.6 A 68-year-old male heavy smoker with a history of poorly differentiated non-small cell lung cancer in the left lower lobe status post chemotherapy, radiation therapy, and recent immunotherapy. He received carboplatin and paclitaxel a year ago, but with poor response. He was on nivolumab in the last 6 months with good response. Repeat FDG PET/CT **(a–c)** demonstrated new diffuse FDG uptake in the GI tract, secondary to recent immunotherapy, which was not seen on prior PET/CT before immunotherapy **(d)**. Increased hip activity is also noted. The tumor mass in the left lower lobe (*arrowhead* in **d**) has significantly decreased in size and no longer FDG avid. (Courtesy of Gang Cheng, MD, Philadelphia, PA.)

References

[1] Friedman KP, Wahl RL. Clinical use of positron emission tomography in the management of cutaneous melanoma. Semin Nucl Med. 2004; 34(4):242–253

[2] Kumar R, Alavi A. Clinical applications of fluorodeoxyglucose–positron emission tomography in the management of malignant melanoma. Curr Opin Oncol. 2005; 17(2):154–159

[3] Bourgeois AC, Chang TT, Fish LM, Bradley YC. Positron emission tomography/computed tomography in melanoma. Radiol Clin North Am. 2013; 51(5):865–879

[4] Bastiaannet E, Oyen WJ, Meijer S, et al. Impact of [18F]fluorodeoxyglucose positron emission tomography on surgical management of melanoma patients. Br J Surg. 2006; 93(2):243–249

[5] Bastiaannet E, Uyl-de Groot CA, Brouwers AH, et al. Cost-effectiveness of adding FDG-PET or CT to the diagnostic work-

up of patients with stage III melanoma. Ann Surg. 2012; 255 (4):771–776

[6] Schröer-Günther MA, Wolff RF, Westwood ME, et al. F-18-fluoro-2-deoxyglucose positron emission tomography (PET) and PET/computed tomography imaging in primary staging of patients with malignant melanoma: a systematic review. Syst Rev. 2012; 1:62

[7] Belhocine TZ, Scott AM, Even-Sapir E, Urbain JL, Essner R. Role of nuclear medicine in the management of cutaneous malignant melanoma. J Nucl Med. 2006; 47(6):957–967

[8] Danielsen M, Kjaer A, Wu M, et al. Prediction of positron emission tomography/computed tomography (PET/CT) positivity in patients with high-risk primary melanoma. Am J Nucl Med Mol Imaging. 2016; 6(5):277–285

[9] Wagner JD. Fluorodeoxyglucose positron emission tomography for melanoma staging: refining the indications. Ann Surg Oncol. 2006; 13(4):444–446

[10] Wagner JD, Schauwecker D, Davidson D, et al. Prospective study of fluorodeoxyglucose-positron emission tomography imaging of lymph node basins in melanoma patients undergoing sentinel node biopsy. J Clin Oncol. 1999; 17(5):1508–1515

[11] Abella-Columna E, Valk PE. Positron emission tomography imaging in melanoma and lymphoma. Semin Roentgenol. 2002; 37(2):129–139

[12] Beasley GM, Parsons C, Broadwater G, et al. A multicenter prospective evaluation of the clinical utility of F-18 FDG-PET/CT in patients with AJCC stage IIIB or IIIC extremity melanoma. Ann Surg. 2012; 256(2):350–356

[13] Francken AB, Fulham MJ, Millward MJ, Thompson JF. Detection of metastatic disease in patients with uveal melanoma using positron emission tomography. Eur J Surg Oncol. 2006; 32(7):780–784

[14] Klingenstein A, Haug AR, Nentwich MM, Tiling R, Schaller UC. Whole-body F-18-fluoro-2-deoxyglucose positron emission tomography/computed tomography imaging in the follow-up of metastatic uveal melanoma. Melanoma Res. 2010; 20(6):511–516

[15] Strobel K, Bode B, Dummer R, et al. Limited value of 18F-FDG PET/CT and S-100B tumour marker in the detection of liver metastases from uveal melanoma compared to liver metastases from cutaneous melanoma. Eur J Nucl Med Mol Imaging. 2009; 36(11):1774–1782

[16] Orcurto V, Denys A, Voelter V, et al. (18)F-fluorodeoxyglucose positron emission tomography/computed tomography and magnetic resonance imaging in patients with liver metastases from uveal melanoma: results from a pilot study. Melanoma Res. 2012; 22(1):63–69

[17] Servois V, Mariani P, Malhaire C, et al. Preoperative staging of liver metastases from uveal melanoma by magnetic resonance imaging (MRI) and fluorodeoxyglucose-positron emission tomography (FDG-PET). Eur J Surg Oncol. 2010; 36(2):189–194

[18] Coit DG, Thompson JA, Algazi A, et al. NCCN Guidelines Insights: Melanoma, Version 3.2016. J Natl Compr Canc Netw. 2016; 14(8):945–958

[19] Bastiaannet E, Hoekstra OS, Oyen WJ, Jager PL, Wobbes T, Hoekstra HJ. Level of fluorodeoxyglucose uptake predicts risk for recurrence in melanoma patients presenting with lymph node metastases. Ann Surg Oncol. 2006; 13(7):919–926

[20] Rodriguez Rivera AM, Alabbas H, Ramjaun A, Meguerditchian AN. Value of positron emission tomography scan in stage III cutaneous melanoma: a systematic review and meta-analysis. Surg Oncol. 2014; 23(1):11–16

[21] Danielsen M, Højgaard L, Kjær A, Fischer BM. Positron emission tomography in the follow-up of cutaneous malignant melanoma patients: a systematic review. Am J Nucl Med Mol Imaging. 2013; 4(1):17–28

[22] Xing Y, Bronstein Y, Ross MI, et al. Contemporary diagnostic imaging modalities for the staging and surveillance of melanoma patients: a meta-analysis. J Natl Cancer Inst. 2011; 103 (2):129–142

[23] Holder WD, Jr, White RL, Jr, Zuger JH, Easton EJ, Jr, Greene FL. Effectiveness of positron emission tomography for the detection of melanoma metastases. Ann Surg. 1998; 227(5):764–769, discussion 769–771

[24] Fuster D, Chiang S, Johnson G, Schuchter LM, Zhuang H, Alavi A. Is 18F-FDG PET more accurate than standard diagnostic procedures in the detection of suspected recurrent melanoma? J Nucl Med. 2004; 45(8):1323–1327

[25] Ghanem N, Altehoefer C, Högerle S, et al. Detectability of liver metastases in malignant melanoma: prospective comparison of magnetic resonance imaging and positron emission tomography. Eur J Radiol. 2005; 54(2):264–270

[26] Falk MS, Truitt AK, Coakley FV, Kashani-Sabet M, Hawkins RA, Franc B. Interpretation, accuracy and management implications of FDG PET/CT in cutaneous malignant melanoma. Nucl Med Commun. 2007; 28(4):273–280

[27] Niederkohr RD, Rosenberg J, Shabo G, Quon A. Clinical value of including the head and lower extremities in 18F-FDG PET/CT imaging for patients with malignant melanoma. Nucl Med Commun. 2007; 28(9):688–695

[28] Lazaga FJ, Oz OK, Adams-Huet B, Anderson J, Mathews D. Comparison of whole-body versus limited whole-body 18F-FDG PET/CT scan in malignant cutaneous melanoma. Clin Nucl Med. 2013; 38(11):882–884

[29] Perng P, Marcus C, Subramaniam RM. (18)F-FDG PET/CT and melanoma: staging, immune modulation and mutation-targeted therapy assessment, and prognosis. AJR Am J Roentgenol. 2015; 205(2):259–270

[30] Wachsmann JW, Ganti R, Peng F. Immune-mediated disease in ipilimumab immunotherapy of melanoma with FDG PET-CT. Acad Radiol. 2017; 24(1):111–115

[31] Essler M, Link A, Belloni B, et al. Prognostic value of [18F]-fluoro-deoxy-glucose PET/CT, S100 or MIA for assessment of cancer-associated mortality in patients with high risk melanoma. PLoS One. 2011; 6(9):e24632

[32] Wieder HA, Tekin G, Rosenbaum-Krumme S, et al. 18FDG-PET to assess recurrence and long term survival in patients with malignant melanoma. Nucl Med (Stuttg). 2013; 52(5):198–203

21 Hepatobiliary Tumors

Eugene C. Lin

21.1 Hepatocellular Carcinoma

The primary value of PET is in detection of extrahepatic disease and monitoring treatment.[1,2] In one report,[3] PET/CT provided additional information in the initial staging of patients with Barcelona Clinic Liver Cancer (BCLC) stages A and B and American Joint Committee on Cancer T2 and T3 classifications.

1. Primary tumor detection:
   a) PET has limited sensitivity for well-differentiated hepatocellular carcinoma (HCC; ▶ Fig. 21.1).
   b) PET has no role in screening for HCC in cirrhotic patients.[4]

2. Extrahepatic disease:
   a) The primary tumor must have fluorodeoxyglucose (FDG) uptake for PET results to be valid.
   b) PET can detect distant disease for staging and recurrence, altering management in up to 30% of patients.[5]
   c) PET may be valuable in patients with treated HCC and a rising serum alpha-fetoprotein and normal conventional imaging. In these cases, the accuracy of PET for detecting recurrence is 74%.[6]

3. **Monitoring therapy**. PET is more accurate than CT (after iodized oil injection) for evaluating tumor viability post-chemoembolization (▶ Fig. 21.2).[7] PET may also detect recurrence after radiofrequency ablation earlier than CT.[8]

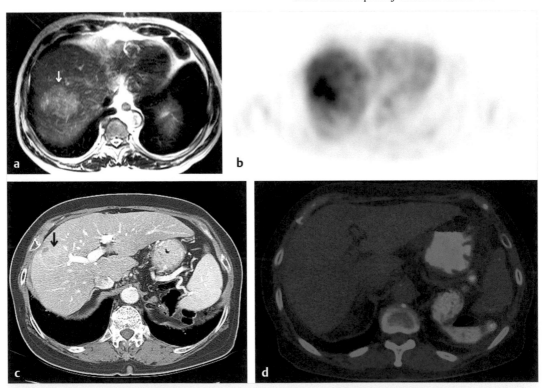

Fig. 21.1 Hepatocellular carcinoma: high-grade versus low grade. **(a)** Axial T2-weighted MRI scan demonstrates a focal area of hyperintensity corresponding to a hepatoma (*arrow*) in the right dome of the liver. **(b)** Axial PET scan demonstrates increased uptake in this high-grade hepatoma. **(c)** Axial CT in a different patient demonstrates a mostly isodense right lobe lesion with an enhancing capsule and a peripheral area of low density (*arrow*). **(d)** Axial PET/CT at the same level demonstrates that this low-grade hepatoma has uptake equal to normal liver.

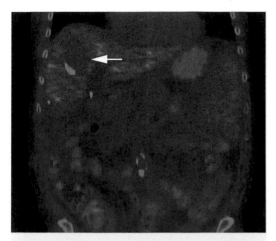

Fig. 21.2 Hepatic chemoembolization. Coronal PET/CT scan demonstrates lack of fluorodeoxyglucose uptake in hepatoma (*arrow*) after chemoembolization.

In a comparison of PET/CT to contrast-enhanced CT after transarterial chemoembolization (TACE), PET/CT was superior to CT in assessing tumor viability in patients with lipiodol deposition in more than 20% of the tumor, and comparable to CT in patients with 20% or less deposition.[9] The ratio of tumor to liver standardized uptake value (SUV) was an independent predictor of response to TACE.

4. **Prognosis.** FDG PET/CT has substantial independent prognostic utility in patient with HCC. It has been shown to predict overall and recurrence-free survival in liver transplantation,[10,11,12] TACE,[13,14] and curative resection.[15]

In a meta-analysis,[16] high tumor SUV/liver SUV ratio was associated with poorer overall and disease-free survival and high tumor SUV was associated with poorer overall survival. FDG uptake in portal venous thrombosis is an independent prognostic factor for progression-free and overall survival in HCC patients without extrahepatic metastases.[17]

The tumor-to-liver standardized uptake ratio is an independent prognostic factor for overall survival for BCLC stage 0 or A HCC patients undergoing curative treatment,[18] and for BCLC stage C HCC patients with intrahepatic disease or extrahepatic disease.[19]

In HCC patients, tumor characteristics such as differentiation and microvascular invasion are independent prognostic factors for overall and disease-free survival after liver transplantation, but cannot be evaluated with conventional imaging modalities. Positive FDG PET/CT findings show a good correlation with differentiation and microvascular invasion, and can be used to predict prognosis after liver transplantation.[20,21] FDG PET findings and the University of California, San Francisco (UCSF) criteria can be combined to predict the risk of HCC recurrence after living donor liver transplantation.[22] In one report,[23] the combination of serum alpha-fetoprotein and FDG PET positivity predicted tumor recurrence better than the Milan criteria in living donor related transplantation (LDLT).

A negative PET can be potentially used to expand the transplant recipient pool. Based upon a retrospective analysis, the National Cancer Center, Korea (NCCK), developed new criteria using negative FDG PET findings and a total tumor size less than 10 cm as significant prognostic factors.[21] In the study of HCC patients undergoing LDLT, the recipient pool was expanded as a greater number of patients fulfilled the NCCK criteria than the Milan criteria. The survival rate of patients fulfilling the NCCK criteria was similar to those of the UCSF and Milan criteria. In a multicenter survey,[24] patients over the Milan criteria with a negative PET and alpha fetoprotein less than 115 ng/mL had a recurrence rate comparable to patients within the Milan criteria.

21.1.1 Accuracy/Comparison to Other Modalities

1. **Primary lesion detection**:
   a) *PET:* sensitivity 50 to 70%[25,26]:
      - Low sensitivity is due to low uptake in well-differentiated HCC.
      - Tumors that are visualized by PET (▶ Fig. 21.1) usually are higher grade and larger in size, with elevated circulating alpha fetoprotein.
   b) PET is less sensitive than CT, MRI, or ultrasound.
   c) In one report, PET most often detected primary HCC lesions in patients with serum alpha-fetoprotein levels greater than 200 ng/mL and beyond the Milan criteria.[27]
2. **Extrahepatic disease**[28]:
   a) *Detection of metastatic HCC* (meta-analysis)[29]: sensitivity of 77% and specificity of 98%:
      - PET has a relatively high detection rate for extrahepatic metastases greater than 1 cm in size but a low detection rate for metastases less than 1 cm.

- PET can detect lesions that are negative or equivocal on conventional imaging.
- Patients with rising tumor markers and negative PET examinations usually do not have extrahepatic metastases; however, HCCs are often detected in the liver within months. Thus, these patients should be closely followed with liver imaging.
- PET is more likely to detect extrahepatic metastases if the primary lesion uptake is high: SUVmax ≥ 4.0 in one report[27] and 3.4 in another.[30] Size greater than 5 cm[30] is another factor.

b) **Bone metastases**: compared to other modalities, PET/CT may be primarily useful in the detection of bone metastases. In a comparison with CT, PET/CT, and bone scintigraphy, CT was more sensitive for the detection of lung metastases, and PET/CT performed better for the detection of bone metastases than CT or bone scintigraphy.[31] CT and PET/CT were comparable for nodal metastases. In two other studies,[32,33] FDG PET/CT had a higher detection rate for bone metastases than bone scintigraphy, on both lesion-based analysis, and patient-based analysis.

3. **Detection of recurrent HCC** (meta-analysis)[29]: sensitivity of 82% and specificity of 89%.

21.1.2 Pearls

1. **SUV.** HCCs usually have lower SUVs than metastases or cholangiocarcinoma.[34] In general, the tumor-to-liver SUV ratio is more useful than the tumor SUV.[9,35]
2. **Fibrolamellar HCC.** Fibrolamellar HCCs that are pathologically low grade can have increased FDG uptake (these tumors have intratumoral fibrous stroma that are associated with increased FDG uptake).[5]
3. **Delayed imaging.** Delayed imaging at 2 or 3 hours may detect more lesions.[36]
4. **Post-TACE.** Patterns of viable tumor post-TACE can manifest as arc-shaped or punctate at the periphery of the tumor. A large rim of activity could be secondary to inflammation, while eccentric foci are more likely to be secondary to tumor.[9]

21.1.3 Pitfalls

1. **Cirrhosis/hepatitis.** Structural changes secondary to cirrhosis have more effect on CT

accuracy than PET/CT accuracy. For example, regenerative nodules do not demonstrate FDG uptake.[37] However, patients with cirrhosis and chronic hepatitis can have slightly increased FDG activity in the liver, which could limit detection of HCC.
2. **Post-TACE.** Highly attenuating materials such as lipiodol can cause false-positive results secondary to attenuation correction artifacts.[35] Therefore, it is necessary to review the non-attenuation-corrected images.
3. **Timing.** PET/CT should be performed at least 1 month after intervention to reduce the incidence of false-positive results secondary to inflammation.[9]

21.2 Gallbladder Cancer and Cholangiocarcinoma

PET can detect the primary tumor, regional lymph nodes (▶ Fig. 21.3), and distant disease (▶ Fig. 21.4). The primary value is in detecting distant disease. In a study of patients with gallbladder cancer and cholangiocarcinoma,[1] PET/CT had a major impact on patient management in 28% of cases.[38] In one study of patients with cholangiocarcinoma and gallbladder carcinoma, PET/CT findings changed management in 17% of patients deemed resectable after initial workup.[39] Data from the National Oncologic PET Registry[40] indicated that FDG PET resulted in a change in management in 41.3% of patients with gallbladder cancer, with an imaging adjusted impact of 14.2%.

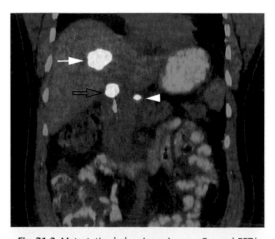

Fig. 21.3 Metastatic cholangiocarcinoma. Coronal PET/CT scan demonstrates both intrahepatic (*arrow*) and extrahepatic (*open arrow*) cholangiocarcinoma and a local nodal metastasis (*arrowhead*).

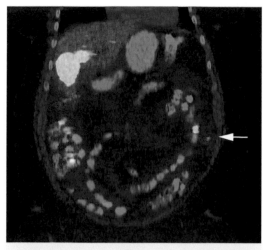

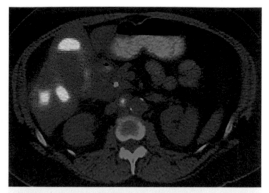

Fig. 21.5 Gallbladder cancer. Axial PET/CT demonstrates increased uptake in a gallbladder cancer with extension into the liver parenchyma and a retroperitoneal nodal metastasis.

Fig. 21.4 Metastatic cholangiocarcinoma. Coronal PET/CT scan demonstrates a large right intrahepatic cholangiocarcinoma with peritoneal metastases (*arrow*) in the left paracolic gutter.

National Comprehensive Cancer Network guidelines[41] for staging gallbladder cancer and cholangiocarcinoma indicate that PET/CT has limited sensitivity but high specificity for the detection of lymph node metastases and can be considered when there is an equivocal finding on CT or MRI as well as in patients with cholangiocarcinoma being considered for resection to evaluate for distant extrahepatic metastases.

1. **Primary tumor.** Although PET/CT is accurate in the diagnosis of primary intrahepatic cholangiocarcinoma and gallbladder cancer, there is conflicting evidence whether it is superior to conventional imaging for the diagnosis of primary tumors. The location of the cholangiocarcinoma is relevant, as PET/CT is more sensitive for the diagnosis of intrahepatic cholangiocarcinoma than hilar or extrahepatic cholangiocarcinoma.[42,43] In one study,[43] the SUVmax and tumor to liver uptake of intrahepatic cholangiocarcinoma was significantly higher than that of hilar cholangiocarcinoma. In one report,[44] PET/CT did not have a significant advantage over CT for the diagnosis of biliary tract cancers, and in another report[45] PET/CT did not have a significant advantage over CT or MRI/MR cholangiopancreatography (MRCP) of the diagnosis of cholangiocarcinoma. In one study,[46] PET/CT detected more primary lesions than contrast-enhanced CT.

a) **Gallbladder carcinoma.** PET is highly sensitive for the detection of gallbladder carcinoma (▶ Fig. 21.5)[47]:
   • However, benign gallbladder polyps can have FDG uptake.
b) PET is particularly useful when other imaging techniques are equivocal.
c) **Primary sclerosing cholangitis.** Limited data suggest PET may be valuable for the detection of cholangiocarcinoma in patients with biliary strictures and/or primary sclerosing cholangitis (▶ Fig. 21.6).[47,48,49] However, in the setting of primary sclerosing cholangitis, false positives secondary to inflammation have been reported.[49] Dynamic scanning with determination of the metabolic clearance of FDG may be helpful in avoiding false positives.[48]
   • An SUV cutoff of 3.6 is helpful in differentiating benign from malignant strictures in the liver hilum.[47]

2. **Metastatic disease.** In one study[44] evaluating patients with both gallbladder cancer and cholangiocarcinoma, PET/CT had a higher positive predictive value than CT (94 vs. 77%) for the diagnosis of regional lymph node metastases and a higher sensitivity for distant metastases (95 vs. 63%). However, the location of the primary tumor is relevant. For example, hilar cholangiocarcinomas are less FDG avid, and PET/CT would rarely change the treatment protocol in hilar cholangiocarcinoma patients in

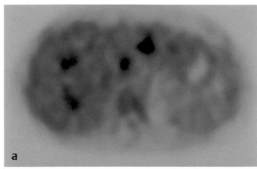

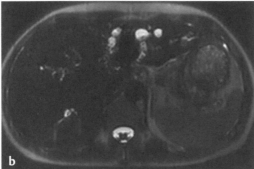

Fig. 21.6 Primary sclerosis cholangitis. **(a)** Axial PET scan demonstrates multiple areas of hepatic uptake that correspond to intrahepatic biliary strictures noted on an axial fat-saturated T2-weighted MRI. **(b)** PET can potentially be helpful in differentiating benign from malignant strictures in primary sclerosing cholangitis based upon degree of fluorodeoxyglucose uptake. In this case, the strictures were benign.

the absence of prior suspicious findings or elevated CA 19–9.[50] PET/CT is more useful for intrahepatic cholangiocarcinomas, where it may result in the identification of occult metastatic disease in up to 20 to 30% of patients.[51]

a) PET is more sensitive for distant metastases than for regional nodal spread.

b) In particular, distant metastases are often detected in peripheral intrahepatic cholangiocarcinoma.[52]

21.2.1 Accuracy/Comparison to Other Modalities

1. **Primary tumor (cholangiocarcinoma**; meta-analysis)[42]: sensitivity of 81% and specificity of 82%:
   a) **Intrahepatic cholangiocarcinoma**: sensitivity of 95% and specificity of 83%.
   b) **Hilar cholangiocarcinoma**: sensitivity of 84% and specificity of 95%.

c) **Extrahepatic cholangiocarcinoma**: sensitivity of 76% and specificity of 74%:
   • Overall PET is more accurate than CT; however, the sensitivity for perihilar cancer is lower than that of CT.[53]

2. **Primary tumor (gallbladder cancer**; meta-analysis)[42]: sensitivity of 87% and specificity of 78%.

3. **Regional lymph nodes** (▶ Table 21.1)[54]:

Table 21.1 Sensitivity and specificity of PET versus CT in the detection of regional lymph node metastases

	Sensitivity %	Specificity %
PET	38	100
CT	59	54

a) PET is less sensitive but more specific than CT for regional lymph node metastases.

b) In one report,[43] PET/CT had a sensitivity and specificity for regional lymph node metastases of 70 and 92%, respectively, compared to 50 and 83%, respectively, for MRI.

4. **Distant disease:** PET/CT is much more sensitive than CT for the detection of distant disease.[39]

21.2.2 Pearls

SUVs of 3.65 and 3.62 have been suggested as cutoffs for biliary tract malignancy.[44,55] For differentiating extrahepatic cholangiocarcinoma from benign stricture, SUV cutoffs of 2.5 and 3.1 have been suggested.[56]

21.2.3 Pitfalls

1. Sensitivity is decreased in extrahepatic, hilar, mucinous, and infiltrating cholangiocarcinomas.
2. Mucinous adenocarcinoma can be false negative.
3. False-positive biliary tract uptake can be seen with recent stent placement (▶ Fig. 7.36).
4. Inflammatory disorders such as primary sclerosing cholangitis, cholangitis from any etiology, and cholecystitis (▶ Fig. 21.7) can cause false positives.
5. Sensitivity for carcinomatosis is limited.[57]
6. The most common type of extrahepatic bile duct cancer is flat and infiltrating. Sensitivity for infiltrative cholangiocarcinoma is much lower than for nodular cholangiocarcinoma.[57]
7. **False-positive gallbladder uptake**. Although most cases of adenomyomatosis do not demonstrate increased FDG uptake, there is one

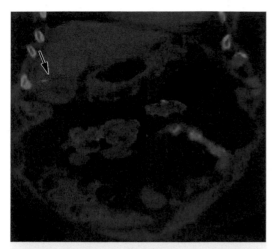

Fig. 21.7 Cholecystitis. Coronal PET/CT demonstrates increased fluorodeoxyglucose uptake in the gallbladder wall (*arrow*) secondary to cholecystitis.

report[58] of focal adenomyomatosis with increased activity. Other reported sources of false-positive gallbladder uptake include xanthogranulomatous cholecystitis and tuberculoid granulomatosis.

8. **Gallbladder polyps**. PET/CT can be helpful in risk stratification of 1- to 2-cm gallbladder polyps. Visual activity ≥ liver, or a cutoff ratio of SUVmax in the polyp to SUVmean in the liver of 1.14 can be used to suggest malignant etiologies.[59]

References

[1] Hustinx R. PET imaging in assessing gastrointestinal tumors. Radiol Clin North Am. 2004; 42(6):1123–1139, ix

[2] Lin EC, Kuni CC. Radionuclide imaging of hepatic and biliary disease. Semin Liver Dis. 2001; 21(2):179–194

[3] Cho Y, Lee DH, Lee YB, et al. Does 18F-FDG positron emission tomography-computed tomography have a role in initial staging of hepatocellular carcinoma? PLoS One. 2014; 9(8): e105679

[4] Teefey SA, Hildeboldt CC, Dehdashti F, et al. Detection of primary hepatic malignancy in liver transplant candidates: prospective comparison of CT, MR imaging, US, and PET. Radiology. 2003; 226(2):533–542

[5] Wudel LJ, Jr, Delbeke D, Morris D, et al. The role of [18F]fluorodeoxyglucose positron emission tomography imaging in the evaluation of hepatocellular carcinoma. Am Surg. 2003; 69(2):117–124, discussion 124–126

[6] Chen YK, Hsieh DS, Liao CS, et al. Utility of FDG-PET for investigating unexplained serum AFP elevation in patients with suspected hepatocellular carcinoma recurrence. Anticancer Res. 2005; 25 6C:4719–4725

[7] Torizuka T, Tamaki N, Inokuma T, et al. Value of fluorine-18-FDG-PET to monitor hepatocellular carcinoma after interventional therapy. J Nucl Med. 1994; 35(12):1965–1969

[8] Paudyal B, Oriuchi N, Paudyal P, et al. Early diagnosis of recurrent hepatocellular carcinoma with 18F-FDG PET after radiofrequency ablation therapy. Oncol Rep. 2007; 18(6):1469–1473

[9] Song HJ, Cheng JY, Hu SL, Zhang GY, Fu Y, Zhang YJ. Value of 18F-FDG PET/CT in detecting viable tumour and predicting prognosis of hepatocellular carcinoma after TACE. Clin Radiol. 2015; 70(2):128–137

[10] Detry O, Govaerts L, Deroover A, et al. Prognostic value of (18)F-FDG PET/CT in liver transplantation for hepatocarcinoma. World J Gastroenterol. 2015; 21(10):3049–3054

[11] Kornberg A, Küpper B, Thrum K, et al. Increased 18F-FDG uptake of hepatocellular carcinoma on positron emission tomography independently predicts tumor recurrence in liver transplant patients. Transplant Proc. 2009; 41(6):2561–2563

[12] Lee JW, Paeng JC, Kang KW, et al. Prediction of tumor recurrence by 18F-FDG PET in liver transplantation for hepatocellular carcinoma. J Nucl Med. 2009; 50(5):682–687

[13] Cho E, Jun CH, Kim BS, Son DJ, Choi WS, Choi SK. 18F-FDG PET CT as a prognostic factor in hepatocellular carcinoma. Turk J Gastroenterol. 2015; 26(4):344–350

[14] Kim BK, Kang WJ, Kim JK, et al. 18F-fluorodeoxyglucose uptake on positron emission tomography as a prognostic predictor in locally advanced hepatocellular carcinoma. Cancer. 2011; 117(20):4779–4787

[15] Han JH, Kim DG, Na GH, et al. Evaluation of prognostic factors on recurrence after curative resections for hepatocellular carcinoma. World J Gastroenterol. 2014; 20(45):17132–17140

[16] Sun DW, An L, Wei F, et al. Prognostic significance of parameters from pretreatment (18)F-FDG PET in hepatocellular carcinoma: a meta-analysis. Abdom Radiol (NY). 2016; 41(1): 33–41

[17] Lee JW, Hwang SH, Kim DY, Han KH, Yun M. Prognostic value of FDG uptake of portal vein tumor thrombosis in patients with locally advanced hepatocellular carcinoma. Clin Nucl Med. 2017; 42(1):e35–e40

[18] Hyun SH, Eo JS, Lee JW, et al. Prognostic value of (18)F-fluorodeoxyglucose positron emission tomography/computed tomography in patients with Barcelona Clinic Liver Cancer stages 0 and A hepatocellular carcinomas: a multicenter retrospective cohort study. Eur J Nucl Med Mol Imaging. 2016; 43(9):1638–1645

[19] Na SJ, Oh JK, Hyun SH, et al. 18F-FDG PET/CT can predict survival of advanced hepatocellular carcinoma patients: a multicenter retrospective cohort study. J Nucl Med. 2017; 58(5): 730–736

[20] Bailly M, Venel Y, Orain I, Salamé E, Ribeiro MJ. 18F-FDG PET in liver transplantation setting of hepatocellular carcinoma: predicting histology? Clin Nucl Med. 2016; 41(3):e126–e129

[21] Lee SD, Lee B, Kim SH, et al. Proposal of new expanded selection criteria using total tumor size and (18)F-fluorodeoxyglucose: positron emission tomography/computed tomography for living donor liver transplantation in patients with hepatocellular carcinoma: the National Cancer Center Korea criteria. World J Transplant. 2016; 6(2):411–422

[22] Hsu CC, Chen CL, Wang CC, et al. Combination of FDG-PET and UCSF criteria for predicting HCC recurrence after living donor liver transplantation. Transplantation. 2016; 100(9): 1925–1932

[23] Hong G, Suh KS, Suh SW, et al. Alpha-fetoprotein and (18)F-FDG positron emission tomography predict tumor recurrence better than Milan criteria in living donor liver transplantation. J Hepatol. 2016; 64(4):852–859

[24] Takada Y, Kaido T, Shirabe K, et al. LTx-PET study group of the Japanese Society of Hepato-Biliary-Pancreatic Surgery and the Japanese Liver Transplantation Society. Significance of

preoperative fluorodeoxyglucose-positron emission tomography in prediction of tumor recurrence after liver transplantation for hepatocellular carcinoma patients: a Japanese multicenter study. J Hepatobiliary Pancreat Sci. 2017; 24(1):49–57

[25] Khan MA, Combs CS, Brunt EM, et al. Positron emission tomography scanning in the evaluation of hepatocellular carcinoma. J Hepatol. 2000; 32(5):792–797

[26] Trojan J, Schroeder O, Raedle J, et al. Fluorine-18 FDG positron emission tomography for imaging of hepatocellular carcinoma. Am J Gastroenterol. 1999; 94(11):3314–3319

[27] Kawamura E, Shiomi S, Kotani K, et al. Positioning of 18F-fluorodeoxyglucose-positron emission tomography imaging in the management algorithm of hepatocellular carcinoma. J Gastroenterol Hepatol. 2014; 29(9):1722–1727

[28] Sugiyama M, Sakahara H, Torizuka T, et al. 18F-FDG PET in the detection of extrahepatic metastases from hepatocellular carcinoma. J Gastroenterol. 2004; 39(10):961–968

[29] Lin CY, Chen JH, Liang JA, Lin CC, Jeng LB, Kao CH. 18F-FDG PET or PET/CT for detecting extrahepatic metastases or recurrent hepatocellular carcinoma: a systematic review and meta-analysis. Eur J Radiol. 2012; 81(9):2417–2422

[30] Lee JE, Jang JY, Jeong SW, et al. Diagnostic value for extrahepatic metastases of hepatocellular carcinoma in positron emission tomography/computed tomography scan. World J Gastroenterol. 2012; 18(23):2979–2987

[31] Kawaoka T, Aikata H, Takaki S, et al. FDG positron emission tomography/computed tomography for the detection of extrahepatic metastases from hepatocellular carcinoma. Hepatol Res. 2009; 39(2):134–142

[32] Seo HJ, Choi YJ, Kim HJ, et al. Evaluation of bone metastasis from hepatocellular carcinoma using (18)F-FDG PET/CT and (99m)Tc-HDP bone scintigraphy: characteristics of soft tissue formation. Nucl Med Mol Imaging. 2011; 45(3):203–211

[33] Seo HJ, Kim GM, Kim JH, Kang WJ, Choi HJ. 18F-FDG PET/CT in hepatocellular carcinoma: detection of bone metastasis and prediction of prognosis. Nucl Med Commun. 2015; 36 (3):226–233

[34] Shiomi S, Nishiguchi S, Ishizu H, et al. Usefulness of positron emission tomography with fluorine-18-fluorodeoxyglucose for predicting outcome in patients with hepatocellular carcinoma. Am J Gastroenterol. 2001; 96(6):1877–1880

[35] Ortega López N. PET/computed tomography in evaluation of transarterial chemoembolization. PET Clin. 2015; 10(4):507–517

[36] Lin WY, Tsai SC, Hung GU. Value of delayed 18F-FDG-PET imaging in the detection of hepatocellular carcinoma. Nucl Med Commun. 2005; 26(4):315–321

[37] Cheung TT, Ho CL, Lo CM, et al. 11C-acetate and 18F-FDG PET/CT for clinical staging and selection of patients with hepatocellular carcinoma for liver transplantation on the basis of Milan criteria: surgeon's perspective. J Nucl Med. 2013; 54 (2):192–200

[38] Albazaz R, Patel CN, Chowdhury FU, Scarsbrook AF. Clinical impact of FDG PET-CT on management decisions for patients with primary biliary tumours. Insights Imaging. 2013; 4(5): 691–700

[39] Petrowsky H, Wildbrett P, Husarik DB, et al. Impact of integrated positron emission tomography and computed tomography on staging and management of gallbladder cancer and cholangiocarcinoma. J Hepatol. 2006; 45(1):43–50

[40] Hillner BE, Siegel BA, Shields AF, et al. Relationship between cancer type and impact of PET and PET/CT on intended management: findings of the national oncologic PET registry. J Nucl Med. 2008; 49(12):1928–1935

[41] Benson AB, III, Abrams TA, Ben-Josef E, et al. NCCN clinical practice guidelines in oncology: hepatobiliary cancers. J Natl Compr Canc Netw. 2009; 7(4):350–391

[42] Annunziata S, Pizzuto DA, Caldarella C, Galiandro F, Sadeghi R, Treglia G. Diagnostic accuracy of fluorine-18-fluorodeoxyglucose positron emission tomography in gallbladder cancer: A meta-analysis. World J Gastroenterol. 2015; 21(40):11481–11488

[43] Jiang L, Tan H, Panje CM, Yu H, Xiu Y, Shi H. Role of 18F-FDG PET/CT Imaging in Intrahepatic Cholangiocarcinoma. Clin Nucl Med. 2016; 41(1):1–7

[44] Lee SW, Kim HJ, Park JH, et al. Clinical usefulness of 18F-FDG PET-CT for patients with gallbladder cancer and cholangiocarcinoma. J Gastroenterol. 2010; 45(5):560–566

[45] Kim JY, Kim MH, Lee TY, et al. Clinical role of 18F-FDG PET-CT in suspected and potentially operable cholangiocarcinoma: a prospective study compared with conventional imaging. Am J Gastroenterol. 2008; 103(5):1145–1151

[46] Elias Y, Mariano AT, Jr, Lu Y. Detection of primary malignancy and metastases with FDG PET/CT in patients with cholangiocarcinomas: lesion-based comparison with contrast enhanced CT. World J Nucl Med. 2016; 15(3):161–166

[47] Reinhardt MJ, Strunk H, Gerhardt T, et al. Detection of Klatskin's tumor in extrahepatic bile duct strictures using delayed 18F-FDG PET/CT: preliminary results for 22 patient studies. J Nucl Med. 2005; 46(7):1158–1163

[48] Prytz H, Keiding S, Björnsson E, et al. Swedish Internal Medicine Liver Club. Dynamic FDG-PET is useful for detection of cholangiocarcinoma in patients with PSC listed for liver transplantation. Hepatology. 2006; 44(6):1572–1580

[49] Wakabayashi H, Akamoto S, Yachida S, et al. Significance of fluorodeoxyglucose PET imaging in the diagnosis of malignancies in patients with biliary stricture. Eur J Surg Oncol. 2005; 31(10):1175–1179

[50] Mansour JC, Aloia TA, Crane CH, Heimbach JK, Nagino M, Vauthey JN. Hilar cholangiocarcinoma: expert consensus statement. HPB. 2015; 17(8):691–699

[51] Weber SM, Ribero D, O'Reilly EM, Kokudo N, Miyazaki M, Pawlik TM. Intrahepatic cholangiocarcinoma: expert consensus statement. HPB. 2015; 17(8):669–680

[52] Kim YJ, Yun M, Lee WJ, Kim KS, Lee JD. Usefulness of 18F-FDG PET in intrahepatic cholangiocarcinoma. Eur J Nucl Med Mol Imaging. 2003; 30(11):1467–1472

[53] Moon CM, Bang S, Chung JB, et al. Usefulness of 18F-fluorodeoxyglucose positron emission tomography in differential diagnosis and staging of cholangiocarcinomas. J Gastroenterol Hepatol. 2008; 23(5):759–765

[54] Kato T, Tsukamoto E, Kuge Y, et al. Clinical role of (18)F-FDG PET for initial staging of patients with extrahepatic bile duct cancer. Eur J Nucl Med Mol Imaging. 2002; 29 (8):1047–1054

[55] Ramos-Font C, Gómez-Rio M, Rodríguez-Fernández A, Jiménez-Heffernan A, Sánchez Sánchez R, Llamas-Elvira JM. Ability of FDG-PET/CT in the detection of gallbladder cancer. J Surg Oncol. 2014; 109(3):218–224

[56] Choi EK, Yoo IeR, Kim SH, et al. The clinical value of dual-time point 18F-FDG PET/CT for differentiating extrahepatic cholangiocarcinoma from benign disease. Clin Nucl Med. 2013; 38(3):e106–e111

[57] Anderson CD, Rice MH, Pinson CW, Chapman WC, Chari RS, Delbeke D. Fluorodeoxyglucose PET imaging in the evaluation of gallbladder carcinoma and cholangiocarcinoma. J Gastrointest Surg. 2004; 8(1):90–97

[58] Maldjian PD, Ghesani N, Ahmed S, Liu Y. Adenomyomatosis of the gallbladder: another cause for a "hot" gallbladder on 18F-FDG PET. AJR Am J Roentgenol. 2007; 189(1):W36–8

[59] Lee J, Yun M, Kim KS, Lee JD, Kim CK. Risk stratification of gallbladder polyps (1–2 cm) for surgical intervention with 18F-FDG PET/CT. J Nucl Med. 2012; 53(3):353–358

22 Pancreatic Cancer

Eugene C. Lin

22.1 Pancreatic Masses

22.1.1 Adenocarcinoma

PET/CT has a potential role in the initial diagnosis of pancreatic cancer in cases where there is a biliary stricture without a mass identified on conventional imaging, or equivocal conventional imaging findings or biopsy. One specific situation in which PET/CT has been evaluated is the differentiation between benign mass-forming focal chronic pancreatitis and pancreatic cancer. However, as the negative predictive value of PET ranges from 65 to 78%,[1] a negative study does not exclude malignancy. However, the positive predictive value is high and lesions with high FDG avidity should generally be resected if possible.

Accuracy/Comparison to Other Modalities

1. *PET/CT for pancreatic adenocarcinoma* (meta-analysis) (▶ Table 22.1, ▶ Table 22.2)[2,3]:

Table 22.1 Sensitivity and specificity of PET/CT versus CT for detection of pancreatic adenocarcinoma

	Sensitivity %	Specificity %
PET/CT	90	76
CT	91	85

Table 22.2 Sensitivity and specificity of PET/CT versus EUS for detection of pancreatic adenocarcinoma

	Sensitivity %	Specificity %
PET/CT	90	80
EUS	82	93

2. *Chronic pancreatitis vs. pancreatic cancer* (meta-analysis): sensitivity 90%; specificity 84%.[2]
3. **Location**. The sensitivity for periampullary neoplasms is less than for neoplasm elsewhere in the pancreas.[4]
4. **Tumor size.** The sensitivity of PET is not substantially affected by tumor size if lesions are greater than 1 cm.
5. *Comparison with CT:*
   a) PET is most helpful compared to CT for lesions less than 2 cm.[5]

b) For lesions greater than 4 cm, CT is superior as large pancreatic tumors often contain areas of low metabolism.
   c) If CT shows no discrete mass, a positive PET is highly predictive of malignancy.[6]
   d) If CT is indeterminate, a positive PET is less specific for malignancy, but is very sensitive.[6]

22.2 Pearls

1. *Clinical history*[7]:
   a) The absence of clinical and laboratory findings of acute pancreatitis does not rule out an inflammatory etiology for a pancreatic mass.
   b) Obtaining a C-reactive protein may be helpful as false-positive results due to inflammation are more likely to occur when C-reactive protein is elevated.
2. *Characteristics of malignant versus inflammatory masses*:
   a) Inflammatory lesions are often more diffuse than focal.
   b) However, acute or chronic pancreatitis secondary to duct obstruction can be seen in conjunction with pancreatic malignancy. In these cases, it is difficult to distinguish tumor from pancreatitis on PET (▶ Fig. 22.1).

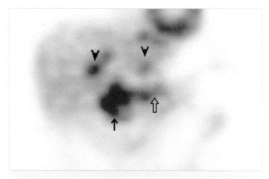

Fig. 22.1 Metastatic pancreatic cancer with chronic pancreatitis. Coronal PET scan demonstrates focal uptake in a pancreatic head adenocarcinoma (*solid arrow*). Increased uptake in the pancreatic body (*open arrow*) is not tumor but secondary to chronic pancreatitis from the obstructing pancreatic head mass. Liver metastases are present in both the right and left lobes (*arrowheads*).

c) Although chronic pancreatitis can cause false-positive results, the majority (87%) of patients with chronic pancreatitis have negative PET examinations. The possibility of malignancy should still be pursued in patients with chronic pancreatitis and positive PET.[8]

3. **SUV**

a) There is no generally agreed upon SUV cutoff for differentiating benign from malignant lesions: published values range from 2.0 to 4.0.[9,10]

b) If the patient has a history of pancreatitis, using SUV cutoff value in the higher range helps avoid false-positive results since pancreatic inflammatory lesions can have substantial uptake.

4. *Autoimmune pancreatitis vs. pancreatic cancer.* Autoimmune pancreatitis can occasionally mimic pancreatic cancer, presenting with focal enlargement of the pancreas and a focal stricture of the pancreatic duct. PET/CT (▶ Fig. 22.2) can be helpful in differentiating autoimmune pancreatitis from pancreatic cancer in these cases. In one study,[11] all patients with autoimmune pancreatitis had increased pancreatic FDG uptake. This uptake was diffuse in more than half of the cases, while patients with pancreatic cancer only had diffuse uptake in 3% of cases. However, if autoimmune pancreatitis presents with focal uptake, it cannot be differentiated from pancreatic cancer. In these cases, increased salivary gland uptake is sometimes seen in conjunction with autoimmune pancreatitis and can be helpful in suggesting the diagnosis. The salivary gland uptake (4.7 mean SUV) is higher than typically seen physiologically (1.9–2.9), and will resolve after steroid treatment.

5. **Delayed imaging**[12]:

a) Delayed imaging at 2 hours can help differentiate between malignant lesions and benign inflammatory lesions.

b) Malignant lesions will have increasing uptake over time, while inflammatory lesions will have a decline in uptake.

c) However, 19% of malignant pancreatic tumors show a decline in uptake from 1 to 2 hours.[13]

22.3 Pitfalls

1. **Hyperglycemia.** Hyperglycemia is a confounding factor for all oncologic PET but is the most problematic in pancreatic PET where it causes a high false-negative rate. PET must be

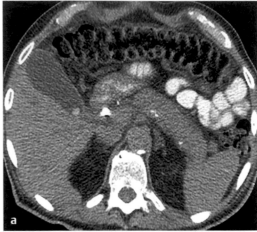

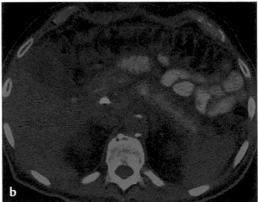

Fig. 22.2 Autoimmune pancreatitis. (a) Axial PET/CT demonstrates diffuse increased fluorodeoxyglucose uptake in the tail of the pancreas secondary to autoimmune pancreatitis. (b) Corresponding axial noncontrast CT demonstrates a rim of increased attenuation around the tail of the pancreas, secondary to inflammatory cell infiltration. This is a characteristic appearance of autoimmune pancreatitis.

interpreted with caution in hyperglycemic patients with a pancreatic mass:

a) In one report,[14] sensitivity was 90% in nondiabetic patients and 82% in patients with a fasting blood glucose between 126 and 200 mg/dL. In another report if plasma glucose was greater than 130 mg/dL, the detection rate of pancreatic malignancies was only 42%.[15]

2. **False positives.** Pancreatitis (chronic, acute, autoimmune) and benign lesions (serous cystadenoma, hemorrhagic pseudocyst).

3. **False negatives.** Early-stage tumors and elevated glucose.

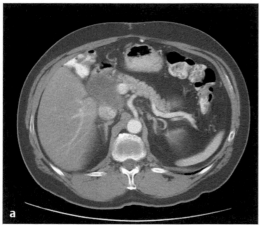

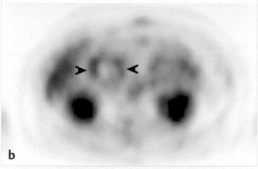

Fig. 22.3 Pancreatic pseudocyst. **(a)** CT scan demonstrates a cystic lesion in the pancreatic head region. **(b)** Axial PET scan at a slightly more inferior level demonstrates uptake around the cyst (*arrowheads*) but no uptake within the cyst. This appearance is consistent with a pseudocyst.

22.4 Cystic Tumors

1. **Overall accuracy.** PET or PET/CT can differentiate benign from malignant cystic tumors (▶ Fig. 22.3) with greater accuracy than CT, using a SUV cutoff of 2.5. (▶ Table 22.3)[16,17]

Table 22.3 Sensitivity and specificity of PET/CT versus CT in the detection of malignant cystic pancreatic tumors

	Sensitivity %	Specificity %
PET/CT	86	91
CT	67–71	87–90

2. **Intraductal papillary mucinous tumor (IPMT).** Patients with IPMTs are often managed using the International Consensus Guidelines (ICG). Two relevant questions are whether the lesion is benign or malignant and the risk of

malignant transformation in benign lesions. The guidelines suggest resection for main duct IPMTs greater than 10 mm in diameter, while branch duct IPMTs are evaluated for resection versus observation on the basis of criteria such as cyst size and mural nodularity. IPMT usually has increased FDG uptake.[18,19] As malignant IPMTs typically have a greater degree of FDG uptake than benign lesions, PET/CT can be helpful for differentiating benign from malignant IPMTs. In two reports,[20,21] PET was less sensitive but substantially more specific, with higher accuracy, than the indocyanine green (ICG) for detecting malignancy. The highest accuracy was achieved by combining PET and the ICG.[21]

In combination with the ICG, PET/CT can increase the accuracy of differentiating benign from malignant IPMNs, but the ICG is more helpful in predicting the risk of malignant transformation. Therefore, PET/CT is primarily helpful in avoiding unnecessary resection of IPMTs in patients who are elderly and/or at moderate to high surgical risk. However, PET/CT may be less useful compared to the ICG in young, fit patients as these patients may undergo resection based upon ICG criteria, even if PET/CT is negative, due to the risk of malignant transformation.

As there is an association between IPMN and extrapancreatic malignancies,[21] PET/CT may be of additional value in detecting unsuspected malignancies.

a) Solid components have more uptake than the cystic components.

b) The cystic component usually has diffuse uptake greater than normal pancreas.

c) **SUV cutoff.** SUV cutoffs ranging from 2.0[22] to 3.0[21] have been employed. As most patients will first be evaluated with a morphologic test, some authors[23] suggest that the morphologic test should maximize sensitivity, while the PET should maximize specificity with a higher SUV cutoff.

d) **Accuracy/comparison to other modalities.** Identifying malignant transformation within IPMN (meta-analysis) (▶ Table 22.4).[24]

Table 22.4 Sensitivity and specificity of PET versus CT/MRI for identification of malignant transformation in intraductal papillary mucinous neoplasms

	Sensitivity %	Specificity %
PET	97	91
CT/MRI	81	76

3. **Solid pseudopapillary tumors (SPTs).** There are limited reports on PET/CT of solid pseudopapillary tumors. Both benign and malignant SPTs can have FDG uptake with SUV greater than 3,[25] and the degree of uptake is typically greater than ductal adenocarcinomas and *neuroendocrine tumors.*[25,26]

22.5 Pancreatic Neuroendocrine Tumors

The sensitivity of PET may be relatively low (► Fig. 22.4) but comparable to CT, MRI, and ultrasound.[19] Small tumors not identified by other imaging methods are also usually not identified by PET.

The degree of FDG uptake in a pancreatic neuroendocrine tumor (PNET) is correlated with WHO tumor grade. Tumors with a higher SUV (≥ 2.5) are typically WHO grade 3 tumors (poorly differentiated).[27] The degree of uptake is also associated with tumor size and TNM (tumor size, node involvement, and metastasis status) stage.[28] Nonfunctioning PNETs can also be detected by PET/CT.[28]

For well-differentiated PNETs, the sensitivity of OctreoScan is higher than FDG PET (80 vs. 60%). However, for poorly differentiated PNETs, the sensitivity of OctreoScan was substantially lower than FDG PET (57 vs. 100%).[29] Thus, FDG PET is often reserved for cases where OctreoScan is negative, the tumors are rapidly progressing, or for high-grade tumors with a high proliferation index (Ki67).

FDG PET/CT has prognostic value in metastatic gastroenteropancreatic NETs. In one report,[30] a tumor/nontumor SUV ratio of 2.5 was associated with poor prognosis (4-year survival rate of 0%).

FDG PET may still be of prognostic utility in patients with a positive OctreoScan, as 25% of patients with a positive OctreoScan had a positive FDG PET and a poor prognosis.

22.6 Staging

PET cannot replace CT as it cannot assess local resectability. PET is most valuable in patients with a higher risk of metastatic disease (e.g., CA 19.9 > 200 U/mL).[31] National Comprehensive Cancer Network guidelines[32] state that PET/CT may be considered after a formal pancreatic CT protocol in high-risk patients (borderline resectable disease, markedly elevated CA 19–9, large primary tumors, or large regional lymph nodes) to detect extrapancreatic disease (► Fig. 22.5, ► Fig. 22.6).

PET is more useful for staging of distant metastases as the detection of local nodal metastases may be poor. In one report, PET/CT had a sensitivity of 30% for N-staging and 88% of M-staging in patients with advanced pancreatic adenocarcinoma.[33] PET can identify distant disease (► Fig. 22.7) not seen on CT and help avoid unnecessary surgery. The use of PET or PET/CT avoids unnecessary surgery by upstaging disease in approximately 17% of patients originally considered resectable by CT and angiography.[34,35] PET is also helpful for evaluating indeterminate liver lesions seen on CT.[36,37]

In the national oncologic PET registry, the use of PET for staging resulted in a change in management in 39.2% of cases, with an imaging-adjusted impact (change in from treatment to nontreatment or nontreatment to treatment) of 13.4%.[38]

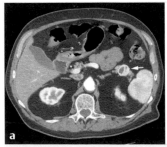 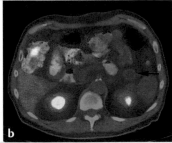 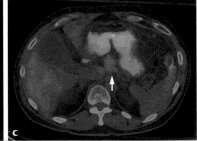

Fig. 22.4 Pancreatic islet cell tumors with variable fluorodeoxyglucose (FDG) uptake. **(a)** Axial CT scan demonstrates a hypervascular islet cell tumor in the tail of the pancreas (*arrow*). **(b)** Axial PET/CT scan demonstrates lack of FDG uptake in the islet cell tumor (*arrow*). **(c)** Axial PET/CT scan in another patient demonstrates moderate FDG uptake in an islet cell tumor (*arrow*) arising from the body of the pancreas.

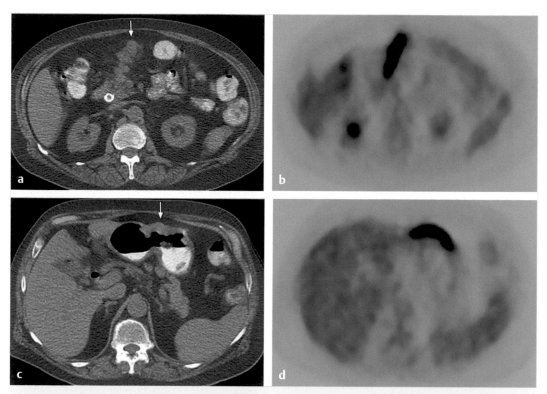

Fig. 22.5 Pancreatic cancer involving the gastrocolic ligament. (a) Axial CT and axial PET (b) demonstrates direct spread (*arrow*) of a pancreatic adenocarcinoma in the gastrocolic ligament. (c) Axial CT and axial PET (d) demonstrate superior extension of the tumor through the gastrocolic ligament to involve the anterior stomach (*arrow*).

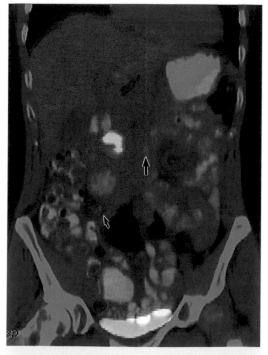

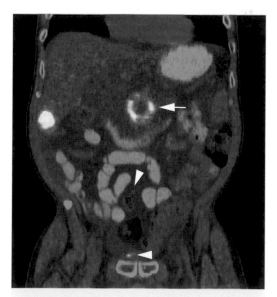

Fig. 22.7 Metastatic pancreatic cancer. Coronal PET/CT demonstrates ringlike uptake in a necrotic pancreatic carcinoma (*arrow*). A liver metastasis is present, as are multiple peritoneal metastases (*arrowheads*).

Fig. 22.6 Pancreatic cancer with nodal metastases. Coronal PET/CT demonstrates peripheral uptake around a necrotic adenocarcinoma in the head of the pancreas, with nodal metastases (*arrows*).

22.7 Accuracy/Comparison to Other Modalities

1. **PET:** Sensitivity 70%, specificity 93%.[39]
2. **Accuracy by site:**
   a) ***PET and PET/CT for liver metastases*** (meta-analysis)[40]: Sensitivity 67%; specificity 96%
      - Very sensitive for metastases greater than 1 cm (97%).[41]
      - Low sensitivity for metastases less than 1 cm (43%).
      - High specificity 95%.
   b) ***PET and PET/CT for lymph node metastases*** (meta-analysis)[40]: sensitivity 64%; specificity 81%.
   c) ***Peritoneal metastasis.*** There is conflicting evidence on the relative sensitivity of PET and CT for peritoneal metastases with reports suggesting a higher sensitivity for CT, while others suggest PET is more sensitive.[1]
3. PET and CT are complementary in the detection of distant metastases in patients with pancreatic cancer. PET can miss liver and lung metastases, but can detect nodal, peritoneal, and osseous metastases missed by CT.[42]

22.8 Pitfalls

1. **Cholestasis.** Cholestasis secondary to intrahepatic biliary dilatation can cause false-positive liver lesions.
2. **Biliary stents.** Recent biliary stent insertion can cause increased uptake along the stent tract. This can mimic nodal or liver metastases, particularly on axial images (▶ Fig. 7.36). It may be difficult to distinguish uptake along a stent from a pancreatic lesion (▶ Fig. 22.8).
3. **Neoadjuvant therapy.** Neoadjuvant therapy is associated with low metabolic activity.[31]

22.9 Therapy Response/Prognosis

1. **Therapy response.** PET can assess response to neoadjuvant chemoradiation and intraoperative radiotherapy.[5,35] PET can predict tumor response before CT.
2. **Postoperative recurrence.** Several studies indicate that PET detects recurrence earlier than CT,[1] although one study[43] suggests the accuracy is comparable. In the national oncologic PET registry, the use of PET resulted in a change in management in 38.3% of cases for restaging and 39.3% of cases for detection of suspected recurrence.[38] The imaging-adjusted impact (change in from treatment to nontreatment or nontreatment to treatment) was 11.3 and 22.1%, respectively.

Specific uses of PET/CT for the detection of recurrence include evaluation of hepatic lesions difficult to biopsy, patients with rising tumor markers and negative conventional workup, and differentiation of fibrosis and tumor in the surgical bed (▶ Fig. 22.9)[44]:
a) PET is valuable in this setting as it is may be difficult to evaluate the pancreatic region on

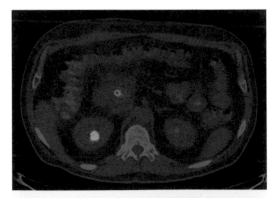

Fig. 22.8 Pancreatic cancer. Uptake is noted in a small pancreatic head cancer. This can be differentiated from inflammatory uptake around the stent by its eccentric location relative to the stent.

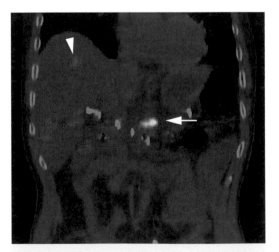

Fig. 22.9 Recurrent pancreatic cancer. Coronal PET/CT demonstrates a recurrence in the pancreatic bed (*arrow*) status post-Whipple procedure. A liver metastasis (*arrowhead*) is present.

CT after surgery and radiation secondary to scarring and inflammation.

b) CT should be the first-line imaging modality for follow-up, with PET performed if CT is equivocal or if CT is negative and tumor markers are rising.

c) PET is superior to CT for detecting local, nonlocoregional, and extra-abdominal recurrences. CT or MRI is superior for the detection of liver metastases.[45]

d) As postoperative inflammatory changes can result in false-positive findings, a delay of at least 6 weeks after surgery is recommended.[1]

3. **Prognosis.** The degree of initial FDG uptake of correlates with survival,[46,47,48] as does the degree of FDG uptake 1 month after chemotherapy.[49] A substantial number of studies have demonstrated that SUVmax is a useful predictor of overall and progression-free survival, in both resectable and unresectable patients.[1] Higher SUVmax is also associated with earlier recurrence after surgery. However, published SUV cutoff have varied substantially, ranging from 3.0 to 10.0.

References

[1] Nunna P, Sheikhbahaei S, Ahn S, Young B, Subramaniam RM. The role of positron emission tomography/computed tomography in management and prediction of survival in pancreatic cancer. J Comput Assist Tomogr. 2016; 40(1):142–151

[2] Rijkers AP, Valkema R, Duivenvoorden HJ, van Eijck CH. Usefulness of F-18-fluorodeoxyglucose positron emission tomography to confirm suspected pancreatic cancer: a meta-analysis. Eur J Surg Oncol. 2014; 40(7):794–804

[3] Tang S, Huang G, Liu J, et al. Usefulness of 18F-FDG PET, combined FDG-PET/CT and EUS in diagnosing primary pancreatic carcinoma: a meta-analysis. Eur J Radiol. 2011; 78(1):142–150

[4] Kalady MF, Clary BM, Clark LA, et al. Clinical utility of positron emission tomography in the diagnosis and management of periampullary neoplasms. Ann Surg Oncol. 2002; 9(8):799–806

[5] Rose DM, Delbeke D, Beauchamp RD, et al. 18Fluorodeoxyglucose-positron emission tomography in the management of patients with suspected pancreatic cancer. Ann Surg. 1999; 229(5):729–737, discussion 737–738

[6] Orlando LA, Kulasingam SL, Matchar DB. Meta-analysis: the detection of pancreatic malignancy with positron emission tomography. Aliment Pharmacol Ther. 2004; 20(10):1063–1070

[7] Shreve PD. Focal fluorine-18 fluorodeoxyglucose accumulation in inflammatory pancreatic disease. Eur J Nucl Med. 1998; 25(3):259–264

[8] van Kouwen MC, Jansen JB, van Goor H, de Castro S, Oyen WJ, Drenth JP. FDG-PET is able to detect pancreatic carcinoma in chronic pancreatitis. Eur J Nucl Med Mol Imaging. 2005; 32(4):399–404

[9] Delbeke D, Rose DM, Chapman WC, et al. Optimal interpretation of FDG PET in the diagnosis, staging and management of pancreatic carcinoma. J Nucl Med. 1999; 40(11):1784–1791

[10] Imdahl A, Nitzsche E, Krautmann F, et al. Evaluation of positron emission tomography with 2-[18F]fluoro-2-deoxy-D-glucose for the differentiation of chronic pancreatitis and pancreatic cancer. Br J Surg. 1999; 86(2):194–199

[11] Lee TY, Kim MH, Park DH, et al. Utility of 18F-FDG PET/CT for differentiation of autoimmune pancreatitis with atypical pancreatic imaging findings from pancreatic cancer. AJR Am J Roentgenol. 2009; 193(2):343–348

[12] Nakamoto Y, Higashi T, Sakahara H, et al. Delayed (18)F-fluoro-2-deoxy-D-glucose positron emission tomography scan for differentiation between malignant and benign lesions in the pancreas. Cancer. 2000; 89(12):2547–2554

[13] Higashi T, Saga T, Nakamoto Y, et al. Diagnosis of pancreatic cancer using fluorine-18 fluorodeoxyglucose positron emission tomography (FDG PET) –usefulness and limitations in "clinical reality". Ann Nucl Med. 2003; 17(4):261–279

[14] Hamidian Jahromi A, Fallahzadeh MK, Takalkar A, Sheng J, Zibari G, Shokouh Amiri H. Impact of plasma glucose level at the time of fluorodeoxyglucose administration on the accuracy of FDG-PET/CT in the diagnosis of pancreatic lesions. Int J Endocrinol Metab. 2014; 12(4):e16429

[15] Diederichs CG, Staib L, Glatting G, Beger HG, Reske SN. FDG PET: elevated plasma glucose reduces both uptake and detection rate of pancreatic malignancies. J Nucl Med. 1998; 39(6):1030–1033

[16] Sperti C, Pasquali C, Decet G, Chierichetti F, Liessi G, Pedrazzoli S. F-18-fluorodeoxyglucose positron emission tomography in differentiating malignant from benign pancreatic cysts: a prospective study. J Gastrointest Surg. 2005; 9(1):22–28, discussion 28–29

[17] Tann M, Sandrasegaran K, Jennings SG, Skandarajah A, McHenry L, Schmidt CM. Positron-emission tomography and computed tomography of cystic pancreatic masses. Clin Radiol. 2007; 62(8):745–751

[18] Yoshioka M, Sato T, Furuya T, et al. Positron emission tomography with 2-deoxy-2-[(18)F] fluoro- d-glucose for diagnosis of intraductal papillary mucinous tumor of the pancreas with parenchymal invasion. J Gastroenterol. 2003; 38(12):1189–1193

[19] Nakamoto Y, Higashi T, Sakahara H, et al. Evaluation of pancreatic islet cell tumors by fluorine-18 fluorodeoxyglucose positron emission tomography: comparison with other modalities. Clin Nucl Med. 2000; 25(2):115–119

[20] Pedrazzoli S, Sperti C, Pasquali C, Bissoli S, Chierichetti F. Comparison of International Consensus Guidelines versus 18-FDG PET in detecting malignancy of intraductal papillary mucinous neoplasms of the pancreas. Ann Surg. 2011; 254(6):971–976

[21] Roch AM, Barron MR, Tann M, et al. Does PET with CT have clinical utility in the management of patients with intraductal papillary mucinous neoplasm? J Am Coll Surg. 2015; 221(1):48–56

[22] Takanami K, Hiraide T, Tsuda M, et al. Additional value of FDG PET/CT to contrast-enhanced CT in the differentiation between benign and malignant intraductal papillary mucinous neoplasms of the pancreas with mural nodules. Ann Nucl Med. 2011; 25(7):501–510

[23] Baiocchi GL, Bertagna F, Gheza F, et al. Searching for indicators of malignancy in pancreatic intraductal papillary mucinous neoplasms: the value of 18FDG-PET confirmed. Ann Surg Oncol. 2012; 19(11):3574–3580

[24] Sultana A, Jackson R, Tim G, et al. What is the best way to identify malignant transformation within pancreatic IPMN: a systematic review and meta-analyses. Clin Transl Gastroenterol. 2015; 6:e130

[25] Guan ZW, Xu BX, Wang RM, Sun L, Tian JH. Hyperaccumulation of (18)F-FDG in order to differentiate solid pseudopapillary tumors from adenocarcinomas and from neuroendocrine pancreatic tumors and review of the literature. Hell J Nucl Med. 2013; 16(2):97–102

[26] Kim YI, Kim SK, Paeng JC, Lee HY. Comparison of F-18-FDG PET/CT findings between pancreatic solid pseudopapillary tumor and pancreatic ductal adenocarcinoma. Eur J Radiol. 2014; 83(1):231–235

[27] Tomimaru Y, Eguchi H, Tatsumi M, et al. Clinical utility of 2-[(18)F] fluoro-2-deoxy-D-glucose positron emission tomography in predicting World Health Organization grade in pancreatic neuroendocrine tumors. Surgery. 2015; 157(2):269–276

[28] Luo G, Liu Z, Guo M, et al. (18)F-FDG PET/CT can be used to detect non-functioning pancreatic neuroendocrine tumors. Int J Oncol. 2014; 45(4):1531–1536

[29] Squires MH, III, Volkan Adsay N, Schuster DM, et al. Octreoscan versus FDG-PET for neuroendocrine tumor staging: a biological approach. Ann Surg Oncol. 2015; 22(7):2295–2301

[30] Bahri H, Laurence L, Edeline J, et al. High prognostic value of 18F-FDG PET for metastatic gastroenteropancreatic neuroendocrine tumors: a long-term evaluation. J Nucl Med. 2014; 55(11):1786–1790

[31] Crippa S, Salgarello M, Laiti S, et al. The role of (18)fluoro-deoxyglucose positron emission tomography/computed tomography in resectable pancreatic cancer. Dig Liver Dis. 2014; 46(8):744–749

[32] Tempero MA, Malafa MP, Behrman SW, et al. Pancreatic adenocarcinoma, version 2.2014: featured updates to the NCCN guidelines. J Natl Compr Canc Netw. 2014; 12(8):1083–1093

[33] Kauhanen SP, Komar G, Seppänen MP, et al. A prospective diagnostic accuracy study of 18F-fluorodeoxyglucose positron emission tomography/computed tomography, multidetector row computed tomography, and magnetic resonance imaging in primary diagnosis and staging of pancreatic cancer. Ann Surg. 2009; 250(6):957–963

[34] Heinrich S, Goerres GW, Schäfer M, et al. Positron emission tomography/computed tomography influences on the management of resectable pancreatic cancer and its cost-effectiveness. Ann Surg. 2005; 242(2):235–243

[35] Kalra MK, Maher MM, Boland GW, Saini S, Fischman AJ. Correlation of positron emission tomography and CT in evaluating pancreatic tumors: technical and clinical implications. AJR Am J Roentgenol. 2003; 181(2):387–393

[36] Hustinx R. PET imaging in assessing gastrointestinal tumors. Radiol Clin North Am. 2004; 42(6):1123–1139, ix

[37] Mertz HR, Sechopoulos P, Delbeke D, Leach SD. EUS, PET, and CT scanning for evaluation of pancreatic adenocarcinoma. Gastrointest Endosc. 2000; 52(3):367–371

[38] Hillner BE, Siegel BA, Shields AF, et al. Relationship between cancer type and impact of PET and PET/CT on intended management: findings of the national oncologic PET registry. J Nucl Med. 2008; 49(12):1928–1935

[39] Gambhir SS, Czernin J, Schwimmer J, Silverman DH, Coleman RE, Phelps ME. A tabulated summary of the FDG PET literature. J Nucl Med. 2001; 42(5) S uppl:1S–93S

[40] Wang Z, Chen JQ, Liu JL, Qin XG, Huang Y. FDG-PET in diagnosis, staging and prognosis of pancreatic carcinoma: a meta-analysis. World J Gastroenterol. 2013; 19(29):4808–4817

[41] Fröhlich A, Diederichs CG, Staib L, Vogel J, Beger HG, Reske SN. Detection of liver metastases from pancreatic cancer using FDG PET. J Nucl Med. 1999; 40(2):250–255

[42] Nishiyama Y, Yamamoto Y, Yokoe K, et al. Contribution of whole body FDG-PET to the detection of distant metastasis in pancreatic cancer. Ann Nucl Med. 2005; 19(6):491–497

[43] Hamidian Jahromi A, Sangster G, Zibari G, et al. Accuracy of multi-detector computed tomography, fluorodeoxyglucose positron emission tomography-CT, and CA 19-9 levels in detecting recurrent pancreatic adenocarcinoma. JOP. 2013; 14(4):466–468

[44] Franke C, Klapdor R, Meyerhoff K, Schauman M. 18-FDG positron emission tomography of the pancreas: diagnostic benefit in the follow-up of pancreatic carcinoma. Anticancer Res. 1999; 19 4A:2437–2442

[45] Ruf J, Lopez Hänninen E, Oettle H, et al. Detection of recurrent pancreatic cancer: comparison of FDG-PET with CT/MRI. Pancreatology. 2005; 5(2–3):266–272

[46] Nakata B, Chung YS, Nishimura S, et al. 18F-fluorodeoxyglucose positron emission tomography and the prognosis of patients with pancreatic adenocarcinoma. Cancer. 1997; 79(4):695–699

[47] Sperti C, Pasquali C, Chierichetti F, Ferronato A, Decet G, Pedrazzoli S. 18-Fluorodeoxyglucose positron emission tomography in predicting survival of patients with pancreatic carcinoma. J Gastrointest Surg. 2003; 7(8):953–959, discussion 959–960

[48] Zimny M, Fass J, Bares R, et al. Fluorodeoxyglucose positron emission tomography and the prognosis of pancreatic carcinoma. Scand J Gastroenterol. 2000; 35(8):883–888

[49] Maisey NR, Webb A, Flux GD, et al. FDG-PET in the prediction of survival of patients with cancer of the pancreas: a pilot study. Br J Cancer. 2000; 83(3):287–293

23 Gynecological Tumors

Eugene C. Lin

23.1 Cervical Cancer

The primary value of PET in cervical cancer is in diagnosis of extrapelvic disease in initial staging and in detection of recurrence.[1,2]

23.1.1 Primary Tumor

PET will detect the majority of primary tumors (▶ Fig. 23.1, ▶ Fig. 23.2), but it is not as accurate as MRI for assessing locoregional involvement.[3] Squamous cell and poorly differentiated tumors generally have more fluorodeoxyglucose (FDG) uptake than nonsquamous cell cancers.[4] The degree of uptake in the primary tumor at diagnosis negatively correlates with treatment response and prognosis.[5]

23.1.2 Staging

National Comprehensive Cancer Network (NCCN) guidelines[6] state that PET/CT could be performed in stage IB2 (clinically visible lesion greater than 4 cm not invading beyond the uterus) patients. However, PET/CT generally has the most value in stage IIA2 or higher patients (clinically visible lesion greater than 4 cm, invading beyond the uterus) as the sensitivity is low and clinical impact minimal in earlier stages.[7,8,9] The primary value of PET/CT is in para-aortic nodal staging in patients with locally advanced cervical cancer (▶ Fig. 23.1, ▶ Fig. 23.2). In particular, PET/CT performs best in patients with a relatively high prevalence of para-aortic nodal metastases (> 15%).[8]

Data from the National Oncologic PET Registry[10] indicated that FDG PET resulted in a change in management in 32.7% of patients with cervical cancer, with an imaging-adjusted impact of 11.9%.

Nodal metastases in patients with locally advanced cervical cancer (along with tumor volume and clinical stage) are the strongest prognostic factor for survival. Pelvic nodes are involved in 30 to 50% of cases, and para-aortic nodes are involved in 10 to 15% of cases.[11] While the pelvic nodes are routinely included in radiation fields, extension of the radiation fields to the para-aortic nodes is associated with increased morbidity. Para-aortic nodes can be staged surgically or by imaging. PET/CT can be a valuable tool in staging if it can preclude invasive surgical staging. PET is particularly useful for evaluating disease in para-aortic nodes when CT and MRI do not demonstrate adenopathy, or when only pelvic adenopathy is demonstrated.[12]

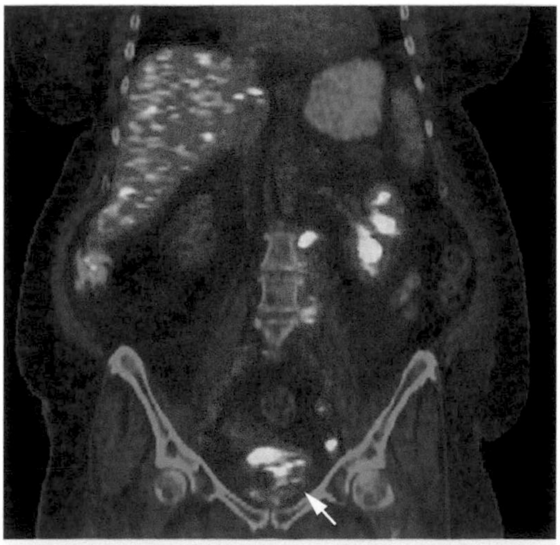

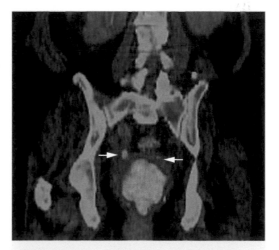

Fig. 23.1 Metastatic cervical cancer. Coronal PET/CT scan demonstrates uptake in a primary cervical carcinoma (*arrow*) with multiple pelvic and retroperitoneal nodal metastases.

Fig. 23.2 Primary cervical cancer with pelvic nodal metastases. Coronal PET/CT demonstrate intense uptake in a primary cervical cancer with pelvic nodal metastases (*arrows*). Given the location of these nodal metastases, ureteral activity if present could potentially decrease sensitivity. (Courtesy of Bruce Higginbotham, MD, Seattle, WA.)

Potential strategies have been proposed for the use of PET/CT in staging cervical cancer.[8,11] The high true-positive rate of PET/CT suggests that surgical staging is unnecessary if the para-aortic nodes are PET positive (or distant metastases are identified). However, surgical staging could be considered in the rare cases where para-aortic nodes are positive but pelvic nodes are negative.

The overall false-negative rate of PET/CT for para-aortic nodal involvement is around 12%, rising to 22% if there is pelvic nodal uptake. Thus, staging surgery should generally be performed in patients with pelvic nodal uptake but no para-aortic nodal uptake. However, if pelvic nodal uptake is absent, the false-negative rate for para-aortic nodal metastases decreases to approximately 9% and the benefit of staging surgery is debatable.[13,14]

Prognosis. SUV ≥ 3.3 in para-aortic lymph nodes is a negative prognostic factor.[15] Increased uptake in lymph nodes on PET even when CT is negative is associated with poor prognosis.[16]

Accuracy/Comparison to Other Modalities

1. **Overall nodal disease** (meta-analysis)[17]: sensitivity of 82% and specificity of 95%.
2. **Para-aortic nodes** (meta-analysis)[8]: sensitivity of 34% (range: 10–72%); specificity of 97% (range: 93–99%):
   a) While the specificity for para-aortic nodal metastases is consistently high, the sensitivity is low and heterogeneous.
3. **CT and MRI.** In a meta-analysis,[17] PET and PET/CT had an overall higher diagnostic performance than CT or MRI in detecting lymph node metastases. There is conflicting evidence on the relative accuracy of PET and MRI for pelvic nodal metastases.[18] One report indicates that PET/CT is more sensitive than MRI for pelvic nodal metastases, but there is no difference in specificity.[19] However, PET is more accurate than MRI for para-aortic nodal metastases.[18]
   Lymph node metastases in cervical cancer (meta-analysis; ▶ Table 23.1).[17]

Table 23.1 Sensitivity and specificity of PET versus CT and MRI for detection of lymph node metastases from cervical cancer

	Sensitivity %	Specificity %
PET	82	95
CT	50	92
MRI	56	891

4. **Early-stage cervical cancer.**
   PET and PET/CT have low to moderate sensitivity but high specificity for the lymph nodes metastases in early-stage cervical cancer. PET has a sensitivity of 53% and specificity of 90% for pelvic lymph node metastases in early-stage (IA–IIA) cervical cancer. The sensitivity for para-aortic nodes is even lower (25%).[20] Therefore, PET may have limited value in early-stage cervical cancer if MRI is negative.[21] PET/CT performs considerably better in early cervical cancer staging, with a sensitivity of 73% and specificity of 97%.[22]

Pearls

1. **Pattern of spread.** Cervical cancer typically spreads through three lymphatic pathways in the pelvis: along the external and internal iliac vessels and presacral along the uterosacral ligament. These pathways drain into the common iliac nodes, para-aortic nodes, and left supraclavicular nodes. An important site to evaluate is the left supraclavicular region, as metastases to this region are associated with poor prognosis. Occult supraclavicular nodal metastases have been identified by PET in 8% of patients. Hematogenous spread, most commonly to the lung, liver, and bones, is rare and unlikely in the absence of pelvic nodal involvement.[23]
2. **Urinary activity.** Minimizing the effects of radioactive urine in the bladder and ureters is important in cervical cancer as the specific areas of concern are the pelvic and para-aortic nodes (▶ Fig. 23.2).
3. **Dual-time imaging.** Dual-time imaging (an additional delayed 3-hour scan) increases accuracy in para-aortic lymph nodes, particularly inferior para-aortic nodes.[22]

Pitfalls

1. In patients with early-stage disease, most of the false-negative results will be seen in the pelvis.
2. In patients with advanced stages of disease, more false-negative results will be noted in para-aortic nodes.
3. Lymphangiography can cause false-positive nodal uptake.[24]
4. A short axis diameter greater than 0.5 cm is the size threshold for accurate identification of metastatic lymph nodes from cervical cancer by PET/CT.[22]

5. Isolated mediastinal nodal uptake is often a false-positive finding.[25]

23.1.3 Recurrence

NCCN guidelines[6] state that in patients at high risk for locoregional (central or para-aortic) failure, a PET/CT scan at 3 to 6 months after chemoradiation may be useful for detecting early or asymptomatic disease that is potentially curable. In one review,[26] the recommended timing of PET/CT was 3 months after radiation.

One analysis[27] suggests that in patients with locally advanced disease treated with chemoradiotherapy, the use of PET/CT after 3 months to triage to completion hysterectomy may be a cost-effective alternative to routine surveillance.

Limited data suggest that PET is more sensitive than conventional imaging for recurrent cervical cancer. PET might be best employed in patients with better prognoses (e.g., determined by squamous cell carcinoma antigen [SCC Ag] levels and symptoms) and possibility of salvage therapies. In these patients, accurate determination of recurrence location can help decide between salvage therapy and chemoradiation.[28,29]

Accuracy/Comparison to Other Modalities

1. **PET/CT** (meta-analysis)[30]: sensitivity of 92% and specificity of 88%.
2. **Locoregional recurrence** (PET and PET/CT; meta-analysis)[31]: sensitivity of 82% and specificity of 98%.
3. **Distant metastases** (PET and PET/CT; meta-analysis): sensitivity of 87% and specificity of 97%.
4. **Body region:** The sensitivity for recurrence is poor in the lung, retrovesical, and para-aortic lymph nodes.[32]
5. **CT/MRI:** PET is more sensitive than CT/MRI, but there is no difference in specificity:
   a) PET is more sensitive than CT/MRI for metastases (89 vs. 39%), but there is no difference in local lesion detection.[29]

Pearls

1. **Symptoms.** PET/CT is more useful for the detection of recurrence in symptomatic patients. In one report, the true-positive rate in asymptomatic patients was 44% compared to 71% in symptomatic patients.[33]

2. **Squamous carcinoma antigen.** PET is useful to detect recurrence if serum squamous carcinoma antigen is elevated.[34] PET/CT is more accurate in patients with SCC Ag elevation than in patients with carcinoembryonic antigen elevation.[35] A negative PET usually indicates absence of disease in patients with SCC Ag elevation.[36]

Pitfalls

Focal rectal activity on PET is a possible cause of false-positive results for recurrent local disease.

23.1.4 Therapy Response/ Prognosis

PET/CT is useful in estimating disease-free survival, overall survival, and time to recurrence. In a meta-analysis,[37] patients with a high SUVmax in the primary tumor or metastatic pelvic or para-aortic lymph nodes had a worse prognosis, with more adverse events and lower survival. The risk of disease recurrence increases on the basis of the most distant level of nodal involvement identified on PET. For example, the hazard ratio is 2.4 with pelvic nodal involvement, and 30.3 for supraclavicular nodal involvement.[38] Preoperative intratumoral FDG uptake heterogeneity is associated with increased risk of recurrence.[39]

In a meta-analysis,[40] metabolic response to therapy was capable of predicting event- and disease-free survival.

Therapy Response

a) **Radiotherapy effect.**[41] Following irradiation, increased FDG activity is common from inflammation and therefore increased FDG activity is sensitive but nonspecific for active tumor.
b) **Neoadjuvant chemotherapy.**[42] Decrease in standardized uptake value (SUV) correlates better with histological response than MRI in patients undergoing neoadjuvant therapy prior to radical hysterectomy.

Prognosis

a) **Pretherapy.** A visual grading system that incorporates the primary tumor size, its shape, the degree of nonuniformity of FDG uptake, and the level of pelvic or para-aortic nodal involvement by PET can estimate prognosis.[43]

b) **Posttherapy.** Persistent FDG uptake following therapy, particularly in para-aortic nodes, is a strong predictor of poor prognosis.[44]

23.2 Ovarian Cancer

23.2.1 Ovarian Masses

PET has little role as a primary modality in the evaluation of primary ovarian masses.[1,2]

1. PET employed alone results in a substantial number of false-positive and false-negative results. While benign tumors typically have faint uptake, endometriomas, fibromas, and teratomas often have mild to moderate uptake. While malignant tumors typically have intense uptake, tumors with a small solid component can have minimal uptake.[45] Among malignant tumors, uptake is lower in mucinous and clear cell adenocarcinomas compared to other subtypes.[46,47]

2. In a meta-analysis, PET alone did not perform as well as CT, MRI, or ultrasound[48] in identifying suspicious ovarian masses. However, in one study,[49] PET/CT had a higher accuracy than CT, MRI, or ultrasound in distinguishing malignant/borderline from benign ovarian tumors. While PET/CT has a reasonably high diagnostic value in differentiating between malignant and benign ovarian tumors[50,51] as well as in distinguishing borderline ovarian tumors from stage 1 malignant ovarian tumors.[52] There is less diagnostic accuracy in distinguishing borderline and benign tumors. However, PET can complement the results of ultrasound and/or MRI findings and improve the overall accuracy of diagnostic imaging in patients with ovarian masses.

Accuracy/Comparison to Other Modalities

Preoperative Identification of Suspicious Adnexal Masses (▶ Table 23.2)[48]

Table 23.2 Sensitivity and specificity of PET versus ultrasound, MRI, and CT for preoperative identification of suspicious adnexal masses

	Sensitivity %	Specificity %
PET	67	79
US	85	87
MRI	92	88
CT	87	84

Pearls

1. **Standardized uptake value (SUV).** There is no established SUV threshold for distinguishing malignant from benign ovarian lesions: published values range from 3.25 to 7.9.[53,54]

2. **Visual threshold.** One arbitrary visual threshold for malignancy includes any uptake equal to or greater than that of the liver.

3. **Postmenopausal uptake.** Ovarian uptake in the postmenopausal woman is much more worrisome than in a premenopausal woman, and malignancy should be strongly suspected.[54]

Pitfalls

1. **False negatives.** Borderline tumors, early-stage ovarian carcinomas, mucinous, and clear cell adenocarcinomas.

2. **False positives:**
   a) Inflammatory processes, endometriomas, benign cystic lesions (e.g., corpus luteum cyst, dermoid cyst, serous cyst), thecoma, physiological uptake.
   b) In premenopausal women, physiologic ovarian uptake is most common around ovulation and during the early luteal phase of the menstrual cycle.[55] Physiologic ovarian uptake can be minimized by scheduling PET just after menstruation.
   Bowel or iliac node activity on PET can sometimes be difficult to differentiate from ovarian activity (▶ Fig. 11.15).

23.2.2 Initial Staging

The primary role of PET is in detection and restaging of recurrent disease rather than in initial staging. The primary role of PET in initial staging is in the detection of extra-abdominal disease, in particular supradiaphragmatic lymph nodes, where it is more accurate than CT.[56,57] A substantial number of patients are upstaged from International Federation of Gynecology and Obstetrics (FIGO) stage III (peritoneum and/or retroperitoneal lymph node involvement) to stage IV (distant disease outside the peritoneum).[58,59] Potentially, PET/CT could be helpful in selecting patients for neoadjuvant chemotherapy. However, PET/CT is currently of unclear clinical utility in this setting, as PET/CT-upstaged patients have a similar prognosis,[58] and PET/CT factors such as SUVmax may not be prognostic variables for complete cytoreduction after primary surgery.[60]

23.2.3 Recurrence

NCCN guidelines[61] indicate that PET/CT can be considered for both monitoring/follow-up and suspicion of recurrent disease.

1. **Cost-effectiveness**. In a cost-effectiveness analysis,[62] in patients with suspected recurrence of ovarian cancer, a CT-only strategy was compared to two PET/CT strategies: PET/CT for negative CT and PET/CT for all. The PET/CT for all strategy was the most cost-effective. While PET/CT for all was more expensive, management was altered in 62% of patients (compared to 31% for PET/CT for negative CT), and more surgeries were avoided.

2. Data from the National Oncologic PET Registry[10] indicated that FDG PET resulted in a change in management in 41.4% of patients with ovarian cancer, with an imaging-adjusted impact of 16.2%.

3. **Second-look laparotomy**. While PET is accurate in the diagnosis of ovarian cancer recurrence (particularly if used in conjunction with conventional imaging techniques), it is still limited because a second-look laparotomy is still necessary if recurrence is strongly suspected. The sensitivity of PET for small-volume disease (< 1 cm) is low compared to second-look laparotomy.[63] In spite of this, PET can change management due to its high positive predictive value[64,65]:

   a) A positive PET scan can preclude the need for invasive surgical assessment.

   b) Tumor deposits large enough to be identified by PET may be considered for surgical resection since these lesions may not respond to chemotherapy.

   c) The small lesions that are missed by PET may be responsive to chemotherapy.

4. **CA-125**. PET is most useful when conventional imaging is inconclusive and CA-125 is elevated. However, there is some evidence[66,67] that PET/CT is valuable even in cases where CA-125 is normal, with a slightly higher sensitivity than CT in these cases:

   a) PET sensitivity is high if there is clinical suspicion of recurrence, particularly if this suspicion is based upon rising CA-125 levels:
   • PET has the highest yield if used when CA-125 is 30 U/mL or greater.[68]

   b) Sensitivity is lower if PET is used in patients who are judged to be disease free based on clinical assessment. However, in a minority of patients with a normal CA-125, recurrence will be identified only with PET.[69]

   c) The sensitivity of combined PET and CA-125 is high (98%).[69]

5. **Prognosis.** There is limited evidence as to the prognostic value of PET in suspected recurrent ovarian cancer. There are conflicting data as to whether semiquantitative metabolic parameters, such as SUVmax, are prognostic factors.[70,71] Patients with localized or no disease identified by PET may have improved survival,[72,73] but CA125 may be more useful for prognosis than PET.[72]

Accuracy/Comparison to Other Modalities

1. **PET/CT** (meta-analysis)[74]: sensitivity of 89% and specificity of 90%.

2. **Clinical situation.** The accuracy of PET depends upon the clinical situation:

   a) *Clinical suspicion of recurrence:* sensitivity of 90% and specificity of 86%.

   b) *Rising CA-125, negative conventional imaging:* sensitivity of 96% and specificity of 80%.

   c) *Negative conventional imaging and CA-125:* sensitivity of 54% and specificity of 73%.

3. PET is most useful when interpreted in conjunction with conventional imaging modalities (CT, MRI)[64]:

   a) The accuracy increases from 79 to 94% when PET is interpreted in conjunction with conventional imaging modalities.[64]

   b) PET is more specific than CT (94 vs. 77%).[75]

4. **Body region**:

   a) *Lymph nodes* (meta-analysis)[76]:
   • Sensitivity: PET and PET/CT, 73%; CT, 43%; MRI, 55%.
   • Specificity: PET and PET/CT, 97%; CT, 95%; MRI, 88%.

   b) *Retroperitoneal nodes.* In ovarian cancer patients, PET is more sensitive in the retroperitoneum than in the peritoneum.[77] However, the sensitivity of PET/CT for isolated retroperitoneal nodal disease is only 41%, with a specificity of 94%.[78] Thus, regional lymphadenectomy may still be necessary with a negative PET study, but PET has a high positive predictive value for retroperitoneal nodal disease with negative or equivocal CT findings.

   c) *Peritoneal metastases*. The majority of published reports[79,80,81] conclude that PET/CT is more sensitive than CT for peritoneal metastases, although a few reports[82,83]

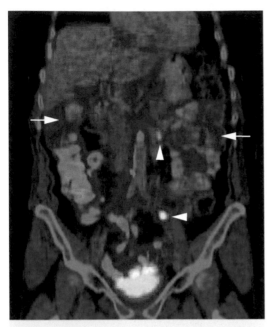

Fig. 23.3 Metastatic ovarian cancer. Coronal PET/CT demonstrates both nodal (*arrowheads*) and peritoneal (*arrows*) metastases from ovarian cancer. PET has better sensitivity for nodal metastases than peritoneal metastases in ovarian cancer. (Courtesy of Carolyn Meltzer MD, Pittsburg, PA.)

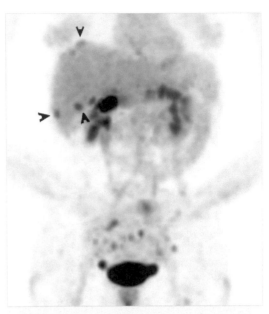

Fig. 23.4 Metastatic ovarian cancer. Coronal PET scan in a patient with ovarian cancer demonstrates multiple serosal metastases around the liver (*arrowheads*) as well as multiple pelvic peritoneal metastases. (Courtesy of Ronald Korn, MD, PhD, Scottsdale, AZ.)

indicate the accuracy is comparable. In one report,[83] PET/CT and MRI had comparable accuracy, although MRI had the higher sensitivity and PET/CT the higher specificity. PET is more sensitive for lymph node metastases than peritoneal metastases (▶ Fig. 23.3, ▶ Fig. 23.4, ▶ Fig. 23.5). With PET/CT, lesions as small as 0.5 cm can be detected,[65] but even with PET/CT imaging, sensitivity for peritoneal metastases less than 1 cm is low.[75]

- Sensitivity is lowest in certain areas in the peritoneal cavity (the right upper abdomen, the small bowel mesentery, and the pelvis).[65]

Pearls

1. It is important to understand the classic patterns of peritoneal spread when evaluating patients with ovarian cancer (see Chapter 11).
2. Supradiaphragmatic lymph node metastases are identified by PET/CT in a substantial number of cases,[56] both in initial staging and in restaging for recurrence. Initial spread is often to the

cardiophrenic lymph nodes, continuing to parasternal lymph nodes.

Pitfalls

Diffuse peritoneal carcinomatosis (▶ Fig. 23.5; ▶ Fig. 11.11) may not cause focal lesions and could be interpreted as a falsely negative study if windowed incorrectly.

23.2.4 Therapy Response

Limited data suggest that PET is useful for early prediction of response to neoadjuvant chemotherapy. Sequential PET studies after the first cycle of neoadjuvant chemotherapy may be more accurate than clinical or histopathological response criteria, including CA-125, in predicting response and survival.[84]

23.3 Endometrial Cancer

NCCN guidelines[85] state that PET/CT can be considered for both staging and follow-up/surveillance of patients with endometrial cancer if metastases are suspected.

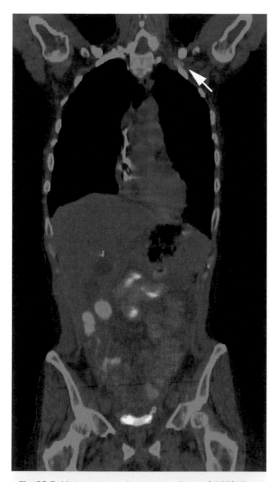

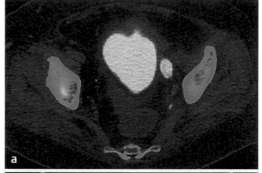

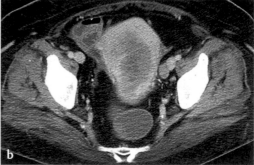

Fig. 23.6 Endometrial carcinoma. Axial PET/CT **(a)** and contrast-enhanced CT **(b)** demonstrates a large endometrial carcinoma with metastases to left external iliac lymph nodes.

Fig. 23.5 Metastatic ovarian cancer. Coronal PET/CT demonstrates extensive peritoneal carcinomatosis secondary to ovarian cancer. This carcinomatosis has both a focal soft tissue component in the central omentum and a diffuse fluid component (not the poor visualization of the inferior border of the liver). There is also a left supraclavicular node metastasis (*arrow*).

The primary tumor is visible on PET in the majority of cases (▶ Fig. 23.6).[86] PET may be helpful for further evaluating equivocal extrauterine lesions seen on CT or MRI. PET may be more useful in primary advanced (stage III or IV) cancer.[87] Data from the National Oncologic PET Registry[10] indicated that FDG PET resulted in a change in management in 36.5% of patients with uterine cancer, with an imaging-adjusted impact of 15.1%.

PET also has prognostic value. In a systematic review,[88] preoperative SUVmax of the primary tumor was an independent prognostic marker for recurrence and death. High FDG uptake has also been reported to predict deep myometrial invasion, cervical stromal invasion, and lymph node metastases.[89]

There is limited data on the applications of FDG PET/CT for other uterine tumors, such as leiomyosarcoma (▶ Fig. 23.7).

23.3.1 Accuracy

1. **Primary tumor** (meta-analysis)[90]: sensitivity of 82% and specificity of 90%.
2. **Preoperative assessment of lymph nodes metastases** (meta-analysis)[91]: sensitivity of 72% and specificity of 94%.
   a) PET/CT is more sensitive than CT or MRI for lymph node metastases from endometrial cancer. In two studies,[92,93] PET/CT had a substantially higher sensitivity (79 vs. 52% and 74 vs. 59%) than MRI. In both studies, MRI and PET/CT had comparably high specificities. In a prospective multicenter trial[94] of patients with high-risk endometrial cancer, the addition of PET to diagnostic CT significantly increased sensitivity for

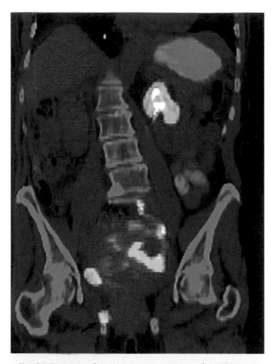

Fig. 23.7 Uterine leiomyosarcoma. Coronal PET/CT demonstrates increased uptake in an uterine leiomyosarcoma with an osseous metastasis (*arrow*).

detection of lymph node metastases in both the abdomen and pelvis (65% compared to 48–50% for CT alone), while maintaining specificity. However, sensitivity is poor for lymph node metastases less than 1 cm.[45]

3. **Distant metastases** (meta-analysis)[90]: sensitivity of 96% and specificity of 95%.

4. **Recurrence** (meta-analysis)[91]: sensitivity of 95% and specificity of 91%.

   a) In posttherapy surveillance, PET may be more accurate than CT or MRI[87,95] and is helpful in both suspected recurrence and detection of asymptomatic recurrent disease.[96] In one report,[97] PET/CT had a higher specificity than conventional imaging (CT and MRI: 96 vs. 62%) with comparable sensitivity (89 vs. 85%).

Pearls

Unlike cervical cancer, endometrial cancer can metastasize to para-aortic and para-caval nodes without pelvic node involvement.

References

[1] Dehdashti F, Siegel BA. Evaluation of breast and gynecologic cancers by positron emission tomography. Semin Roentgenol. 2002; 37(2):151–168

[2] Zimny M, Siggelkow W. Positron emission tomography scanning in gynecologic and breast cancers. Curr Opin Obstet Gynecol. 2003; 15(1):69–75

[3] Belhocine T, Thille A, Fridman V, et al. Contribution of whole-body 18FDG PET imaging in the management of cervical cancer. Gynecol Oncol. 2002; 87(1):90–97

[4] Mirpour S, Mhlanga JC, Logeswaran P, Russo G, Mercier G, Subramaniam RM. The role of PET/CT in the management of cervical cancer. AJR Am J Roentgenol. 2013; 201(2):W192–W205

[5] Kidd EA, Siegel BA, Dehdashti F, Grigsby PW. The standardized uptake value for F-18 fluorodeoxyglucose is a sensitive predictive biomarker for cervical cancer treatment response and survival. Cancer. 2007; 110(8):1738–1744

[6] Koh WJ, Greer BE, Abu-Rustum NR, et al. Cervical cancer, version 2.2015. J Natl Compr Canc Netw. 2015; 13(4):395–404, quiz 404

[7] Bansal V, Damania K, Sharma AR. Fluorodeoxyglucose positron emission tomography-computed tomography in evaluation of pelvic and para-aortic nodal involvement in early stage and operable cervical cancer: comparison with surgicopathological findings. Indian J Nucl Med. 2011; 26(4):177–180

[8] Kang S, Kim SK, Chung DC, et al. Diagnostic value of (18)F-FDG PET for evaluation of paraaortic nodal metastasis in patients with cervical carcinoma: a metaanalysis. J Nucl Med. 2010; 51(3):360–367

[9] Signorelli M, Guerra L, Montanelli L, et al. Preoperative staging of cervical cancer: is 18-FDG-PET/CT really effective in patients with early stage disease? Gynecol Oncol. 2011; 123(2):236–240

[10] Hillner BE, Siegel BA, Shields AF, et al. Relationship between cancer type and impact of PET and PET/CT on intended management: findings of the national oncologic PET registry. J Nucl Med. 2008; 49(12):1928–1935

[11] Gouy S, Morice P, Narducci F, et al. Nodal-staging surgery for locally advanced cervical cancer in the era of PET. Lancet Oncol. 2012; 13(5):e212–e220

[12] Lin WC, Hung YC, Yeh LS, Kao CH, Yen RF, Shen YY. Usefulness of (18)F-fluorodeoxyglucose positron emission tomography to detect para-aortic lymph nodal metastasis in advanced cervical cancer with negative computed tomography findings. Gynecol Oncol. 2003; 89(1):73–76

[13] Margulies AL, Peres A, Barranger E, et al. Selection of patients with advanced-stage cervical cancer for para-aortic lymphadenectomy in the era of PET/CT. Anticancer Res. 2013; 33(1):283–286

[14] Takayanagi I, Goromaru N, Koike K, et al. Interaction of newly synthesized N-cyclopropylmethyl derivatives of (-)-6 beta-acetylthionormorphine with opioid receptors. Gen Pharmacol. 1990; 21(4):541–546

[15] Yen TC, See LC, Lai CH, et al. Standardized uptake value in para-aortic lymph nodes is a significant prognostic factor in patients with primary advanced squamous cervical cancer. Eur J Nucl Med Mol Imaging. 2008; 35(3):493–501

[16] Grigsby PW, Siegel BA, Dehdashti F. Lymph node staging by positron emission tomography in patients with carcinoma of the cervix. J Clin Oncol. 2001; 19(17):3745–3749

[17] Choi HJ, Ju W, Myung SK, Kim Y. Diagnostic performance of computer tomography, magnetic resonance imaging, and positron emission tomography or positron emission tomog-

raphy/computer tomography for detection of metastatic lymph nodes in patients with cervical cancer: meta-analysis. Cancer Sci. 2010; 101(6):1471–1479

[18] Monteil J, Maubon A, Leobon S, et al. Lymph node assessment with (18)F-FDG-PET and MRI in uterine cervical cancer. Anticancer Res. 2011; 31(11):3865–3871

[19] Choi HJ, Roh JW, Seo SS, et al. Comparison of the accuracy of magnetic resonance imaging and positron emission tomography/computed tomography in the presurgical detection of lymph node metastases in patients with uterine cervical carcinoma: a prospective study. Cancer. 2006; 106(4):914–922

[20] Wright JD, Dehdashti F, Herzog TJ, et al. Preoperative lymph node staging of early-stage cervical carcinoma by [18F]-fluoro-2-deoxy-D-glucose-positron emission tomography. Cancer. 2005; 104(11):2484–2491

[21] Chou HH, Chang TC, Yen TC, et al. Low value of [18F]-fluoro-2-deoxy-D-glucose positron emission tomography in primary staging of early-stage cervical cancer before radical hysterectomy. J Clin Oncol. 2006; 24(1):123–128

[22] Sironi S, Buda A, Picchio M, et al. Lymph node metastasis in patients with clinical early-stage cervical cancer: detection with integrated FDG PET/CT. Radiology. 2006; 238(1):272–279

[23] Grant P, Sakellis C, Jacene HA. Gynecologic oncologic imaging with PET/CT. Semin Nucl Med. 2014; 44(6):461–478

[24] Reinhardt MJ, Ehritt-Braun C, Vogelgesang D, et al. Metastatic lymph nodes in patients with cervical cancer: detection with MR imaging and FDG PET. Radiology. 2001; 218(3):776–782

[25] Onal C, Oymak E, Findikcioglu A, Reyhan M. Isolated mediastinal lymph node false positivity of [18F]-fluorodeoxyglucose-positron emission tomography/computed tomography in patients with cervical cancer. Int J Gynecol Cancer. 2013; 23(2):337–342

[26] Amit A, Person O, Keidar Z. FDG PET/CT in monitoring response to treatment in gynecological malignancies. Curr Opin Obstet Gynecol. 2013; 25(1):17–22

[27] Phippen NT, Havrilesky LJ, Barnett JC, Hamilton CA, Stany MP, Lowery WJ. Does routine posttreatment PET/CT add value to the care of women with locally advanced cervical cancer? Int J Gynecol Cancer. 2016; 26(5):944–950

[28] Belhocine TZ. 18F-FDG PET imaging in posttherapy monitoring of cervical cancers: from diagnosis to prognosis. J Nucl Med. 2004; 45(10):1602–1604

[29] Yen TC, See LC, Chang TC, et al. Defining the priority of using 18F-FDG PET for recurrent cervical cancer. J Nucl Med. 2004; 45(10):1632–1639

[30] Meads C, Auguste P, Davenport C, et al. Positron emission tomography/computerised tomography imaging in detecting and managing recurrent cervical cancer: systematic review of evidence, elicitation of subjective probabilities and economic modelling. Health Technol Assess. 2013; 17(12):1–323

[31] Chu Y, Zheng A, Wang F, et al. Diagnostic value of 18F-FDG-PET or PET-CT in recurrent cervical cancer: a systematic review and meta-analysis. Nucl Med Commun. 2014; 35(2):144–150

[32] Ryu SY, Kim MH, Choi SC, Choi CW, Lee KH. Detection of early recurrence with 18F-FDG PET in patients with cervical cancer. J Nucl Med. 2003; 44(3):347–352

[33] Mittra E, El-Maghraby T, Rodriguez CA, et al. Efficacy of 18F-FDG PET/CT in the evaluation of patients with recurrent cervical carcinoma. Eur J Nucl Med Mol Imaging. 2009; 36(12):1952–1959

[34] Chang TC, Law KS, Hong JH, et al. Positron emission tomography for unexplained elevation of serum squamous cell carcinoma antigen levels during follow-up for patients with cervical malignancies: a phase II study. Cancer. 2004; 101(1):164–171

[35] Chong A, Ha JM, Jeong SY, et al. Clinical usefulness of (18)F-FDG PET/CT in the detection of early recurrence in treated cervical cancer patients with unexplained elevation of serum tumor markers. Chonnam Med J. 2013; 49(1):20–26

[36] Jao MS, Chang TC, Chang HP, Wu TI, Chao A, Lai CH. Long-term follow up of cervical cancer patients with unexplained squamous cell carcinoma antigen elevation after post-therapy surveillance using positron emission tomography. J Obstet Gynaecol Res. 2010; 36(5):1003–1008

[37] Sarker A, Im HJ, Cheon GJ, et al. Prognostic implications of the SUVmax of primary tumors and metastatic lymph node measured by 18F-FDG PET in patients with uterine cervical cancer: a meta-analysis. Clin Nucl Med. 2016; 41(1):34–40

[38] Kidd EA, Siegel BA, Dehdashti F, et al. Lymph node staging by positron emission tomography in cervical cancer: relationship to prognosis. J Clin Oncol. 2010; 28(12):2108–2113

[39] Chung HH, Kang SY, Ha S, et al. Prognostic value of preoperative intratumoral FDG uptake heterogeneity in early stage uterine cervical cancer. J Gynecol Oncol. 2016; 27(2):e15

[40] Zhao Q, Feng Y, Mao X, Qie M. Prognostic value of fluorine-18-fluorodeoxyglucose positron emission tomography or PET-computed tomography in cervical cancer: a meta-analysis. Int J Gynecol Cancer. 2013; 23(7):1184–1190

[41] Nakamoto Y, Eisbruch A, Achtyes ED, et al. Prognostic value of positron emission tomography using F-18-fluorodeoxyglucose in patients with cervical cancer undergoing radiotherapy. Gynecol Oncol. 2002; 84(2):289–295

[42] Yoshida Y, Kurokawa T, Kawahara K, et al. Metabolic monitoring of advanced uterine cervical cancer neoadjuvant chemotherapy by using [F-18]-Fluorodeoxyglucose positron emission tomography: preliminary results in three patients. Gynecol Oncol. 2004; 95(3):597–602

[43] Miller TR, Pinkus E, Dehdashti F, Grigsby PW. Improved prognostic value of 18F-FDG PET using a simple visual analysis of tumor characteristics in patients with cervical cancer. J Nucl Med. 2003; 44(2):192–197

[44] Grigsby PW, Siegel BA, Dehdashti F, Mutch DG. Posttherapy surveillance monitoring of cervical cancer by FDG-PET. Int J Radiat Oncol Biol Phys. 2003; 55(4):907–913

[45] Kitajima K, Ueno Y, Maeda T, et al. Spectrum of fluorodeoxyglucose-positron emission tomography/computed tomography and magnetic resonance imaging findings of ovarian tumors. Jpn J Radiol. 2011; 29(9):605–608

[46] Tanizaki Y, Kobayashi A, Shiro M, et al. Diagnostic value of preoperative SUVmax on FDG-PET/CT for the detection of ovarian cancer. Int J Gynecol Cancer. 2014; 24(3):454–460

[47] Tsuboyama T, Tatsumi M, Onishi H, et al. Assessment of combination of contrast-enhanced magnetic resonance imaging and positron emission tomography/computed tomography for evaluation of ovarian masses. Invest Radiol. 2014; 49(8):524–531

[48] Dodge JE, Covens AL, Lacchetti C, et al. Gynecology Cancer Disease Site Group. Preoperative identification of a suspicious adnexal mass: a systematic review and meta-analysis. Gynecol Oncol. 2012; 126(1):157–166

[49] Nam EJ, Yun MJ, Oh YT, et al. Diagnosis and staging of primary ovarian cancer: correlation between PET/CT, Doppler US, and CT or MRI. Gynecol Oncol. 2010; 116(3):389–394

[50] Kitajima K, Suzuki K, Senda M, et al. FDG-PET/CT for diagnosis of primary ovarian cancer. Nucl Med Commun. 2011; 32(7):549–553

[51] Yamamoto Y, Oguri H, Yamada R, Maeda N, Kohsaki S, Fukaya T. Preoperative evaluation of pelvic masses with combined 18F-fluorodeoxyglucose positron emission tomography and computed tomography. Int J Gynaecol Obstet. 2008; 102(2):124–127

[52] Kim C, Chung HH, Oh SW, Kang KW, Chung JK, Lee DS. differential diagnosis of borderline ovarian tumors from stage i malignant ovarian tumors using FDG PET/CT. Nucl Med Mol Imaging. 2013; 47(2):81–88

[53] Hubner KF, McDonald TW, Niethammer JG, Smith GT, Gould HR, Buonocore E. Assessment of primary and metastatic ovarian cancer by positron emission tomography (PET) using 2-[18F]deoxyglucose (2-[18F]FDG). Gynecol Oncol. 1993; 51 (2):197–204

[54] Lerman H, Metser U, Grisaru D, Fishman A, Lievshitz G, Even-Sapir E. Normal and abnormal 18F-FDG endometrial and ovarian uptake in pre- and postmenopausal patients: assessment by PET/CT. J Nucl Med. 2004; 45(2):266–271

[55] Kim SK, Kang KW, Roh JW, Sim JS, Lee ES, Park SY. Incidental ovarian 18F-FDG accumulation on PET: correlation with the menstrual cycle. Eur J Nucl Med Mol Imaging. 2005; 32(7): 757–763

[56] Hynninen J, Auranen A, Carpén O, et al. FDG PET/CT in staging of advanced epithelial ovarian cancer: frequency of supradiaphragmatic lymph node metastasis challenges the traditional pattern of disease spread. Gynecol Oncol. 2012; 126 (1):64–68

[57] Hynninen J, Kemppainen J, Lavonius M, et al. A prospective comparison of integrated FDG-PET/contrast-enhanced CT and contrast-enhanced CT for pretreatment imaging of advanced epithelial ovarian cancer. Gynecol Oncol. 2013; 131 (2):389–394

[58] Fruscio R, Sina F, Dolci C, et al. Preoperative 18F-FDG PET/CT in the management of advanced epithelial ovarian cancer. Gynecol Oncol. 2013; 131(3):689–693

[59] Risum S, Høgdall C, Loft A, et al. Does the use of diagnostic PET/CT cause stage migration in patients with primary advanced ovarian cancer? Gynecol Oncol. 2010; 116(3):395–398

[60] Risum S, Loft A, Høgdall C, et al. Standardized FDG uptake as a prognostic variable and as a predictor of incomplete cytoreduction in primary advanced ovarian cancer. Acta Oncol. 2011; 50(3):415–419

[61] Morgan RJ, Jr, Armstrong DK, Alvarez RD, et al. Ovarian cancer, version 1.2016, NCCN Clinical Practice Guidelines in Oncology. J Natl Compr Canc Netw. 2016; 14(9):1134–1163

[62] Mansueto M, Grimaldi A, Mangili G, et al. Positron emission tomography/computed tomography introduction in the clinical management of patients with suspected recurrence of ovarian cancer: a cost-effectiveness analysis. Eur J Cancer Care (Engl). 2009; 18(6):612–619

[63] Rose PG, Faulhaber P, Miraldi F, Abdul-Karim FW. Positive emission tomography for evaluating a complete clinical response in patients with ovarian or peritoneal carcinoma: correlation with second-look laparotomy. Gynecol Oncol. 2001; 82(1):17–21

[64] Nakamoto Y, Saga T, Ishimori T, et al. Clinical value of positron emission tomography with FDG for recurrent ovarian cancer. AJR Am J Roentgenol. 2001; 176(6):1449–1454

[65] Sironi S, Messa C, Mangili G, et al. Integrated FDG PET/CT in patients with persistent ovarian cancer: correlation with histologic findings. Radiology. 2004; 233(2):433–440

[66] Bhosale P, Peungjesada S, Wei W, et al. Clinical utility of positron emission tomography/computed tomography in the evaluation of suspected recurrent ovarian cancer in the setting of normal CA-125 levels. Int J Gynecol Cancer. 2010; 20 (6):936–944

[67] Evangelista L, Palma MD, Gregianin M, et al. Diagnostic and prognostic evaluation of fluorodeoxyglucose positron emission tomography/computed tomography and its correlation with serum cancer antigen-125 (CA125) in a large cohort of ovarian cancer patients. J Turk Ger Gynecol Assoc. 2015; 16 (3):137–144

[68] Menzel C, Döbert N, Hamscho N, et al. The influence of CA 125 and CEA levels on the results of (18)F-deoxyglucose positron emission tomography in suspected recurrence of epithelial ovarian cancer. Strahlenther Onkol. 2004; 180(8):497–501

[69] Murakami M, Miyamoto T, Iida T, et al. Whole-body positron emission tomography and tumor marker CA125 for detection of recurrence in epithelial ovarian cancer. Int J Gynecol Cancer. 2006; 16 Suppl 1:99–107

[70] Caobelli F, Alongi P, Evangelista L, et al. Young AIMN Working Group. Predictive value of (18)F-FDG PET/CT in restaging patients affected by ovarian carcinoma: a multicentre study. Eur J Nucl Med Mol Imaging. 2016; 43(3):404–413

[71] Kim CY, Jeong SY, Chong GO, et al. Quantitative metabolic parameters measured on F-18 FDG PET/CT predict survival after relapse in patients with relapsed epithelial ovarian cancer. Gynecol Oncol. 2015; 136(3):498–504

[72] Kurosaki H, Oriuchi N, Okazaki A, et al. Prognostic value of FDG-PET in patients with ovarian carcinoma following surgical treatment. Ann Nucl Med. 2006; 20(3):171–174

[73] Simcock B, Neesham D, Quinn M, Drummond E, Milner A, Hicks RJ. The impact of PET/CT in the management of recurrent ovarian cancer. Gynecol Oncol. 2006; 103(1):271–276

[74] Limei Z, Yong C, Yan X, Shuai T, Jiangyan X, Zhiqing L. Accuracy of positron emission tomography/computed tomography in the diagnosis and restaging for recurrent ovarian cancer: a meta-analysis. Int J Gynecol Cancer. 2013; 23(4): 598–607

[75] Pannu HK, Cohade C, Bristow RE, Fishman EK, Wahl RL. PET-CT detection of abdominal recurrence of ovarian cancer: radiologic-surgical correlation. Abdom Imaging. 2004; 29(3): 398–403

[76] Yuan Y, Gu ZX, Tao XF, Liu SY. Computer tomography, magnetic resonance imaging, and positron emission tomography or positron emission tomography/computer tomography for detection of metastatic lymph nodes in patients with ovarian cancer: a meta-analysis. Eur J Radiol. 2012; 81(5):1002–1006

[77] Drieskens O, Stroobants S, Gysen M, Vandenbosch G, Mortelmans L, Vergote I. Positron emission tomography with FDG in the detection of peritoneal and retroperitoneal metastases of ovarian cancer. Gynecol Obstet Invest. 2003; 55(3):130–134

[78] Bristow RE, Giuntoli RL, II, Pannu HK, Schulick RD, Fishman EK, Wahl RL. Combined PET/CT for detecting recurrent ovarian cancer limited to retroperitoneal lymph nodes. Gynecol Oncol. 2005; 99(2):294–300

[79] Kim HW, Won KS, Zeon SK, Ahn BC, Gayed IW. Peritoneal carcinomatosis in patients with ovarian cancer: enhanced CT versus 18F-FDG PET/CT. Clin Nucl Med. 2013; 38(2):93–97

[80] Panagiotidis E, Datseris IE, Exarhos D, Skilakaki M, Skoura E, Bamias A. High incidence of peritoneal implants in recurrence of intra-abdominal cancer revealed by 18F-FDG PET/CT in patients with increased tumor markers and negative findings on conventional imaging. Nucl Med Commun. 2012; 33 (4):431–438

[81] Rubini G, Altini C, Notaristefano A, et al. Role of 18F-FDG PET/CT in diagnosing peritoneal carcinomatosis in the restaging of patient with ovarian cancer as compared to contrast enhanced CT and tumor marker Ca-125. Rev Esp Med Nucl Imagen Mol. 2014; 33(1):22–27

[82] Funicelli L, Travaini LL, Landoni F, Trifirò G, Bonello L, Bellomi M. Peritoneal carcinomatosis from ovarian cancer: the role of CT and [18F]FDG-PET/CT. Abdom Imaging. 2010; 35(6):701–707

[83] Schmidt S, Meuli RA, Achtari C, Prior JO. Peritoneal carcinomatosis in primary ovarian cancer staging: comparison between MDCT, MRI, and 18F-FDG PET/CT. Clin Nucl Med. 2015; 40(5):371–377

[84] Avril N, Sassen S, Schmalfeldt B, et al. Prediction of response to neoadjuvant chemotherapy by sequential F-18-fluoro-deoxyglucose positron emission tomography in patients with advanced-stage ovarian cancer. J Clin Oncol. 2005; 23(30): 7445–7453

[85] Koh WJ, Greer BE, Abu-Rustum NR, et al. Uterine neoplasms, version 1.2014. J Natl Compr Canc Netw. 2014; 12(2):248–280

[86] Suzuki R, Miyagi E, Takahashi N, et al. Validity of positron emission tomography using fluoro-2-deoxyglucose for the preoperative evaluation of endometrial cancer. Int J Gynecol Cancer. 2007; 17(4):890–896

[87] Chao A, Chang TC, Ng KK, et al. 18F-FDG PET in the management of endometrial cancer. Eur J Nucl Med Mol Imaging. 2006; 33(1):36–44

[88] Ghooshkhanei H, Treglia G, Sabouri G, Davoodi R, Sadeghi R. Risk stratification and prognosis determination using (18)F-FDG PET imaging in endometrial cancer patients: a systematic review and meta-analysis. Gynecol Oncol. 2014; 132(3): 669–676

[89] Haldorsen IS, Salvesen HB. What is the best preoperative imaging for endometrial cancer? Curr Oncol Rep. 2016; 18 (4):25

[90] Kakhki VR, Shahriari S, Treglia G, et al. Diagnostic performance of fluorine 18 fluorodeoxyglucose positron emission tomography imaging for detection of primary lesion and staging of endometrial cancer patients: systematic review and meta-analysis of the literature. Int J Gynecol Cancer. 2013; 23(9):1536–1543

[91] Bollineni VR, Ytre-Hauge S, Bollineni-Balabay O, Salvesen HB, Haldorsen IS. High diagnostic value of 18F-FDG PET/CT in endometrial cancer: systematic review and meta-analysis of the literature. J Nucl Med. 2016; 57(6):879–885

[92] Antonsen SL, Jensen LN, Loft A, et al. MRI, PET/CT and ultrasound in the preoperative staging of endometrial cancer: a multicenter prospective comparative study. Gynecol Oncol. 2013; 128(2):300–308

[93] Kim HJ, Cho A, Yun M, Kim YT, Kang WJ. Comparison of FDG PET/CT and MRI in lymph node staging of endometrial cancer. Ann Nucl Med. 2016; 30(2):104–113

[94] Atri M, Zhang Z, Dehdashti F, et al. Utility of PET/CT to evaluate retroperitoneal lymph node metastasis in high-risk endometrial cancer: results of ACRIN 6671/GOG 0233 trial. Radiology. 2017; 283(2):450–459

[95] Saga T, Higashi T, Ishimori T, et al. Clinical value of FDG-PET in the follow up of post-operative patients with endometrial cancer. Ann Nucl Med. 2003; 17(3);197–203

[96] Belhocine T, De Barsy C, Hustinx R, Willems-Foidart J. Usefulness of (18)F-FDG PET in the post-therapy surveillance of endometrial carcinoma. Eur J Nucl Med Mol Imaging. 2002; 29 (9):1132–1139

[97] Sharma P, Kumar R, Singh H, et al. Carcinoma endometrium: role of 18-FDG PET/CT for detection of suspected recurrence. Clin Nucl Med. 2012; 37(7):649–655

24 Urological Tumors

Eugene C. Lin and Evan Sirc

24.1 Renal Cell Carcinoma[1]

24.1.1 Renal Masses

The role of PET in evaluation of renal masses is somewhat limited. Both solid and cystic renal masses can be evaluated. Renal masses are sometimes detected incidentally on PET images.

1. **Solid lesions.** FDG PET imaging is of limited value in solid lesions demonstrated by conventional imaging techniques since resection is usually necessary. In a systematic review,[2] the sensitivity for solid renal masses ranged from 22 to 77%, with low median SUVmax levels (2.6–2.9; ► Fig. 24.1). In addition, the sensitivity of fluorodeoxyglucose (FDG) PET is lower than that of CT.
2. **Indeterminate renal cysts:**
   a) A positive PET scan in an indeterminate renal cyst (► Fig. 24.2) is very specific for malignancy and further diagnostic tests such as cyst aspiration can be avoided before resection.[3]
   b) However, a negative PET scan does not completely rule out malignancy.
3. **Renal metastases:** Limited data suggest that PET can detect renal metastases.[4] Primary and metastatic renal tumors have a similar degree of FDG uptake.[5]

Accuracy/Comparison to Other Modalities

FDG PET is fairly specific for the diagnosis of malignancy in renal masses, but sensitivity will vary depending upon lesion size and location.

1. **PET and PET/CT for renal lesions** (meta-analysis)[6]: sensitivity of 62% and specificity of 88%.
2. **PET versus CT** (► Table 24.1).[7]

Table 24.1 Sensitivity and specificity of PET versus CT in the detection of renal tumors

	Sensitivity %	Specificity %
PET	60	100
CT	92	100

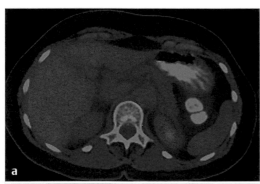
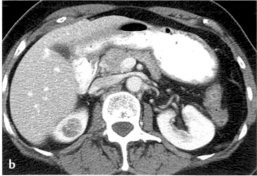

Fig. 24.1 Renal cell carcinoma. Axial PET/CT **(a)** and contrast-enhanced CT **(b)** demonstrate a clear cell carcinoma in the upper pole of the right kidney without increased fluorodeoxyglucose uptake.

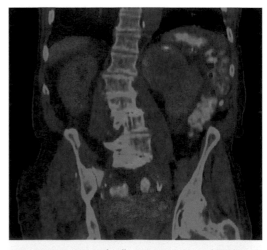

Fig. 24.2 Cystic renal cell carcinoma. Coronal PET/CT demonstrates focal areas of peripheral uptake in a large left upper pole renal cyst, consistent with cystic renal cell carcinoma. However, the lack of fluorodeoxyglucose in a complex renal cyst would not exclude renal cell carcinoma.

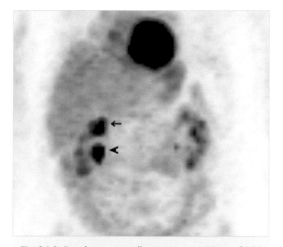

Fig. 24.3 Renal mass or collecting system. Coronal PET scan demonstrates focal activity in the upper pole of the right kidney (*arrow*). Note the similarity of appearance to renal collecting system activity (*arrowhead*). In this case, it is difficult to determine whether this is uptake in a renal mass or stasis in the upper pole collecting system. In this case, the uptake was secondary to a renal cell carcinoma.

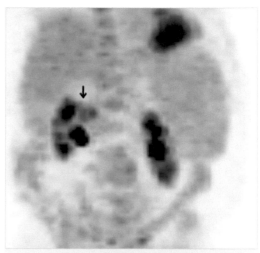

Fig. 24.4 Subtle renal cell carcinoma. Coronal PET scan demonstrates a subtle medial right upper pole renal mass (*arrow*). Note that this is only slightly more intense than normal renal parenchyma and can only be diagnosed by the contour deformity. Most renal cell carcinomas are more intense than this.

Pearls/Pitfalls

1. **Necessity of diuresis.** Diuresis is extremely important if PET is performed to evaluate a renal mass.
   a) False-negative results can result from the presence of urinary activity adjacent to and obscuring the lesion (▶ Fig. 24.3).
   b) False-positive results can occur from focal collections of urine, which mimic a lesion.
2. **Adjacent lesions.** Lesions outside but adjacent to the kidney can sometimes appear to be exophytic renal masses on PET (▶ Fig. 8.5).
   a) Correlation with anatomic imaging is necessary before a diagnosis of an exophytic renal mass is made.
3. **Degree of uptake.** FDG uptake greater than that of renal parenchyma is noted in the majority of renal cell carcinomas (RCCs), but the degree of uptake is sometimes only minimally more than the surrounding tissues and may be difficult to differentiate from normal parenchyma (▶ Fig. 24.4). FDG uptake in a renal mass greater than normal kidney suggests a high-grade clear cell or papillary RCC.[8] The standardized uptake values (SUVs) of low-grade clear cell and chromophobe RCCs may overlap with normal renal tissue.

4. **Oncocytomas.** Oncocytomas are usually isointense with the adjacent renal parenchyma, although false-positive increased uptake has been reported.[9,10,11] Adrenocortical oncocytomas have also been reported to have intense activity.[12,13]
5. **Angiomyolipomas.** In the largest reported series[14] of 21 patients with renal angiomyolipomas, none of the lesions had an SUVmax greater than 1.98. However, there have been two reported cases[15] of false-positive increased uptake in renal angiomyolipomas.
6. **Inflammatory lesions.** Inflammatory lesions such as xanthogranulomatous pyelonephritis can have false-positive increased uptake.[16]
7. **Prognosis.** Pretreatment SUVmax[17,18,19] predicts tumor grade and survival.

24.1.2 Staging/Restaging

Data from the National Oncologic PET Registry[20] indicated that FDG PET resulted in a change in management in 35.8% of patients with kidney cancer, with an imaging-adjusted impact of 16%.
1. PET is primarily useful in the following:
   a) Identifying distant metastases (▶ Fig. 24.5).

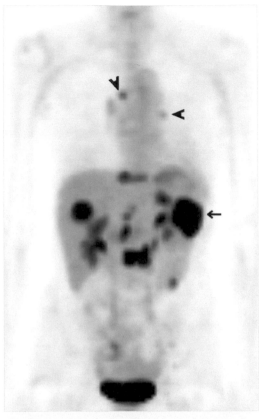

Fig. 24.5 Metastatic renal cell carcinoma. Coronal PET scan demonstrates a left renal cell carcinoma (*arrow*) metastatic to the bone, liver, abdominal nodes, and mediastinum (*arrowheads*).

   b) Evaluating indeterminate lesions seen on anatomic imaging techniques.
   c) Solitary metastasis being considered for resection.
2. PET is unlikely to be helpful in tumors with a low histological grade and limited local stage (≤ T2).[9]
3. **Restaging.** PET is most helpful in further evaluating patients with indeterminate lesions seen on anatomic imaging modalities.

Accuracy/Comparison with Other Modalities

1. **PET/CT for extrarenal lesions** (meta-analysis)[6]: sensitivity of 91% and specificity of 88%.
2. **PET for restaging:** sensitivity of 71% and specificity of 75%.[21]
3. ***Bone metastases.*** *There is conflicting literature on the accuracy of FDG PET for bone metastases*

compared to other modalities. In one report,[22] FDG PET was more sensitive and accurate than bone scan. In another report,[7] FDG PET was less sensitive but more specific than combined CT and bone scan.

4. **Prognosis.** FDG uptake is higher in RCC patients with a higher Furman grade, TNM (tumor size, node involvement, and metastasis status) stage, and venous and lymphatic invasion. A higher SUVmax and increased number of PET-positive lesions is associated with shorter overall and disease-free survival.[23]

Therapy Follow-up

FDG PET/CT may be useful in response assessment after treatment with tyrosine-kinase inhibitors in patients with advanced RCCs.[24] Metabolism assessed by FDG PET after treatment can predict overall and progression-free survival. However, the role is currently not well defined, as there is heterogeneity in the literature regarding the timing of imaging after treatment,[25,26,27] as well as method of measuring metabolic response (SUVmax vs. SUVpeak and total lesion glycolysis).[25]

24.2 Testicular Cancer

The primary value of PET/CT in testicular cancer is in the evaluation of postchemotherapy residual masses, particularly in patients with seminomas and masses greater than 3 cm in size.

Other potential applications include initial staging, identification of suspected recurrence with elevated tumor markers, and predicting response to treatment.

24.2.1 Staging

The accuracy of PET in detected testicular neoplasms is unknown, but PET can sometimes detect unsuspected testicular neoplasms (▶ Fig. 24.6). Although PET has achieved slightly better results than CT for primary staging of stage I and II disease,[28] there is limited value in routine clinical practice as most patients with subsequent recurrence can still be cured by chemotherapy.[29] In addition, although PET identifies some patients with disease not detected by CT, small-volume and microscopic disease is still often present as the relapse rate in PET negative patients is fairly high.[30] PET may be of value in primary staging in cases of equivocal CT results, or patients suspected of having distant metastases at initial presentation.

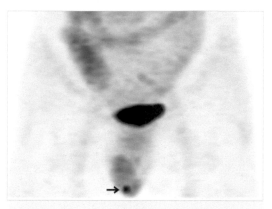

Fig. 24.6 Testicular tumor. Focal testicular uptake is noted (*arrow*) on a coronal PET scan. This was an incidentally detected right testicular seminoma.

PET has more value in staging stage II testicular germ cell tumors (▶ Fig. 24.7) and less value in stage I tumors.[31]

Accuracy/Comparison to Other Modalities

1. **PET:** sensitivity of 82% and specificity of 94%.[32]
2. **Retroperitoneal lymph nodes**. The sensitivity of PET in the detection of retroperitoneal lymph node metastases in seminomatous and nonseminomatous testicular cancer varies between 67 and 91%.[29]
3. The primary value of PET compared to CT is in reducing false-positive results.
4. In a multicenter trial of patients with clinical stage I/II nonseminomatous germ cell tumor (NSGCT),[28] both PET and CT had high specificity, while false-negative findings were more frequent with CT. PET achieved correct nodal staging in 83% of patients compared to 71% for CT.

Pitfalls

1. Both PET and CT will miss disease in small retroperitoneal nodes (≤ 1 cm).
2. PET cannot detect mature teratoma.

24.2.2 Recurrence

It is important to know whether the primary tumor was a seminoma or NSGCT. Mature teratoma does not have increased uptake. Because mature teratoma is present in more than 40% of resected masses in NSGCT, it is a major source of

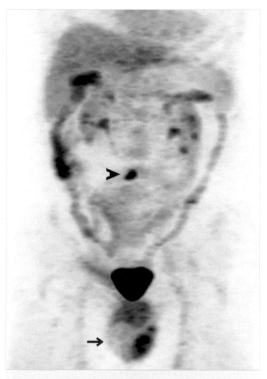

Fig. 24.7 Metastatic testicular cancer. Coronal PET scan demonstrates uptake in a metastatic retroperitoneal node (*arrowhead*). The patient is status post right orchiectomy (*arrow*) for testicular cancer.

false-negative results (mature teratoma is benign but is removed due to risk of malignant transformation). In seminomas, only 4% of residual lesions are mature teratoma. Thus, FDG PET has a greater role in evaluating tumor recurrence in seminoma than in NSGCT.[33,34]

Seminomas

In patients presenting with advanced-stage seminoma, detectable residual masses will be present in approximately 60% after therapy. These residual masses often represent fibrosis and necrosis, but cannot be differentiated from tumor by CT. Lesions smaller than 3 cm are usually followed by imaging. The management of residual masses greater than 3 cm is controversial, and both surgery and continued observation have been recommended. National Comprehensive Cancer Network (NCCN) guidelines[35] recommend a PET scan in patients with seminoma, a mass greater than 3 cm and normal level of markers approximately 6 weeks after chemotherapy to decide between surveillance and resumed treatment. The European Consensus Conference on Diagnosis and Treatment of Germ Cell Cancer (European Consensus)[36] recommends PET in patients with seminomas ≥ 3 cm not earlier than 8 weeks after chemotherapy. Given the high negative predictive value (NPV) of PET, both the NCCN and European Consensus guidelines indicate that patients with negative PET scan can be followed, irrespective of the size of the residual lesion. While the NCCN guidelines suggest that resection should be considered in patients with a positive PET, the European Consensus guidelines suggest that the positive predictive value (PPV) of PET is less reliable, and biopsy, or close observation with serial CT scans or repeat PET/CT scans, should be considered. Decoene et al[37] have suggested that only a minority of patients with positive PET results require surgery (e.g., patients at a high risk for recurrence, ureteral compression, or unclear initial histology). In other cases, the authors suggest a repeat PET study at least 6 weeks after the initial PET scan, with continued active surveillance unless there is progressive disease or increased SUVs.

In the largest prospective trial (SEMPET),[33,34] PET was significantly more accurate than CT in the evaluation of masses greater than 3 cm. However, a retrospective review[38] found that while negative PET studies indicated no residual disease, false-positive PET scans were not uncommon. However, in the largest series evaluating PET in postchemotherapy seminoma residual masses (a retrospective validation of the SEMPET trial),[39] the accuracy of PET improved from 73 to 88% if performed more than 6 weeks after the last chemotherapy cycle, indicating that performing PET too soon after therapy is a substantial contributor to false-positive results. Correctly timed PET scans had a PPV of 78%. This same study did not support the use of PET in masses less than 3 cm as the sensitivity was only 67% even with proper timing.

Therefore, in lesions greater than 3 cm, PET performed more than 6 weeks after chemotherapy is substantially more accurate than CT in differentiating fibrosis/necrosis from residual tumor (▶ Fig. 24.8). Patients with a negative PET scan can be observed (NPV 96%), while patients with a positive scan are candidates for surgery, although the false-positive rate (PPV 78%) suggests that biopsy and follow-up imaging are other options. Anecdotal reports[39] have suggested that equivocal or false-positive PET studies may be negative on repeat studies.

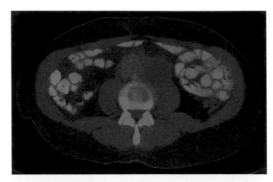

Fig. 24.8 Seminoma with retroperitoneal mass. Axial PET/CT in a patient with seminoma demonstrates a large retroperitoneal mass. The right aspect has fluorodeoxyglucose (FDG) uptake consistent with tumor and the left aspect is cystic appearing without FDG uptake.

Nonseminomatous Germ Cell Tumors

In one report,[40] the NPV of a negative postchemotherapy PET scan in patients with NSGCTs was 81.7%. In another report,[41] the sensitivity of PET/CT for nonseminoma lesion detection was lower than for seminoma lesions (77 vs. 92%). However, in one study high-risk (lymphovascular invasion positive) patients with clinical stage I NSGSTs and a negative PET had a high risk of relapse.[42] Thus, PET may not be sufficiently sensitive in this setting. Although NCCN and European guidelines do not suggest a routine role for PET in NSGSTs, PET can be helpful in detecting recurrence in patients with rising tumor markers and negative CT scans.[43]

Elevated Tumor Markers

PET is helpful in patients with elevated tumor markers whether or not a residual mass is seen on CT. In patients with elevated markers and a residual mass, the NPV is low (50%), but PET is often the first modality to identify the recurrence on follow-up studies.[44]

Accuracy/Comparison to Other Modalities

1. **PET and PET/CT for postchemotherapy management of seminomas** (meta-analysis)[45]: sensitivity of 78% and specificity of 86%.
   a) There was a better diagnostic accuracy for residual/recurrent lesions greater than 3 cm compared to lesions less than 3 cm.

Table 24.2 Sensitivity and specificity of PET versus CT in the detection of recurrent seminomas

	Sensitivity %	Specificity %
PET	80	100
CT	70	74

2. **PET versus CT for seminomas** (▶ Table 24.2)[34]:
   a) PET is more accurate than CT, primarily due to the higher specificity of PET.
   b) However, there have been reported cases of residual masses, some greater than 3 cm, with false-positive uptake secondary to necrosis or inflammation[38]
3. **PET for NSGST (stage I):** sensitivity of 70% and specificity of 100%.[46]

Pearls

1. *SUV*:
   a) Seminomas usually have higher SUVs than nonseminomatous lesions.[47]
   b) If SUV is greater than 5 in a lesion, it is much more likely to be viable tumor than mature teratoma or necrosis/fibrosis.[48]

Pitfalls

1. PET does not detect mature teratomas.
2. False positives secondary to necrosis or inflammation are possible in residual masses, some greater than 3 cm in size.

24.3 Bladder Cancer

PET can detect both regional lymph node disease (▶ Fig. 24.9) and distant metastases from muscle invasive bladder cancer. A major obstacle to detecting regional lymph node disease is bladder activity, and therefore bladder catheterization and/or forced diuresis is often necessary. Potential uses include preoperative staging, treatment optimization, restaging, evaluation of metastatic disease response, early assessment of treatment response, and prognostication.[23]

Data from the National Oncologic PET Registry[20] indicated that FDG PET resulted in a change in management in 37.9% of patients with prostate cancer, with an imaging-adjusted impact of 15.4%.

For preoperative staging, PET is more sensitive than CT with comparable high specificity.[49,50] In one report,[51] PET detected all bone metastases detected by bone scintigraphy. Soubra et al[50]

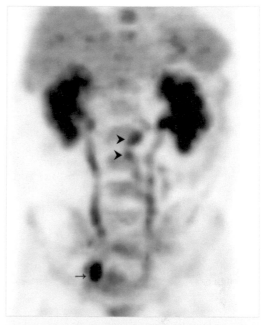

Fig. 24.9 Metastatic bladder cancer. Coronal PET scan demonstrates a right bladder cancer (*arrow*) metastatic to retroperitoneal nodes (*arrowheads*). The bladder cancer is only visualized because the bladder is empty from Foley catheter placement.

suggest that the main utility of PET for staging would be in patients at low risk for metastatic disease in whom a positive PET-CT scan would alter care. Based on their meta-analysis, a hypothetical patient with a high pretest probability (50%) of positive lymph nodes would still have a posttest probability of 33% after a negative PET. Although PET has reasonable accuracy for the detection of bladder lesions if techniques such as forced diuresis are employed, it is not superior to CT or MRI for this purpose.[52]

PET may have prognostic value as patients with PET positive disease during preoperative staging have lower median survival time. In one report,[53] the presence of extravesical FDG-avid lesions was an independent predictor of mortality.

24.3.1 Accuracy

1. **PET and PET/CT for detection of bladder cancer** (meta-analysis)[52]: sensitivity of 80% and specificity of 84%.
2. **Preoperative staging for lymph node metastases** (meta-analysis; ▶ Table 24.3).[50]

Table 24.3 Sensitivity and specificity of PET/CT versus CT for preoperative staging for lymph node metastases from bladder cancer

	Sensitivity %	Specificity %
PET/CT	57	95
CT	35	95

3. In one report,[51] PET was slightly more sensitive but less specific than CT for presurgical staging and monitoring.
4. In one report,[54] there was no statistically significant difference between PET/CT and MRI for N staging of urothelial bladder cancer, although the trend indicated an advantage for PET/CT.

24.3.2 Pitfalls

Although prior chemotherapy diminished sensitivity in one study,[55] another study[56] did not find a difference in accuracy if the study was performed at least 2 months after chemotherapy.

24.4 Prostate Cancer

24.4.1 Incidentally Noted Prostate FDG Uptake

In a meta-analysis,[57] the pooled prevalence of incidental prostate uptake was 1.8%. The risk of malignancy is difficult to determine as many patients are not further evaluated, but in the meta-analysis, the pooled risk of malignancy in patients who were further evaluated was 17%. However, the risk of malignancy in patients undergoing biopsy was 62%. In one report,[58] cases of incidentally detected prostate hypermetabolism with abnormal digital rectal examination (DRE) and/or prostate-specific antigen (PSA) showed high rates of positivity by biopsy. A higher mean age and peripheral location are predictors of malignancy. Although one report[59] indicates that an SUVmax of 6 is helpful for identifying malignant prostatic uptake and there is a trend toward higher SUVs in malignancies compared to benign etiologies, SUV cutoffs are not reliable for differentiating benign from malignant uptake.

There is conflicting evidence about whether the absence of calcification in an area of uptake is associated with malignancy. Two reports[60,61] have suggested that the absence of calcification increases the risk of malignancy, while no association was found in two other reports.[57,62] Multiplicity was not significantly different between benign and malignant lesions.[62]

Therefore, further workup with DRE and/or PSA should be considered in patients with incidental prostate uptake in the peripheral gland, with patient age, SUV, and absence of calcification other factors that could potentially be taken into account. If DRE and/or PSA is abnormal, biopsy should be considered.

24.4.2 Staging/Restaging

FDG PET is of limited value in prostate cancer due to the low FDG avidity of most prostate cancer cells. In addition, urinary activity limits pelvic evaluation unless bladder catheterization and diuresis are used. FDG can also accumulate in benign prostatic hyperplasia (BPH) and inflammation. There is more robust evidence for amino acid PET/CT for restaging of patients with biochemical relapse of prostate cancer.[63] In a meta-analysis of the diagnostic accuracy of four radiotracers,[64] ^{18}F-fluorocholine had the highest area under the curve, followed by ^{11}C-choline, ^{11}C-acetate, and ^{18}F-FDG. However, there are other labeled compounds that may have superior accuracy than the naturally occurring amino acids, specifically the synthetic amino acid anti-1-amino3-F-18-flurocylcobutane1-carboxylic acid (FACBC or fluciclovine; ▶ Fig. 24.10) and labeled prostate-specific membrane antigen (PMSA). Only the former is currently approved by the U.S. Food and Drug Administration.

[18]F-Flucicovine and ^{68}Ga-PMSA

Amino acid transport is upregulated in prostate cancer. Prostate cancer can be imaged with radiolabeled natural and synthetic amino acids. Fluciclovine is a synthetic amino acid. Fluciclovine transport most closely mirrors glutamine and has higher uptake in prostate cancer cell lines than methionine, glutamine, choline, and acetate.[65]

PMSA is a transmembrane protein that is expressed in the apical epithelium of the secretory ducts in benign prostatic tissue. Prostatic malignancy results in upregulation and migration of PMSA to the plasma membrane, particularly during the transition to hormone refractory disease. PMSA expression in prostate cancer cell membranes is 100- to 1000-fold that in normal cells. Increased PMSA expression is associated with higher grade and increased risk of tumor progression.[66,67,68] The most studied ligand is gallium-68 (^{68}Ga).

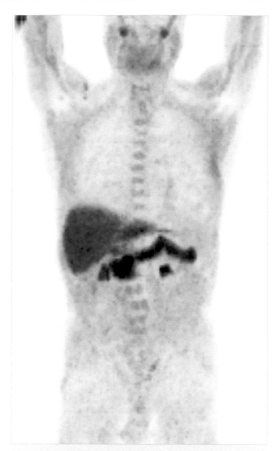

Fig. 24.10 ^{18}F-fluciclovine normal distribution. Maximum intensity projection (MIP) image from a normal ^{18}F-fluciclovine scan demonstrates activity in the liver, pancreas, bone marrow, skeletal muscle, and renal collecting systems. (This image is provided courtesy of Evan Sirc MD, Walnut Creek, CA.)

24.4.3 Biochemical Recurrence

The primary use of both ^{18}F-fluciclovine (▶ Fig. 24.11) and ^{68}Ga-PMSA PET is in the setting of biochemical recurrence after radical prostatectomy, particularly in patients with low PSA values (< 10 ng/mL).[65,66] This is significant as most guidelines do not recommend conventional imaging when the PSA is less than 10.

^{18}F-fluciclovine and ^{68}Ga PMSA PET have not been directly compared. However, it is possible that ^{68}Ga-PMSA PET may be superior for detection of recurrence at very low PSA levels (e.g., < 1 ng/mL), as well as for detection of bone metastases.

In a multisite study of 596 patients with biochemical recurrence,[69] the ^{18}F fluciclovine was positive in 68% of patients. In the lowest PSA quartile (≤ 0.79 ng/mL), the positivity rate was 41%. In another report,[70] fluciclovine PET was positive in 37% of patients for PSA levels less than 1 ng/mL. The positivity rate of fluciclovine PET will increase with increasing PSA and more rapid doubling time.[65] In a meta-analysis,[71] ^{68}Ga-PMSA PET was positive in 76% of patients with biochemical recurrence. The rate of positivity increased with shorter PSA doubling time. For PSA levels of 0 to 0.2, 0.2 to 1, 1 to 2, and greater than 2 ng/mL, the positive scan rates were 42, 58, 76, and 95%, respectively. Shorter PSA doubling time also increased positivity. One report[72] indicates that the optimal cutoff values for performing PMSA PET are a PSA of 0.83 ng/mL and a PSA doubling time of 6.5 months.

In a study of bone scan negative patients with suspected recurrent prostate cancer,[70] fluciclovine PET/CT had a sensitivity of 89% and specificity of 56% in the prostate/bed compared to 11 and 87%, respectively, for CT. In extraprostatic regions, fluciclovine PET had a sensitivity of 46% and specificity of 100% compared to 11 and 100%, respectively, for CT. In a study of patients with biochemical recurrence (median PSA 1.31 ng/mL),[73] PMSA PET detected 78% of pathologically proven lymph node metastases, while morphologic imaging (CT or MRI) detected only 27%.

In prospective comparison of ^{18}F-fluciclovine and ^{11}C-choline,[74] at PSA levels of less than 1, 1 to less than 2, 3 to less than 3, and ≥ 3, the detection rates for choline PET were 14, 29, 36, and 50%, respectively, and 21, 29, 45, and 59%, respectively, for fluciclovine PET. In a prospective comparison of ^{18}F-fluoromethycholine and ^{68}Ga-PMSA PET,[75] at PSA levels of less than 0.5, 0.5 to 2, and greater than 2 ng/mL, the detection rates for fluoromethylcholine PET were 12.5, 31, and 57%, respectively, and 50, 69, and 86%, respectively, for PMSA PET.

In a prospective study of patients with suspected recurrent prostate carcinoma,[76] ^{18}F-fluciclovine had a sensitivity of 90% and specificity of 40% in the prostate/bed compared to 67 and 57% for ^{111}In-capromab pendetide. For extraprostatic disease, ^{18}F-fluciclovine had a sensitivity of 55% and specificity of 97% compared to 10 and 87%, respectively, for ^{111}In-capromab pendetide.

24.4.4 Primary Staging

Neither ^{18}F-fluciclovine nor ^{68}Ga-PMSA PET is well established for primary staging, although one review indicates that PMSA PET is of high clinical yield for primary staging in high-risk disease.[66]

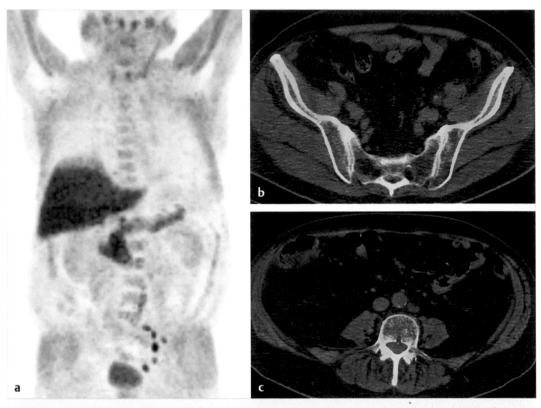

Fig. 24.11 Metastatic prostate cancer. ^{18}F-fluciclovine maximum intensity projection (MIP; **a**) and axial PET/CT **(b,c)** in a patient with biochemical recurrence of prostate cancer (prostate-specific antigen [PSA]: 42.2 ng/mL) demonstrates increased uptake in pelvic and retroperitoneal nodal metastases. (These images are provided courtesy of Jonathan Posin, MD, Walnut Creek, CA.)

In a meta-analysis,[71] PMSA PET was positive in 40% of patients for primary staging. However, in the largest study of 130 patients with intermediate- to high-risk prostate cancer prior to radical prostatectomy and lymph node dissection,[77] the sensitivity and specificity of ^{68}Ga PMSA PET were 66 and 99%, respectively, compared to 44 and 85% for morphologic imaging.

24.4.5 Bone Metastases

One report[78] compared bone scintigraphy and ^{68}Ga-PMSA PET prostate cancer patients for primary staging, biochemical recurrence, and metastatic castration-resistant prostate cancer. The region-based sensitivity and specificity of PET were 99% and 99 to 100%, respectively, and 82 to 87% and 92 to 98%, respectively, for bone scintigraphy. PET performed better than bone scintigraphy in primary staging and biochemical recurrence. There have been little data on the accuracy of ^{18}F-fluciclovine for bone metastases (▶ Fig. 24.12) as patients with known bone metastases demonstrated by bone scintigraphy were excluded from initial trials. However, some authors[65] note that in their experience, fluciclovine demonstrates intense uptake in lytic lesions but may have absent uptake in dense sclerotic lesions, and thus they do not recommend replacing bone scintigraphy with fluciclovine.

24.4.6 ^{18}F-Fluciclovine Interpretation[79]

[68]Ga PMSA interpretation will be discussed in Chapter 28.

Physiologic Uptake

• The most intense radiotracer activity is visualized in the pancreas and the liver, with pancreatic uptake more intense than hepatic uptake.[76]

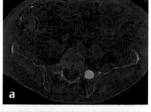

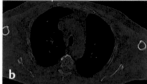

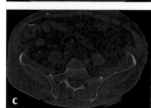

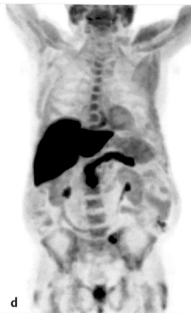

Fig. 24.12 Bone metastases demonstrated by ^{18}F-fluciclovine. An 88-year-old male 8 years status post prostatectomy for Gleason 9 prostate cancer with rise in prostate-specific antigen to 12.42. An initial ^{18}F NaF scan showed increased foci of activity in the sacrum (**a**) and left scapula (**b**), called indeterminate since no corresponding sclerotic foci were present on localizer CT. Axial fused (**c**) and maximum intensity projection (MIP; **d**) Axumin study shows positivity in the sacral lesion but suggests that the scapular lesion may be false positive due to lack of uptake. (These images are provided courtesy of Barry Engelstad, MD, Walnut Creek, CA.)

- There is typically mild to moderate activity in the spleen, renal parenchyma, and bowels.
- During early time point scanning, there is usually minimal excreted radiotracer activity in the renal pelvis or bladder; however, a minority of patients can show mild to moderate uptake.
- Mild to moderate adrenal gland uptake is a normal variant.
- Bone marrow activity is moderate and can be heterogeneous.
- Mild activity is usually present in skeletal muscle when scanned during an early acquisition with increasing skeletal muscle activity over time.
- Cardiac muscle displays mild to moderate uptake.
- Mild symmetric activity can be seen as a normal variant involving inguinal, distal external iliac, hilar, and axillary lymph nodes.
- Brain and lung parenchymal activity is minimal (less than blood pool). Moderate activity can be visualized in the pituitary gland.

Inflammatory Uptake

- Fluciclovine imaging generally demonstrates less uptake in regions of inflammation than does FDG.
- Mild activity can still be seen, however, due to the increased cellular expression of amino acid transporters associated with inflammation.

Lymph Node Metastases

- Most closely inspect pelvic and retroperitoneal lymph nodes in sites typical for metastatic spread of prostate cancer.
- For larger lymph nodes (> 1 cm in size), nodal uptake greater than uptake in the bone marrow is concerning for metastatic disease. For smaller lymph nodes (< 1 cm in size), nodal uptake greater than blood pool activity is concerning for metastatic disease.[79]
- Mild activity can be seen as a normal variant involving inguinal, distal external iliac, hilar, and axillary lymph nodes.

Prostatectomy Bed

- Focal uptake greater than bone marrow activity is suspicious for recurrent disease (or uptake greater than blood pool activity for small lesions).[79]
- Do not confuse normal physiologic activity in the rectum with activity in the prostate bed.
- Inspection of the coronal and sagittal PET may be helpful to differentiate physiologic from pathological activity in this region.

Non-Prostatectomy

- Focal uptake greater than bone marrow activity is suspicious for malignancy (or uptake greater than blood pool activity for small lesions).[79]

- Heterogeneous uptake is more suspicious than homogeneous activity.
- Benign uptake can be seen with prostatitis and BPH that can simulate prostate cancer.

Skeletal Metastases

- A focus of osseous activity that is conspicuous on the maximum intensity projection (MIP) imaging must be closely inspected to assess for a skeletal metastasis.
- Uptake is often greater in lucent or faintly sclerotic lesions and may be low-level or imperceptible in more densely sclerotic lesions.[79]
- A bone lesion visualized on the CT portion of the examination that does not display increased fluciclovine activity is indeterminate. Dedicated bone imaging with conventional bone scanning, F-18 NaF PET imaging, or MRI should be recommended.
- Skeletal uptake associated with degenerative joint disease is less frequently seen than with FDG.

FDG PET for Staging/Restaging

Despite the relatively limited value of FDG in comparison to other tracers, data from the National Oncologic PET Registry[20] indicated that FDG PET resulted in a change in management in 35.1% of patients with prostate cancer, with an imaging-adjusted impact of 15%.

Specific situations in which FDG PET may be of value include patients with poorly differentiated primary tumors (Gleason score > 7) and higher PSA levels.[80] In one report,[81] FDG PET/CT was studied for preoperative staging and prognostic stratification of patients with Gleason sum ≥ 8 at biopsy, and improved pretreatment prognostic stratification. Restaging in cases of biochemical recurrence[82] and evaluation of treatment response[80] are other potential applications.

FDG PET is primarily useful in castrate-resistant disease. It has better concordance with other imaging modalities in castrate-resistant metastases compared to castrate-sensitive disease,[83] and has prognostic value in castrate-resistant patients.[84,85] It may also be helpful in predicting the transition from castrate-sensitive to castrate-resistant states.

1. Primary tumor:
   a) Most (81%) primary prostate tumors (▶ Fig. 24.13) have low FDG uptake.[86]
2. Preoperative staging:
   a) FDG PET is insensitive for staging pelvic lymph nodes prior to surgery.

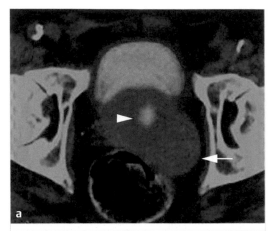

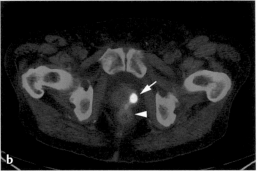

Fig. 24.13 Variable uptake in prostate cancer. **(a)** Axial PET/CT scan demonstrates a large exophytic left prostate carcinoma (*arrow*) with no fluorodeoxyglucose uptake. Central prostatic activity (*arrowhead*) is in the urethra. (This image is provided courtesy of Bruce Higginbotham, MD, Seattle, WA.) **(b)** Axial PET/CT demonstrates focal uptake is present in a left prostate cancer (*arrow*). Many prostate carcinomas do not demonstrate this degree of uptake. Note the proximity of the prostate to rectal activity (*arrowhead*), which is a common cause of false-positive results when evaluating for local recurrence.

   b) FDG PET is not useful for evaluating organ-confined prostate cancer defined by conventional workup.
3. Recurrence:
   a) *Clinical/imaging factors.* FDG PET has potential value where the following are applicable[87,88,89]:
      - PSA greater than 4 ng/mL or increases greater than 0.2 ng/mL per month.
      - Advanced cancer.
      - Untreated patient.
      - Incomplete or lack of response to treatment.

- Negative bone scan.
- Equivocal pelvic CT findings.

b) Local recurrence:
- FDG PET has poor accuracy for differentiating local recurrence and scar.[90]

c) Metastatic disease:
- FDG PET has limited sensitivity for metastatic disease.
- However, FDG PET is more likely to detect distant metastases than local recurrence.[91]

4. Prognosis. FDG PET has prognostic value in castrate-resistant patients with prostate cancer. In patients with castrate-resistant prostate cancer, the number of bone lesions on PET and the sum of the maximum SUVs[84,85] predict overall survival. In patients with a Gleason sum ≥ 8 at biopsy, intraprostatic FDG uptake predict pathological grade of the primary tumor and survival following radical prostatectomy.[81]

5. Therapy response. FDG PET may have some role as a surrogate marker of response to chemotherapy in hormone-resistant disease.[92] FDG PET may have some value in monitoring anti-androgenic treatment.[91] Androgen ablation decreases tumor glucose utilization.[93] PET is less sensitive in patients who are being treated with anti-androgenic hormones. However, PET may have value in predicting response to anti-androgenic treatment. As FDG uptake in prostate tumors depends upon the presence and activity of androgen, PET may be helpful in predicting the time to reach an androgen refractory state.[94]

a) Patients with a flare phenomenon seen on bone scan may be more accurately assessed with PET.

Accuracy/Comparison to Other Modalities

1. **Recurrence (FDG PET):** sensitivity of 79% and specificity of 66%.[91]
   a) These values were obtained at PSA levels greater than 2.4 ng/mL.
   b) Overall FDG PET detects local or systemic disease in 31% of patients with a PSA relapse.[95]
   c) FDG PET is superior to CT but inferior to MRI for detection of recurrence in the prostate bed.
   d) FDG PET may be able to replace CT in the setting of suspected recurrence, but other modalities such as endorectal MRI for local

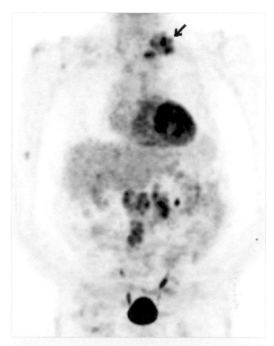

Fig. 24.14 Metastatic prostate cancer. Coronal PET scan demonstrates metastatic disease from prostate cancer to retroperitoneal and left supraclavicular nodes (*arrow*). The left supraclavicular nodes are a common area of nonregional nodal spread (via the thoracic duct) from prostate cancer. (This image is provided courtesy of Ronald Korn, MD, PhD, Scottsdale, AZ.)

recurrence and bone scan for bone metastases would still be necessary.

2. **Body region.** PET is more useful for soft tissue and nodal metastases than for bone metastases (▶ Fig. 24.14, ▶ Fig. 24.15, ▶ Fig. 24.16).

3. **Bone metastasis:**
   a) FDG PET is significantly less sensitive but more specific than bone scan for sclerotic prostate cancer metastasis.
   b) The reported sensitivity of FDG PET is as low as 18% (androgen-independent disease) relative to bone scan.[96]
   c) Lesions seen on bone scan only are usually quiescent (stable compared to prior scans).[7]
   d) Lesions seen on FDG PET scan only are usually active (and become positive on subsequent bone scans).

4. **Comparison to CT.** FDG PET is as sensitive or more sensitive than CT for overall detection of metastatic disease (however, CT has poor sensitivity in prostate cancer).

5. **Comparison to monoclonal antibodies.** In patients with high PSA levels (> 4 ng/mL) or high

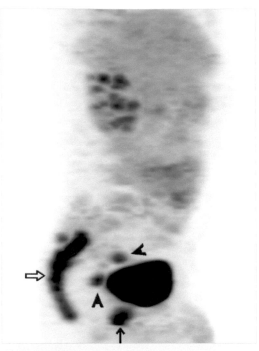

Fig. 24.15 Metastatic prostate cancer. Saglttal PET scan demonstrates uptake in a primary prostate carcinoma (*arrow*) with sacral (*open arrow*) and pelvic nodal (*arrowheads*) metastases.

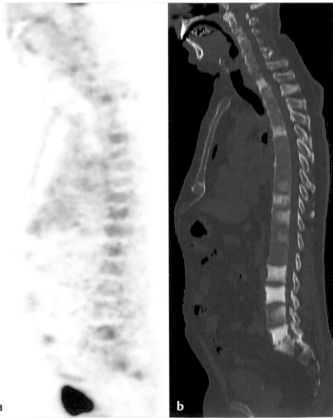

Fig. 24.16 Bone metastases from prostate cancer. **(a)** Sagittal PET and CT **(b)** demonstrate mild fluorodeoxyglucose uptake corresponding to sclerotic bone metastases from prostate cancer. (These images are provided courtesy of Evan Sirc MD, Walnut Creek, CA.)

PSA velocity, FDG PET has a higher detection rate for metastatic disease than ^{111}In-capromab pendetide.[88]

References

[1] Mathews D, Oz OK. Positron emission tomography in prostate and renal cell carcinoma. Curr Opin Urol. 2002; 12(5): 381–385

[2] Gofrit ON, Orevi M. Diagnostic challenges of kidney cancer: a systematic review of the role of positron emission tomography-computerized tomography. J Urol. 2016; 196(3):648–657

[3] Goldberg MA, Mayo-Smith WW, Papanicolaou N, Fischman AJ, Lee MJ. FDG PET characterization of renal masses: preliminary experience. Clin Radiol. 1997; 52(7):510–515

[4] Kaneta T, Hakamatsuka T, Yamada T, et al. FDG PET in solitary metastastic/secondary tumor of the kidney: a report of three cases and a review of the relevant literature. Ann Nucl Med. 2006; 20(1):79–82

[5] Kumar R, Chauhan A, Lakhani P, Xiu Y, Zhuang H, Alavi A. 2-Deoxy-2-[F-18]fluoro-D-glucose-positron emission tomography in characterization of solid renal masses. Mol Imaging Biol. 2005; 7(6):431–439

[6] Wang HY, Ding HJ, Chen JH, et al. Meta-analysis of the diagnostic performance of [18F]FDG-PET and PET/CT in renal cell carcinoma. Cancer Imaging. 2012; 12:464–474

[7] Kang DE, White RL, Jr, Zuger JH, Sasser HC, Teigland CM. Clinical use of fluorodeoxyglucose F 18 positron emission tomography for detection of renal cell carcinoma. J Urol. 2004; 171 (5):1806–1809

[8] Takahashi M, Kume H, Koyama K, et al. Preoperative evaluation of renal cell carcinoma by using 18F-FDG PET/CT. Clin Nucl Med. 2015; 40(12):936–940

[9] Aide N, Cappele O, Bottet P, et al. Efficiency of [(18)F]FDG PET in characterising renal cancer and detecting distant metastases: a comparison with CT. Eur J Nucl Med Mol Imaging. 2003; 30(9):1236–1245

[10] Raman A, Campbell T, McLeod N. An interesting case of F-18 fluorodeoxyglucose positron emission tomography avid renal oncocytoma. ANZ J Surg. 2016; 86(1–2):99–100

[11] Ramdave S, Thomas GW, Berlangieri SU, et al. Clinical role of F-18 fluorodeoxyglucose positron emission tomography for detection and management of renal cell carcinoma. J Urol. 2001; 166(3):825–830

[12] Kim DJ, Chung JJ, Ryu YH, Hong SW, Yu JS, Kim JH. Adrenocortical oncocytoma displaying intense activity on 18F-FDG-PET: a case report and a literature review. Ann Nucl Med. 2008; 22(9):821–824

[13] Sato N, Nakamura Y, Takanami K, et al. Case report: adrenal oncocytoma associated with markedly increased FDG uptake and immunohistochemically positive for GLUT1. Endocr Pathol. 2014; 25(4):410–415

[14] Lin CY, Chen HY, Ding HJ, Yen KY, Kao CH. FDG PET or PET/CT in evaluation of renal angiomyolipoma. Korean J Radiol. 2013; 14(2):337–342

[15] Arnold RT, Myers DT. Visualization of renal angiomyolipoma on F-18 FDG PET/CT. Clin Nucl Med. 2009; 34(8):539–540

[16] Ak I, Can C. F-18 FDG PET in detecting renal cell carcinoma. Acta Radiol. 2005; 46(8):895–899

[17] Ferda J, Ferdova E, Hora M, et al. 18F-FDG-PET/CT in potentially advanced renal cell carcinoma: a role in treatment decisions and prognosis estimation. Anticancer Res. 2013; 33 (6):2665–2672

[18] Nakaigawa N, Kondo K, Tateishi U, et al. FDG PET/CT as a prognostic biomarker in the era of molecular-targeting therapies: max SUVmax predicts survival of patients with advanced renal cell carcinoma. BMC Cancer. 2016; 16:67

[19] Ozülker T, Ozülker F, Ozbek E, Ozpaçaci T. A prospective diagnostic accuracy study of F-18 fluorodeoxyglucose-positron emission tomography/computed tomography in the evaluation of indeterminate renal masses. Nucl Med Commun. 2011; 32(4):265–272

[20] Hillner BE, Siegel BA, Shields AF, et al. Relationship between cancer type and impact of PET and PET/CT on intended management: findings of the national oncologic PET registry. J Nucl Med. 2008; 49(12):1928–1935

[21] Jadvar H, Kherbache HM, Pinski JK, Conti PS. Diagnostic role of [F-18]-FDG positron emission tomography in restaging renal cell carcinoma. Clin Nephrol. 2003; 60(6):395–400

[22] Wu HC, Yen RF, Shen YY, Kao CH, Lin CC, Lee CC. Comparing whole body 18F-2-deoxyglucose positron emission tomography and technetium-99 m methylene diphosphate bone scan to detect bone metastases in patients with renal cell carcinomas - a preliminary report. J Cancer Res Clin Oncol. 2002; 128(9):503–506

[23] Kitajima K, Yamamoto S, Fukushima K, Minamimoto R, Kamai T, Jadvar H. Update on advances in molecular PET in urological oncology. Jpn J Radiol. 2016; 34(7):470–485

[24] Caldarella C, Muoio B, Isgrò MA, Porfiri E, Treglia G, Giovanella L. The role of fluorine-18-fluorodeoxyglucose positron emission tomography in evaluating the response to tyrosine-kinase inhibitors in patients with metastatic primary renal cell carcinoma. Radiol Oncol. 2014; 48(3):219–227

[25] Farnebo J, Grybäck P, Harmenberg U, et al. Volumetric FDG-PET predicts overall and progression-free survival after 14 days of targeted therapy in metastatic renal cell carcinoma. BMC Cancer. 2014; 14:408

[26] Kayani I, Avril N, Bomanji J, et al. Sequential FDG-PET/CT as a biomarker of response to Sunitinib in metastatic clear cell renal cancer. Clin Cancer Res. 2011; 17(18):6021–6028

[27] Ueno D, Yao M, Tateishi U, et al. Early assessment by FDG-PET/CT of patients with advanced renal cell carcinoma treated with tyrosine kinase inhibitors is predictive of disease course. BMC Cancer. 2012; 12:162

[28] de Wit M, Brenner W, Hartmann M, et al. [18F]-FDG-PET in clinical stage I/II non-seminomatous germ cell tumours: results of the German multicentre trial. Ann Oncol. 2008; 19 (9):1619–1623

[29] Avril N, Dambha F, Murray I, Shamash J, Powles T, Sahdev A. The clinical advances of fluorine-2-D-deoxyglucose–positron emission tomography/computed tomography in urological cancers. Int J Urol. 2010; 17(6):501–511

[30] Sohaib SA, Cook G, Koh DM. Imaging studies for germ cell tumors. Hematol Oncol Clin North Am. 2011; 25(3):487–502, vii

[31] Albers P, Bender H, Yilmaz H, Schoeneich G, Biersack HJ, Mueller SC. Positron emission tomography in the clinical staging of patients with stage I and II testicular germ cell tumors. Urology. 1999; 53(4):808–811

[32] Gambhir SS, Czernin J, Schwimmer J, Silverman DH, Coleman RE, Phelps ME. A tabulated summary of the FDG PET literature. J Nucl Med. 2001; 42(5) Suppl:1S–93S

[33] De Santis M, Bokemeyer C, Becherer A, et al. Predictive impact of 2-18fluoro-2-deoxy-D-glucose positron emission tomography for residual postchemotherapy masses in patients with bulky seminoma. J Clin Oncol. 2001; 19 (17):3740–3744

[34] De Santis M, Becherer A, Bokemeyer C, et al. 2-18fluoro-deoxy-D-glucose positron emission tomography is a reliable predictor for viable tumor in postchemotherapy seminoma:

an update of the prospective multicentric SEMPET trial. J Clin Oncol. 2004; 22(6):1034–1039

[35] Motzer RJ, Jonasch E, Agarwal N, et al. Testicular cancer, version 2.2015. J Natl Compr Canc Netw. 2015; 13(6):772–799

[36] Beyer J, Albers P, Altena R, et al. Maintaining success, reducing treatment burden, focusing on survivorship: highlights from the third European consensus conference on diagnosis and treatment of germ-cell cancer. Ann Oncol. 2013; 24(4):878–888

[37] Decoene J, Winter C, Albers P. False-positive fluorodeoxyglucose positron emission tomography results after chemotherapy in patients with metastatic seminoma. Urol Oncol. 2015; 33(1):23.e15–23.e21

[38] Lewis DA, Tann M, Kesler K, McCool A, Foster RS, Einhorn LH. Positron emission tomography scans in postchemotherapy seminoma patients with residual masses: a retrospective review from Indiana University Hospital. J Clin Oncol. 2006; 24 (34):e54–e55

[39] Bachner M, Loriot Y, Gross-Goupil M, et al. 2-18fluoro-deoxy-D-glucose positron emission tomography (FDG-PET) for postchemotherapy seminoma residual lesions: a retrospective validation of the SEMPET trial. Ann Oncol. 2012; 23(1):59–64

[40] Buchler T, Simonova K, Fencl P, Jarkovsky J, Abrahamova J. Clinical outcomes of patients with nonseminomatous germ cell tumours and negative postchemotherapy positron emission tomography. Cancer Invest. 2012; 30(6):487–492

[41] Ambrosini V, Zucchini G, Nicolini S, et al. 18F-FDG PET/CT impact on testicular tumours clinical management. Eur J Nucl Med Mol Imaging. 2014; 41(4):668–673

[42] Huddart RA, O'Doherty MJ, Padhani A, et al. NCRI Testis Tumour Clinical Study Group. 18fluorodeoxyglucose positron emission tomography in the prediction of relapse in patients with high-risk, clinical stage I nonseminomatous germ cell tumors: preliminary report of MRC Trial TE22: the NCRI Testis Tumour Clinical Study Group. J Clin Oncol. 2007; 25(21):3090–3095

[43] Cook GJ, Sohaib A, Huddart RA, Dearnaley DP, Horwich A, Chua S. The role of 18F-FDG PET/CT in the management of testicular cancers. Nucl Med Commun. 2015; 36(7):702–708

[44] Hain SF, O'Doherty MJ, Timothy AR, Leslie MD, Harper PG, Huddart RA. Fluorodeoxyglucose positron emission tomography in the evaluation of germ cell tumours at relapse. Br J Cancer. 2000; 83(7):863–869

[45] Treglia G, Sadeghi R, Annunziata S, Caldarella C, Bertagna F, Giovanella L. Diagnostic performance of fluorine-18-fluorodeoxyglucose positron emission tomography in the postchemotherapy management of patients with seminoma: systematic review and meta-analysis. BioMed Res Int. 2014; 2014:852681

[46] Lassen U, Daugaard G, Eigtved A, Højgaard L, Damgaard K, Rørth M. Whole-body FDG-PET in patients with stage I nonseminomatous germ cell tumours. Eur J Nucl Med Mol Imaging. 2003; 30(3):396–402

[47] Cremerius U, Effert PJ, Adam G, et al. FDG PET for detection and therapy control of metastatic germ cell tumor. J Nucl Med. 1998; 39(5):815–822

[48] Stephens AW, Gonin R, Hutchins GD, Einhorn LH. Positron emission tomography evaluation of residual radiographic abnormalities in postchemotherapy germ cell tumor patients. J Clin Oncol. 1996; 14(5):1637–1641

[49] Goodfellow H, Viney Z, Hughes P, et al. Role of fluorodeoxyglucose positron emission tomography (FDG PET)-computed tomography (CT) in the staging of bladder cancer. BJU Int. 2014; 114(3):389–395

[50] Soubra A, Hayward D, Dahm P, et al. The diagnostic accuracy of 18-fluorodeoxyglucose positron emission tomography and computed tomography in staging bladder cancer: a single-institution study and a systematic review with meta-analysis. World J Urol. 2016; 34(9):1229–1237

[51] Lodde M, Lacombe L, Friede J, Morin F, Saourine A, Fradet Y. Evaluation of fluorodeoxyglucose positron-emission tomography with computed tomography for staging of urothelial carcinoma. BJU Int. 2010; 106(5):658–663

[52] Wang N, Jiang P, Lu Y. Is fluorine-18 fluorodeoxyglucose positron emission tomography useful for detecting bladder lesions? A meta-analysis of the literature. Urol Int. 2014; 92(2):143–149

[53] Mertens LS, Mir MC, Scott AM, et al. 18F-fluorodeoxyglucose–positron emission tomography/computed tomography aids staging and predicts mortality in patients with muscle-invasive bladder cancer. Urology. 2014; 83(2):393–398

[54] Jensen TK, Holt P, Gerke O, et al. Preoperative lymph-node staging of invasive urothelial bladder cancer with 18F-fluorodeoxyglucose positron emission tomography/computed axial tomography and magnetic resonance imaging: correlation with histopathology. Scand J Urol Nephrol. 2011; 45(2):122–128

[55] Liu IJ, Lai YH, Espiritu JI, et al. Evaluation of fluorodeoxyglucose positron emission tomography imaging in metastatic transitional cell carcinoma with and without prior chemotherapy. Urol Int. 2006; 77(1):69–75

[56] Yang Z, Pan L, Cheng J, et al. Clinical value of whole body fluorine-18 fluorodeoxyglucose positron emission tomography/computed tomography in the detection of metastatic bladder cancer. Int J Urol. 2012; 19(7):639–644

[57] Bertagna F, Sadeghi R, Giovanella L, Treglia G. Incidental uptake of 18F-fluorodeoxyglucose on positron emission tomography in the prostate gland. Systematic review and meta-analysis on prevalence and risk of malignancy. Nucl Med (Stuttg). 2014; 53(6):249–258

[58] Hwang I, Chong A, Jung SI, et al. Is further evaluation needed for incidental focal uptake in the prostate in 18-fluoro-2-deoxyglucose positron emission tomography-computed tomography images? Ann Nucl Med. 2013; 27(2):140–145

[59] Brown AM, Lindenberg ML, Sankineni S, et al. Does focal incidental 18F-FDG PET/CT uptake in the prostate have significance? Abdom Imaging. 2015; 40(8):3222–3229

[60] Han EJ, H O J, Choi WH, Yoo IR, Chung SK. Significance of incidental focal uptake in prostate on 18-fluoro-2-deoxyglucose positron emission tomography CT images. Br J Radiol. 2010; 83(995):915–920

[61] Seino H, Ono S, Miura H, et al. Incidental prostate 18F-FDG uptake without calcification indicates the possibility of prostate cancer. Oncol Rep. 2014; 31(4):1517–1522

[62] Cho SK, Choi JY, Yoo J, et al. Incidental focal (18)F-FDG uptake in the prostate: clinical significance and differential diagnostic criteria. Nucl Med Mol Imaging. 2011; 45(3):192–196

[63] Jadvar H. Positron emission tomography in prostate cancer: summary of systematic reviews and meta-analysis. Tomography. 2015; 1(1):18–22

[64] Liu J, Chen Z, Wang T, et al. Influence of four radiotracers in PET/CT on diagnostic accuracy for prostate cancer: a bivariate random-effects meta-analysis. Cell Physiol Biochem. 2016; 39(2):467–480

[65] Savir-Baruch B, Zanoni L, Schuster DM. Imaging of prostate cancer using fluciclovine. PET Clin. 2017; 12(2):145–157

[66] Hofman MS, Iravani A. Gallium-68 prostate-specific membrane antigen PET imaging. PET Clin. 2017; 12(2):219–234

[67] Maurer T, Eiber M, Schwaiger M, Gschwend JE. Current use of PSMA-PET in prostate cancer management. Nat Rev Urol. 2016; 13(4):226–235

[68] Sathianathen NJ, Lamb A, Nair R, et al. Updates of prostate cancer staging: Prostate-specific membrane antigen. Investig Clin Urol. 2016; 57 Suppl 2:S147–S154

[69] Bach-Gansmo T, Nanni C, Nieh PT, et al. Multisite experience of the safety, detection rate and diagnostic performance of fluciclovine (18F) positron emission tomography/computerized tomography imaging in the staging of biochemically recurrent prostate cancer. J Urol. 2017; 197(3, Pt 1):676–683

[70] Odewole OA, Tade FI, Nieh PT, et al. Recurrent prostate cancer detection with anti-3-[(18)F]FACBC PET/CT: comparison with CT. Eur J Nucl Med Mol Imaging. 2016; 43(10):1773–1783

[71] Perera M, Papa N, Christidis D, et al. Sensitivity, specificity, and predictors of positive 68Ga-prostate-specific membrane antigen positron emission tomography in advanced prostate cancer: a systematic review and meta-analysis. Eur Urol. 2016; 70(6):926–937

[72] Ceci F, Uprimny C, Nilica B, et al. (68)Ga-PSMA PET/CT for restaging recurrent prostate cancer: which factors are associated with PET/CT detection rate? Eur J Nucl Med Mol Imaging. 2015; 42(8):1284–1294

[73] Rauscher I, Maurer T, Beer AJ, et al. Value of 68Ga-PSMA HBED-CC PET for the assessment of lymph node metastases in prostate cancer patients with biochemical recurrence: comparison with histopathology after salvage lymphadenectomy. J Nucl Med. 2016; 57(11):1713–1719

[74] Nanni C, Zanoni L, Pultrone C, et al. (18)F-FACBC (anti1-amino-3-(18)F-fluorocyclobutane-1-carboxylic acid) versus (11)C-choline PET/CT in prostate cancer relapse: results of a prospective trial. Eur J Nucl Med Mol Imaging. 2016; 43(9):1601–1610

[75] Morigi JJ, Stricker PD, van Leeuwen PJ, et al. Prospective comparison of 18F-fluoromethylcholine versus 68Ga-PSMA PET/CT in prostate cancer patients who have rising PSA after curative treatment and are being considered for targeted therapy. J Nucl Med. 2015; 56(8):1185–1190

[76] Schuster DM, Nieh PT, Jani AB, et al. Anti-3-[(18)F]FACBC positron emission tomography-computerized tomography and (111)In-capromab pendetide single photon emission computerized tomography-computerized tomography for recurrent prostate carcinoma: results of a prospective clinical trial. J Urol. 2014; 191(5):1446–1453

[77] Maurer T, Gschwend JE, Rauscher I, et al. Diagnostic efficacy of (68)gallium-PSMA positron emission tomography compared to conventional imaging for lymph node staging of 130 consecutive patients with intermediate to high risk prostate cancer. J Urol. 2016; 195(5):1436–1443

[78] Pyka T, Okamoto S, Dahlbender M, et al. Comparison of bone scintigraphy and 68Ga-PSMA PET for skeletal staging in prostate cancer. Eur J Nucl Med Mol Imaging. 2016; 43(12):2114–2121

[79] SNMMI. Axumin (Fluciclovine F 18) Image Interpretation Training. 2016. Available at: https://www.snmmilearningcenter.org/Activity/4521746/Detail.aspx. Accessed May 23, 2017

[80] Jadvar H. Imaging evaluation of prostate cancer with 18F-fluorodeoxyglucose PET/CT: utility and limitations. Eur J Nucl Med Mol Imaging. 2013; 40 Suppl 1:S5–S10

[81] Beauregard JM, Blouin AC, Fradet V, et al. FDG-PET/CT for pre-operative staging and prognostic stratification of patients with high-grade prostate cancer at biopsy. Cancer Imaging. 2015; 15:2

[82] Öztürk H, Karapolat I. 18F-fluorodeoxyglucose PET/CT for detection of disease in patients with prostate-specific antigen relapse following radical treatment of a local-stage prostate cancer. Oncol Lett. 2016; 11(1):316–322

[83] Jadvar H. Molecular imaging of prostate cancer: PET radiotracers. AJR Am J Roentgenol. 2012; 199(2):278–291

[84] Jadvar H, Desai B, Ji L, et al. Baseline 18F-FDG PET/CT parameters as imaging biomarkers of overall survival in castrate-resistant metastatic prostate cancer. J Nucl Med. 2013; 54(8):1195–1201

[85] Vargas HA, Wassberg C, Fox JJ, et al. Bone metastases in castration-resistant prostate cancer: associations between morphologic CT patterns, glycolytic activity, and androgen receptor expression on PET and overall survival. Radiology. 2014; 271(1):220–229

[86] Effert PJ, Bares R, Handt S, Wolff JM, Büll U, Jakse G. Metabolic imaging of untreated prostate cancer by positron emission tomography with 18fluorine-labeled deoxyglucose. J Urol. 1996; 155(3):994–998

[87] Chang CH, Wu HC, Tsai JJ, Shen YY, Changlai SP, Kao A. Detecting metastatic pelvic lymph nodes by 18F-2-deoxyglucose positron emission tomography in patients with prostate-specific antigen relapse after treatment for localized prostate cancer. Urol Int. 2003; 70(4):311–315

[88] Seltzer MA, Barbaric Z, Belldegrun A, et al. Comparison of helical computerized tomography, positron emission tomography and monoclonal antibody scans for evaluation of lymph node metastases in patients with prostate specific antigen relapse after treatment for localized prostate cancer. J Urol. 1999; 162(4):1322–1328

[89] Sung J, Espiritu JI, Segall GM, Terris MK. Fluorodeoxyglucose positron emission tomography studies in the diagnosis and staging of clinically advanced prostate cancer. BJU Int. 2003; 92(1):24–27

[90] Hofer C, Laubenbacher C, Block T, Breul J, Hartung R, Schwaiger M. Fluorine-18-fluorodeoxyglucose positron emission tomography is useless for the detection of local recurrence after radical prostatectomy. Eur Urol. 1999; 36(1):31–35

[91] Schöder H, Larson SM. Positron emission tomography for prostate, bladder, and renal cancer. Semin Nucl Med. 2004; 34(4):274–292

[92] Powles T, Murray I, Brock C, Oliver T, Avril N. Molecular positron emission tomography and PET/CT imaging in urological malignancies. Eur Urol. 2007; 51(6):1511–1520, discussion 1520–1521

[93] Oyama N, Akino H, Suzuki Y, et al. FDG PET for evaluating the change of glucose metabolism in prostate cancer after androgen ablation. Nucl Med Commun. 2001; 22(9):963–969

[94] Jadvar H. Prostate cancer: PET with 18F-FDG, 18F- or 11C-acetate, and 18F- or 11C-choline. J Nucl Med. 2011; 52(1):81–89

[95] Schöder H, Herrmann K, Gönen M, et al. 2-[18F]fluoro-2-deoxyglucose positron emission tomography for the detection of disease in patients with prostate-specific antigen relapse after radical prostatectomy. Clin Cancer Res. 2005; 11(13):4761–4769

[96] Morris MJ, Akhurst T, Osman I, et al. Fluorinated deoxyglucose positron emission tomography imaging in progressive metastatic prostate cancer. Urology. 2002; 59(6):913–918

25 Colorectal Cancer

Eugene C. Lin

25.1 Primary Colonic Neoplasms

Positron emission tomography/computed tomography (PET/CT) colonography[1] has been described; some of the advantages of PET/CT colonography over CT colonography are that it can be performed without bowel preparation and it has a higher positive predictive value for polyps. However in general, PET/CT has little role in screening for colonic neoplasm, but colonic lesions may be detected incidentally on PET/CT scans performed for other indications (▶ Fig. 25.1). Although the sensitivity of PET/CT for colorectal neoplasms is variable, the specificity and positive predictive value is high enough that colonoscopy is warranted in patients with focal colonic uptake, if the detection of a premalignant or malignant lesion would impact management.

In a meta-analysis,[2] the pooled risk of malignant or premalignant lesions in patients with focal colorectal incidental uptake was 68%. The risk was lower in Asia-Oceania compared to Europe and America.

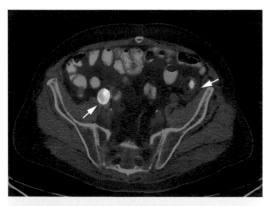

Fig. 25.1 Colon polyps. Axial PET/CT scan demonstrates uptake in two colonic polyps (*arrows*). Focal uptake colonic uptake should usually be further evaluated. However, focal colonic uptake on PET/CT will be false positive in approximately 30% of cases. standardized uptake value is not helpful in distinguishing pathologic from physiologic uptake. Focal uptake in the ascending colon or cecum is more likely to be physiologic than elsewhere in the colon.

25.2 Accuracy/Comparison to Other Modalities

1. The published detection rates for PET/CT has ranged widely, from 20 to 90%.[3] One study suggests that PET is unlikely to miss a colon cancer, while another suggests that the sensitivity of PET for colon cancers less than 2 cm is limited.[4] However, PET/CT will detect the primary tumor in most patients with a known colorectal cancer.

2. **PET:** Sensitivity is 74% and specificity is 84% for colonic neoplasm (adenomas or carcinoma) compared to colonoscopy.[5]
   a) Factors influencing detection rate are size, presence of a villous component, shape (decreased sensitivity for flat morphology, highest for pedunculated polyps), and histologic grade, with histologic grade being the strongest factor.[6]
   b) For polyps ≥ 11 mm, detection rates have ranged from 59 to 85%.[6,7]

25.3 Pearls/Pitfalls

1. **Degree of uptake**. Both adenomas (▶ Fig. 25.1) and carcinomas (▶ Fig. 25.2) may appear with increased uptake on PET/CT. While the degree of uptake tends to be higher in malignant lesions[8] and tumor size and depth of invasion are associated with higher standardized uptake values (SUVs),[9] published SUV cutoffs for evaluating colonic uptake range from 4.35 to 11.4,[8,10] suggesting that no specific cutoffs are useful in general clinical practice. One group suggests that to avoid missing a malignancy or high-grade dysplasia, a colonoscopy should be performed at a maximum SUV (SUVmax) of 2.5, although the optimal cutoff is higher.[11] In a meta-analysis,[2] there was a significant overlap in average SUV between malignant, premalignant, and benign etiologies (▶ Fig. 25.3) of focal colonic uptake.

2. **Nonmalignant causes of uptake**[12]:
   a) Focal physiologic uptake can cause false-positive findings:
      • With PET/CT, focal bowel uptake is false positive approximately one-third of the time.[13] The false-positive rate is higher with PET alone.

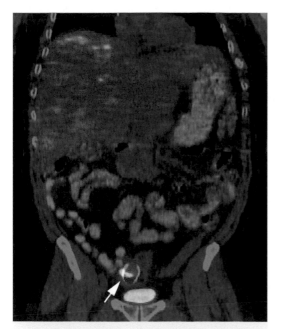

Fig. 25.2 Metastatic primary colon cancer. Coronal PET/CT demonstrates a primary sigmoid colon cancer (*arrow*) with extensive hepatic metastases. A stent has been placed in the region of the tumor to relieve obstruction.

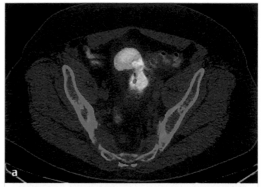

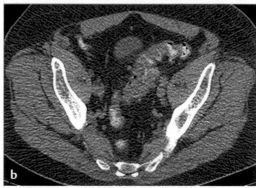

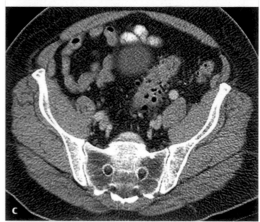

- SUV values cannot distinguish between focal physiological uptake and neoplasm.[13]
  b) Hemorrhoids can have increased uptake likely secondary to inflammation.
  c) Hyperplastic polyps usually do not have fluorodeoxyglucose (FDG) uptake, although uptake has been described in rare cases.
3. **Uptake pattern.** The pattern of uptake is helpful in differential diagnosis:
  a) Nodular colonic uptake is often due to a focal lesion.
  b) Segmental uptake is often secondary to inflammation.
  c) Diffuse uptake is usually normal. There is usually more uptake normally in the right colon, particularly in the cecum.[14]
4. **Location of uptake.** A higher false-positive rate is observed in the right colon compared to the distal colon.[15,16] This is particularly true in the cecum, where focal uptake can be seen from factors such as lymphoid uptake.
5. **Colonoscopy and colonic FDG uptake.** If focal FDG uptake is confined to the left colon, a complete colonic evaluation by colonoscopy is still necessary as advanced adenomas and

Fig. 25.3 Diverticulitis mimicking colon cancer. (a) Axial PET/CT in a patient with Hodgkin's disease demonstrates intense uptake in the sigmoid colon, corresponding to an area of diverticulosis and wall thickening noted on the CT (b). This was more suspicious for colon cancer than diverticulitis given the lack of surrounding inflammatory changes on CT. However, colonoscopy did not demonstrate malignancy and was consistent with very mild diverticulitis. A follow-up CT approximately 3 months later (c) demonstrates resolution of the wall thickening.

cancers can also be found in the right colon in these patients.[17] However, if patients have had a recent colonoscopy with no lesion identified in the region of the FDG uptake, an additional colonoscopy is generally not necessary to reevaluate the area of unmatched FDG uptake.[18]

6. **KRAS mutations**. KRAS gene mutations, occurring in approximately 40% of colorectal cancers, are associated with resistance to anti-epidermal growth factor receptor antibody therapy. The majority of studies[19,20,21,22] indicate that FDG accumulation is higher in colorectal cancer with KRAS mutations, suggesting that PET/CT could supplement genomic analysis, which can be limited by tumor heterogeneity or discordance between the primary and metastases.

25.4 Initial Staging

1. **Colon cancer**. National Comprehensive Cancer Network (NCCN) guidelines[23] indicate that PET/CT should only be used in initial staging to evaluate equivocal findings on CT, or in patients with a contraindication to IV contrast. Most patients who are surgical candidates do not have metastatic disease at presentation, particularly if cross-sectional imaging is negative, and the additional yield of PET in these patients is low. In addition, patients will often undergo colectomy to relieve obstruction, and intraoperative staging can be done during surgery. Evidence-based guidelines[24] do not recommend the routine use of PET/CT in the staging for clinical stage I to III colorectal cancers. However, PET/CT could potentially be useful in patients with stage IV disease who are candidates for resection. An international consensus panel[25] suggests that PET/CT may be useful in the detection of extrahepatic disease in patients with synchronous liver metastases at initial diagnosis, particularly if there is a high tumor load or a difficult hepatic resection is planned. PET/CT may also be helpful in patients with normal CT and high carcinoembryonic antigen (CEA) where demonstration of metastatic disease may preclude surgery. In patients with advanced disease (▶ Fig. 25.2), PET may allow optimal staging compared to findings during surgery.

   a) PET/CT colonography is more accurate in defining TNM (*t*umor size, *n*ode involvement, and *m*etastasis status) stage than CT alone, primarily due to more accurate definition of T stage. Bowel distention during PET/CT colonography is helpful for evaluating the bowel wall and surrounding soft tissue. However, T stage is often of minor clinical relevance in colon cancer (accurate assessment of T-stage preoperatively is more important in rectal cancer). Thus, the change in patient management from PET/CT in colorectal cancer staging is often due to detection of synchronous tumors.[26] In one report,[27] PET/CT had a high sensitivity and negative predictive value for the detection of proximal synchronous lesions in patients with obstructive colorectal cancer.

2. **Rectal cancer**. NCCN guidelines[28] state that PET/CT should only be used for initial staging to evaluate an equivocal finding on CT, or in patients with contraindications to IV contrast. PET may have value in advanced primary rectal cancer, particularly as a baseline study if neoadjuvant chemoradiation is being considered. In these patients, it can detect distant metastatic or synchronous disease and upstage disease in 8 to 24% of patients.[29,30,31]

   a) Discordant findings (usually lymph node metastases) between PET/CT and CT are more common in low rectal cancers than in mid or high rectal cancers; thus, PET/CT will more frequently add additional staging information in low rectal cancers.[32]

   b) Patients with adverse features on rectal MRI increase the risk for synchronous metastatic disease, and these patients may benefit from additional PET/CT evaluation.[33]

25.4.1 Accuracy/Comparison to Other Modalities

Lymph node staging (meta-analysis)[34]: sensitivity of 43% and specificity of 88%.

   Liver metastases (meta-analysis):
   • Sensitivity of 93% and specificity of 93% (patient-based analysis).
   • Sensitivity of 60% and specificity of 79% (lesion-based analysis).

Less sensitive, but more specific than MRI or CT.

25.5 Recurrence/Restaging

PET is a standard modality for evaluating colon cancer recurrence.[35,36] The primary uses are as follows:

1. **Rising CEA**. PET/CT is valuable in patients with rising CEA and suspected recurrent disease,

when anatomic imaging is equivocal or negative (▶ Fig. 25.4, ▶ Fig. 25.5, ▶ Fig. 25.6). In one study[37] of patients with an elevated CEA level, 55% of patient with PET/CT-detected relapsed disease were deemed eligible for further curative therapy. Detection of recurrence by PET is not associated with CA 19–9 levels.[38]

a) The exact utility of PET depends upon the level of CEA elevation. If CEA is less than 25 ng/mL, PET is helpful for triaging patients for appropriate management. If CEA is greater than 25 ng/mL, PET is mainly helpful in confirming the presence of advanced disease and occasionally in identifying potentially

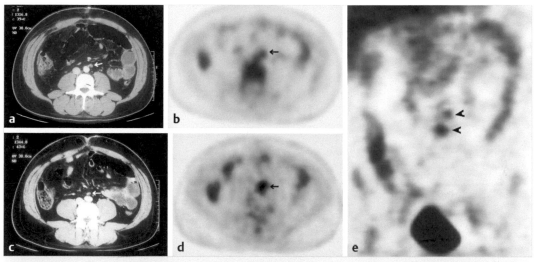

Fig. 25.4 Small metastatic nodes from colon cancer. **(a,c)** Axial CT scans in a patient with colon cancer demonstrate small retroperitoneal nodes (*arrows*). These measure approximately 5 mm in short axis dimension and would be considered normal by CT. **(b,d)** Axial PET scans demonstrate focal increased uptake (*arrows*) corresponding to these nodes. This degree of uptake in nodes of this small size is highly suggestive for malignancy. A low SUV value would not change the diagnosis of malignancy as partial volume effects could lower SUV substantially. **(e)** Coronal PET scan demonstrates uptake in the two nodes (*arrowheads*). Note that even though the nodes are less than 1 cm on CT, the contrast-to-noise ratio is great on PET and the nodes are very clearly seen. Lesion detection on PET is improved in regions with little motion and surrounding physiologic activity (e.g., the retroperitoneum). Although the superior node to the left of midline is comparable in size to the midline inferior node on the CT, the inferior node is more intense and appears "larger" on PET. PET is not accurate for size determination.

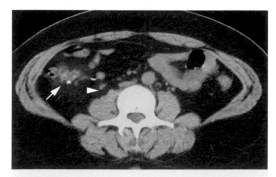

Fig. 25.5 Recurrent colon cancer. Axial PET/CT scan in a patient with colon cancer demonstrates recurrent disease (*arrow*) near an anastomosis. A small medial focus of activity (*arrowhead*) is in the ureter.

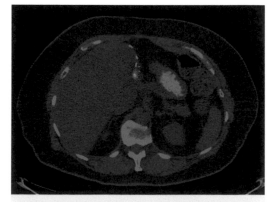

Fig. 25.6 Recurrent colon cancer. Axial PET/CT in a patient with colon cancer demonstrates recurrence at the margin of a prior hepatic resection.

resectable disease.[39] A cost-effective cutoff for utilizing PET to evaluate unexplained CEA elevation may be 10 ng/mL, although one study[38] indicates that the best compromise between sensitivity and specificity was achieved for CEA levels of 3.5 ng/mL.

2. PET/CT may also detect recurrence in patients with normal or low CEA values but suspicious of clinical symptoms or imaging findings.[40,41]

3. **Restaging in patients with apparently resectable hepatic metastases.** The primary value of PET/CT in patients with known hepatic metastases from colorectal cancer in whom surgery is being contemplated is in the detection of extrahepatic metastases, reducing futile laparotomies and to a lesser extent futile hepatectomies. The detection of extrahepatic metastases may preclude surgery, although in some cases PET/CT can be used to plan resection of extrahepatic disease, as additional resection of portal lymph nodes and peritoneal metastases in patients with hepatic metastases could potentially improve survival.[42] In one review[42] of 10 studies, the findings on PET altered management in 25% of patients, in about two-thirds of cases due to the detection of extrahepatic disease. However, there have only been two randomized studies. In one study,[43] unnecessary surgery was prevented by the addition of PET in one out of six patients. Another randomized study[44] is an outlier from previous studies, as change in management occurred in only 8.7% of cases as a result of PET, with 2.7% of patients avoiding futile surgery. However, about half the patients in this study received chemotherapy within 12 weeks of the surgery, which can decrease the sensitivity of PET.[45]

   a) In patients screened with preoperative PET before hepatic resection, PET detects unsuspected tumor in 25% and reduces the number of unnecessary laparotomies.[46] The overall 5-year survival after hepatic resection is 58% in colon cancer patients who have been examined with PET (compared to 30% in patients who have been assessed by conventional techniques).[47]

4. **Differentiation of posttreatment changes from recurrence**. This is a common problem in rectal cancer as both recurrence and postradiation scars cause can result in abnormal soft-tissue masses in the presacral space (▶ Fig. 25.7).

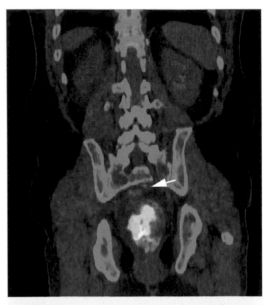

Fig. 25.7 Recurrent rectal cancer. Coronal PET/CT demonstrates a large presacral recurrence of rectal cancer. A small local nodal metastasis (*arrow*) is present.

25.5.1 Accuracy

1. **PET (hepatic):** sensitivity of 80% and specificity of 92%.[48]

   PET (extrahepatic): sensitivity of 91% and specificity of 98%:

   a) *Lesion size.* Sensitivity of PET is much lower for liver lesions less than 1 cm in size.

   b) *Mucinous tumors.* Sensitivity is low for mucinous tumors (58%), possibly due to hypocellularity of the malignant mass.[49]

   c) *Body region.* The specificity is very high in the liver and in local pelvic recurrence, and lower elsewhere in the body.

2. **PET/CT for local recurrence** (meta-analysis)[50]: sensitivity of 94% and specificity of 94%.

3. **PET/CT with elevated CEA** (meta-analysis): sensitivity of 94% and specificity of 77%[51]:

   a) PET/CT increases the accuracy to 90 from 75% for PET alone.[52]

   b) The primary advantage of PET/CT over PET is in increasing specificity for extra-abdominal and hepatic recurrences.

4. Local recurrence versus scar:

   a) **PET:** Sensitivity of 84% and specificity of 88%[53]:

   • The best results are obtained when PET is performed more than 12 months after radiation.

- PET is more accurate than immunoscintigraphy, with equal or greater sensitivity than MRI.
b) **PET/CT**: PET/CT increases accuracy in differentiating benign from malignant uptake in the pelvis and in presacral masses compared to PET alone (▶ Fig. 25.3).[54]
c) **Pelvic uptake**: sensitivity of 96% and specificity of 90%.
d) **Presacral mass**: sensitivity of 100% and specificity of 96%.

Comparison to Other Modalities

1. **Liver metastases.** In a meta-analysis[55] of patients with colorectal liver metastases, PET had a slightly lower sensitivity than MRI and CT on both patient- and lesion-based analyses, but was more specific than MRI and CT:
   a) CT portography has a higher degree of sensitivity but much lower degree of specificity for identifying liver metastases than PET.[56]
   b) MRI with liver-specific contrast agents such as mangafodipir trisodium, superparamagnetic iron oxide particles, or Eovist (gadolinium-EOB-DTPA, Schering AG) can detect more liver lesions than PET (▶ Fig. 25.8).[57,58]

2. **Extrahepatic metastases**:
   PET: sensitivity of 91% and specificity of 98%.[48]
   CT: sensitivity of 61% and specificity of 91%.
   a) **Peritoneal recurrence**: PET sensitivity of 88% and CT sensitivity of 38%.[48,59]
   b) **Body region**: PET is more sensitive than CT in the abdomen, pelvis, and retroperitoneum, and is comparable to CT in the lungs.[48,60]
   c) **Immunoscintigraphy:** Compared to immunoscintigraphy (technetium-99 m anti-CEA antibody), PET is significantly superior for the detection of distant metastases.[61]

3. **Local and distant recurrence.**[62] PET/CT is superior to CT for detecting both extrahepatic metastases and local recurrence. In a meta-analysis[63] of imaging for patients with suspected local or distant recurrence of colorectal cancer, PET and PET/CT was more accurate than CT, with an area under the curve of 0.94 compared to 0.83 for CT.
   a) **Extrahepatic metastases** (sensitivity): PET/CT, 89%; CT, 64%.
   b) **Local recurrence at primary colorectal resection site** (sensitivity): PET/CT, 93%; CT, 53%.

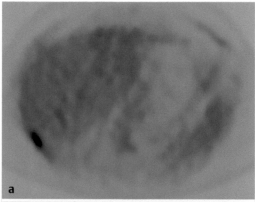
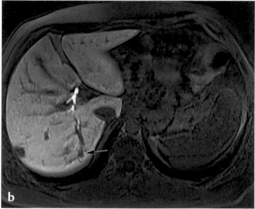

Fig. 25.8 Liver metastases. **(a)** Axial PET scan in a patient with rectal adenocarcinoma demonstrates a liver metastasis. **(b)** Axial hepatobiliary phase MRI performed with the hepatocellular contrast agent Eovist (gadolinium-EOB-DTPA, Schering AG), demonstrates the same metastasis in the peripheral right liver seen on PET, as well as an additional metastasis (*arrow*) not identified on PET.

   c) PET/CT changes management in 21% of patients.

Pearls

1. In patients with known liver metastases by anatomic imaging, PET can detect additional liver metastases but is most useful in detecting extrahepatic metastases and therefore precluding liver resection.
2. If hepatic resection is planned, it is difficult to localize liver lesions to specific segments on PET, as anatomic landmarks such as the hepatic veins are not visualized. Thus, correlation with anatomic imaging is necessary before surgery. PET/CT is ideally suited for this purpose.

3. **Prognosis.** Primary tumor grade and SUV of liver metastases are prognostic variables in patients undergoing liver resection after PET imaging:

a) Standard prognostic variables for outcome after liver metastases resection such as number of lesions, size, and synchronicity may be less important if PET is performed. These prognostic variables are a surrogate for extrahepatic disease, but PET can often detect this extrahepatic disease. However, primary tumor grade may be more valuable as a prognostic variable if PET is performed since poor differentiation could suggest a greater likelihood of small-volume disease not detectable by PET. Therefore, patients who have poorly differentiated primary tumors may still have a high chance of recurrence and poor outcome even if PET is negative for extrahepatic disease.[47]

b) Survival is significantly longer in patients with a low SUV in liver metastases than for patients with a high SUV.[64]

25.5.2 Pitfalls

1. **Normal CEA.** Positive PET findings in patients with normal CEA, even if symptoms suggest recurrence, should be interpreted with caution since most often no disease is found on follow-up examinations.

2. **Postsurgical.** A common cause of false-positive results in evaluating pelvic recurrence of rectal cancer is posterior displacement of pelvic contents following surgery. PET/CT is very helpful in reducing false-positive findings as a result of this type of intervention.[54] Minimizing bladder activity by voiding/catheterization is also helpful.

3. **Neoadjuvant chemotherapy.** The sensitivity of PET in detecting colorectal hepatic metastases decreases following neoadjuvant chemotherapy.[65] This is true even if PET imaging is performed with a minimal interval of 2 weeks following chemotherapy and may be related to decreased size of the metastases and reduction of uptake due to downregulation of glycolytic enzyme. In a meta-analysis,[45] the sensitivity of PET/CT for liver metastases in chemo-naïve patients was 71% compared to 52% after neoadjuvant chemotherapy.

4. **Mucinous tumors.** PET/CT is limited for the evaluation of mucinous colorectal tumors due to low FDG uptake. However, in one report,[66] FDG uptake was similar between mucinous and nonmucinous rectal adenocarcinomas.

25.6 Therapy Response[67]

In a meta-analysis,[68] PET/CT for evaluating metabolic response to therapy predicted event-free and overall survival in patients with liver metastases from colorectal carcinoma. Nonresponders had a risk of death approximately 2.5 times as high as responders. In addition, the pretreatment SUV was an independent prognostic factor for overall survival. However, posttreatment SUV did not predict overall survival.

PET has multiple uses in assessing therapy response in colorectal carcinomas[69]:

1. **Chemotherapy response in advanced colorectal cancer.** PET is useful for predicting response to chemotherapy in patients with unresectable colorectal cancer liver metastases.

a) *Interim PET.* PET can differentiate responders from nonresponders early in the course of chemotherapy for hepatic metastases. PET should be performed at least 4 weeks after initiating therapy as false-positive results from inflammation can be seen in the first 2 weeks of treatment.[70]

b) *End of therapy PET.* After completion of therapy, PET findings correlate better with pathological response than the findings on CT. However, one study suggests that liver metastases that have a complete metabolic response on PET and disappear on CT or MRI can still contain viable tumor.[71] Thus, if patients with unresectable liver metastases are treated to render them resectable, PET findings should not preclude curative resection.

c) *Prognosis.* There is a significant survival benefit in patients with low FDG uptake in colorectal cancer metastases.[72] This is true for both patients who undergo resection and those who are treated with chemotherapy.

2. **Monitoring response to local ablative therapy for liver metastases.** PET can be used to monitor the results of minimally invasive therapies such as radiofrequency ablation (RFA) and interarterial ^{90}Y microsphere radioembolization. Several reports[73,74,75] indicate that PET is more accurate than contrast-enhanced CT for evaluation of treatment success after RFA, and also more cost-effective.[73] In a meta-analysis,[76] PET/CT had a higher sensitivity than CT for detecting

disease progression after radiotherapy (85 and 53%, respectively), while specificity was similar (92 and 96%, respectively). PET/CT provides a more accurate and earlier assessment of therapy response to ^{90}Y radioembolization than does CT.[77] As local tumor progression secondary to residual tumor is most common in tumors greater than 3 cm, PET/CT is of less value in lesions less than 2 cm.[11] PET/CT may be most valuable in patients with multiple and bilobar tumors[75]:

a) On CT and MRI, a nonpathological rim of increased contrast enhancement is found immediately after RFA, which often cannot be differentiated from residual tumor.[78] After RFA, inflammation and tissue regeneration at the periphery of the necrotic zone can result in a peripheral rind of low- to moderate-intensity FDG uptake, typically starting 2 to 3 days after RFA but decreasing to background in about 6 months.[79,80] This uptake can mask foci of residual disease. Thus, PET/CT is most accurate when performed within 2 days after RFA. However, in one report,[81] circumferential FDG uptake was occasionally noted in completely ablated tumors 24 hours after RFA, suggesting that imaging should be performed as soon as possible after RFA. In a meta-analysis,[82] the sensitivity and specificity of PET and PET/CT for detecting residual tumor after RFA were 79 and 84%, respectively, if performed within 2 days of RFA. If imaging was performed 1 week after treatment, the sensitivity and specificity were 48 and 94%, respectively, and 52 and 94%, respectively, at 3 months. PET negative lesions after ablation are very unlikely to develop local recurrence.

b) The most specific pattern for local tumor progression is focal nodular uptake around the ablation zone.[81]

3. **Response evaluation in preoperative chemoradiotherapy for primary rectal cancer.** Neoadjuvant chemoradiotherapy (CRT) followed by total mesorectal excision surgery is the standard treatment for locally advanced mid and lower rectal carcinoma. Approximately 20% of patients will achieve a complete pathologic response, which is predictive of improved local control and disease-free survival. Tumor regression is also a prognostic factor. PET performed as early as 12 days after preoperative CRT predicts pathologic response.[83] One meta-analysis suggests that PET is more suitable for the prediction of tumor regression than pathologic complete response.[84] Accurate response assessment to CRT could potentially help in optimizing the surgical approach or choosing a nonoperative approach, identifying nonresponders who are not candidates for organ preservation, and predicting long-term prognosis. Morphologic imaging modalities such as CT or MRI are limited in response assessment as it may be difficult to distinguish treatment-related inflammation and fibrosis from viable tumor cells in residual masses.[84] In one report,[85] PET had a greater impact on patient management postneoadjuvant CRT than CT or conventional MRI. However, diffusion-weighted MRI may be an alternative or supplement to PET/CT in these settings. In one report,[86] diffusion-weighted MRI was superior to PET/CT in predicting pathologic response, and a few reports[87,88] suggest that PET/CT and diffusion-weighted MRI are most useful when combined. However, European Society of Medical Oncology guidelines indicate that currently the extent of surgery should not be modified on the basis of PET or MRI.

In a meta-analysis,[55] the pooled sensitivity and specificity of PET for predicting response to neoadjuvant therapy were 73 and 77%, respectively. However, there is substantial variability in the timing of PET scans and methods of analysis in the published literature. In the previous meta-analysis, if PET was performed at 1 to 2 weeks after the start of CRT, the pooled sensitivity and specificity were 84 and 81%, respectively. This is consistent with the results of other meta-analyses,[84,89] which suggest that the accuracy of PET is higher when performed during rather than after the completion of therapy.

Parameters that can be used to evaluate response include change in SUVmax, SUVmax posttherapy, and visual analysis. A systematic review[90] indicates that both the change in SUV and SUV posttherapy are strongly associated with disease-free and overall survival and predicts pathologic complete response. In a meta-analysis, the pooled value for SUV change was 63% and the pooled value for SUV posttherapy was 4.4%.[55]

References

[1] Taylor SA, Bomanji JB, Manpanzure L, et al. Nonlaxative PET/CT colonography: feasibility, acceptability, and pilot performance in patients at higher risk of colonic neoplasia. J Nucl Med. 2010; 51(6):854–861

[2] Treglia G, Taralli S, Salsano M, Muoio B, Sadeghi R, Giovanella L. Prevalence and malignancy risk of focal colorectal incidental uptake detected by (18)F-FDG-PET or PET/CT: a meta-analysis. Radiol Oncol. 2014; 48(2):99–104

[3] Huang SW, Hsu CM, Jeng WJ, Yen TC, Su MY, Chiu CT. A comparison of positron emission tomography and colonoscopy for the detection of advanced colorectal neoplasms in subjects undergoing a health check-up. PLoS One. 2013; 8(7): e69111

[4] Friedland S, Soetikno R, Carlisle M, Taur A, Kaltenbach T, Segall G. 18-Fluorodeoxyglucose positron emission tomography has limited sensitivity for colonic adenoma and early stage colon cancer. Gastrointest Endosc. 2005; 61(3):395–400

[5] Drenth JP, Nagengast FM, Oyen WJ. Evaluation of (pre-)malignant colonic abnormalities: endoscopic validation of FDG-PET findings. Eur J Nucl Med. 2001; 28(12):1766–1769

[6] Nakajo M, Jinnouchi S, Tashiro Y, et al. Effect of clinicopathologic factors on visibility of colorectal polyps with FDG PET. AJR Am J Roentgenol. 2009; 192(3):754–760

[7] Hirakawa T, Kato J, Okumura Y, et al. Detectability of colorectal neoplasia with fluorine-18-2-fluoro-2-deoxy-D-glucose positron emission tomography and computed tomography (FDG-PET/CT). J Gastroenterol. 2012; 47(2):127–135

[8] van Hoeij FB, Keijsers RG, Loffeld BC, Dun G, Stadhouders PH, Weusten BL. Incidental colonic focal FDG uptake on PET/CT: can the maximum standardized uptake value (SUVmax) guide us in the timing of colonoscopy? Eur J Nucl Med Mol Imaging. 2015; 42(1):66–71

[9] Gu J, Yamamoto H, Fukunaga H, et al. Correlation of GLUT-1 overexpression, tumor size, and depth of invasion with 18F-2-fluoro-2-deoxy-D-glucose uptake by positron emission tomography in colorectal cancer. Dig Dis Sci. 2006; 51(12): 2198–2205

[10] Cho SH, Kim SW, Kim WC, et al. Incidental focal colorectal 18F-fluorodeoxyglucose uptake on positron emission tomography/computed tomography. World J Gastroenterol. 2013; 19(22):3453–3458

[11] Na SY, Kim KJ, Han S, et al. Who should undergo a colonoscopy among patients with incidental colon uptake on PET-CT? Scand J Gastroenterol. 2015; 50(8):1045–1053

[12] Kamel EM, Thumshirn M, Truninger K, et al. Significance of incidental 18F-FDG accumulations in the gastrointestinal tract in PET/CT: correlation with endoscopic and histopathologic results. J Nucl Med. 2004; 45(11):1804–1810

[13] Gutman F, Alberini JL, Wartski M, et al. Incidental colonic focal lesions detected by FDG PET/CT. AJR Am J Roentgenol. 2005; 185(2):495–500

[14] Tatlidil R, Jadvar H, Bading JR, Conti PS. Incidental colonic fluorodeoxyglucose uptake: correlation with colonoscopic and histopathologic findings. Radiology. 2002; 224(3):783–787

[15] Peng J, He Y, Xu J, Sheng J, Cai S, Zhang Z. Detection of incidental colorectal tumours with 18F-labelled 2-fluoro-2-deoxyglucose positron emission tomography/computed tomography scans: results of a prospective study. Colorectal Dis. 2011; 13(11):e374–e378

[16] Seivert M, Plomteux O, Colard A, et al. Endoscopic findings in case of incidental colonic uptake in PET-CT how to improve PET-CT specificity? Acta Gastroenterol Belg. 2014; 77(4): 413–417

[17] Lee C, Koh SJ, Kim JW, et al. Incidental colonic 18F-fluorodeoxyglucose uptake: do we need colonoscopy for patients with focal uptake confined to the left-sided colon? Dig Dis Sci. 2013; 58(1):229–235

[18] Yun CY, Jung JO, Suh SO, et al. Is it useful to perform additional colonoscopy to detect unmatched lesion between positron emission tomography/computed tomography and colonoscopy? Korean J Gastroenterol. 2013; 61(6):319–326

[19] Iwamoto M, Kawada K, Nakamoto Y, et al. Regulation of 18F-FDG accumulation in colorectal cancer cells with mutated KRAS. J Nucl Med. 2014; 55(12):2038–2044

[20] Kawada K, Nakamoto Y, Kawada M, et al. Relationship between 18F-fluorodeoxyglucose accumulation and KRAS/BRAF mutations in colorectal cancer. Clin Cancer Res. 2012; 18(6):1696–1703

[21] Kawada K, Toda K, Nakamoto Y, et al. Relationship between 18F-FDG PET/CT scans and KRAS mutations in metastatic colorectal cancer. J Nucl Med. 2015; 56(9):1322–1327

[22] Lee JH, Kang J, Baik SH, et al. Relationship between 18F-fluorodeoxyglucose uptake and V-Ki-ras2 Kirsten rat sarcoma viral oncogene homolog mutation in colorectal cancer patients: variability depending on C-reactive protein level. Medicine (Baltimore). 2016; 95(1):e2236

[23] Benson AB, III, Venook AP, Bekaii-Saab T, et al. National Comprehensive Cancer Network. Colon cancer, version 3.2014. J Natl Compr Canc Netw. 2014; 12(7):1028–1059

[24] Chan K, Welch S, Walker-Dilks C, Raifu A, Ontario provincial Gastrointestinal Disease Site Group. Evidence-based guideline recommendations on the use of positron emission tomography imaging in colorectal cancer. Clin Oncol (R Coll Radiol). 2012; 24(4):232–249

[25] Adam R, de Gramont A, Figueras J, et al. of the EGOSLIM (Expert Group on OncoSurgery management of LIver Metastases) group. Managing synchronous liver metastases from colorectal cancer: a multidisciplinary international consensus. Cancer Treat Rev. 2015; 41(9):729–741

[26] Veit-Haibach P, Kuehle CA, Beyer T, et al. Diagnostic accuracy of colorectal cancer staging with whole-body PET/CT colonography. JAMA. 2006; 296(21):2590–2600

[27] Kim WS, Lee HS, Lee JM, et al. Fluoro-2-deoxy-d-glucose positron emission tomography/computed tomography for the detection of proximal synchronous lesions in patients with obstructive colorectal cancer. J Gastroenterol Hepatol. 2017; 32(2):401–408

[28] Benson AB, III, Venook AP, Bekaii-Saab T, et al. Rectal Cancer, Version 2.2015. J Natl Compr Canc Netw. 2015; 13(6):719–728, quiz 728

[29] Heriot AG, Hicks RJ, Drummond EG, et al. Does positron emission tomography change management in primary rectal cancer? A prospective assessment. Dis Colon Rectum. 2004; 47 (4):451–458

[30] Nahas CS, Akhurst T, Yeung H, et al. Positron emission tomography detection of distant metastatic or synchronous disease in patients with locally advanced rectal cancer receiving preoperative chemoradiation. Ann Surg Oncol. 2008; 15(3):704–711

[31] Muthusamy VR, Chang KJ. Optimal methods for staging rectal cancer. Clin Cancer Res. 2007; 13(22, Pt 2):6877s–6884s

[32] Gearhart SL, Frassica D, Rosen R, Choti M, Schulick R, Wahl R. Improved staging with pretreatment positron emission tomography/computed tomography in low rectal cancer. Ann Surg Oncol. 2006; 13(3):397–404

[33] Hunter CJ, Garant A, Vuong T, et al. Adverse features on rectal MRI identify a high-risk group that may benefit from more intensive preoperative staging and treatment. Ann Surg Oncol. 2012; 19(4):1199–1205

[34] Lu YY, Chen JH, Ding HJ, Chien CR, Lin WY, Kao CH. A systematic review and meta-analysis of pretherapeutic lymph node staging of colorectal cancer by 18F-FDG PET or PET/CT. Nucl Med Commun. 2012; 33(11):1127–1133

[35] Vitola J, Delbeke D. Positron emission tomography for evaluation of colorectal carcinoma. Semin Roentgenol. 2002; 37(2): 118–128

[36] Chin BB, Wahl RL. 18F-Fluoro-2-deoxyglucose positron emission tomography in the evaluation of gastrointestinal malignancies. Gut. 2003; 52 Suppl 4:iv23–iv29

[37] Khan K, Athauda A, Aitken K, et al. Survival outcomes in asymptomatic patients with normal conventional imaging but raised carcinoembryonic antigen levels in colorectal cancer following positron emission tomography-computed tomography imaging. Oncologist. 2016; 21(12):1502–1508

[38] Chiaravalloti A, Fiorentini A, Palombo E, et al. Evaluation of recurrent disease in the re-staging of colorectal cancer by 18F-FDG PET/CT: use of CEA and CA 19-9 in patient selection. Oncol Lett. 2016; 12(5):4209–4213

[39] Liu FY, Chen JS, Changchien CR, et al. Utility of 2-fluoro-2-deoxy-D-glucose positron emission tomography in managing patients of colorectal cancer with unexplained carcinoembryonic antigen elevation at different levels. Dis Colon Rectum. 2005; 48(10):1900–1912

[40] Agarwal A, Marcus C, Xiao J, Nene P, Kachnic LA, Subramaniam RM. FDG PET/CT in the management of colorectal and anal cancers. AJR Am J Roentgenol. 2014; 203(5):1109–1119

[41] Laurens ST, Oyen WJ. Impact of fluorodeoxyglucose PET/computed tomography on the management of patients with colorectal cancer. PET Clin. 2015; 10(3):345–360

[42] Strasberg SM, Dehdashti F. Role of FDG-PET staging in selecting the optimum patient for hepatic resection of metastatic colorectal cancer. J Surg Oncol. 2010; 102(8):955–959

[43] Ruers TJ, Wiering B, van der Sijp JR, et al. Improved selection of patients for hepatic surgery of colorectal liver metastases with (18)F-FDG PET: a randomized study. J Nucl Med. 2009; 50(7):1036–1041

[44] Moulton CA, Gu CS, Law CH, et al. Effect of PET before liver resection on surgical management for colorectal adenocarcinoma metastases: a randomized clinical trial. JAMA. 2014; 311(18):1863–1869

[45] van Kessel CS, Buckens CF, van den Bosch MA, van Leeuwen MS, van Hillegersberg R, Verkooijen HM. Preoperative imaging of colorectal liver metastases after neoadjuvant chemotherapy: a meta-analysis. Ann Surg Oncol. 2012; 19(9):2805–2813

[46] Wiering B, Krabbe PF, Dekker HM, Oyen WJ, Ruers TJ. The role of FDG-PET in the selection of patients with colorectal liver metastases. Ann Surg Oncol. 2007; 14(2):771–779

[47] Fernandez FG, Drebin JA, Linehan DC, Dehdashti F, Siegel BA, Strasberg SM. Five-year survival after resection of hepatic metastases from colorectal cancer in patients screened by positron emission tomography with F-18 fluorodeoxyglucose (FDG-PET). Ann Surg. 2004; 240(3):438–447, discussion 447–450

[48] Wiering B, Krabbe PF, Jager GJ, Oyen WJ, Ruers TJ. The impact of fluor-18-deoxyglucose-positron emission tomography in the management of colorectal liver metastases. Cancer. 2005; 104(12):2658–2670

[49] Whiteford MH, Whiteford HM, Yee LF, et al. Usefulness of FDG-PET scan in the assessment of suspected metastatic or recurrent adenocarcinoma of the colon and rectum. Dis Colon Rectum. 2000; 43(6):759–767, discussion 767–770

[50] Yu T, Meng N, Chi D, Zhao Y, Wang K, Luo Y. Diagnostic value of (18)F-FDG PET/CT in detecting local recurrent colorectal cancer: a pooled analysis of 26 individual studies. Cell Biochem Biophys. 2015; 72(2):443–451

[51] Lu YY, Chen JH, Chien CR, et al. Use of FDG-PET or PET/CT to detect recurrent colorectal cancer in patients with elevated CEA: a systematic review and meta-analysis. Int J Colorectal Dis. 2013; 28(8):1039–1047

[52] Votrubova J, Belohlavek O, Jaruskova M, et al. The role of FDG-PET/CT in the detection of recurrent colorectal cancer. Eur J Nucl Med Mol Imaging. 2006; 33(7):779–784

[53] Moore HG, Akhurst T, Larson SM, Minsky BD, Mazumdar M, Guillem JG. A case-controlled study of 18-fluorodeoxyglucose positron emission tomography in the detection of pelvic recurrence in previously irradiated rectal cancer patients. J Am Coll Surg. 2003; 197(1):22–28

[54] Even-Sapir E, Parag Y, Lerman H, et al. Detection of recurrence in patients with rectal cancer: PET/CT after abdominoperineal or anterior resection. Radiology. 2004; 232(3):815–822

[55] Maffione AM, Marzola MC, Capirci C, Colletti PM, Rubello D. Value of (18)F-FDG PET for predicting response to neoadjuvant therapy in rectal cancer: systematic review and meta-analysis. AJR Am J Roentgenol. 2015; 204(6):1261–1268

[56] Delbeke D, Vitola JV, Sandler MP, et al. Staging recurrent metastatic colorectal carcinoma with PET. J Nucl Med. 1997; 38(8):1196–1201

[57] Sahani DV, Kalva SP, Fischman AJ, et al. Detection of liver metastases from adenocarcinoma of the colon and pancreas: comparison of mangafodipir trisodium-enhanced liver MRI and whole-body FDG PET. AJR Am J Roentgenol. 2005; 185 (1):239–246

[58] Rappeport ED, Loft A, Berthelsen AK, et al. Contrast-enhanced FDG-PET/CT vs. SPIO-enhanced MRI vs. FDG-PET vs. CT in patients with liver metastases from colorectal cancer: a prospective study with intraoperative confirmation. Acta Radiol. 2007; 48(4):369–378

[59] Tanaka T, Kawai Y, Kanai M, Taki Y, Nakamoto Y, Takabayashi A. Usefulness of FDG-positron emission tomography in diagnosing peritoneal recurrence of colorectal cancer. Am J Surg. 2002; 184(5):433–436

[60] Valk PE, Abella-Columna E, Haseman MK, et al. Whole-body PET imaging with [18F]fluorodeoxyglucose in management of recurrent colorectal cancer. Arch Surg. 1999; 134(5):503–511, discussion 511–513

[61] Willkomm P, Bender H, Bangard M, Decker P, Grünwald F, Biersack HJ. FDG PET and immunoscintigraphy with 99mTc-labeled antibody fragments for detection of the recurrence of colorectal cancer. J Nucl Med. 2000; 41(10):1657–1663

[62] Selzner M, Hany TF, Wildbrett P, McCormack L, Kadry Z, Clavien PA. Does the novel PET/CT imaging modality impact on the treatment of patients with metastatic colorectal cancer of the liver? Ann Surg. 2004; 240(6):1027–1034, discussion 1035–1036

[63] Maas M, Rutten IJ, Nelemans PJ, et al. What is the most accurate whole-body imaging modality for assessment of local and distant recurrent disease in colorectal cancer? A meta-analysis : imaging for recurrent colorectal cancer. Eur J Nucl Med Mol Imaging. 2011; 38(1):1560–1571

[64] Riedl CC, Akhurst T, Larson S, et al. 18F-FDG PET scanning correlates with tissue markers of poor prognosis and predicts mortality for patients after liver resection for colorectal metastases. J Nucl Med. 2007; 48(5):771–775

[65] Lubezky N, Metser U, Geva R, et al. The role and limitations of 18-fluoro-2-deoxy-D-glucose positron emission tomography (FDG-PET) scan and computerized tomography (CT) in restaging patients with hepatic colorectal metastases following neoadjuvant chemotherapy: comparison with operative and pathological findings. J Gastrointest Surg. 2007; 11(4):472–478

[66] Dos Anjos DA, Habr-Gama A, Vailati BB, et al. (18)F-FDG uptake by rectal cancer is similar in mucinous and nonmucinous histological subtypes. Ann Nucl Med. 2016; 30(8):513–517

[67] Kostakoglu L, Goldsmith SJ. 18F-FDG PET evaluation of the response to therapy for lymphoma and for breast, lung, and colorectal carcinoma. J Nucl Med. 2003; 44(2):224–239

[68] Xia Q, Liu J, Wu C, et al. Prognostic significance of (18)FDG PET/CT in colorectal cancer patients with liver metastases: a meta-analysis. Cancer Imaging. 2015; 15:19

[69] de Geus-Oei LF, Ruers TJ, Punt CJ, Leer JW, Corstens FH, Oyen WJ. FDG-PET in colorectal cancer. Cancer Imaging. 2006; 6: S71–S81

[70] Findlay M, Young H, Cunningham D, et al. Noninvasive monitoring of tumor metabolism using fluorodeoxyglucose and positron emission tomography in colorectal cancer liver metastases: correlation with tumor response to fluorouracil. J Clin Oncol. 1996; 14(3):700–708

[71] Tan MC, Linehan DC, Hawkins WG, Siegel BA, Strasberg SM. Chemotherapy-induced normalization of FDG uptake by colorectal liver metastases does not usually indicate complete pathologic response. J Gastrointest Surg. 2007; 11(9):1112–1119

[72] de Geus-Oei LF, Wiering B, Krabbe PF, Ruers TJ, Punt CJ, Oyen WJ. FDG-PET for prediction of survival of patients with metastatic colorectal carcinoma. Ann Oncol. 2006; 17(11):1650–1655

[73] Chen W, Zhuang H, Cheng G, Torigian DA, Alavi A. Comparison of FDG-PET, MRI and CT for post radiofrequency ablation evaluation of hepatic tumors. Ann Nucl Med. 2013; 27(1): 58–64

[74] Cornelis F, Sotirchos V, Violari E, et al. 18F-FDG PET/CT is an immediate imaging biomarker of treatment success after liver metastasis ablation. J Nucl Med. 2016; 57(7):1052–1057

[75] Sahin DA, Agcaoglu O, Chretien C, Siperstein A, Berber E. The utility of PET/CT in the management of patients with colorectal liver metastases undergoing laparascopic radiofrequency thermal ablation. Ann Surg Oncol. 2012; 19(3):850–855

[76] Samim M, Molenaar IQ, Seesing MF, et al. The diagnostic performance of 18F-FDG PET/CT, CT and MRI in the treatment evaluation of ablation therapy for colorectal liver metastases: A systematic review and meta-analysis. Surg Oncol. 2017; 26 (1):37–45

[77] Bienert M, McCook B, Carr BI, et al. 90Y microsphere treatment of unresectable liver metastases: changes in 18F-FDG uptake and tumour size on PET/CT. Eur J Nucl Med Mol Imaging. 2005; 32(7):778–787

[78] Antoch G, Vogt FM, Veit P, et al. Assessment of liver tissue after radiofrequency ablation: findings with different imaging procedures. J Nucl Med. 2005; 46(3):520–525

[79] Purandare NC, Rangarajan V, Shah SA, et al. Therapeutic response to radiofrequency ablation of neoplastic lesions: FDG PET/CT findings. Radiographics. 2011; 31(1):201–213

[80] Sainani NI, Gervais DA, Mueller PR, Arellano RS. Imaging after percutaneous radiofrequency ablation of hepatic tumors: part 1, normal findings. AJR Am J Roentgenol. 2013; 200(1): 184–193

[81] Vandenbroucke F, Vandemeulebroucke J, Ilsen B, et al. Predictive value of pattern classification 24 hours after radiofrequency ablation of liver metastases on CT and positron emission tomography/CT. J Vasc Interv Radiol. 2014; 25(8): 1240–1249

[82] Zheng JH, Chang ZH, Han CB, et al. Detection of residual tumor following radiofrequency ablation of liver metastases using 18F-FDG PET/PET-CT: a systematic review and meta-analysis. Nucl Med Commun. 2014; 35(4):339–346

[83] Cascini GL, Avallone A, Delrio P, et al. 18F-FDG PET is an early predictor of pathologic tumor response to preoperative radiochemotherapy in locally advanced rectal cancer. J Nucl Med. 2006; 47(8):1241–1248

[84] Li C, Lan X, Yuan H, Feng H, Xia X, Zhang Y. 18F-FDG PET predicts pathological response to preoperative chemoradiotherapy in patients with primary rectal cancer: a meta-analysis. Ann Nucl Med. 2014; 28(5):436–446

[85] Schneider DA, Akhurst TJ, Ngan SY, et al. Relative value of restaging MRI, CT, and FDG-PET scan after preoperative chemoradiation for rectal cancer. Dis Colon Rectum. 2016; 59(3):179–186

[86] Li YL, Wu LM, Chen XX, Delproposto Z, Hu JN, Xu JR. Is diffusion-weighted MRI superior to FDG-PET or FDG-PET/CT in evaluating and predicting pathological response to preoperative neoadjuvant therapy in patients with rectal cancer? J Dig Dis. 2014; 15(10):525–537

[87] Ippolito D, Fior D, Trattenero C, et al. Combined value of apparent diffusion coefficient-standardized uptake value max in evaluation of post-treated locally advanced rectal cancer. World J Radiol. 2015; 7(12):509–520

[88] Song I, Kim SH, Lee SJ, Choi JY, Kim MJ, Rhim H. Value of diffusion-weighted imaging in the detection of viable tumour after neoadjuvant chemoradiation therapy in patients with locally advanced rectal cancer: comparison with T2 weighted and PET/CT imaging. Br J Radiol. 2012; 85(1013):577–586

[89] Zhang C, Tong J, Sun X, Liu J, Wang Y, Huang G. 18F-FDG-PET evaluation of treatment response to neo-adjuvant therapy in patients with locally advanced rectal cancer: a meta-analysis. Int J Cancer. 2012; 131(11):2604–2611

[90] Memon S, Lynch AC, Akhurst T, et al. Systematic review of FDG-PET prediction of complete pathological response and survival in rectal cancer. Ann Surg Oncol. 2014; 21(11): 3598–3607

26 Musculoskeletal Tumors

Eugene C. Lin

26.1 Distinguishing Benign from Malignant Tumors

In a known bone or soft-tissue lesion, positron emission tomography (PET) is of some value in determining whether the lesion is benign or malignant, and in grading malignant lesions. Also, bone or soft-tissue lesions are detected incidentally on PET performed for other indications. The degree of fluorodeoxyglucose (FDG) uptake in the lesion can aid in differential diagnosis when correlated with conventional imaging (CI) modalities.

26.2 Benign versus Malignant Bone Tumors

Although malignant bone tumors tend to be more FDG avid than benign tumors, this primarily applies for histologically similar tumors (e.g., chondroid tumors). This may not apply when comparing tumors of different histological groups. Benign aggressive lesions, such as giant cell tumors, can have a similar if not greater degree of FDG uptake than high-grade malignancies. Many highly FDG-avid benign tumors contain a substantial number of histiocytic or giant cells[1]:

1. **Low uptake.** A low level of uptake suggests that a bone lesion is likely benign (although there are false-negative results in plasmacytoma and low-grade chondrosarcoma).
2. **High uptake.** A high level of uptake is less specific. While lesions with high uptake are more likely to represent malignancy (primary or metastatic), high uptake can be seen in a large number of benign lesions (see pitfalls section).
3. **Chondrosarcoma versus enchondroma**[2]:
   a) Chondrosarcomas (▶ Fig. 26.1) usually have less uptake than other sarcomas but more uptake than enchondromas.
   b) PET cannot distinguish between benign tumors and grade I chondrosarcomas.
   c) Grade II and III chondrosarcomas have higher glucose metabolism than low-grade cartilage tumors:
      • A standardized uptake value (SUV) cutoff of 2.3 is helpful in differentiating grade II and III chondrosarcomas from low-grade tumors.

4. **Chondrosarcoma versus osteochondroma.**[3] Limited data suggest a SUV cutoff of 2.0 may differentiate benign from malignant osteochondromas.[3]

26.2.1 Accuracy

PET and PET/CT for differentiating primary bone sarcomas form benign lesions (meta-analysis)[4]: sensitivity of 96% and specificity of 79%.

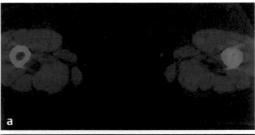
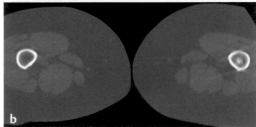
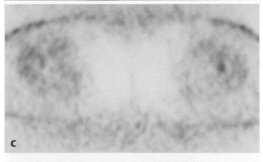

Fig. 26.1 Chondrosarcoma. (a) Axial PET/CT demonstrates uptake in a low-grade chondrosarcoma of the left femur. As the CT (b) demonstrates a dense chondroid matrix in this region, the non-attenuation-corrected images (c) should be reviewed to determine that the visualized activity is not artifactual. However, it is unlikely that the degree of increased attenuation from a chondroid matrix would be enough to result in artifactually increased activity.

26.2.2 Pearls

1. In general, malignant bone lesions have higher FDG uptake than benign lesions.
2. Metastases have the highest uptake, usually more than primary malignant bone lesions.[5]
3. However, benign bone tumors can have substantial FDG accumulation (> 2.0 SUV):
   a) Particularly true for histiocytic or giant cell–containing lesions (▶ Fig. 26.2).
4. Greater intratumoral heterogeneity of FDG uptake is associated with malignancy.[6]

26.2.3 Pitfalls

1. *False negatives*.[7,8] Low-grade chondrosarcoma, osteosarcoma, Ewing's sarcoma, plasmacytoma, and myxoid tumors.
2. *False positives*.[1,9,10] Giant cell tumor, chondroblastoma, fibrous dysplasia (▶ Fig. 26.3), sarcoidosis, Langerhans cell histiocytosis, nonossifying fibroma, osteoblastoma, osteoid osteomas aneurysmal bone cyst, Paget's disease (active; ▶ Fig. 26.4), enchondroma, chondromyxoid fibroma, desmoplastic fibroma, brown tumor (prior to treatment), fibro-osseous defects, nonossifying fibroma, aneurysmal bone cyst, osteomyelitis, bone infarct, and acute or subacute fracture.

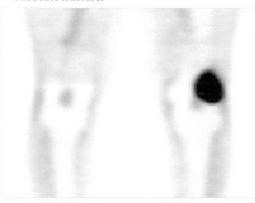

Fig. 26.2 Giant cell tumor. Coronal PET scan demonstrates intense uptake (standardized uptake value [SUV] 10.8) in a giant cell tumor of the left knee. This is a classic location for giant cell tumor involving the metaphysis with subarticular extension. Many benign bone tumors can have high levels of fluorodeoxyglucose uptake. (This image is provided courtesy of Janet Eary, MD, Seattle, WA.)

26.2.4 Benign versus Malignant Soft-Tissue Tumors

1. *Low uptake.* Low FDG uptake is of limited value in differentiating benign from malignant soft-tissue tumors as it could represent either a nonmalignant lesion or a low-grade sarcoma.
2. *High uptake.* High uptake is more useful as it usually indicates intermediate- or high-grade malignancy. While some benign lesions can have high uptake, radiographic correlation can often differentiate these lesions from sarcomas.
3. *Liposarcoma versus lipoma.* Limited data suggest that an SUV cutoff of 0.81 may differentiate liposarcomas (▶ Fig. 26.5) from lipomas.[11]

26.2.5 Accuracy

PET and PET/CT (meta-analysis)[12]: sensitivity of 96% and specificity of 77%.

26.2.6 Pearls/Pitfalls

1. *Tumor grade.* FDG uptake correlates with tumor grade[13]:
   a) SUV ≥ 1.6 or SUV peak/SUV liver greater than 2.4[14] suggests high-grade tumors. However, the degree of FDG uptake may not reliably indicate high-grade sarcomas at recurrence.[14]
   b) Lesions with SUV less than 1.6 are usually low grade or benign.

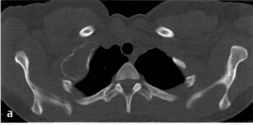
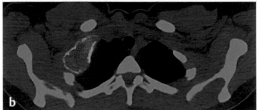

Fig. 26.3 Fibrous dysplasia. (a) Axial CT image demonstrates an expansile right rib lesion in a 28-year-old man without a history of cancer. (b) Axial PET/CT demonstrates moderate fluorodeoxyglucose uptake in the rib lesion with a maximum standardized uptake value (SUVmax) of 4.0. After resection, this was diagnosed as fibrous dysplasia.

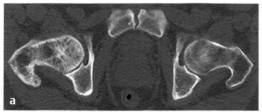

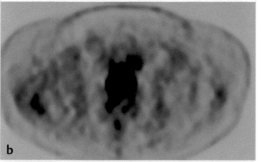

Fig. 26.4 Paget's disease. **(a)** Axial CT demonstrates cortical and trabecular thickening consistent with the mixed phase of Paget's disease. Fluorodeoxyglucose uptake in Paget's disease is variable, and on an axial PET scan **(b)**, uptake is noted only in a portion of the CT abnormality (in the trochanter).

2. **Benign lesions.** Benign soft-tissue lesions usually do not have substantial FDG uptake[15]:
   a) Lipomas and hemangiomas have the lowest uptake.
   b) *False positives.* High uptake can be seen in giant cell tumor of the tendon sheath, sarcoid, desmoid, and schwannomas. Uptake in a hibernoma can mimic a liposarcoma (▶ Fig. 26.6).[16]
   c) *False negatives.* Malignant myxoid lesion and well-differentiated liposarcoma can have low FDG uptake.[17]
3. **Delayed imaging.** Delayed imaging can help differentiate benign from malignant tumors as malignant lesions show an increase in uptake on delayed images.
   a) Benign lesions reach maximum uptake early (30 minutes), while high-grade malignant lesions reach maximum uptake late (4 hours).[18]

26.3 Evaluation of Known Musculoskeletal Tumors

PET is valuable in both osseous and soft-tissue malignancies. The primary uses are as follows:

Fig. 26.5 Liposarcomas. Coronal PET scans demonstrate fluorodeoxyglucose uptake in liposarcomas in the thigh **(a)** and abdomen **(b)**. The abdominal liposarcoma is heterogeneous with a standardized uptake value (SUV) of 11.7 consistent with a poor prognosis tumor. Given the heterogeneity of uptake, the PET scan would be helpful in guiding biopsy. The thigh liposarcoma has a much lower SUV of 2.7 consistent with a better prognosis tumor. However, there is some degree of heterogeneity suggesting myxoid degeneration and a poorer prognosis than might be predicted by the SUV alone. (Courtesy of Janet Eary, MD, Seattle, WA.)

a) Staging.
b) Guiding biopsy.
c) Detecting recurrence.
d) Therapy response.
e) Tumor grading.

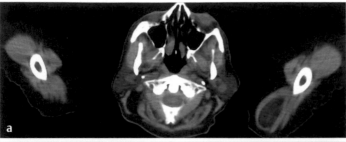

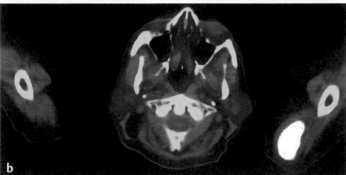

Fig. 26.6 Hibernoma. An 80-year-old female with history of uterine cancer. Axial CT (a) and PET/CT (b) images demonstrate a fluorodeoxyglucose avid fat-containing lesion in the left deltoid musculature, stable for more than 2 years. The clinical diagnosis is hibernoma. Well-differentiated liposarcoma should be among the differential especially when there is no prior comparison. (These images are provided courtesy of Gang Cheng, MD, Philadelphia, PA.)

26.3.1 Osteosarcoma and Soft-Tissue Sarcomas[19,20]

The primary applications of PET are in guiding biopsy, therapy monitoring, and diagnosing local recurrence.

1. **Staging.** PET has some value in staging osteosarcoma (▶ Fig. 26.7):
   a) PET/CT is more sensitive and accurate than bone scan in detection of bone metastases from osteosarcoma.[21,22,23]
   b) PET cannot substitute for CT in detecting lung metastases from osteosarcoma.[24] Although PET/CT is less sensitive than CT for detection of lung metastases (84 vs. 94%), PET/CT has slightly greater specificity (79 vs. 71%)[23] and can differentiate between metastases and benign lesions.[23]
2. **Tumor grading:**
   a) In known sarcomas, high SUV correlates with high histologic tumor grade (▶ Fig. 26.5) and tumor necrosis.[1] Within the subset of high-grade sarcomas, the degree of FDG uptake (baseline SUVmax) at the time of diagnosis is an adverse prognostic factor for patient outcome.[25]
   b) Benign lesions can occasionally have uptake levels comparable to those of sarcomas.
3. **Guiding biopsy in heterogeneous tumors** (▶ Fig. 26.5). Fusion with CT or MRI is helpful.

PET may have additional value compared to MRI as areas of signal heterogeneity on MRI do not necessarily correlate with the highest metabolic activity, and biopsy of areas of high metabolic activity has the highest diagnostic yield.[26]

4. **Therapy monitoring:**
   a) PET predicts tumor response to preoperative neoadjuvant chemotherapy and eventual outcome (▶ Fig. 26.8).[19] In a meta-analysis,[27] a posttherapy SUV ≤ 2.5, and a 50% or greater decrease in SUV were valuable in predicting histological response to neoadjuvant chemotherapy. SUV ≤ 2.5 had better predictive performance, with a sensitivity of 73% and specificity of 86%. In one report,[28] PET was superior to MRI for response assessment in patients with osteosarcoma.
   b) PET may be superior to bone scintigraphy in monitoring osteosarcoma therapy.[29]
   c) *Osteosarcoma versus Ewing's sarcoma.* The FDG PET response to neoadjuvant therapy is different for osteosarcoma and Ewing's sarcoma. In one report,[30] a 50% reduction in metabolic tumor volume correlated with a favorable histologic response for overall survival in patients with osteosarcoma, while a 90% reduction was necessary in patients with Ewing's sarcoma.

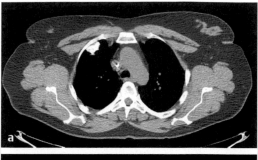

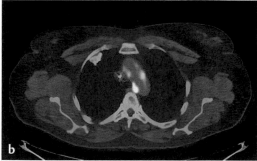

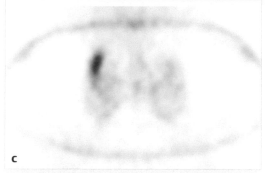

c

Fig. 26.7 Osteosarcoma lung metastasis. (a) CT scan in a patient with osteosarcoma demonstrates a calcified right upper lobe lesion. (b) Axial PET/CT scan demonstrates uptake in this lesion consistent with metastasis. In this case, it is important to review the non-attenuation-corrected images (c) to determine that the uptake is not artifactual secondary to the increased density of the lesion. Although PET can detect lung metastases from osteosarcoma, CT is more sensitive for this purpose.

5. **Diagnosis of local recurrence** (▶ Fig. 26.9). PET/CT is more accurate than CT or MRI for the detection of local recurrence in patients with osteosarcoma, as CT and MRI have difficulty in differentiating posttherapy tissue changes and fibrosis from local relapse.[25] In a meta-analysis,[4] the overall sensitivity and specificity for detecting recurrence from all bone sarcomas was 92 and 93%, respectively.

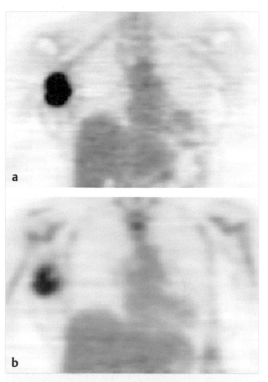

a

b

Fig. 26.8 Sarcoma response to therapy. Coronal PET scans demonstrate therapy response in a right axillary soft-tissue sarcoma pretherapy (a) and posttherapy (b). Courtesy of Janet Eary, MD, Seattle, WA.)

6. **Prognosis.** FDG uptake in sarcomas correlates negatively with survival and positively with disease progression.[31] In a meta-analysis of studies involving patients with bone and soft-tissue sarcomas,[32] prechemotherapy SUV, postchemotherapy SUV, SUV ratio, total lesion glycolysis, and metabolic tumor volume had prognostic significance for event-free and overall survival. Total lesion glycolysis had the highest hazard ratios, and prechemotherapy SUV was also significantly associated with higher rate of metastases and local recurrence.

Accuracy/Comparison to Other Modalities

Staging

Combined PET/CT and CI results in correct N staging in 97% and correct M staging in 93% of patients.[33] The accuracy is significantly higher than PET alone.

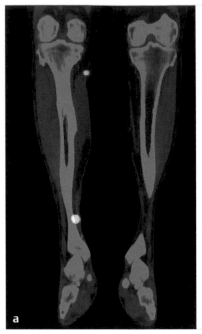
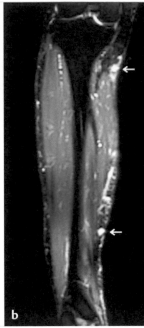

Fig. 26.9 Recurrent sarcoma. **(a)** Coronal PET/CT demonstrates two foci of uptake in the soft tissue of the medial right calf secondary to recurrent sarcoma. **(b)** Coronal short tau inversion recovery (STIR) MRI in the same patient demonstrates two hyperintense foci (*arrows*) corresponding to the fluorodeoxyglucose uptake.

Tumor Recurrence

1. *CI.* PET has a small advantage compared to CI for detection of soft-tissue and bone metastases (▶ Table 26.1).[34]

Table 26.1 Sensitivity and specificity of PET versus conventional imaging in the detection of soft tissue and bone metastases in recurrent sarcomas

	Sensitivity %	Specificity %
PET	96	81
CT	100	56

2. *MRI.* PET is useful for the evaluation of potential recurrence when MRI is equivocal[35]:
   a) One specific situation where PET is valuable is when metallic prosthesis artifact will limit MRI.
   b) PET has the additional advantage over MRI for evaluating the whole body for distant metastatic sites.
3. *Sestamibi.* PET is more accurate than sestamibi (▶ Table 26.2).[36]

Table 26.2 Sensitivity and specificity of PET versus sestamibi in recurrent sarcomas

	Sensitivity %	Specificity %
PET	98	90
Sestamibi	82	80

Pitfalls

1. **Lung metastases.** A negative PET scan in the presence of suspicious CT findings does not exclude metastases as a significant percentage of pulmonary metastases less than 1 cm that are negative on PET.[37]
2. **Postamputation Evaluation**[38]:
   a) *Diffuse uptake*: Diffuse increased uptake can be seen in the stump up to 18 months postamputation.
   b) *Focal uptake*: Focal areas of uptake can be seen in areas of skin breakdown from pressure. Clinical correlation is necessary as focal areas of uptake without correlative skin breakdown usually represent recurrence.
3. **Therapy response.**[15] Lesions that respond completely sometimes have a peripheral rim of FDG uptake, which corresponds to a fibrous pseudocapsule containing inflammatory tissue.

26.3.2 Ewing's Sarcoma

PET/CT scan is used for the staging, restaging, and assessment of therapy response in patients with Ewing's sarcoma.

Prognosis

The pretreatment SUVmax can predict overall survival in patients with Ewing's sarcoma. In one report,[39] an SUVmax greater than 5.8 was associated with worse overall survival.

Recurrence

In a meta-analysis,[4] the overall sensitivity and specificity for detecting recurrence from all bone sarcomas were 92 and 93%, respectively. In one report,[40] PET/CT had a sensitivity of 95% and specificity of 87% for the detection of recurrence of skeletal Ewing's sarcoma. In another report,[23] PET/CT in patients with Ewing's sarcoma performed better at follow-up than initial staging. In addition, there was a greater diagnostic benefit for follow-up of patients with Ewing's sarcoma than with osteosarcoma. This is in concordance with the known pattern of metastatic recurrence: primarily in the lung in osteosarcoma and in the lung and bone in Ewing's sarcoma.

Therapy Response

The FDG PET response to neoadjuvant therapy is different for osteosarcoma and Ewing's sarcoma. In one report,[30] a 50% reduction in metabolic tumor volume correlated with a favorable histologic response for overall survival in patients with osteosarcoma, while a 90% reduction was necessary in patients with Ewing's sarcoma.

Accuracy/Comparison to Other Modalities

1. **PET and PET/CT** (meta-analysis)[41]: sensitivity of 96% and specificity of 92%.
2. **Bone metastases.** In a prospective multicenter trial,[42] PET was more sensitive than CI modalities (bone scan, CT, and MRI) for detection of bone metastases. However, in one study,[43] bone scan detected osseous metastases not detected by PET/CT when the metastases were sclerotic. The authors suggest initial staging with FDG PET/CT. If the osseous lesions are lytic, bone scan is not necessary, while an additional bone scan is performed for patients with sclerotic osseous lesions.
3. **Lung metastases.** PET is less sensitive than CT for lung metastases.[42,44] However, PET is more specific,[23] and is capable of distinguishing metastases from benign lesions.[45]
4. **Lymph node metastases.** PET is more sensitive than CT for lymph node metastases.[42]

26.3.3 Multiple Myeloma

PET is useful in evaluating initial extent of disease and treatment response. PET/CT may be especially useful in patients with nonsecretory myeloma, elevated lactate dehydrogenase, Bence Jones protein escape, suspected extramedullary plasmacytoma, or otherwise rapidly recurrent disease.[46] PET is also useful in the posttransplant setting where patients are nonsecretors, but the lesions still have FDG uptake.[47]

Monoclonal Gammopathy of Undetermined Significance and Smoldering Multiple Myeloma

Patients with monoclonal gammopathy of undetermined significance (MGUS) typically do not have areas of increased FDG uptake. A negative FDG PET reliably predicts stable MGUS.[48] In addition, the majority of patients with low-level smoldering multiple myeloma (SMM) do not have increased FDG uptake.[49] The International Myeloma Working Group (IMWG) recommends that either PET/CT, low-dose whole-body CT, or MRI be done in all patients with suspected SMM. The IMWG criteria[50] indicate that one of more sites of osteolytic bone destruction ≥ 5 mm in size identified by PET/CT or CT fulfills the criteria for bone disease in multiple myeloma. However, in the IMWG criteria, increased FDG uptake alone in the absence of underlying osteolytic bone destruction is not adequate for the diagnosis of bone disease. However, in one study[51] patients with SMM and focal FDG uptake without osteolytic lesions had a 58% probability of progression to multiple myeloma in 2 years, compared to 33% for PET-negative patients.

Prognosis

Baseline FDG positivity is associated with poor outcome (event-free and overall survival). In the largest study[52] comparing bone survey, MRI, and PET, the presence of more than three FDG-avid lesions was the leading independent parameter associated with poor outcome. Extramedullary disease and high SUVs (> 4.2) also have independent negative prognostic value.[53]

Response to Treatment

PET/CT may be helpful in assessing response to treatment. Compared to CT or MRI, PET has the advantage of distinguishing between metabolically

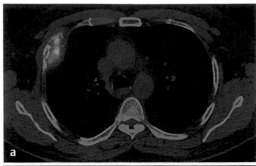

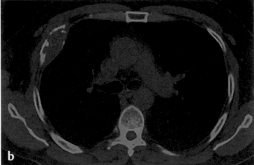

Fig. 26.10 Multiple myeloma therapy response. **(a)** Axial PET/CT demonstrates intense uptake in an expansile rib lesion secondary to myeloma. **(b)** Follow-up posttherapy axial PET/CT demonstrates a substantial decrease in the fluorodeoxyglucose uptake with minimal change in appearance of the CT.

active and inactive lytic lesions (▶ Fig. 26.10). Osteolytic lesions secondary to MM identified by CT or radiograph rarely heal completely. MRI response is delayed as marrow signal abnormalities can take weeks to years to resolve, and MRI also has low specificity in differentiating viable disease from bone remodeling.[54] Due to a high number of false-positive results, an IMWG consensus statement[55] does not recommend MRI for treatment follow-up and suggests that PET/CT may be of more value in this setting. In one study,[56] approximately two-thirds of patients with a response to therapy had a faster normalization of findings on PET/CT than MRI. PET/CT detected recurrence in 80% of patients compared to 50% by MRI. Currently, the data on treatment response is primarily in transplant-eligible patients. In patients undergoing induction therapy and autologous stem cell transplantation (ASCT), FDG positivity at baseline and persistence after therapy is associated with shorter overall and progression-free survival.[53] A negative PET after therapy is associated with a favorable outcome. Complete normalization of the

FDG PET scan after ASCT correlates with improved progression-free and overall survival.[57] PET/CT after ASCT retains its prognostic significance for risk of progression and death even among patients achieving conventionally defined complete response.[51] In one analysis,[58] PET CT had an overall accuracy of 74% for determination of remission status after ASCT compared to 52% for MRI.

Pathologic Fracture

In one study of myeloma patients,[59] an SUV greater than 3.2 could discriminate between old and new pathologic fractures, while a combination of SUV greater than 3.5 and MRI findings of diffuse or multifocal vertebral body involvement predicted impending fracture.

Accuracy/Comparison to Other Modalities

1. ***PET and PET/CT*** (meta-analysis)[60]:
   a) Intramedullary lesions: sensitivity of 61% and specificity of 94%.
   b) Extramedullary lesions: sensitivity of 96% and specificity of 78%.
2. ***Plain radiographs***. Concordance between PET and radiography has been assessed in seven studies.[61] in six of these, PET demonstrated more lytic lesions (▶ Fig. 26.11). The use of PET/CT may obviate the need for a skeletal survey. However, as PET/CT, CT, and MRI may have limitations in detecting skull and rib lesions, some authors have suggested additional radiographs of these regions[62]:
   a) In addition, PET can identify extramedullary disease.
   b) The one area where PET does not detect more lytic lesions is the skull; this may be secondary to high FDG uptake in the brain.
3. ***MRI***. Concordance between PET and MRI has been assessed in five studies.[61] in four studies, PET was inferior to MRI, primarily in the detection of diffuse marrow infiltration in the spine and pelvis (▶ Fig. 26.12). However, PET/CT is more sensitive in detecting extramedullary disease not included in the field of view of MRI, as well as rib and appendicular lesions.
4. ***Extramedullary disease***. Extramedullary myelomatous disease is associated with advanced disease and poor prognosis. It can affect any organ system and the imaging features are often nonspecific. PET/CT is more sensitive than other imaging modalities for

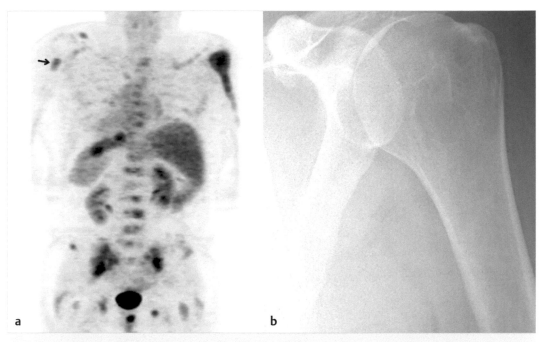

a   b

Fig. 26.11 Multiple myeloma: PET versus plain film. **(a)** Coronal PET scan (posterior projection) in a patient with multiple myeloma demonstrates multiple osseous lesions. Although there is a lesion of the proximal left humeral shaft seen on PET (*arrow*), the corresponding radiograph **(b)** is negative.

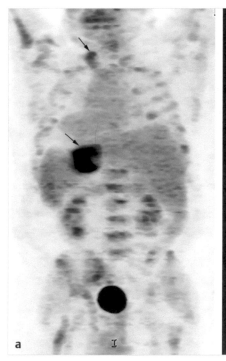

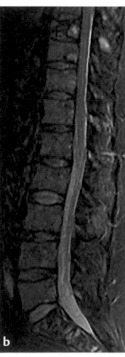

a   b

Fig. 26.12 Multiple myeloma. **(a)** Maximum intensity projection PET demonstrates uptake in two foci of extraosseous myeloma (*arrows*) along with uptake in multiple osseous lesions. **(b)** Sagittal T2-weighted MRI in the same patient demonstrates diffuse vertebral marrow involvement, substantially greater than demonstrated on the PET.

identifying extramedullary disease
(▶ Fig. 26.12), revealing additional lesions in
almost 30% of patients diagnosed with solitary
plasmacytoma by MRI.[63]

5. **Sestamibi**. There are conflicting data as to
whether sestamibi or PET identifies more
lesions.[64,65] In a systematic review, there was no
statistically significant difference in sensitivity
or specificity between sestamibi and FDG PET[66]:
   a) Sestamibi uptake correlates with extent of
   marrow infiltration better than PET.
   b) FDG uptake correlates with active disease
   progression.

Pitfalls

1. If PET/CT is used as the sole imaging modality in
myeloma, it will miss some small lytic bone
lesions and could miss diffuse spine
involvement.[67] In patients with newly
diagnosed multiple myeloma, 24% will have a
negative FDG PET scan.[57] MRI may be superior
to PET/CT in diagnosing infiltrative disease in
the spine.[68]

2. PET is limited when there is diffuse bone
marrow activity as widespread disease is
difficult to differentiate from activated normal
marrow.

3. False-negative findings can result within 10
days after the administration of high-dose
steroids.[54]

4. FDG PET will be negative in 25% of patients with
relapsing disease despite the presence of active
disease.[57]

References

[1] Costelloe CM, Chuang HH, Madewell JE. FDG PET/CT of primary bone tumors. AJR Am J Roentgenol. 2014; 202(6): W521–W531

[2] Lee FY, Yu J, Chang SS, Fawwaz R, Parisien MV. Diagnostic value and limitations of fluorine-18 fluorodeoxyglucose positron emission tomography for cartilaginous tumors of bone. J Bone Joint Surg Am. 2004; 86-A(12):2677–2685

[3] Feldman F, Vanheertum R, Saxena C. 18Fluoro-deoxyglucose positron emission tomography evaluation of benign versus malignant osteochondromas: preliminary observations. J Comput Assist Tomogr. 2006; 30(5):858–864

[4] Liu F, Zhang Q, Zhu D, et al. Performance of positron emission tomography and positron emission tomography/computed tomography using fluorine-18-fluorodeoxyglucose for the diagnosis, staging, and recurrence assessment of bone sarcoma: a systematic review and meta-analysis. Medicine (Baltimore). 2015; 94(36):e1462

[5] Watanabe H, Shinozaki T, Yanagawa T, et al. Glucose metabolic analysis of musculoskeletal tumours using 18fluorine-FDG PET as an aid to preoperative planning. J Bone Joint Surg Br. 2000; 82(5):760–767

[6] Nakajo M, Nakajo M, Jinguji M, et al. The value of intratumoral heterogeneity of (18)F-FDG uptake to differentiate between primary benign and malignant musculoskeletal tumours on PET/CT. Br J Radiol. 2015; 88(1055):20150552

[7] Schulte M, Brecht-Krauss D, Heymer B, et al. Grading of tumors and tumorlike lesions of bone: evaluation by FDG PET. J Nucl Med. 2000; 41(10):1695–1701

[8] Hicks RJ, Toner GC, Choong PF. Clinical applications of molecular imaging in sarcoma evaluation. Cancer Imaging. 2005; 5: 66–72

[9] Aoki J, Watanabe H, Shinozaki T, et al. FDG PET of primary benign and malignant bone tumors: standardized uptake value in 52 lesions. Radiology. 2001; 219(3):774–777

[10] Goodin GS, Shulkin BL, Kaufman RA, McCarville MB. PET/CT characterization of fibroosseous defects in children: 18F-FDG uptake can mimic metastatic disease. AJR Am J Roentgenol. 2006; 187(4):1124–1128

[11] Suzuki R, Watanabe H, Yanagawa T, et al. PET evaluation of fatty tumors in the extremity: possibility of using the standardized uptake value (SUV) to differentiate benign tumors from liposarcoma. Ann Nucl Med. 2005; 19(8):661–670

[12] Etchebehere EC, Hobbs BP, Milton DR, et al. Assessing the role of 18F-FDG PET and 18F-FDG PET/CT in the diagnosis of soft tissue musculoskeletal malignancies: a systematic review and meta-analysis. Eur J Nucl Med Mol Imaging. 2016; 43(5): 860–870

[13] Adler LP, Blair HF, Makley JT, et al. Noninvasive grading of musculoskeletal tumors using PET. J Nucl Med. 1991; 32(8): 1508–1512

[14] Fendler WP, Chalkidis RP, Ilhan H, et al. Evaluation of several FDG PET parameters for prediction of soft tissue tumour grade at primary diagnosis and recurrence. Eur Radiol. 2015; 25(8):2214–2221

[15] Aoki J, Endo K, Watanabe H, et al. FDG-PET for evaluating musculoskeletal tumors: a review. J Orthop Sci. 2003; 8(3): 435–441

[16] Lin D, Jacobs M, Percy T, Dowdy Y, Mantil J. High 2-deoxy-2 [F-18]fluoro-D-glucose uptake on positron emission tomography in hibernoma originally thought to be myxoid liposarcoma. Mol Imaging Biol. 2005; 7(3):201–202

[17] Nose H, Otsuka H, Otomi Y, et al. Correlations between F-18 FDG PET/CT and pathological findings in soft tissue lesions. J Med Invest. 2013; 60(3–4):184–190

[18] Lodge MA, Lucas JD, Marsden PK, Cronin BF, O'Doherty MJ, Smith MA. A PET study of 18FDG uptake in soft tissue masses. Eur J Nucl Med. 1999; 26(1):22–30

[19] Brenner W, Bohuslavizki KH, Eary JF. PET imaging of osteosarcoma. J Nucl Med. 2003; 44(6):930–942

[20] Jadvar H, Gamie S, Ramanna L, Conti PS. Musculoskeletal system. Semin Nucl Med. 2004; 34(4):254–261

[21] Byun BH, Kong CB, Lim I, et al. Comparison of (18)F-FDG PET/CT and (99 m)Tc-MDP bone scintigraphy for detection of bone metastasis in osteosarcoma. Skeletal Radiol. 2013; 42 (12):1673–1681

[22] Hurley C, McCarville MB, Shulkin BL, et al. Comparison of (18) F-FDG-PET-CT and bone scintigraphy for evaluation of osseous metastases in newly diagnosed and recurrent osteosarcoma. Pediatr Blood Cancer. 2016; 63(8):1381–1386

[23] Quartuccio N, Treglia G, Salsano M, et al. The role of fluorine-18-Fluorodeoxyglucose positron emission tomography in staging and restaging of patients with osteosarcoma. Radiol Oncol. 2013; 47(2):97–102

[24] Franzius C, Daldrup-Link HE, Sciuk J, et al. FDG-PET for detection of pulmonary metastases from malignant primary bone tumors: comparison with spiral CT. Ann Oncol. 2001; 12(4): 479–486

[25] Schuetze SM. Utility of positron emission tomography in sarcomas. Curr Opin Oncol. 2006; 18(4):369–373

[26] Becher S, Oskouei S. PET imaging in sarcoma. Orthop Clin North Am. 2015; 46(3):409–415, xi

[27] Hongtao L, Hui Z, Bingshun W, et al. 18F-FDG positron emission tomography for the assessment of histological response to neoadjuvant chemotherapy in osteosarcomas: a meta-analysis. Surg Oncol. 2012; 21(4):e165–e170

[28] Denecke T, Hundsdörfer P, Misch D, et al. Assessment of histological response of paediatric bone sarcomas using FDG PET in comparison to morphological volume measurement and standardized MRI parameters. Eur J Nucl Med Mol Imaging. 2010; 37(10):1842–1853

[29] Franzius C, Sciuk J, Brinkschmidt C, Jürgens H, Schober O. Evaluation of chemotherapy response in primary bone tumors with F-18 FDG positron emission tomography compared with histologically assessed tumor necrosis. Clin Nucl Med. 2000; 25(11):874–881

[30] Gaston LL, Di Bella C, Slavin J, Hicks RJ, Choong PF. 18F-FDG PET response to neoadjuvant chemotherapy for Ewing sarcoma and osteosarcoma are different. Skeletal Radiol. 2011; 40 (8):1007–1015

[31] Eary JF, O'Sullivan F, Powitan Y, et al. Sarcoma tumor FDG uptake measured by PET and patient outcome: a retrospective analysis. Eur J Nucl Med Mol Imaging. 2002; 29(9):1149–1154

[32] Li YJ, Dai YL, Cheng YS, Zhang WB, Tu CQ. Positron emission tomography (18)F-fluorodeoxyglucose uptake and prognosis in patients with bone and soft tissue sarcoma: A meta-analysis. Eur J Surg Oncol. 2016; 42(8):1103–1114

[33] Tateishi U, Yamaguchi U, Seki K, Terauchi T, Arai Y, Kim EE. Bone and soft-tissue sarcoma: preoperative staging with fluorine 18 fluorodeoxyglucose PET/CT and conventional imaging. Radiology. 2007; 245(3):839–847

[34] Franzius C, Daldrup-Link HE, Wagner-Bohn A, et al. FDG-PET for detection of recurrences from malignant primary bone tumors: comparison with conventional imaging. Ann Oncol. 2002; 13(1):157–160

[35] Bredella MA, Caputo GR, Steinbach LS. Value of FDG positron emission tomography in conjunction with MR imaging for evaluating therapy response in patients with musculoskeletal sarcomas. AJR Am J Roentgenol. 2002; 179(5):1145–1150

[36] Garcia R, Kim EE, Wong FC, et al. Comparison of fluorine-18-FDG PET and technetium-99m-MIBI SPECT in evaluation of musculoskeletal sarcomas. J Nucl Med. 1996; 37(9):1476–1479

[37] Iagaru A, Chawla S, Menendez L, Conti PS. 18F-FDG PET and PET/CT for detection of pulmonary metastases from musculoskeletal sarcomas. Nucl Med Commun. 2006; 27(10):795–802

[38] Mulligan ME, Badros AZ. PET/CT and MR imaging in myeloma. Skeletal Radiol. 2007; 36(1):5–16

[39] Hwang JP, Lim I, Kong CB, et al. Prognostic value of SUVmax measured by pretreatment fluorine-18 fluorodeoxyglucose positron emission tomography/computed tomography in patients with Ewing sarcoma. PLoS One. 2016; 11(4):e0153281

[40] Sharma P, Khangembam BC, Suman KC, et al. Diagnostic accuracy of 18F-FDG PET/CT for detecting recurrence in patients with primary skeletal Ewing sarcoma. Eur J Nucl Med Mol Imaging. 2013; 40(7):1036–1043

[41] Treglia G, Salsano M, Stefanelli A, Mattoli MV, Giordano A, Bonomo L. Diagnostic accuracy of 18F-FDG-PET and PET/CT in patients with Ewing sarcoma family tumours: a systematic review and a meta-analysis. Skeletal Radiol. 2012; 41(3):249–256

[42] Völker T, Denecke T, Steffen I, et al. Positron emission tomography for staging of pediatric sarcoma patients: results of a prospective multicenter trial. J Clin Oncol. 2007; 25(34):5435–5441

[43] Ulaner GA, Magnan H, Healey JH, Weber WA, Meyers PA. Is methylene diphosphonate bone scan necessary for initial staging of Ewing sarcoma if 18F-FDG PET/CT is performed? AJR Am J Roentgenol. 2014; 202(4):859–867

[44] Györke T, Zajic T, Lange A, et al. Impact of FDG PET for staging of Ewing sarcomas and primitive neuroectodermal tumours. Nucl Med Commun. 2006; 27(1):17–24

[45] Cistaro A, Lopci E, Gastaldo L, Fania P, Brach Del Prever A, Fagioli F. The role of 18F-FDG PET/CT in the metabolic characterization of lung nodules in pediatric patients with bone sarcoma. Pediatr Blood Cancer. 2012; 59(7):1206–1210

[46] Dimopoulos M, Kyle R, Fermand JP, et al. International Myeloma Workshop Consensus Panel 3. Consensus recommendations for standard investigative workup: report of the International Myeloma Workshop Consensus Panel 3. Blood. 2011; 117(18):4701–4705

[47] Hain SF, O'Doherty MJ, Lucas JD, Smith MA. Fluorodeoxyglucose PET in the evaluation of amputations for soft tissue sarcoma. Nucl Med Commun. 1999; 20(9):845–848

[48] Mihailovic J, Goldsmith SJ. Multiple myeloma: 18F-FDG-PET/CT and diagnostic imaging. Semin Nucl Med. 2015; 45(1):16–31

[49] Dammacco F, Rubini G, Ferrari C, Vacca A, Racanelli V. 18F-FDG PET/CT: a review of diagnostic and prognostic features in multiple myeloma and related disorders. Clin Exp Med. 2015; 15(1):1–18

[50] Rajkumar SV, Dimopoulos MA, Palumbo A, et al. International Myeloma Working Group updated criteria for the diagnosis of multiple myeloma. Lancet Oncol. 2014; 15(12):e538–e548

[51] Zamagni E, Nanni C, Gay F, et al. 18F-FDG PET/CT focal, but not osteolytic, lesions predict the progression of smoldering myeloma to active disease. Leukemia. 2016; 30(2):417–422

[52] Bartel TB, Haessler J, Brown TL, et al. F18-fluorodeoxyglucose positron emission tomography in the context of other imaging techniques and prognostic factors in multiple myeloma. Blood. 2009; 114(10):2068–2076

[53] Caers J, Withofs N, Hillengass J, et al. The role of positron emission tomography-computed tomography and magnetic resonance imaging in diagnosis and follow up of multiple myeloma. Haematologica. 2014; 99(4):629–637

[54] Mesguich C, Fardanesh R, Tanenbaum L, Chari A, Jagannath S, Kostakoglu L. State of the art imaging of multiple myeloma: comparative review of FDG PET/CT imaging in various clinical settings. Eur J Radiol. 2014; 83(12):2203–2223

[55] Dimopoulos MA, Hillengass J, Usmani S, et al. Role of magnetic resonance imaging in the management of patients with multiple myeloma: a consensus statement. J Clin Oncol. 2015; 33(6):657–664

[56] Spinnato P, Bazzocchi A, Brioli A, et al. Contrast enhanced MRI and 18F-FDG PET-CT in the assessment of multiple myeloma: a comparison of results in different phases of the disease. Eur J Radiol. 2012; 81(12):4013–4018

[57] de Waal EG, Glaudemans AW, Schröder CP, Vellenga E, Slart RH. Nuclear medicine imaging of multiple myeloma, particularly in the relapsed setting. Eur J Nucl Med Mol Imaging. 2017; 44(2):332–341

[58] Derlin T, Peldschus K, Münster S, et al. Comparative diagnostic performance of 18F-FDG PET/CT versus whole-body MRI for determination of remission status in multiple myeloma after stem cell transplantation. Eur Radiol. 2013; 23(2):570–578

[59] Mulligan M, Chirindel A, Karchevsky M. Characterizing and predicting pathologic spine fractures in myeloma patients with FDG PET/CT and MR imaging. Cancer Invest. 2011; 29 (5):370–376

[60] Lu YY, Chen JH, Lin WY, et al. FDG PET or PET/CT for detecting intramedullary and extramedullary lesions in multiple myeloma: a systematic review and meta-analysis. Clin Nucl Med. 2012; 37(9):833–837

[61] van Lammeren-Venema D, Regelink JC, Riphagen II, Zweegman S, Hoekstra OS, Zijlstra JM. 18F-fluoro-deoxyglucose positron emission tomography in assessment of myeloma-related bone disease: a systematic review. Cancer. 2012; 118 (8):1971–1981

[62] Regelink JC, Minnema MC, Terpos E, et al. Comparison of modern and conventional imaging techniques in establishing multiple myeloma-related bone disease: a systematic review. Br J Haematol. 2013; 162(1):50–61

[63] Dimopoulos M, Terpos E, Comenzo RL, et al. IMWG. International myeloma working group consensus statement and guidelines regarding the current role of imaging techniques in the diagnosis and monitoring of multiple myeloma. Leukemia. 2009; 23(9):1545–1556

[64] Hung GU, Tsai CC, Tsai SC, Lin WY. Comparison of Tc-99 m sestamibi and F-18 FDG-PET in the assessment of multiple myeloma. Anticancer Res. 2005; 25 6C:4737–4741

[65] Mileshkin L, Blum R, Seymour JF, Patrikeos A, Hicks RJ, Prince HM. A comparison of fluorine-18 fluoro-deoxyglucose PET and technetium-99 m sestamibi in assessing patients with multiple myeloma. Eur J Haematol. 2004; 72(1):32–37

[66] Weng WW, Dong MJ, Zhang J, et al. A systematic review of MRI, scintigraphy, FDG-PET and PET/CT for diagnosis of multiple myeloma related bone disease–which is best? Asian Pac J Cancer Prev. 2014; 15(22):9879–9884

[67] Breyer RJ, III, Mulligan ME, Smith SE, Line BR, Badros AZ. Comparison of imaging with FDG PET/CT with other imaging modalities in myeloma. Skeletal Radiol. 2006; 35(9):632–640

[68] Nanni C, Zamagni E, Farsad M, et al. Role of 18F-FDG PET/CT in the assessment of bone involvement in newly diagnosed multiple myeloma: preliminary results. Eur J Nucl Med Mol Imaging. 2006; 33(5):525–531

27 ^{18}F Sodium Fluoride PET/CT in Bone

Alireza Rezaee, Poul Høilund-Carlsen, Søren Hess, Werner Langsteger, and Mohsen Beheshti

27.1 Introduction

1. Sodium ^{18}F sodium fluoride (^{18}F-NaF) is a highly sensitive bone-seeking PET radiotracer and its uptake reflects blood flow and bone remodeling status. Its first pass clearance is about 100% at low flow rates and down below 50% at high flow rates.[1,2,3]
2. ^{18}F-fluoride is produced by cyclotron with a half-life of approximately 110 minutes.[2,4]
3. The advantages of ^{18}F-NaF PET/CT over ^{99m}Tc methylene diphosphonate (MDP) bone scan are its much higher sensitivity and a higher accuracy, a better spatial resolution, improved bone-to-background ratio, as well as semiquantitative potentials.[3,5]
4. The mechanism of localization to bone is deemed to be due to chemosorption of ^{18}F-NaF to the hydroxyapatite structure at the site of new bone formation.[6]
5. Patients need to be well hydrated to quickly excrete radiopharmaceutical by kidneys in order to limit radiation exposure and improve image quality. The urinary bladder should be emptied right before imaging. Patients do not need to fast, and may take all their usual medications.[1]
6. Several characteristics make this modality attractive in assessment of bone lesions. Higher sensitivity and higher accuracy with similar overall radiation dose compared with bone scintigraphy, better differentiation of bone and soft-tissue structures, quantifying possibility, a rapidly increasing availability of PET/CT scanners, shorter imaging process, which is more convenient for patients with potential to reduce the cost for health care system, and not least the ability to show both blastic and lytic lesions (▶ Fig. 27.1).[1,7,8,9]

27.2 Indications[1,9]

27.2.1 Malignant Osseous Disease

1. Initial diagnosis/staging, localization, and determination of the extent of bone metastatic disease (▶ Fig. 27.2).
2. Restaging and evaluation of recurrent disease.

3. Assessment of response to radiation therapy, systemic chemotherapy, or combined treatment.

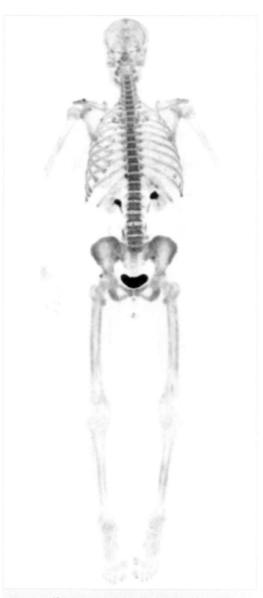

Fig. 27.1 ^{18}F-NaF PET. Maximum intensity projection (MIP) view shows physiologic ^{18}F-NaF distribution with symmetrical radiotracer uptake in the skeleton and excellent bone/soft-tissue contrast.

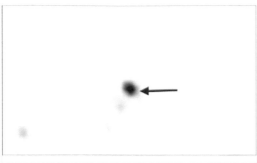

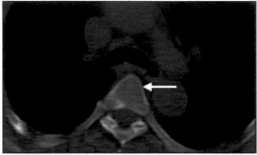

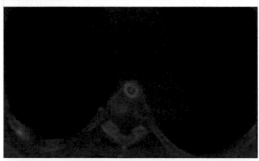

Fig. 27.2 ¹⁸F-NaF PET/CT of a breast cancer patient. Transaxial view of a thoracic spine (upper: PET; middle: CT; lower: fusion PET/CT). Focal-increased tracer uptake is evident on ¹⁸F-NaF PET (upper, *arrow*) suggestive of bone metastasis with only faint sclerotic change on CT (middle, *arrow*), which emphasizes on the impact of functional imaging in early detection of bone metastasis.

Accuracy/Comparison to Other Modalities

1. Overall ¹⁸F-NaF PET/CT: sensitivity = 96%; specificity = 93%.[10]
2. Overall ¹⁸F-FDG PET/CT: sensitivity = 67%; specificity = 96%.[10]
3. Overall ⁹⁹ᵐTc MDP bone scintigraphy: sensitivity = 88%; specificity = 93%.[10]
4. ¹⁸F-NaF PET/CT is a sensitive and specific method to detect metastases to skeleton,

particularly from prostate, breast, and lung cancers.[1,11,12,13,14]

5. It is also an accurate modality to differentiate benign from malignant lesions.[11]
6. ¹⁸F-NaF PET/CT is capable of detecting bone metastases earlier than ⁹⁹ᵐTc-MDP planar whole-body bone scintigraphy.[15]
7. ¹⁸F-NaF PET/CT is useful in detection of occult osseous metastases at lower prostate-specific antigen (PSA) levels when compared with conventional imaging.[16]
8. More investigations are warranted to define the role of ¹⁸F-NaF PET/CT in evaluation of primary osseous disease.[11]
9. ¹⁸F-fluorocholine (¹⁸F-FCH) PET/CT: sensitivity = 79%; specificity = 97% in bone metastases from prostate cancer[17] and 91 and 87%, respectively, in spinal metastases from prostate cancer.[18]
10. There is no significant difference in accuracy between ¹⁸F-NaF and ¹⁸F-FCH PET/CT in evaluation of skeletal metastasis from prostate cancer (86 vs. 85%). However, the latter is the superior method in detecting bone marrow metastases.[19]
11. In patients with non-¹⁸F-FCH and ¹⁸F-FDG avid sclerotic lesions on CT, correlation with PET/CT with a bone-seeking agent like ¹⁸F-NaF is recommended (▶ Fig. 27.3).[19]
12. ⁶⁸Ga prostate-specific membrane antigen (⁶⁸Ga-PSMA) PET/CT: sensitivity = 99 to 100%; specificity = 88 to 100% in bone metastases from prostate cancer.[20]
13. The ¹⁸F-NaF PET/CT is also superior to MRI and CT for detection of osseous metastases:
    a) ¹⁸F-NaF PET/CT: sensitivity = 96%; specificity = 93%.[10]
    b) MRI: sensitivity = 95%; specificity = 90%.[21]
    c) CT: sensitivity = 74%; specificity = 56%.[21]

Pitfalls

1. Tracer avid benign osseous lesions such as degenerative changes, facet arthropathy, recent trauma and fractures, inflammatory processes including arthritis and osteomyelitis as well as Paget's disease may be misinterpreted as metastasis (false positive).[5,22] Morphologic correlation and anatomic localization with dedicated CT improve the specificity (▶ Fig. 27.4).
2. SUV$_{max}$ of skeletal metastases from castrate-resistant prostate cancer on ¹⁸F-NaF PET/CT seem to be significantly higher compared with

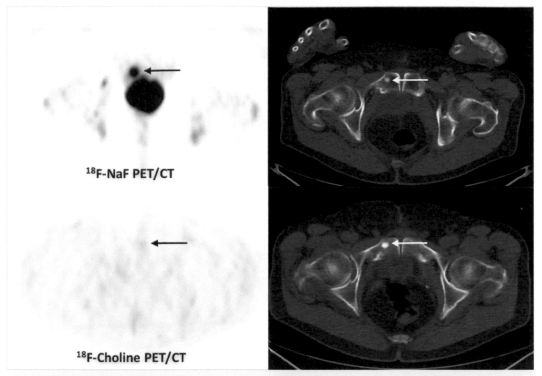

Fig. 27.3 ^{18}F-NaF PET/CT (upper row) and ^{18}F-Choline PET/CT (lower row) with 1-week interval from a prostate cancer patient (Gleason score: 7; primary prostate-specific antigen [PSA]: 5.6 ng/mL) with biochemical recurrence after radical prostatectomy and adjuvant radiotherapy and trigger PSA of 0.25 ng/mL. ^{18}F-NaF PET reveals focal increased tracer uptake on the right pubic bone corresponding with sclerotic lesion on CT (upper row, *arrows*) suggestive of bone metastasis. ^{18}F-choline PET shows no uptake in the sclerotic lesion on the right pubic bone (lower row, *arrows*), which may be due to its limited sensitivity on densely sclerotic lesions (e.g., Hounsfield unit > 800).

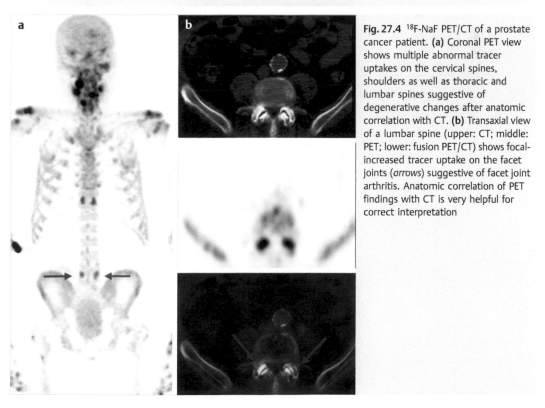

Fig. 27.4 ^{18}F-NaF PET/CT of a prostate cancer patient. **(a)** Coronal PET view shows multiple abnormal tracer uptakes on the cervical spines, shoulders as well as thoracic and lumbar spines suggestive of degenerative changes after anatomic correlation with CT. **(b)** Transaxial view of a lumbar spine (upper: CT; middle: PET; lower: fusion PET/CT) shows focal-increased tracer uptake on the facet joints (*arrows*) suggestive of facet joint arthritis. Anatomic correlation of PET findings with CT is very helpful for correct interpretation

degenerative lesions. However, there is no clear cutoff for SUV to differentiate benign from malignant lesions.[23,24]

3. Limited sensitivity for small purely lytic lesions (false negative).[5]

4. As with [99mTc]-MDP, [18F]-NaF PET/CT reveals only indirect evidence for skeletal metastases as a relatively late event occurring only when the number of cancer cells homing in red marrow has become sufficiently large to cause bone remodeling.[1,12,13,14]

5. The mechanism and line of events mentioned earlier also explain why [99mTc]-MDP, [18F]-NaF avid focal bone lesions may persist long after active cancer cells are gone and create a false impression of still active metastasizing disease.[1,12,13,14]

27.2.2 Assessment of Response to Therapy

Accuracy/Comparison to Other Modalities

1. [18F]-NaF PET/CT has performed excellent and is superior to conventional [99mTc]-MDP bone scintigraphy in assessment of skeletal metastatic disease in different cancers.[22]

2. The impact of [18F]-NaF PET/CT used for treatment monitoring was high in patients with evidence of progressive osseous metastasis (▶ Fig. 27.5).[22]

3. The modality gave rise to change in treatment plan in approximately 40% of cases with osseous metastatic disease.[22]

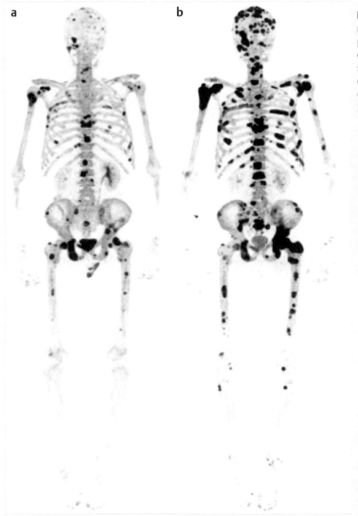

Fig. 27.5 [18F]-NaF PET/CT in therapy monitoring of a prostate cancer patient. Multiple bone metastases are evident on primary [18F]-NaF PET/CT study (a). Follow-up [18F]-NaF PET/CT examination 4 weeks after beginning of the therapy shows significant progression of the disease (b).

4. ^{18}F-NaF PET/CT may have a prognostic value in patients with skeletal metastases.[15]
5. Overall survival correlates significantly with the number of osseous lesions on primary and changes in SUV on follow-up ^{18}F-NaF PET/CT images (► Fig. 27.6). Further prospective studies are still warranted.[15]

Pearls/Pitfalls

1. Utilization of granulocyte colony–stimulating factor (G-CSF) for myelosuppression in the course of chemotherapy may cause a false-positive uptake of ^{18}F-FDG or ^{18}F-FCH but not ^{18}F-NaF, which is encouraging for its use in patients who received those agents.[25]
2. Treatment with bisphosphonates affect readability of ^{99m}Tc-MDP bone scintigraphy, but not ^{18}F-NaF PET/CT in spite of reducing ^{18}F-NaF uptake.[25]
3. ^{18}F-NaF PET/CT is able to monitor response to therapy; nevertheless, the interpreters should be aware of "flare phenomenon" after a favorable response to hormonal therapy in breast or prostate cancer.[25] It normally starts soon (7–10 days) after therapy commencement and could last for up to 6 months.[21]
4. The fact that ^{18}F-NaF PET/CT depicts bone tissue changes and not cancer cell accumulation is an inborn source of error. It limits the detection of early small bone (marrow) metastases and may give a false impression of persisting bone metastases, when active cancer cells have long gone.[1,14]

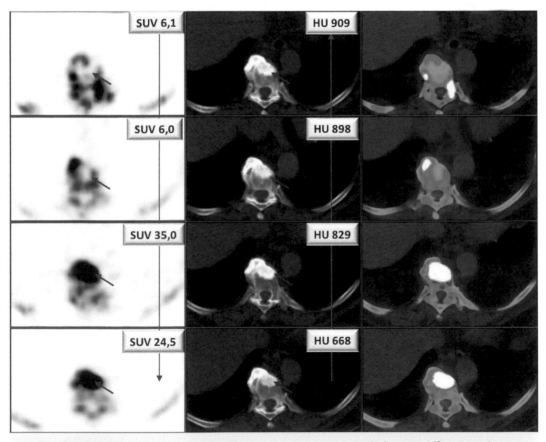

SUV 6,1   HU 909

SUV 6,0   HU 898

SUV 35,0   HU 829

SUV 24,5   HU 668

Fig. 27.6 ^{18}F-NaF PET/CT in therapy monitoring of a prostate cancer patient. Marked increased ^{18}F-NaF uptake is seen on a thoracic spine corresponding with sclerotic lesion on CT (lower row, *arrows*), suggestive of bone metastases. Improvement of the disease is evident after therapy with decreasing pattern of tracer intensity on ^{18}F-NaF PET (upper row, left). However, reverse correlation is evident between ^{18}F-NaF intensity on PET and density of sclerotic lesions on CT, which emphasizes on the superior value of functional to morphological imaging in therapy monitoring of metastatic bone disease. HU, Hounsfield unit; SUV, standardized uptake value.

Benign Osseous Disease [26]

1. Metabolic bone disease:
   a) Hyperparathyroidism: very sensitive method for detection of increased osseous turnover and insufficiency fractures as well as evaluation of brown tumor extension.
   b) Renal osteodystrophy: to differentiate high- from low-turnover lesions.
   c) Osteoporosis: can detect insufficiency fractures.
2. *Inflammatory and rheumatologic bone disease:*
   a) Sacroiliitis: ^{18}F-NaF PET/CT is superior to bone scintigraphy with sensitivity of 80 versus 47%, respectively.
3. Trauma:
   a) ^{18}F-NaF PET/CT is highly sensitive in discovering all kinds of fractures such as occult, insufficiency, and pathologic types. The radiotracer accumulates at the site of fracture 3 hours after injury.[2] It is able to detect rib and spinal fractures sooner than conventional X-ray studies.[27]
4. Assessment of prosthetic joints:
   a) Three-phase bone scan provides a very high negative predictive value in evaluation of loosening or infection of prosthetic joints; however, it has a low specificity.
   b) The SUV$_{max}$ of aseptic and septic joint loosening on ^{18}F-NaF PET/CT are significantly different. Using this semiquantitative measures improves specificity of modality compared with conventional bone scintigraphy.
   c) Diagnostic value of ^{18}F-NaF PET/CT for septic loosening is high in patients with major uptake extending over half of the bone–implant interface, that is, sensitivity and specificity of 95 and 98%, respectively.
   d) ^{18}F-NaF PET/CT is a quite promising method to differentiate loosening from an infectious process.
5. Benign bone tumors:
   a) MRI could be misleading in evaluation of osteoid osteoma.
   b) ^{18}F-NaF PET/CT can be utilized as an alternative to whole-body bone scan to detect this tumor in complex skeleton such as spine, foot, and wrist.
   c) Enchondroma presents with intense uptake on ^{18}F-NaF PET/CT. Correlation with CT is recommended to prevent misinterpretation.

6. Evaluation of bone graft and its viability:
   a) Jaw osteonecrosis: ^{18}F-NaF is more sensitive than ^{18}F-FDG PET/CT.
   b) Hip osteonecrosis: ^{18}F-NaF PET/CT can detect more foci in acetabulum compared with MRI and single-photon emission computed tomography (SPECT) and its uptake could be a predictor for disease progression.
   c) Bone grafts: ^{18}F-NaF PET/CT is a promising modality to evaluate the normal healing process.
7. *Degenerative joint disease (DJD):*
   a) ^{18}F-NaF PET/CT is a highly sensitive method, particularly for complex bone DJDs (foot and wrist) where the planar bone scan or radiographs have limited value.
   b) It suffers from insufficient specificity, which can be improved by CT correlation to avoid overdiagnosis.
8. Back pain and failed back surgery:
   a) ^{18}F-NaF PET/CT is an encouraging tool in:
      • Patients with back pain of unclear origin and inconclusive conventional imaging.
      • Discovery of reasons for persistent or recurrent pain after spinal surgery.
9. *Mandibular condylar hyperplasia:* ^{18}F-NaF PET/CT is a valid method for assessment.

27.3 Pediatric Bone Scanning with ^{18}F-NaF PET/CT[28]

1. The modality is used to delineate benign and malignant bone lesions in children.
2. Skeletal survey is presently the gold standard for assessment of child abuse; however, ^{18}F-NaF PET/CT is superior to skeletal survey with better sensitivity (85 vs. 72%) and comparable specificity (97 vs. 98%) for detection of fractures.
3. It is the optimal modality to detect rib fractures, which are the most common fractures in child abuse with an overall sensitivity of 92 versus 68% for skeletal survey. It is capable of depicting posterior rib fractures, which are extremely hard to detect on plain X-ray films.
4. In detection of classic metaphyseal lesion, which is a series of fractures seen in child abuse, ^{18}F-NaF PET/CT is more sensitive (67%) than conventional ^{99m}Tc-MDP bone scintigraphy (35%). However, this is the only type of fracture in child abuse that is better detected with skeletal survey than with PET/CT.

27.4 Quantitative 18F-NaF PET/CT Imaging in the Assessment of Metabolic Bone Disease[29]

1. Dynamic 18F-NaF PET/CT provides a new method for evaluation of bone metabolism that can measure the effects of treatment for osteoporosis at specific sites such as the spine and hip.
2. It is in opposition of laboratory bone markers that measure the integrated response to therapy over the whole skeleton.

27.5 Conclusion

The authors believe that 18F-NaF PET/CT will replace the conventional 99mTc-MDP whole-body bone scintigraphy in the evaluation of multiple malignant and benign skeletal diseases in the near future.[30] This is mainly due to higher accuracy with similar overall radiation doses, more availability of PET/CT clinics, and shorter imaging process, which is more convenient for patients and may reduce the cost for the health care system. However, despite the many advantages of 18F-NaF PET/CT compared to conventional bone imaging, being indirect, 18F-NaF is not the ideal tracer for demonstrating bone metastases. Therefore, we estimate that its clinical use will eventually be more in benign than in malignant disorders.

References

[1] Basu S, Torigian D, Alavi A. Evolving concept of imaging bone marrow metastasis in the twenty-first century: critical role of FDG-PET. Eur J Nucl Med Mol Imaging. 2008; 35(3):465–471

[2] Czernin J, Satyamurthy N, Schiepers C. Molecular mechanisms of bone 18F-NaF deposition. J Nucl Med. 2010; 51(12):1826–1829

[3] Minamimoto R, Loening A, Jamali M, et al. Prospective comparison of 99mTc-MDP scintigraphy, combined 18F-NaF and 18F-FDG PET/CT, and whole-body MRI in patients with breast and prostate cancer. J Nucl Med. 2015; 56(12):1862–1868

[4] Fogelman I. Skeletal uptake of diphosphonate: a review. Eur J Nucl Med. 1980; 5(6):473–476

[5] Bastawrous S, Bhargava P, Behnia F, Djang DS, Haseley DR. Newer PET application with an old tracer: role of 18F-NaF skeletal PET/CT in oncologic practice. Radiographics. 2014; 34(5):1295–1316

[6] Wong KK, Piert M. Dynamic bone imaging with 99mTc-labeled diphosphonates and 18F-NaF: mechanisms and applications. J Nucl Med. 2013; 54(4):590–599

[7] Araz M, Aras G, Küçük ON. The role of 18F-NaF PET/CT in metastatic bone disease. J Bone Oncol. 2015; 4(3):92–97

[8] Lim R, Fahey FH, Drubach LA, Connolly LP, Treves ST. Early experience with fluorine-18 sodium fluoride bone PET in young patients with back pain. J Pediatr Orthop. 2007; 27(3):277–282

[9] Beheshti M, Mottaghy FM, Payche F, et al. (18)F-NaF PET/CT: EANM procedure guidelines for bone imaging. Eur J Nucl Med Mol Imaging. 2015; 42(11):1767–1777

[10] Iagaru A, Mittra E, Dick DW, Gambhir SS. Prospective evaluation of (99m)Tc MDP scintigraphy, (18)F NaF PET/CT, and (18)F FDG PET/CT for detection of skeletal metastases. Mol Imaging Biol. 2012; 14(2):252–259

[11] Mosci C, Iagaru A. 18F NaF PET/CT in the assessment of malignant bone disease. In: Beheshti M, ed. PET CLINICS. Clinical Utility of 18F NaF PET/CT in Benign and Malignant Disorders. Vol. 7. Philadelphia, PA: Saunders; 2012:263–274

[12] Caglar M, Kupik O, Karabulut E, Høilund-Carlsen PF. Detection of bone metastases in breast cancer patients in the PET/CT era: Do we still need the bone scan? Rev Esp Med Nucl Imagen Mol. 2016; 35(1):3–11

[13] Hildebrandt MG, Gerke O, Baun C, et al. [18F]Fluorodeoxyglucose (FDG)-positron emission tomography (PET)/computed tomography (CT) in suspected recurrent breast cancer: a prospective comparative study of dual-time-point FDG-PET/CT, contrast-enhanced CT, and bone scintigraphy. J Clin Oncol. 2016; 34(16):1889–1897

[14] Raynor W, Houshmand S, Gholami S, et al. Evolving role of molecular imaging with (18)F-sodium fluoride PET as a biomarker for calcium metabolism. Curr Osteoporos Rep. 2016; 14(4):115–125

[15] Apolo AB, Lindenberg L, Shih JH, et al. Prospective study evaluating Na18F PET/CT in predicting clinical outcomes and survival in advanced prostate cancer. J Nucl Med. 2016; 57(6):886–892

[16] Jadvar H, Desai B, Ji L, et al. Prospective evaluation of 18F-NaF and 18F-FDG PET/CT in detection of occult metastatic disease in biochemical recurrence of prostate cancer. Clin Nucl Med. 2012; 37(7):637–643

[17] Beheshti M, Vali R, Waldenberger P, et al. The use of F-18 choline PET in the assessment of bone metastases in prostate cancer: correlation with morphological changes on CT. Mol Imaging Biol. 2009; 11(6):446–454

[18] Poulsen MH, Petersen H, Høilund-Carlsen PF, et al. Spine metastases in prostate cancer: comparison of technetium-99m-MDP whole-body bone scintigraphy, [(18) F]choline positron emission tomography(PET)/computed tomography (CT) and [(18) F]NaF PET/CT. BJU Int. 2014; 114(6):818–823

[19] Beheshti M, Vali R, Waldenberger P, et al. Detection of bone metastases in patients with prostate cancer by 18F fluorocholine and 18F fluoride PET-CT: a comparative study. Eur J Nucl Med Mol Imaging. 2008; 35(10):1766–1774

[20] Pyka T, Okamoto S, Dahlbender M, et al. Comparison of bone scintigraphy and 68Ga-PSMA PET for skeletal staging in prostate cancer. Eur J Nucl Med Mol Imaging. 2016; 43(12):2114–2121

[21] O'Sullivan GJ, Carty FL, Cronin CG. Imaging of bone metastasis: an update. World J Radiol. 2015; 7(8):202–211

[22] Hillner BE, Siegel BA, Hanna L, Duan F, Quinn B, Shields AF. 18F-fluoride PET used for treatment monitoring of systemic cancer therapy: results from the National Oncologic PET Registry. J Nucl Med. 2015; 56(2):222–228

[23] Muzahir S, Jeraj R, Liu G, et al. Differentiation of metastatic vs degenerative joint disease using semi-quantitative analysis with (18)F-NaF PET/CT in castrate resistant prostate cancer patients. Am J Nucl Med Mol Imaging. 2015; 5(2):162–168

[24] Vali R, Beheshti M, Waldenberger P, Langsteger W. Assessment of malignant and benign bone lesions by static F-18 fluoride PET-CT: additional value of SUV. J Nucl Med. 2008; 49:150

[25] Lecouvet FE, Talbot JN, Messiou C, Bourguet P, Liu Y, de Souza NM, EORTC Imaging Group. Monitoring the response of bone metastases to treatment with magnetic resonance imaging and nuclear medicine techniques: a review and position statement by the European Organisation for Research and Treatment of Cancer imaging group. Eur J Cancer. 2014; 50(15):2519–2531

[26] Strobel K, Vali R. 18F-NaF PET/CT versus conventional bone scanning in the assessment of benign bone disease. In: Beheshti M, ed. PET Clinics. Clinical Utility of 18F NaF PET/CT in Benign and Malignant Disorders. Vol. 7. Philadelphia, PA: Saunders; 2012:249–261

[27] Drubach LA, Johnston PR, Newton AW, Perez-Rossello JM, Grant FD, Kleinman PK. Skeletal trauma in child abuse: detection with 18F-NaF PET. Radiology. 2010; 255(1):173–181

[28] Drubach L. Pediatric bone scanning, clinical indication of 18F-NaF PET/CT. In: Beheshti M, ed. PET Clinics. Clinical Utility of 18F NaF PET/CT in Benign and Malignant Disorders. Vol. 7. Philadelphia, PA: Saunders; 2012:293–301

[29] Blake G, Siddique M, Frost M, Moore A, Fogelman I. Quantitative PET imaging using 18F sodium fluoride in the assessment of metabolic bone disease and the monitoring of their response to therapy. In: Beheshti M, ed. PET Clinics. Clinical Utility of 18F NaF PET/CT in Benign and Malignant Disorders. Vol. 7. Philadelphia, PA: Saunders; 2012:275–291

[30] Langsteger W, Heinisch M, Fogelman I. The role of fluorodeoxyglucose, 18F-dihydroxyphenylalanine, 18F-choline, and 18F-fluoride in bone imaging with emphasis on prostate and breast. Semin Nucl Med. 2006; 36(1):73–92

28 68Ga-Based Imaging Techniques

Paolo Castellucci, Cristina Nanni, and Valentina Ambrosini

28.1 68Ga Prostate-Specific Membrane Antigen

28.1.1 Introduction[1,2,3,4,5]

1. Prostate cancer (PCa) is the third leading cause of cancer death in men.[1]
2. Different imaging methods can be used in the natural history of the disease.[1,2]
3. PET/CT (with 11C-choline or 18F-choline) is currently the most used imaging method.[1]
4. Main limitation of choline PET/CT is the low sensitivity in nodal staging and PSA values lower than 1 ng/mL in case of biochemical recurrence (BCR).[2]
5. New probes such 68Ga-PSMA have been recently proposed.[3,4,5]

In this chapter, we will briefly present an overview of the advantages and limitations of the new molecular probe targeting the prostate specific membrane antigen (PSMA) that seems to be the most promising radiopharmaceutical for an extensive clinical use (▶ Fig. 28.1).

Technical Aspects[6,7,8,9]

1. PSMA is the glutamate carboxy-peptidase II (GCPII), a membrane bound metallopeptidase physiologically expressed in several tissues. Human GCPII contains 750 amino acids and weighs approximately 84 kDa.[6]
2. In PCa tissue, PSMA is involved in angiogenesis, as increased PSMA expression has been found in the stroma adjacent to neovasculature of solid tumors.
3. PSMA is not specific for PCa only, since it is overexpressed in many other cancers.[7]
4. PSMA is an ideal target for tumor-specific imaging and therapy since it is overexpressed in more than 90% of PCa lesions.[7]
5. PSMA is very versatile since it offers a wide range of opportunity: it can be labeled with different radioactive emitters such as gamma emitters (99Tc or 111In) and beta emitters like 68Ga (PSMA-11, PSMA I&T, and PSMA-617) or 18F (PSMA-1007 a compound with hepatobiliary excretion and no urinary excretion, which showed very promising results).[8]

6. For therapeutic purposes, PSMA can be labeled with high energy and long half-life emitters such as 177Lu or 131I or even alpha emitters such as 225Ac.[9]

28.1.2 Imaging with PSMA PET/CT in the Natural History of PCa[10,11,12,13,14,15,16,17,18,19,20,21]

Main indications for Ga-PSMA PET/CT imaging are diagnosis, guide biopsy, staging the disease before primary treatment, detecting the site or sites of

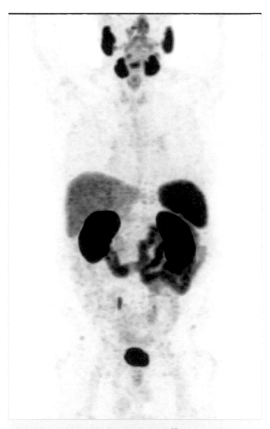

Fig. 28.1 Normal biodistribution of 68Ga prostate-specific membrane antigen 11 (PSMA-11), 60 minutes after the administration of 150 MBq (2 MBq/kg). Maximum intensity projection to note the intense uptake in the salivary glands, spleen, proximal small bowel, and kidneys.

recurrence in case of BCR, addressing patients to personalized therapies, and assessing therapy response.

Intraprostatic Diagnosis and Staging

PSMA PET/CT or PET/MRI can guide subsequent rebiopsies in patients at high risk of PCa but with negative findings at first biopsy:

1. In 21 patients with newly diagnosed PCa, ^{68}Ga-PSMA PET/CT showed a suboptimal sensitivity of 67% but a specificity and accuracy of 92 and 72%, respectively, a positive predictive value (PPV) of 97%, and a negative predictive value (NPV) of 42%.[10]
2. In seven patients with newly diagnosed PCa candidates of radical prostatectomy, ^{68}Ga-PSMA PET and MRI alone gave complementary results. Using both information to delineate the extent of intraprostatic PCa foci, sensitivity of 82% and specificity of 89% have been reached.[11]
3. In 53 patients with simultaneous ^{68}Ga-PSMA PET/MRI acquisition, the information provided by the two methods statistically outperformed the ones of multiparametric MRI and ^{68}Ga-PSMA PET imaging alone for a precise localization of intraprostatic PCa foci.[12]

Lymph Nodal Staging

^{68}Ga-PSMA PET/CT or ^{68}Ga-PSMA PET/MRI can be used for the assessment of lymph-node metastases (LNM) in patients at high risk of nodal involvement at staging.

1. It is possible to grade the individual risk of LNM using preoperative nomograms.[13]
2. A risk of nodal metastases greater than 5% is an indication to perform an extended pelvic nodal dissection (ePLND).
3. An accurate staging may guide surgeons in performing image-guided ePLND or to exclude from surgery patients who already show distant metastatic spread of the disease.
4. In 130 intermediate- and high-risk patients with, a presurgical ^{68}Ga-PSMA PET/CT assessed the presence of LNM in 117/734 (15.9%) lymph node templates. A sensitivity of 65.9%, a specificity of 98.9%, and accuracy of 88.5% were found. On a per-side-based analysis, the sensitivity, specificity, and accuracy were 68.3, 99.1, and 95.2%, respectively.[14]
5. In 30 patients with intermediate- and high-risk PCa, ^{68}Ga-PSMA PET/CT showed a sensitivity of

64%, specificity of 95%, PPV of 88%, and NPV of 82% on a patient basis. On a lymph node region-based analysis, the sensitivity dropped down to 56%, but the specificity was 98%, the PPV was 90%, and the NPV was 94%. The mean size of the missed lymph nodes at ^{68}Ga-PSMA PET/CT was equal to 2.7 mm.[15]

In conclusion, ^{68}Ga-PSMA PET/CT imaging showed suboptimal sensitivity in the detection of small LNM. In order to minimize this limitation, only patients showing high or very high risk of LNs or distant lesions should be studied with PSMA PET/CT before primary treatment. This approach could reduce false-negative results, increase the percentage of patients in whom unusual location of the disease could be detected by PSMA PET/CT, and finally exclude from aggressive treatments patients showing multiple distant lesions at presentation (▶ Fig. 28.2).

Recurrence after Primary Treatment

Restaging the disease in case of BCR is the main application of ^{68}Ga-PSMA PET/CT and nowadays it could be considered the best imaging modality for the precise individualization of the site of recurrence especially in the early phases of BCR when PSA levels are still relatively low.

1. An accurate imaging procedure may help physicians in addressing patients to a tailored salvage therapy.
2. Choline PET/CT has some limitations since the sensitivity in case of low PSA values is still suboptimal.[16]
3. The optimal timing for salvage therapies would be when the PSA levels are low. This should correspond to a limited cancer burden and, hopefully, to the presence of single or few (oligometastatic) metastatic lesions.[17]
4. In a population of 248 recurrent PCa patients (median PSA: 1.99 ng/mL), the authors reported a positivity rate of 89.5% in the whole population. In other subgroups, they reported a positivity rate of 93.0% for PSA values between 1 and 2 ng/mL; a positivity rate of 72.7% for PSA values between 0.5 and 1 ng/mL; and a positivity rate of 57.9% for PSA values between 0.2 and 0.5 ng/mL.[18]
5. In a cohort of 70 patients (median PSA 1.7 ng/mL), a positivity rate of 74.2% has been found in the whole population. A PSA level of 0.83 ng/mL and a PSA doubling time (PSAdt) of 6.5 months were found to be valuable cutoff values for

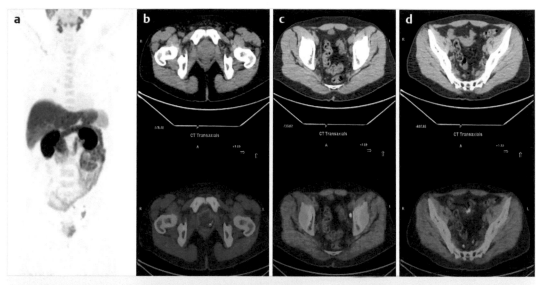

Fig. 28.2 A 65-year-old patient with prostate cancer at presentation with very high risk for nodal metastasis (Gleason score 4 + 4; T3a; prostate-specific antigen [PSA] 21 ng/mL). 68Ga prostate-specific membrane antigen 11 (PSMA-11) PET/CT, 60 minutes after the administration of 140 MBq (2 MBq/kg). **(a)** Maximum intensity projection. **(b)** Fused images showing intense 68Ga-PSMA uptake in the prostate especially in the left lobe (maximum standardized uptake value [SUVmax] = 10). **(c)** Fused images showing intense 68Ga-PSMA uptake in a left external iliac lymph node (LN). **(d)** Fused images showing intense 68Ga-PSMA uptake in pararectal LNs. According to 68Ga-PSMA-11 PET/CT, an extended pelvic nodal dissection has been performed including presacral and pararectal LNs.

predicting with high probability a positive or negative 68Ga-PSMA PET/CT scan result.[19]

6. In a cohort of 131 PCa patients (median PSA 2.2 ng/mL), the authors found an overall positivity rate for 68Ga-PSMA PET/CT of 75%. The clinical impact of 68Ga-PSMA PET/CT on subsequent management has been observed in 99/131 patients (76% of the whole population). 68Ga-PSMA PET/CT changed therapeutic strategy addressing patients to salvage radiotherapy, salvage node dissection, or salvage local treatments, but also to androgen deprivation therapy (ADT) administration. In all the 34 oligometastasis patients at 68Ga-PSMA PET/CT, the authors observed an impact on clinical management.[20]

7. In 126 patients who underwent 68Ga-PSMA PET/CT or 68Ga-PSMA PET/RM in a single institution, 103 (82%) of patients had disease detected on 68Ga-PSMA PET/CT. Based on survey results, there were 67 (53.2%) patients with major changes, and 8 (6.4%) patients with minor changes in management.[21]

In conclusion, 68Ga PSMA PET/CT may have a significant impact on patient management, mainly in the early phases of BCR in order to guide metastasis-directed therapy performed with curative intent. However, the influence of parameters such as PSA values at the time of the PET scan, PSA kinetics, time to relapse (TTR), and the administration of ADT at the time of investigation on PSMA PET/CT detection rate should be more deeply investigated since they may lead to a better patient selection with an improvement in accuracy (▶ Fig. 28.3).

Ga-PSMA Conclusion

68Ga-PSMA radiopharmaceuticals proved to be superior to 11C or 18F choline and conventional radiological imaging for either stage or restage PCa. In selected patient populations, it proved to have a significant impact on patient management. This would help in optimizing the use of lesion-targeted approach and improve outcome, especially in patients with recurrent PCa.

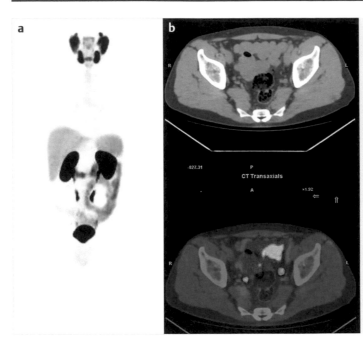

Fig. 28.3 A 64-year-old patient with prostate cancer (Gleason score 4 + 4; T3a, prostate-specific antigen [PSA] 21 ng/mL). The patient showed a biochemical recurrence 24 months after primary treatment with radical intent (radical prostatectomy). At the time of PET investigation, PSA was 0.6 ng/mL and PSA doubling time (PSAdt) of 6 months. ^{68}Ga-PSMA-11 PET/CT, 60 minutes after the administration of 136 MBq (2 MBq/kg). **(a)** Maximum intensity projection. **(b)** Fused images showing intense ^{68}Ga PSMA uptake in a 9-mm right obturator lymph node (maximum standardized uptake value [SUVmax] = 6). The patient has been addressed to a salvage lymph nodal dissection.

28.2 ^{68}Ga-Labeled Somatostatin Analogs

28.2.1 Introduction[22,23]

1. ^{68}Ga-labeled SA comprise a group of radiopharmaceuticals that bind to somatostatin receptors (SR).[22]
2. The currently clinically employed compounds (DOTA-TATE, DOTA-TOC, DOTA-NOC) show different binding affinity to the SR subtypes[23]: DOTA-TATE shows the higher affinity for SR2, while DOTA-NOC shows the wider SR-subtypes affinity profile (binding to SR2, 3, and 5).
3. Clinical evidence suggests that differences in SR binding affinity are not clinically relevant, although SUVmax values are not directly comparable.

28.2.2 Indications to SR Imaging with PET/CT[22,24,25,26,27]

1. The main indication to the use of ^{68}Ga-SA PET/CT is the assessment of patients with NEN.
2. NEN comprise a large variety of rare (incidence: 3–5/100,000/y) and very heterogeneous tumors[24] that can arise in virtually every internal organ, but mainly occur in the gastroenteropancreatic and bronchopulmonary

systems. NEN are mostly nonfunctioning although some patients may present with symptoms related to hormone hypersecretion. The disease course is influenced by the primary site and international guidelines indicate the need of a site-specific management.

3. NEN are classified according to the WHO 2010[25] in three grades (grades 1–3) based on the ki-67 values and the cells morphology: well-differentiated NEN (grades 1 and 2) show a high expression of SR.
4. ^{68}Ga-SA PET/CT is included in the routine diagnostic workup of NEN patients for staging (▶ Fig. 28.4), restaging, identification of the unknown primary site, and selection of candidates for target therapy (PRRT).[22]
5. Less strong evidence supports ^{68}Ga-SA PET/CT employment for the assessment of therapy response (a decreased uptake in a given lesion may indicate a reduction in both receptor number and lesion volume, but it cannot rule out the concomitant presence of undifferentiated clones that may not express SR).[22]
6. The role of ^{68}Ga-SA PET/CT in cases presenting a suspicious neuroendocrine lesion is debatable and strongly influenced by the pretest probability of disease. For example, among the various biochemical markers employed for the assessment of NEN (e.g., chromogranin A), a

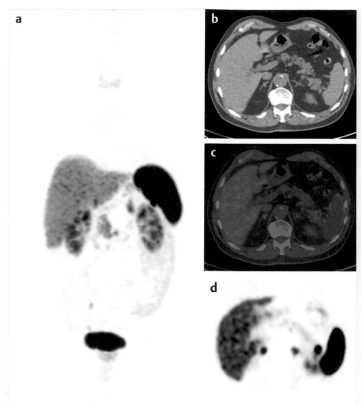

Fig. 28.4 (a-d) 68Ga-NOC PET/CT images of a patient with a well-differentiated G1NEN lesion of the pancreatic tail (SUVmax = 57, corresponding to high expression of SR).

careful estimation of concomitant conditions other than NEN that could determine their increase should be performed (e.g., treatment with pump inhibitors, chronic gastritis).[22]

7. In Europe, 68Ga-SA PET/CT is the gold standard functional imaging modality to study well-differentiated NEN. It has replaced somatostatin receptor scintigraphy (SRS) and is included in European guidelines.[22,26,27]

8. In the United States, DOTA-TATE has been recently approved by the Food and Drug Administration (FDA).

28.2.3 68Ga-SA PET/CT Accuracy/Comparison to Other Modalities[22,28,29,30,31,32,33,34,35,36,37,38]

1. Many reports[22,28,29,30,31,32,33,34,35] indicate the higher diagnostic accuracy of 68Ga-SA PET/CT over both scintigraphy (also when including SPECT/CT acquisitions) and PET/CT with metabolic radiopharmaceuticals (18F-FDG or 18F-DOPA).

2. In a recent prospective trial[34] including 131 patients with gastroenteropancreatic NEN and unknown primary NEN, 68Ga-DOTA-TATE showed a higher detection rate (95.2%) as compared to 111In-pentetreotide SPECT/CT (30.9%) and CT or MRI (45.6%).

3. Although current European Neuroendocrine Tumor Society (ENETS) 2016 guidelines still include SRS for SR imaging,[27] due to its worldwide availability and low costs, it is going to be progressively replaced by 68Ga-SA PET/CT due to the well-known advantages of the latter (higher diagnostic accuracy and spatial resolution, the possibility to perform semiquantitative analysis, more favorable biodistribution with lower physiologic uptake in bowel and liver, and overall lower costs).

4. The overall sensitivity and specificity of 68Ga-SA PET/CT (with either TATE, NOC, or TOC) for the detection of well-differentiated NEN are very high (> 90%) at both the primary and the metastatic sites.[29,35]

5. The largest published study[32] included 728 patients and 1,258 PET/CT scans and reported

high sensitivity (> 94%) and specificity (> 92%) of TATE for tumor lesion detection.

6. Three meta-analyses reported high diagnostic accuracy of ^{68}Ga-SA PET/CT for the detection of NEN lesions, particularly for well-differentiated forms.[28,36,37] Treglia et al[28] reported the following findings: sensitivity range, 72 to 100%; pooled, 93% (95% confidence interval [CI]: 91–95%); specificity range, 67 to 100%; pooled, 91% (95% CI: 82–97%). Geijer et al[36] found the following: sensibility range, 70 to 100%; pooled, 93% (95% CI: 91–94%); specificity range, 67 to 100%; pooled, 96% (95% CI: 95–98%). Graham et al[37] found the following: sensibility, 92% (95% CI: 85–96%); specificity, 82% (95% CI: 69–90%).

7. A recent meta-analysis reported the higher diagnostic accuracy of ^{68}Ga-DOTA-TATE as compared to octreotide and conventional imaging (sensitivity range: 87–100%; specificity range: 86–100%).[38]

28.2.4 ^{68}Ga-SA PET/CT Impact on Management[39,40,41,42]

1. ^{68}Ga-SA PET/CT PET/CT-derived data impact on clinical management: the presence of SR-positive lesions is a prerequisite for target therapy with either cold or hot (PRRT) SA.

2. A recently published systematic review[39] (including data from 1,561 patients) reported an overall change in management in 44% (range: 16–71%) after ^{68}Ga-SA PET/CT (with DOTATOC, DOTATATE, or DOTANOC).

3. This is in line with what was reported in previous studies in smaller patient samples.[40]

4. Although hampered by well-known technical limitations, the ^{68}Ga-SA PET/CT SUVmax can be used as an indirect marker of tumor differentiation (higher SUVmax correlates to higher SR expression and therefore lower tumor grade): patients with higher SUVmax have a better prognosis.[41,42]

28.2.5 The Combined Use of ^{68}Ga-SA PET/CT and ^{18}F-FDG: Grading, Guidelines, and Clinical Evidence[43, 44,45,46,47,48]

1. Although generally characterized by an indolent behavior, NEN patients presenting ^{18}F-FDG-avid lesions show a more aggressive clinical course.

2. There is no agreement on the added role of routinely performing ^{18}F-FDG in combination with ^{68}Ga-SA PET/CT in the well-differentiated grade 1 and 2 NEN group.[43,44,45,46,47]

3. ENETS 2016 guidelines indicate a role for ^{18}F-FDG only in the grade 3 (undifferentiated) group.

4. Recently published evidence[45] also supports the potential role of ^{18}F-FDG in the well-differentiated grade 2 group (especially if presenting with high ki-67 levels or ^{68}Ga-SA-negative lesions), while in the grade 1 group, it should be reserved to selected cases with a clinical suspicion of more aggressive disease.

5. The clinical relevance of performing ^{68}Ga-SAPET/CT in the grade 3 NEN is less clear. Current evidence[48] suggests that the grade 3 group comprises both patients (ki-67 < 50%) who present a clinical behavior more similar to the G2 group and patients with very aggressive tumors (ki-67 > 50%), mostly ^{18}F-FDG positive. In this latter clinical setting, considering the aggressiveness of the tumor, the detection of SR, again generally low, is not likely to impact the clinical management.

28.2.6 Synthesis and Image Acquisition[22,49]

1. The synthesis and labeling process of ^{68}Ga-DOTA peptides is quite easy and economic: gallium can be easily eluted from a commercially available ^{68}Ge/^{68}Ga generator and therefore there is no need for an onsite cyclotron. ^{68}Ga (t1/2 = 68 minutes) presents an 89% positron emission and negligible gamma emission (1,077 keV) of 3.2%. The long half-life of the mother radionuclide ^{68}Ge (270.8 days) makes it possible to use the generator for approximately 9 to 12 months depending upon the requirement, rendering the whole procedure relatively economic.

2. In 2010, the European Association of Nuclear Medicine (EANM) published the first practical guidelines[22] for ^{68}Ga-labeled peptide PET/CT imaging. ^{68}Ga-SA PET/CT acquisition starts at 60 minutes after intravenous injection of approximately 100 MBq (75–250 MBq) of the radiolabeled peptide (such as ^{68}Ga-DOTA-NOC, ^{68}Ga-DOTA-TOC, etc.). The amount of injected radioactivity strictly depends on the daily production of the generator for each single elution (usually ranging between 300 and 700 MBq) and, of course, by the number of patients scanned per day.

3. There is no absolute indication regarding whether specific patient preparation is required.

4. The issue of the need of SA treatment discontinuation is still under debate. Performing PET/CT while on SA treatment was even reported to increase image contrast by reducing the uptake at physiologic sites with unchanged tumor lesions uptake in a small population of patients studied on and off treatment in two consecutive days.[49] When discontinuation is clinically feasible and performed, short-acting analogs should be stopped for at least 48 hours, while long-acting formulations should be stopped for 4 to 6 weeks.[22] The use of contrast media is not routinely recommended.

28.2.7 68GA-SA Image Interpretation and Pitfalls[22]

1. Physiologic uptake (**Box 28.1**) may be observed at the pituitary gland, spleen, liver, adrenals, pancreatic head/uncinate process, thyroid, and urinary tract (kidneys and urinary bladder) (▶ Fig. 28.5, ▶ Fig. 28.6).

2. False positives are the most frequently encountered pitfalls[22]: sites of inflammation or infection (including posttherapy findings and concomitant inflammatory/infectious disorders), the presence of accessory spleens or lymphoma (due to the presence of switch substrate retrovector [SSR] on activated lymphocytes and macrophages), increased tracer uptake at the head of the pancreas (observed in 30–60% of cases), is not necessarily associated with the presence of disease; its correct interpretation requires a careful evaluation and correlation of PET findings with morphological imaging features, especially in cases presenting with a focal pattern.

3. False-negative findings include small lesions dimension (< 5 mm) and tumors presenting with low or variable expression of SR (e.g., medullary thyroid carcinoma, neuroblastoma, insulinoma, pheochromocytoma, high-grade NEN).

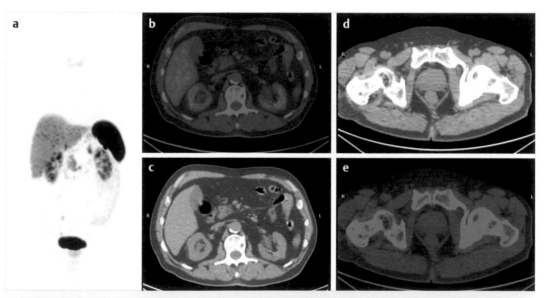

Fig. 28.5 68Ga-DOTA-NOC PET/CT maximum intensity projection (MIP; **a**) images of the same patient of ▶ Fig. 28.1, showing the presence of collateral findings. (**b**) Faint and diffuse uptake in the pancreatic head. 68Ga-somatostatin analog uptake in the pancreatic head/uncinate process, especially if diffuse, can be observed without the presence of disease. Pancreatic head uptake should always be carefully evaluated and correlated with CT findings (**c**) in order to exclude the presence of a neuroendocrine tumor nodule. Faint tracer uptake can be observed in the normal prostate (**d,e**) and the thyroid (**a**).

Fig. 28.6 (a-c) ^{68}Ga-DOTA-NOC PET/CT maximum intensity projection and transaxial PET and low-dose CT images of a patient with right frontal meningioma showing intense tracer uptake (maximum standardized uptake value [SUVmax] = 59). Physiological uptake in the hypophysis and spleen is also evident.

Box 28.1 ^{68}Ga-SA PET/CT Pitfalls

False Positives
1. Accessory spleens.
2. Inflammation.
3. Infection.
4. Lymphoma.
5. Head of the pancreas.

False Negatives
1. Small lesions size (< 5 mm).
2. Low/variable SR expression:
   a) Medullary thyroid.
   b) Cancer.
   c) Neuroblastoma.
   d) Pheochromocytoma.
   e) Insulinoma.
   f) High-grade NEN.

Beyond NEN: Tumor that may also present SR expression
1. Sarcoma.
2. Melanoma.
3. Lymphomas.
4. Breast carcinoma.
5. Prostate carcinoma.
6. Non-small-cell lung cancer.
7. Renal cell carcinoma.
8. Differentiated thyroid carcinoma.
9. Astrocytoma.
10. Ependymoma.

28.2.8 ^{68}Ga-SA PET/CT Conclusions

Many reports in the literature indicate the crucial role of ^{68}Ga-SA PET/CT in the workup of patients with NEN, for both the diagnostic assessment of well-differentiated NEN lesions and the selection of patients that may benefit from target therapy. In the clinical setting of G1 and G2 patients, ^{68}Ga-SA PET/CT is more accurate than SRS, morphological imaging, and PET/CT with other tracers. Many reports indicate that ^{68}Ga-SA PET/CT impacts the clinical management in about half the cases. The role of ^{68}Ga-SA PET/CT in patients with G3 (undifferentiated) tumor is to be considered in selected cases based on the clinical therapeutic plan in case of PET/CT positivity.

28.3 Emerging ^{68}Ga-Labeled Radiopharmaceuticals

28.3.1 ^{68}Ga-Somatostatin Antagonists[50,51,52]

1. Although mostly experimental and available only in selected centers, some Somatostatin antagonists (SANTs) labeled with ^{68}Ga have been employed to study NEN patients.
2. The reported data indicate very promising results. Ginj et al[50] reported that SANT bind to more SR binding sites than SA in animal studies, resulting in higher affinity, with potential relevance if applied in NEN forms that show lower/variable expression of SR (neuroblastoma, medullary thyroid carcinoma, insulinoma, pheochromocytoma).[51]
3. Moreover, the added value of compounds with higher SR binding affinity could find clinically relevant applications in the therapeutic setting: four patients with NEN were successfully treated with ^{177}Lu-labeled ANT (^{177}Lu-DOTA-JR11).[52]

28.3.2 ^{68}Ga-Exendin[53,54]

1. ^{68}Ga-exendin is a novel radiopharmaceutical that binds to glucagonlike peptide 1 receptor (GLP-1R) and has been employed to detect the presence of insulinoma lesions.
2. Insulinoma is rare but has a major clinical impact on patients' lives due to insulin incretion that leads to difficult-to-treat hypoglycemia crisis. Diagnosis is usually hampered by small dimensions and by the fact that only approximately 20% express SR.
3. Preliminary but increasing evidence supports the role of ^{68}Ga-exendin for the detection of insulinoma. Although the number of cases studied is limited, the authors agree[53,54] that this novel radiopharmaceutical is accurate for the preoperative detection of hidden insulinoma (reported sensitivity of 97.7%).

References

[1] Mottet N, Bellmunt J, Bolla M, et al. EAU-ESTRO-SIOG guidelines on prostate cancer. Part 1: screening, diagnosis, and local treatment with curative intent. Eur Urol. 2017; 71:618–629

[2] Cornford P, Bellmunt J, Bolla M, et al. EAU-ESTRO-SIOG guidelines on prostate cancer. Part II: treatment of relapsing, metastatic, and castration-resistant prostate cancer. Eur Urol. 2017; 71:630–642

[3] Afshar-Oromieh A, Malcher A, Eder M, et al. PET imaging with a [68Ga]gallium-labelled PSMA ligand for the diagnosis of prostate cancer: biodistribution in humans and first evaluation of tumour lesions. Eur J Nucl Med Mol Imaging. 2013; 40(4):486–495

[4] Schuster DM, Nanni C, Fanti S. Evaluation of prostate cancer with radiolabeled amino acid analogs. J Nucl Med. 2016; 57 Suppl 3:61S–66S

[5] Wieser G, Popp I, Christian Rischke H, et al. Diagnosis of recurrent prostate cancer with PET/CT imaging using the gastrin-releasing peptide receptor antagonist 68Ga-RM2: preliminary results in patients with negative or inconclusive [18F]fluoroethylcholine-PET/CT. Eur J Nucl Med Mol Imaging. 2017; 44(9):1463–1472

[6] Israeli RS, Powell CT, Fair WR, Heston WD. Molecular cloning of a complementary DNA encoding a prostate-specific membrane antigen. Cancer Res. 1993; 53(2):227–230

[7] Silver DA, Pellicer I, Fair WR, Heston WD, Cordon-Cardo C. Prostate-specific membrane antigen expression in normal and malignant human tissues. Clin Cancer Res. 1997; 3(1): 81–85

[8] Giesel FL, Hadaschik B, Cardinale J, et al. F-18 labelled PSMA-1007: biodistribution, radiation dosimetry and histopathological validation of tumor lesions in prostate cancer patients. Eur J Nucl Med Mol Imaging. 2017; 44(4):678–688

[9] Rowe SP, Drzezga A, Neumaier B, et al. Prostate-specific membrane antigen-targeted radiohalogenated PET and therapeutic agents for prostate cancer. J Nucl Med. 2016; 57 Suppl 3:90S–96S

[10] Fendler WP, Schmidt DF, Wenter V, et al. 68Ga-PSMA PET/CT detects the location and extent of primary prostate cancer. J Nucl Med. 2016; 57(11):1720–1725

[11] Zamboglou C, Drendel V, Jilg CA, et al. Comparison of 68Ga-HBED-CC PSMA-PET/CT and multiparametric MRI for gross tumour volume detection in patients with primary prostate cancer based on slice by slice comparison with histopathology. Theranostics. 2017; 7(1):228–237

[12] Eiber M, Weirich G, Holzapfel K, et al. Simultaneous 68Ga-PSMA HBED-CC PET/MRI improves the localization of primary prostate cancer. Eur Urol. 2016; 70(5):829–836

[13] Briganti A, Larcher A, Abdollah F, et al. Updated nomogram predicting lymph node invasion in patients with prostate cancer undergoing extended pelvic lymph node dissection: the essential importance of percentage of positive cores. Eur Urol. 2012; 61(3):480–487

[14] Maurer T, Gschwend JE, Rauscher I, et al. Diagnostic efficacy of (68)gallium-PSMA positron emission tomography compared to conventional imaging for lymph node staging of 130 consecutive patients with intermediate to high risk prostate cancer. J Urol. 2016; 195(5):1436–1443

[15] van Leeuwen PJ, Emmett L, Ho B, et al. Prospective evaluation of 68gallium-prostate-specific membrane antigen positron emission tomography/computed tomography for preoperative lymph node staging in prostate cancer. BJU Int. 2017; 119(2):209–215

[16] Castellucci P, Ceci F, Graziani T, et al. Early biochemical relapse after radical prostatectomy: which prostate cancer patients may benefit from a restaging 11C-choline PET/CT scan before salvage radiation therapy? J Nucl Med. 2014; 55(9): 1424–1429

[17] Stephenson AJ, Scardino PT, Kattan MW, et al. Predicting the outcome of salvage radiation therapy for recurrent prostate cancer after radical prostatectomy. J Clin Oncol. 2007; 25 (15):2035–2041

[18] Eiber M, Maurer T, Souvatzoglou M, et al. Evaluation of hybrid 68Ga-PSMA-ligand PET/CT in 248 patients with bio-

chemical recurrence after radical prostatectomy. J Nucl Med. 2015; 56(5):668–674

[19] Ceci F, Uprimny C, Nilica B, et al. (68)Ga-PSMA PET/CT for restaging recurrent prostate cancer: which factors are associated with PET/CT detection rate? Eur J Nucl Med Mol Imaging. 2015; 42(8):1284–1294

[20] Albissini S, Artigas C, Aoun F, et al. Clinical impact of 68Ga-prostate-specific membrane antigen (PSMA) positron emission tomography/computed tomography (PET/CT) in patients with prostate cancer with rising prostate-specific antigen after treatment with curative intent: preliminary analysis of a multidisciplinary approach. BJU Int. 2017; 120:197–203

[21] Hope TA, Aggarwal R, Chee B. Impact of Ga-68 PSMA-11 PET on management in patients with biochemically recurrent prostate cancer. J Nucl Med. 2017; 58(12):1956–1961

[22] Virgolini I, Ambrosini V, Bomanji JB, et al. Procedure guidelines for PET/CT tumour imaging with 68Ga-DOTA-conjugated peptides: 68Ga-DOTA-TOC, 68Ga-DOTA-NOC, 68Ga-DOTA-TATE. Eur J Nucl Med Mol Imaging. 2010; 37(10): 2004–2010

[23] Antunes P, Ginj M, Zhang H, et al. Are radiogallium-labelled DOTA-conjugated somatostatin analogues superior to those labelled with other radiometals? Eur J Nucl Med Mol Imaging. 2007; 34(7):982–993

[24] Yao JC, Hassan M, Phan A, et al. One hundred years after "carcinoid": epidemiology of and prognostic factors for neuroendocrine tumors in 35,825 cases in the United States. J Clin Oncol. 2008; 26(18):3063–3072

[25] Bosman F, Carneiro F, Hruban R, et al. WHO Classification of Tumours of the Digestive System. Lyon, France: IARC press; 2010

[26] Krenning EP, Kwekkeboom DJ, Bakker WH, et al. Somatostatin receptor scintigraphy with [111 In-DTPA-D-Phe1]- and [123I-Tyr3]-octreotide: the Rotterdam experience with more than 1000 patients. Eur J Nucl Med. 1993; 20(8):716–731

[27] Falconi M, Eriksson B, Kaltsas G, et al. Vienna Consensus Conference participants. ENETS consensus guidelines update for the management of patients with functional pancreatic neuroendocrine tumors and non-functional pancreatic neuroendocrine tumors. Neuroendocrinology. 2016; 103(2):153–171

[28] Treglia G, Castaldi P, Rindi G, Giordano A, Rufini V. Diagnostic performance of gallium-68 somatostatin receptor PET and PET/CT in patients with thoracic and gastroenteropancreatic neuroendocrine tumours: a meta-analysis. Endocrine. 2012; 42(1):80–87

[29] Gabriel M, Decristoforo C, Kendler D, et al. 68Ga-DOTA-Tyr3-octreotide PET in neuroendocrine tumors: comparison with somatostatin receptor scintigraphy and CT. J Nucl Med. 2007; 48(4):508–518

[30] Ambrosini V, Tomassetti P, Castellucci P, et al. Comparison between 68Ga-DOTA-NOC and 18F-DOPA PET for the detection of gastro-entero-pancreatic and lung neuro-endocrine tumours. Eur J Nucl Med Mol Imaging. 2008; 35(8):1431–1438

[31] Srirajaskanthan R, Kayani I, Quigley AM, Soh J, Caplin ME, Bomanji J. The role of 68Ga-DOTATATE PET in patients with neuroendocrine tumors and negative or equivocal findings on 111 In-DTPA-octreotide scintigraphy. J Nucl Med. 2010; 51(6):875–882

[32] Skoura E, Michopoulou S, Mohmaduvesh M, et al. The impact of 68Ga-DOTATATE PET/CT imaging on management of patients with neuroendocrine tumors: experience from a National Referral Center in the United Kingdom. J Nucl Med. 2016; 57(1):34–40

[33] Ambrosini V, Campana D, Tomassetti P, Fanti S. 68Ga-labelled peptides for diagnosis of gastroenteropancreatic NET. Eur J Nucl Med Mol Imaging. 2012; 39(39) Suppl 1:S52–S60

[34] Sadowski SM, Neychev V, Millo C, et al. Prospective Study of 68Ga-DOTATATE positron emission tomography/computed tomography for detecting gastro-entero-pancreatic neuroendocrine tumors and unknown primary sites. J Clin Oncol. 2016; 34(6):588–596

[35] Ambrosini V, Nanni C, Zompatori M, et al. (68)Ga-DOTA-NOC PET/CT in comparison with CT for the detection of bone metastasis in patients with neuroendocrine tumours. Eur J Nucl Med Mol Imaging. 2010; 37(4):722–727

[36] Geijer H, Breimer LH. Somatostatin receptor PET/CT in neuroendocrine tumours: update on systematic review and meta-analysis. Eur J Nucl Med Mol Imaging. 2013; 40(11):1770–1780

[37] Graham MM, Gu X, Ginader T, Breheny P, Sunderland JJ. 68Ga-DOTATOC imaging of neuroendocrine tumors: a systematic review and metaanalysis. J Nucl Med. 2017; 58(9): 1452–1458

[38] Deppen SA, Blume J, Bobbey AJ, et al. 68Ga-DOTATATE compared with 111 In-DTPA-octreotide and conventional imaging for pulmonary and gastroenteropancreatic neuroendocrine tumors: a systematic review and meta-analysis. J Nucl Med. 2016; 57(6):872–878

[39] Barrio M, Czernin J, Fanti S, et al. The impact of somatostatin receptor-directed PET/CT on the management of patients with neuroendocrine tumor: a systematic review and meta-analysis. J Nucl Med. 2017; 58(5):756–761

[40] Ambrosini V, Campana D, Bodei L, et al. 68Ga-DOTANOC PET/CT clinical impact in patients with neuroendocrine tumors. J Nucl Med. 2010; 51(5):669–673

[41] Campana D, Ambrosini V, Pezzilli R, et al. Standardized uptake values of (68)Ga-DOTANOC PET: a promising prognostic tool in neuroendocrine tumors. J Nucl Med. 2010; 51(3):353–359

[42] Ambrosini V, Campana D, Polverari G, et al. Prognostic value of 68Ga-DOTANOC PET/CT SUVmax in patients with neuroendocrine tumors of the pancreas. J Nucl Med. 2015; 56(12): 1843–1848

[43] Partelli S, Rinzivillo M, Maurizi A, et al. The role of combined Ga-DOTANOC and (18)FDG PET/CT in the management of patients with pancreatic neuroendocrine tumors. Neuroendocrinology. 2014; 100(4):293–299

[44] Kundu P, Lata S, Sharma P, Singh H, Malhotra A, Bal C. Prospective evaluation of (68)Ga-DOTANOC PET-CT in differentiated thyroid cancer patients with raised thyroglobulin and negative (131)I-whole body scan: comparison with (18)F-FDG PET-CT. Eur J Nucl Med Mol Imaging. 2014; 41(7):1354–1362

[45] Bahri H, Laurence L, Edeline J, et al. High prognostic value of 18F-FDG PET for metastatic gastroenteropancreatic neuroendocrine tumors: a long-term evaluation. J Nucl Med. 2014; 55(11):1786–1790

[46] Nilica B, Waitz D, Stevanovic V, et al. Direct comparison of (68)Ga-DOTA-TOC and (18)F-FDG PET/CT in the follow-up of patients with neuroendocrine tumour treated with the first full peptide receptor radionuclide therapy cycle. Eur J Nucl Med Mol Imaging. 2016; 43(9):1585–1592

[47] Panagiotidis E, Alshammari A, Michopoulou S, et al. Comparison of the impact of 68Ga-DOTATATE and 18F-FDG PET/CT on clinical management in patients with neuroendocrine tumors. J Nucl Med. 2017; 58(1):91–96

[48] Fazio N, Milione M. Gastroenteropancreatic neuroendocrine carcinomas: the NET G3 subcategory is a reality. Oncologist. 2017; 22(3):359

[49] Interim results on the influence of lanreotide on uptake of [68Ga]-DOTATATE in patients with metastatic or unresectable NET: no evidence for discontinuation of lanreotide be-

fore [68Ga]-DOTATATE PET/CT. Clin Adv Hematol Oncol. 2016; 14(5) Suppl 7:13–15

[50] Ginj M, Zhang H, Waser B, et al. Radiolabeled somatostatin receptor antagonists are preferable to agonists for in vivo peptide receptor targeting of tumors. Proc Natl Acad Sci U S A. 2006; 103(44):16436–16441

[51] Reubi JC, Waser B, Mäcke H, Rivier J. Highly increased 125I–JR11 antagonist binding in vitro reveals novel indications for sst2 targeting in human cancers. J Nucl Med. 2017; 58(2): 300–306

[52] Wild D, Fani M, Fischer R, et al. Comparison of somatostatin receptor agonist and antagonist for peptide receptor radionuclide therapy: a pilot study. J Nucl Med. 2014; 55(8):1248–1252

[53] Luo Y, Pan Q, Yao S, et al. Glucagon-like peptide-1 receptor PET/CT with 68Ga-NOTA-exendin-4 for detecting localized insulinoma: a prospective cohort study. J Nucl Med. 2016; 57 (5):715–720

[54] Antwi K, Fani M, Nicolas G, et al. Localization of hidden insulinomas with 68Ga-DOTA-exendin-4 PET/CT: a pilot study. J Nucl Med. 2015; 56(7):1075–1078

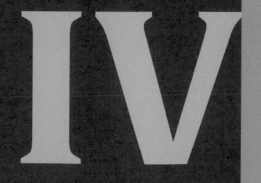

Part IV

Nononcologic Applications

29 Pediatric PET/CT   *324*

30 PET/CT in Radiation Therapy
Planning   *331*

31 FDG-PET/CT in the Evaluation
of Infection and Inflammation   *338*

32 Neurological Applications of
Fluorodeoxyglucose PET   *352*

33 Neurological Applications of
Nonfluorodeoxyglucose
Tracers   *360*

34 Cardiac PET and PET/CT   *372*

IV

29 Pediatric PET/CT

M. Beth McCarville

29.1 Introduction

The use of positron emission tomography/computed tomography (PET/CT) in children requires consideration of several unique technical and logistic issues. Young children often require sedation for PET/CT, and personnel trained in the management of children are vital to patient safety. Pregnant guardians of young patients should not be allowed in the fluorodeoxyglucose (FDG) uptake room, and arrangements must be made for the supervision of such patients. Before administration of the radioisotope, young female patients themselves must be questioned regarding their childbearing potential. This delicate subject is best handled by a technologist with experience working with young girls. Additionally, interpretation

of pediatric PET/CT imaging requires familiarity with pediatric anatomy and physiology because, compared with adults, children have more metabolically active brown fat and less retroperitoneal fat (▶ Fig. 29.1).[1] PET/CT is becoming an increasingly important adjunct to the care of the pediatric oncology patient. Several indications for its use in children are discussed herein.

29.2 Bone Tumors

29.2.1 Clinical Indication

PET/CT has shown value in detecting bone metastases from primary Ewing sarcoma of bone and in the response evaluation of primary Ewing sarcoma and osteosarcoma.

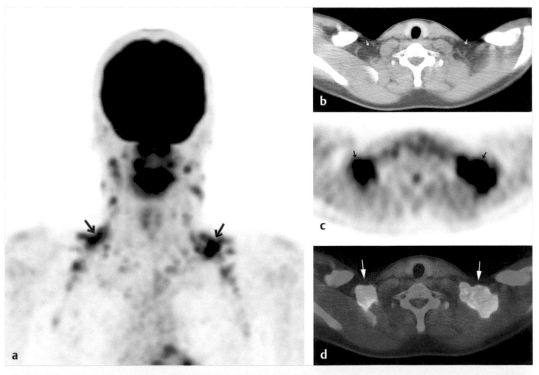

Fig. 29.1 A 16-year-old boy previously treated for Hodgkin lymphoma. **(a)** Maximum intensity projection (MIP) PET image showing intense fluorodeoxyglucose (FDG) activity in the supraclavicular areas (*arrows*) that is difficult to accurately localize by PET alone. Co-registered axial **(b)** CT, **(c)** PET, and **(d)** fused PET/CT images allow confident localization of FDG activity to brown fat (*arrows*). Children often have abundant metabolically active brown fat, such as shown here.

29.2.2 Accuracy

1. In one study, on an examination-based analysis, the sensitivity, specificity, and accuracy of PET for detecting bone metastases from Ewing sarcoma of bone were 1.00, 0.96, and 0.97, respectively.[2]
2. A study evaluating the maximum standardized uptake value (SUV) of primary tumors before initiation of neoadjuvant chemotherapy (SUV1) and after neoadjuvant chemotherapy (SUV2) in patients with either osteosarcoma ($n = 18$) or Ewing sarcoma of bone ($n = 15$) found that the positive predictive value (PPV) for a favorable response ($\geq 90\%$ tumor necrosis) of an SUV2 less than 2 was 93%, and the negative predictive value (NPV) for unfavorable response ($< 90\%$ necrosis) was 75%. The PPV and NPV for favorable and unfavorable response using an SUV2:SUV1 cut point of 0.5 were 78 and 63%, respectively.[3]

29.2.3 Pearls

1. It is postulated that bone marrow metastases, such as commonly seen in Ewing sarcoma, are FDG avid but often lack avidity for the bone-seeking agent, technetium-99 m methylene diphosphonate (^{99m}Tc MDP). PET has the additional potential advantage of demonstrating extraosseous metastases.[2]

29.2.4 Pitfalls

1. On PET alone, skull metastases may be obscured by intense brain FDG activity. Evaluation of the skull in the bone window setting on correlative CT imaging, obtained during PET/CT, may increase the sensitivity for detection of skull metastases.[2,4]
2. In children, benign fibro-osseous lesions can mimic bone metastases on PET imaging. Furthermore, maximum SUVs of these benign lesions overlap those of malignant lesions. Information gained from correlative CT or MR images is useful in determining the benign nature of such lesions (▶ Fig. 29.2).[5,6]
3. Maximum SUVs of primary Ewing sarcoma and osteosarcoma may not accurately reflect overall tumor necrosis because small metabolically active foci may be present within tumor that is greater than 90% necrotic.[3,7]
4. After chemotherapy or radiation therapy, SUVs may remain high within primary bone tumors due to inflammation or reactive fibrosis rather than viable tumor.[3,7]

29.3 Soft-Tissue Tumors

29.3.1 Clinical Indication

In children with soft-tissue malignancies, PET/CT has shown value in identifying the site of an

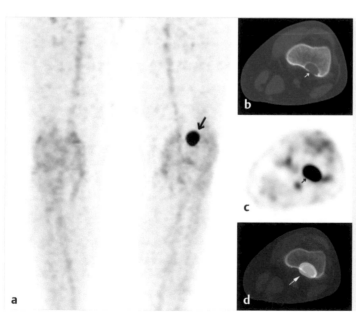

Fig. 29.2 A 19-year-old boy under treatment for metastatic paraganglioma. (a) Maximum intensity projection (MIP) image of the knees shows intense fluorodeoxyglucose (FDG) activity in the distal left femur (*arrow*), worrisome for metastatic deposit. Co-registered axial (b) CT, (c) PET, and (d) fused PET/CT images, viewed in a bone window setting, allow identification of a benign nonossifying fibroma (*arrows*). Benign fibro-osseous lesions, such as this, are relatively common in children and can demonstrate minimal to intense FDG avidity.

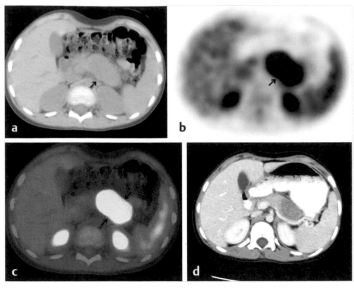

Fig. 29.3 A 10-year-old girl with metastatic alveolar rhabdomyosarcoma. Co-registered axial (a) CT, (b) PET, and (c) fused PET/CT images demonstrate an intensely fluorodeoxyglucose-avid pancreas metastasis (arrows) that was not clinically suspected. (d) This diagnostic CT, with oral and intravenous contrast, confirms the pancreatic location of the mass. PET/CT is useful in detecting clinically occult sites of metastatic disease in children with a variety of soft-tissue and bone sarcomas.

unknown primary tumor, staging, monitoring response to therapy, and detecting recurrence.

29.3.2 Accuracy

1. Because soft-tissue malignancies in children are rare, there have been no formal studies of the accuracy of PET or PET/CT in the diagnosis or follow-up of these tumors.

29.3.3 Pearls

1. About 4% of rhabdomyosarcoma (RMS) will present with widely metastatic disease and unknown primary site.[8] PET/CT allows examination of the entire body in one sitting and can reveal the primary RMS as well as metastatic foci.[9]
2. One retrospective review showed that, in children with a variety of soft-tissue malignancies, PET/CT detected sites of metastatic disease missed by physical examination and conventional imaging, including ^{99m}Tc MDP bone scintigraphy and CT. PET/CT appears to be especially valuable in the assessment of children with alveolar RMS, which has a propensity to metastasize to unusual soft-tissue sites (▶ Fig. 29.3).[9]
3. After chemotherapy, FDG avidity of primary and metastatic foci, from childhood soft-tissue malignancies, appears to reflect tumor viability (▶ Fig. 29.4).[9]

4. About 25 to 35% of children with sarcomas experience recurrence after therapy.[10] PET/CT is sensitive to recurrent disease in children with a variety of soft-tissue sarcomas, particularly those with alveolar RMS.[9]

29.3.4 Pitfalls

1. In children with soft-tissue malignancies, PET/CT cannot reliably distinguish benign from malignant lymph nodes. Enlarged nodes due to follicular hyperplasia and sinus histiocytosis can appear intensely FDG avid (▶ Fig. 29.5).[9] Conversely, enlarged, malignant lymph nodes may show only minimal FDG avidity.[11]

29.4 Langerhans Cell Histiocytosis
29.4.1 Clinical Indications

PET/CT may be useful in the baseline evaluation, response to therapy, and detection of reactivation of Langerhans cell histiocytosis (LCH).[12,13,14]

29.4.2 Accuracy

1. Because of the rarity of LCH, there has been no systematic investigation of the accuracy of PET/CT in its diagnosis and management.

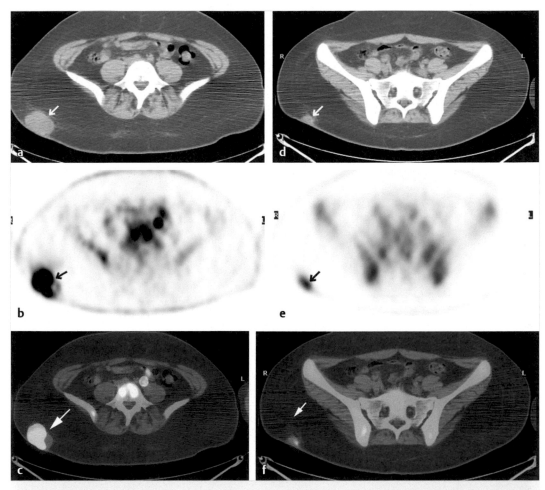

Fig. 29.4 An 18-year-old girl with extraosseous Ewing sarcoma family of tumor. Baseline co-registered, axial **(a)** CT, **(b)** PET, and **(c)** fused PET/CT images show the intensely fluorodeoxyglucose (FDG) avid primary tumor in the right buttock. **(d–f)** At completion of chemotherapy, the tumor had become smaller but remained intensely FDG avid (*arrows*). Histology confirmed the majority of this residual tumor was viable.

29.4.3 Pearls

1. At baseline, PET/CT may detect sites of disease not evident on physical examination or conventional imaging examinations (▶ Fig. 29.6).[12,13,14]

2. During therapy, FDG PET/CT may be more sensitive to LCH disease activity than plain film radiography and [99mTc] MDP bone scintigraphy.[12,13,14,15]

3. After therapy, patients with solitary bone lesions have a 10% risk of disease reactivation, whereas those with multiple bone lesions are seven times more likely to recur. Risk of reactivation also depends on site of bone lesions; 39% of patients with multiple lesions that include the skull will have disease reactivation compared with 18% of those without skull lesions.[12] PET/CT may be more sensitive to disease reactivation than plain radiography.

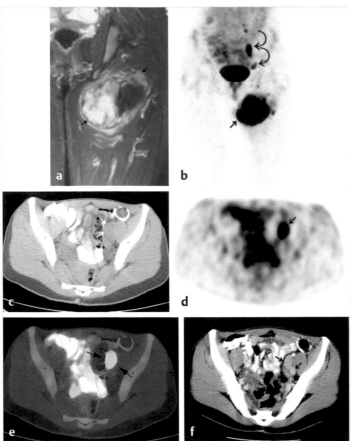

Fig. 29.5 A 19-year-old girl with malignant peripheral nerve sheath tumor. **(a)** Coronal short tau inversion recovery (STIR) MRI shows the primary left thigh tumor (*arrows*) at diagnosis. **(b)** This baseline maximum intensity projection (MIP) PET image demonstrates intense fluorodeoxyglucose (FDG) activity in the primary tumor (*straight arrow*) and several foci of intense FDG activity in the left pelvis (*curved arrows*). Co-registered axial **(c)** CT, **(d)** PET, and **(e)** fused PET/CT images localize the left pelvic activity to enlarged iliac nodes (*arrows*). **(f)** This diagnostic CT with oral and intravenous contrast confirms the presence of enlarged left iliac nodes (*arrows*). These were worrisome for nodal spread from the left thigh malignancy, but on pathologic inspection they contained only follicular hyperplasia and sinus histiocytosis.

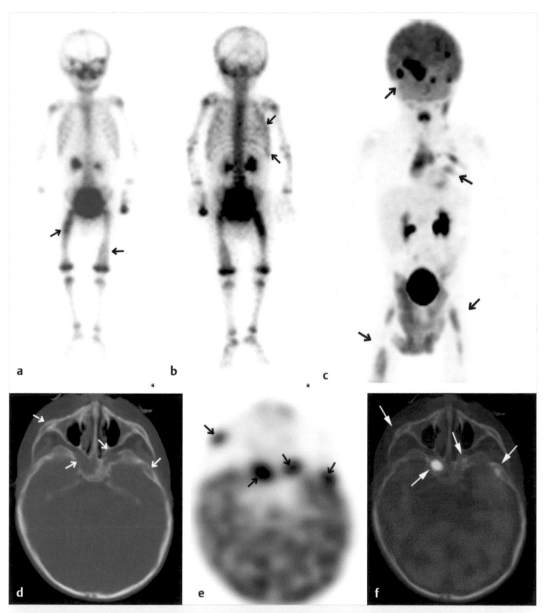

Fig. 29.6 A 17-month-old boy presented with right proptosis and was suspected to have neuroblastoma. **(a)** This baseline anterior technetium-99 m (⁹⁹ᵐTc) bone scan image shows abnormal activity in both femora (*arrows*). **(b)** This posterior ⁹⁹ᵐTc bone scan image shows subtle activity in several posterior right ribs (*arrows*). **(c)** This baseline maximum intensity projection (MIP) image shows abnormal fluorodeoxyglucose (FDG) activity in both femora, in several left ribs, and in the head (*arrows*). The foci of abnormal activity in the head were localized to the skull by these co-registered axial **(d)** CT, **(e)** PET, and **(f)** fused PET/CT images (*arrows*). The skull lesions and left rib abnormalities were not well seen on the ⁹⁹ᵐTc bone scan.

References

[1] Kaste SC. Issues specific to implementing PET-CT for pediatric oncology: what we have learned along the way. Pediatr Radiol. 2004; 34(3):205–213

[2] Franzius C, Sciuk J, Daldrup-Link HE, Jürgens H, Schober O. FDG-PET for detection of osseous metastases from malignant primary bone tumours: comparison with bone scintigraphy. Eur J Nucl Med. 2000; 27(9):1305–1311

[3] Hawkins DS, Rajendran JG, Conrad EU, III, Bruckner JD, Eary JF. Evaluation of chemotherapy response in pediatric bone sarcomas by [F-18]-fluorodeoxy-D-glucose positron emission tomography. Cancer. 2002; 94(12):3277–3284

[4] Kushner BH, Yeung HW, Larson SM, Kramer K, Cheung NK. Extending positron emission tomography scan utility to high-risk neuroblastoma: fluorine-18 fluorodeoxyglucose positron emission tomography as sole imaging modality in follow-up of patients. J Clin Oncol. 2001; 19(14):3397–3405

[5] Aoki J, Watanabe H, Shinozaki T, et al. FDG PET of primary benign and malignant bone tumors: standardized uptake value in 52 lesions. Radiology. 2001; 219(3):774–777

[6] Goodin GS, Shulkin BL, Kaufman RA, McCarville MB. PET/CT characterization of fibroosseous defects in children: 18F-FDG uptake can mimic metastatic disease. AJR Am J Roentgenol. 2006; 187(4):1124–1128

[7] Hawkins DS, Schuetze SM, Butrynski JE, et al. [18F]Fluorodeoxyglucose positron emission tomography predicts outcome for Ewing sarcoma family of tumors. J Clin Oncol. 2005; 23(34):8828–8834

[8] Etcubanas E, Peiper S, Stass S, Green A. Rhabdomyosarcoma, presenting as disseminated mallgnancy from an unknown primary site: a retrospective study of ten pediatric cases. Med Pediatr Oncol. 1989; 17(1):39–44

[9] McCarville MB, Christie R, Daw NC, Spunt SL, Kaste SC. PET/CT in the evaluation of childhood sarcomas. AJR Am J Roentgenol. 2005; 184(4):1293–1304

[10] Pizzo PA, Poplack DG, eds. Section IV: management of common cancers of childhood. In: Principles and Practice of Pediatric Oncology. Philadelphia, PA: Lippincott, Williams & Wilkins; 2002:489–1176

[11] Ben Arush MW, Bar Shalom R, Postovsky S, et al. Assessing the use of FDG-PET in the detection of regional and metastatic nodes in alveolar rhabdomyosarcoma of extremities. J Pediatr Hematol Oncol. 2006; 28(7):440–445

[12] Kaste SC, Rodriguez-Galindo C, McCarville ME, Shulkin BL. PET-CT in pediatric Langerhans cell histiocytosis. Pediatr Radiol. 2007; 37(7):615–622

[13] Lee HJ, Ahn BC, Lee SW, Lee J. The usefulness of F-18 fluorodeoxyglucose positron emission tomography/computed tomography in patients with Langerhans cell histiocytosis. Ann Nucl Med. 2012; 26(9):730–737

[14] Obert J, Vercellino L, Van Der Gucht A, et al. 18F-fluorodeoxyglucose positron emission tomography-computed tomography in the management of adult multisystem Langerhans cell histiocytosis. Eur J Nucl Med Mol Imaging. 2017; 44(4):598–610

[15] Koç ZP, Şimşek S, Akarsu S, Balcı TA, Onur MR, Kepenek F. Insufficiency of bone scintigraphy in vertebral lesions of Langerhans cell histiocytosis compared to f-18 fluorodeoxyglucose positron emission tomography/computed tomography and diagnostic computed tomography. Mol Imaging Radionucl Ther. 2015; 24(1):21–24

30 PET/CT in Radiation Therapy Planning

Sandip Basu and Guobin Song

30.1 PET-CT in Radiotherapy Planning: What Are We Looking for?

Individualized radiation treatment planning based upon (1) better disease staging and thereby appropriate selection and delineation of target volumes and organs at risk; (2) multitracer PET to image the pathophysiological pathways and heterogeneity within the tumor (tracers of metabolism, proliferation, hypoxia, apoptosis, gene expression); and (3) theragnostic imaging through PET during the course of treatment.

The introduction of PET/CT-based combined structure-function imaging and integrating multimodality imaging data into the radiation therapy planning (RTP) process has been a major step toward advancing RTP in cancer patients. The impact of this new development can be viewed from the following three standpoints:

1. Accurate staging.
2. Delineating the accurate volume and the extent of the disease.
3. Dose painting and theragnostic imaging.

30.2 Effect of Accurate Staging by FDG-PET/CT

PET allows better staging not only at the primary site but also at the locoregional level and distant regions. Conventional imaging technique may result in false up- or under-staging in a variety of cancers. When radiation therapy is employed for optimal management of the diseased sites, understaging may result in partial treatment and overstaging may lead to unnecessary radiation toxicity to the site(s) without disease. Staging with fluorodeoxyglucose (FDG) PET (FDG-PET) may change the intent of treatment from curative to palliative in 10 to 26% of cases when new distant metastasis is detected. Several studies have documented that the improved staging with FDG-PET can be used to improve patient management and significantly impact radiation therapy planning and therefore improve outcome and minimize toxicity.[1,2,3,4]

30.3 Tumor Volume Delineation

1. The functional information from PET images can be fused to the anatomic data from CT and/or MRI within the RTP system to aid in detecting tumor and delineating the target volume for RTP. There is a considerable interest on the impact of such combined information on treatment planning as the interobserver variability is substantially reduced compared to when these modalities are individually used.
2. Thresholding is the most commonly adopted method to determine volumes automatically from PET images. Most algorithms have been derived from the study of spheres of various sizes with differing levels of background signal. Some investigators have chosen to use a threshold based upon a percentage of the maximum standardized uptake values (SUVmax), while others have relied on a threshold based on an absolute SUVmax value.[5] Contours are based upon the maximum in the lesion of interest with values ranging from 30 to 50% of the SUVmax used by various investigators (methodologies detailed in the following section).
3. In lung cancer, incorporation of PET data improves tumor volume and dose coverage, and spares normal tissues leading to less toxicity with the potential option of escalating dose to tumor tissue (▶ Fig. 30.1). In esophageal cancer and lymphoma, PET scan can be used to include PET-positive lymph nodes in the target volume.
4. In most other tumor sites, not enough data are currently available to draw definitive conclusions, though a few studies demonstrate its promise.
5. Daisne et al[6] compared CT, MRI, and PET with pathologic findings in head and neck cancer patients. Smaller gross tumor volume (GTV) was observed with FDG-PET for oropharyngeal, laryngeal, and hypopharyngeal tumors.
6. Three major issues that require to be addressed and on which the majority of the studies are presently focused are (1) whether it allows accurate tumor delineation; (2) whether its incorporation influences GTV, clinical target volume (CTV), and planning target volume (PTV); and, lastly, (3) whether there is an improvement of treatment outcome.[6,7,8]

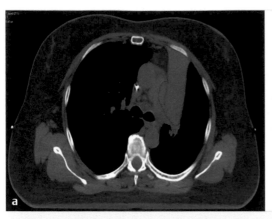
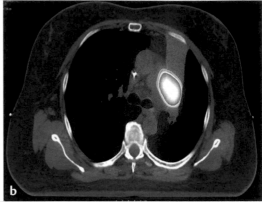

Fig. 30.1 **(a)** A CT image taken for radiotherapy planning purpose showing the gross tumor volume (GTV) including the collapsed lung volume (*in pink*). **(b)** Modification and delineating the GTV (*in blue*) using the metabolically avid volume of the fused PET/CT image.

30.4 Target Volumes in Radiation Therapy Planning

1. **Gross tumor volume (GTV):** Derived from the gross demonstrable extent and location of tumor identified with the CT or simulator images.
2. **Clinical target volume (CTV):** Expanded GTV to include subclinical disease based on additional clinical information.
3. **Planning target volume (PTV):** Expanded CTV by the addition of a variable margin to take into account internal organ movement as well as patient-motion and setup uncertainties.[9,10]
4. **Biological target volumes (BTV):** Derived from the biological information about tumors and surrounding normal tissue obtained from the PET component of PET/CT.[11] BTV can have different implications based upon PET radiotracer used for scanning, for example, BTV determined from an FDG might be considered to represent the viable tumor cells and can be used for determining a minimum dose for the entire tumor, whereas a BTV resulting from fluoromisonidazole (FMISO; a PET tracer for hypoxia) would represent a smaller tumor subvolume where the maximum tumor dose requires delivery to the hypoxic cells associated with radio resistance.

30.4.1 Thresholding for Target Delineation with PET

Delineation of target volumes on PET images can be undertaken by two approaches: (1) visual assessment (drawn by hand) and (2) automated segmentation methods.

Delineation by Visual Assessment

The shortcomings of this modality pertain to high level of operator dependence and include the following: (1) blurred boundaries related to the limitation of resolution and (2) variable boundaries related to the image display settings in PET (windowing level and width). The quality of delineation depends on both these aforementioned factors. Hence, expertise and strict operator guidelines are needed for the display device. Combining PET and CT images can help.

Automated/Semiautomated Segmentation Methods

This could be accomplished by the following methods:
1. Thresholding:
   a) Hard thresholding: The binary decision of target versus nontarget is undertaken on the principle that any voxel with an SUV higher than the threshold value is the target.
   b) Soft thresholding: This consists of histogram approximation by a mixture of several probability density functions, and subsequently adjusting density parameters using expectation–maximization algorithm.
2. Clustering methods: Useful when target is surrounded by healthy tissues, air, inflammation, and so on, and involves gathering pixels with close values, either by hard

boundaries or by soft or probabilistic ones or by mixtures of multivariate distributions.

With respect to the search for the most appropriate technique for bettering the resolution of images, edge-preserving tools would be more preferred compared to the Gaussian postreconstruction smoothing.

30.5 Clinical Applications

Integration of PET images in radiotherapy planning has been primarily studied in non–small-cell lung cancer (NSCLC),[12,13,14] with some studies published in esophageal carcinoma,[15] head and neck cancer,[16] and rectal carcinoma.[17]

30.5.1 Recent Study Results

Lung Cancer

1. A recent survey of the published findings shows that treatment volumes are significantly altered in 30 to 60% of patients with non–small-cell lung carcinoma with the addition of biologic targeting with FDG-PET.[18]
2. In a series of 44 patients with NSCLC, FDG-PET altered the stage of the disease in 25% of the cases by downstaging the disease in the majority of them.[19] GTV based on FDG-PET was on average smaller than the GTV defined by CT. Also, in a different study, it was found that for the same radiotoxicity to the lungs, spinal cord, and esophagus, the dose to the tumor can be enhanced by 25%; this resulted in a potentially higher tumor control probability (24% for PET/CT planning compared with 6.3% for CT-only planning).[20]
3. FDG-PET also alters the delineation of the GTV by discriminating tumor tissue from atelectasis (▶ Fig. 30.1) or necrosis.[18,21,22] Modifications in target volume delineation allows delivering a tumoricidal dose to the target while minimizing the radiation dose to the uninvolved tissue.
4. Particularly, at the locoregional level, the use of PET/CT for fused images with planning CT (pCT) may allow adequate tumor visualization and nodal staging: selective mediastinal node irradiation based on FDG-PET-based better mediastinal nodal staging in patients with NSCLC resulted in low isolated nodal failure rates.[23]

Head and Neck Carcinoma

Recent studies have shown excellent treatment outcomes in head and neck carcinoma (HNC) patients treated with intensity-modulated radiation therapy (IMRT),[24,25] in which many small pencil beams are used to conform to the volume irradiated to any irregular shape. IMRT has the ability to deliver high doses of radiation to the tumor target with very high precision; thus, accurate tumor targeting and delineation is required more than ever.

Recent studies in patients with locally advanced head and neck squamous cell carcinoma demonstrated that PET/CT-based radiation treatment would significantly change the dose distribution.[26,27]

PET/CT has also been found helpful in the management of occult primary head and neck tumors by determining a site of origin of the primary tumor in 60% of cases.[28] This translates into reduced dose distribution to uninvolved mucosal site compared with the results of CT scan–only based plans.

Brain Tumors

Non-FDG PET tracers, for example, amino acid (AA) based PET agents such as ^{11}C-abelled methionine (MET) and ^{18}F-labeled O-2-fluoroethyl-L-tyrosine (FET) has found important place in brain tumor delineation. Similarly, meningiomas and glomus tumors demonstrate overexpression of somatostatin-receptor subtype 2 (SSTR2) receptors and can be imaged with somatostatin receptor–based PET agents such as ^{68}Ga-labeled somatostatin derivatives, for example, 1,4,7,10-tetraazacyclododecane-N,N′,N″,N‴-tetraacetic-acid-DPhe1-Tyr3-octreotide (DOTATOC) and 1,4,7,10-tetraazacyclododecane-N,N′,N″,N‴-tetraacetic-acid-D-Phe1-Tyr3-octreotate (DOTATATE). PET images are particularly useful in delineating borders in infiltrating tumors. Visualization of tumor biology by fluorothymidine (FLT) PET, FMISO-PET, and arginine-glycine-aspartic acid (RGD) PET are also promising areas for RT planning in brain tumor.[29,30,31]

30.6 The Concept of "Dose Painting" and "Theragnostic" Imaging

These novel concepts are primarily based upon the results of scanning with novel imaging markers of tumor hypoxia or proliferation and variations in tumor volume and viability during radiotherapy that could modify the delineation of target volumes.

30.6.1 "Dose Painting"

Information obtained from other novel tracers like those of hypoxia, proliferation, apoptosis, and receptor expression can be integrated to that of FDG-PET imaging, which provides greater insight of the biologic pathways involved in radiation responses.[32,33,34,35,36,37] Taken together, these can be utilized by the new sophisticated software planning algorithms to deliver IMRT treatments[38,39,40,41,42] where the intensity through the treatment beam is varied. Combining several IMRT treatment portals can result in complex cross-sectional dose distributions being achieved and even the delivery of high-dose areas within the target, a technique that has been referred to as "dose painting."[11] This concept depends on the ability to visualize tumor subvolumes that are potentially radioresistant and then paint some additional dose restricted to those subvolumes.

Methodologies for Dose Painting

1. **Dose painting by contours (DPBC).** This principle is based upon delineating active/resistant subregions of the PTV, based upon specific functional characteristics, such as the metabolically active part of the tumor depicted by FDG-PET (► Fig. 30.2) or hypoxic fraction depicted by hypoxia-specific tracers (e.g., FMISO, fluoroazomycin arabinoside [FAZA], or Copper(II)-diacetyl-bis(N(4)-methylthiosemicarbazone) [Cu-ATSM]), and prescribing additional dose to the part or adopting dose escalation to the part while keeping the mean tumor dose constant.[43,44,45,46]
2. **Dose painting by numbers (DPBN).** Dose painting by numbers entails spatially varying dose delivery as per the specific functional/molecular characteristics of the tumor.[47]

30.6.2 PET/CT for Adaptive Radiotherapy during Course of Treatment: The "Theragnostic" Imaging

This is based upon calculation of the mean dose delivery during the early part of the treatment and the tumor response during this initial period of therapy and revise the subsequent treatment plan.[48,49,50,51] This replanning of the radiotherapy during the course of treatment can help in substantial sparing of the surrounding nontarget tissues and is the major advantage of "theragnostic" imaging, a term coined by Bentzen.[51]

30.7 Respiratory Gating of PET/CT

1. **Respiratory gating of PET/CT (RG-PET/CT)** is investigated as a tool for improving (1) image quality, (2) quantitative accuracy of PET/CT, and (3) to assess and measure tumor and organ motion for radiotherapy planning. The aim is to accurately target the dose of radiation to the "diseased" tissue volume with relative sparing of the surrounding normal tissue.
2. The essential prerequisites are (1) a respiratory monitoring system and (2) dedicated acquisition/processing protocols in addition to a state-of-the-art PET-CT scanner.
3. Gating systems that can be coupled with the development of treatment plans and target volumes in equivalent physiological state are under active research. These will allow the radiation to be delivered in synchrony with physiological motion such as respiration.[52,53,54,55]

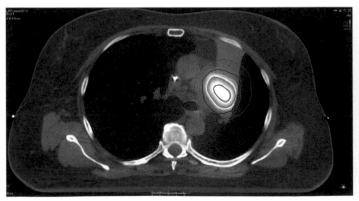

Fig. 30.2 Radiotherapy dose painting. Incorporation of the FDG-PET data enables dose modification of the radiation therapy plan with different dose levels (70 Gy, *pink line*; 60 Gy, *red line*; 45 Gy, *purple line*) to subvolumes of different standardized uptake value range.

4. The clinical advantages of 4D-PET/CT envisaged are as follows: (1) better tumor tissue characterization (particularly small lesions) due to better lesion to background contrast, (2) better assessment of response to therapy and follow-up due to more accurate quantification and, importantly, (3) its potential for individualized target volume delineation through better assessment of target movement.

5. The advantages are especially relevant to the treatment of the thoracic neoplasms, but the indications have been extended to recurrences/metastases (< 50 mm/less than 5 lesions).

30.8 Working Principle of RG 4D-PET/CT for RT Planning

1. The information from 4D-PET/CT regarding possible movement of the lesion helps to define internal target volume (ITV).

2. Both ITV$_{BTV}$ and ITV$_{CTV}$ generated from the respiratory gating are combined through Boolean union to generate "anatomical/functional" ITV.

3. Following corrections for setup margins generates 4D-PTV (PTV$_{4D}$).[56,57,58,59]

30.9 Future Challenges for Incorporating PET into RT Planning on a Routine Basis

1. Interpretation of PET images for contouring target volumes.

2. Proper co-registration of PET and CT images.

3. Computer software for easy image transfer to and acceptance by treatment planning systems from the PET systems.

4. Mechanisms to account for tumor motion.

30.10 Promising Approaches

1. Use of 4D-PET/CT can correct for respiratory motion artifacts seen in conventional PET/CT imaging. It has potential to reduce smearing and improve the accuracy in PET/CT co-registration.

2. Employing PET/CT for radiosurgery treatment planning for the purpose of improved local control rates following radiosurgery and reduce subsequent tumor recurrence rates.

30.11 Summary

The literature with regard to the clinical impact and patient outcome of using PET/CT to modify dose in metabolically active tumor cells continues to be evolving at this time and further clinical studies are needed. The detailed structural and functional imaging information potentially improves RTP by minimizing unnecessary irradiation of normal tissues and by reducing the risk of geographic miss. The potential of PET to quantify metabolism and identify new imaging targets within tumor tissue such as cellular proliferation, hypoxia, tumor receptors, and gene expression, and thereby helping in the biological optimization of dose delivery is an exciting area of research.[53,54,55,60,61] However, the impact of PET/CT-based IMRT dose painting RTP on tumor control and final clinical outcome can only be determined with prospective research studies of patients.

References

[1] Mah K, Caldwell CB, Ung YC, et al. The impact of (18)FDG-PET on target and critical organs in CT-based treatment planning of patients with poorly defined non-small-cell lung carcinoma: a prospective study. Int J Radiat Oncol Biol Phys. 2002; 52(2):339–350

[2] Ciernik IF, Dizendorf E, Baumert BG, et al. Radiation treatment planning with an integrated positron emission and computer tomography (PET/CT): a feasibility study. Int J Radiat Oncol Biol Phys. 2003; 57(3):853–863

[3] Dizendorf EV, Baumert BG, von Schulthess GK, Lütolf UM, Steinert HC. Impact of whole-body 18F-FDG PET on staging and managing patients for radiation therapy. J Nucl Med. 2003; 44(1):24–29

[4] Kalff V, Hicks RJ, MacManus MP, et al. Clinical impact of (18)F fluorodeoxyglucose positron emission tomography in patients with non-small-cell lung cancer: a prospective study. J Clin Oncol. 2001; 19(1):111–118

[5] Black QC, Grills IS, Kestin LL, et al. Defining a radiotherapy target with positron emission tomography. Int J Radiat Oncol Biol Phys. 2004; 60(4):1272–1282

[6] Daisne J-F, Sibomana M, Bol A, Doumont T, Lonneux M, Grégoire V. Tri-dimensional automatic segmentation of PET volumes based on measured source-to-background ratios: influence of reconstruction algorithms. Radiother Oncol. 2003; 69(3):247–250

[7] Erdi YE, Mawlawi O, Larson SM, et al. Segmentation of lung lesion volume by adaptive positron emission tomography image thresholding. Cancer. 1997; 80(12) Suppl:2505–2509

[8] Yaremko B, Riauka T, Robinson D, Murray B, McEwan A, Roa W. Threshold modification for tumour imaging in non-small-cell lung cancer using positron emission tomography. Nucl Med Commun. 2005; 26(5):433–440

[9] International Commission on Radiation Units and Measurements. Prescribing, Recording and Reporting Photon Beam Therapy. ICRU Report 50. Bethesda, MD: ICRU; 1993

[10] International Commission on Radiation Units and Measurements. Prescribing, Recording and Reporting Photon Beam Therapy (Supplement to ICRU Report 50). ICRU Report 62. Bethesda, MD: ICRU; 1999

[11] Ling CC, Humm J, Larson S, et al. Towards multidimensional radiotherapy (MD-CRT): biological imaging and biological

conformality. Int J Radiat Oncol Biol Phys. 2000; 47(3):551–560

[12] Caldwell CB, Mah K, Ung YC, et al. Observer variation in contouring gross tumor volume in patients with poorly defined non-small-cell lung tumors on CT: the impact of 18FDG-hybrid PET fusion. Int J Radiat Oncol Biol Phys. 2001; 51(4):923–931

[13] Erdi YE, Rosenzweig K, Erdi AK, et al. Radiotherapy treatment planning for patients with non-small cell lung cancer using positron emission tomography (PET). Radiother Oncol. 2002; 62(1):51–60

[14] Fox JL, Rengan R, O'Meara W, et al. Does registration of PET and planning CT images decrease interobserver and intraobserver variation in delineating tumor volumes for non-small-cell lung cancer? Int J Radiat Oncol Biol Phys. 2005; 62(1):70–75

[15] Moureau-Zabotto L, Touboul E, Lerouge D, et al. Impact of CT and 18F-deoxyglucose positron emission tomography image fusion for conformal radiotherapy in esophageal carcinoma. Int J Radiat Oncol Biol Phys. 2005; 63(2):340–345

[16] Scarfone C, Lavely WC, Cmelak AJ, et al. Prospective feasibility trial of radiotherapy target definition for head and neck cancer using 3-dimensional PET and CT imaging. J Nucl Med. 2004; 45(4):543–552

[17] Roels S, Duthoy W, Haustermans K, et al. Definition and delineation of the clinical target volume for rectal cancer. Int J Radiat Oncol Biol Phys. 2006; 65(4):1129–1142

[18] Bradley JD, Perez CA, Dehdashti F, Siegel BA. Implementing biologic target volumes in radiation treatment planning for non-small cell lung cancer. J Nucl Med. 2004; 45 Suppl 1:96S–101S

[19] De Ruysscher D, Wanders S, van Haren E, et al. Selective mediastinal node irradiation based on FDG-PET scan data in patients with non-small-cell lung cancer: a prospective clinical study. Int J Radiat Oncol Biol Phys. 2005; 62(4):988–994

[20] De Ruysscher D, Wanders S, Minken A, et al. Effects of radiotherapy planning with a dedicated combined PET-CT-simulator of patients with non-small cell lung cancer on dose limiting normal tissues and radiation dose-escalation: a planning study. Radiother Oncol. 2005; 77(1):5–10

[21] Nestle U, Walter K, Schmidt S, et al. 18F-deoxyglucose positron emission tomography (FDG-PET) for the planning of radiotherapy in lung cancer: high impact in patients with atelectasis. Int J Radiat Oncol Biol Phys. 1999; 44(3):593–597

[22] Bradley J, Thorstad WL, Mutic S, et al. Impact of FDG-PET on radiation therapy volume delineation in non-small-cell lung cancer. Int J Radiat Oncol Biol Phys. 2004; 59(1):78–86

[23] De Ruysscher D, Wanders S, van Haren E, et al. Selective mediastinal node irradiation based on FDG-PET scan data in patients with non-small-cell lung cancer: a prospective clinical study. Int J Radiat Oncol Biol Phys. 2005; 62(4):988–994

[24] Chao KS, Deasy JO, Markman J, et al. A prospective study of salivary function sparing in patients with head-and-neck cancers receiving intensity-modulated or three-dimensional radiation therapy: initial results. Int J Radiat Oncol Biol Phys. 2001; 49(4):907–916

[25] Lee N, Xia P, Quivey JM, et al. Intensity-modulated radiotherapy in the treatment of nasopharyngeal carcinoma: an update of the UCSF experience. Int J Radiat Oncol Biol Phys. 2002; 53(1):12–22

[26] Schwartz DL, Ford E, Rajendran J, et al. FDG-PET/CT imaging for preradiotherapy staging of head-and-neck squamous cell carcinoma. Int J Radiat Oncol Biol Phys. 2005; 61(1):129–136

[27] Schwartz DL, Ford EC, Rajendran J, et al. FDG-PET/CT-guided intensity modulated head and neck radiotherapy: a pilot investigation. Head Neck. 2005; 27(6):478–487

[28] Wong WL, Saunders M. The impact of FDG PET on the management of occult primary head and neck tumours. Clin Oncol (R Coll Radiol). 2003; 15(8):461–466

[29] Milker-Zabel S, Zabel-du Bois A, Henze M, et al. Improved target volume definition for fractionated stereotactic radiotherapy in patients with intracranial meningiomas by correlation of CT, MRI, and [68Ga]-DOTATOC-PET. Int J Radiat Oncol Biol Phys. 2006; 65(1):222–227

[30] Gehler B, Paulsen F, Oksüz MÖ, et al. [68Ga]-DOTATOC-PET/CT for meningioma IMRT treatment planning. Radiat Oncol. 2009; 4:56

[31] Astner ST, Bundschuh RA, Beer AJ, et al. Assessment of tumor volumes in skull base glomus tumors using Gluc-Lys[(18)F]-TOCA positron emission tomography. Int J Radiat Oncol Biol Phys. 2009; 73(4):1135–1140

[32] Fujibayashi Y, Taniuchi H, Yonekura Y, Ohtani H, Konishi J, Yokoyama A. Copper-62-ATSM: a new hypoxia imaging agent with high membrane permeability and low redox potential. J Nucl Med. 1997; 38(7):1155–1160

[33] Shields AF, Grierson JR, Dohmen BM, et al. Imaging proliferation in vivo with [F-18]FLT and positron emission tomography. Nat Med. 1998; 4(11):1334–1336

[34] Borbath I, Grégoire V, Bergström M, Laryea D, Långström B, Pauwels S. Use of 5-[(76)Br]bromo-2'-fluoro-2'-deoxyuridine as a ligand for tumour proliferation: validation in an animal tumour model. Eur J Nucl Med Mol Imaging. 2002; 29(1):19–27

[35] Grönroos T, Bentzen L, Marjamäki P, et al. Comparison of the biodistribution of two hypoxia markers [18F]FETNIM and [18F]FMISO in an experimental mammary carcinoma. Eur J Nucl Med Mol Imaging. 2004; 31(4):513–520

[36] Mahy P, De Bast M, Leveque PH, et al. Preclinical validation of the hypoxia tracer 2-(2-nitroimidazol-1-yl)- N-(3,3,3-[(18)F]trifluoropropyl)acetamide, [[(18)F]EF3. Eur J Nucl Mol Imaging. 2004; 31(9):1263–1272

[37] Mishani E, Abourbeh G, Jacobson O, et al. High-affinity epidermal growth factor receptor (EGFR) irreversible inhibitors with diminished chemical reactivities as positron emission tomography (PET)-imaging agent candidates of EGFR overexpressing tumors. J Med Chem. 2005; 48(16):5337–5348

[38] Chao KS, Bosch WR, Mutic S, et al. A novel approach to overcome hypoxic tumor resistance: Cu-ATSM-guided intensity-modulated radiation therapy. Int J Radiat Oncol Biol Phys. 2001; 49(4):1171–1182

[39] Douglas JG, Stelzer KJ, Mankoff DA, et al. [F-18]-fluorodeoxyglucose positron emission tomography for targeting radiation dose escalation for patients with glioblastoma multiforme: clinical outcomes and patterns of failure. Int J Radiat Oncol Biol Phys. 2006; 64(3):886–891

[40] Mutic S, Malyapa RS, Grigsby PW, et al. PET-guided IMRT for cervical carcinoma with positive para-aortic lymph nodes-a dose-escalation treatment planning study. Int J Radiat Oncol Biol Phys. 2003; 55(1):28–35

[41] Vanuytsel LJ, Vansteenkiste JF, Stroobants SG, et al. The impact of (18)F-fluoro-2-deoxy-D-glucose positron emission tomography (FDG-PET) lymph node staging on the radiation treatment volumes in patients with non-small cell lung cancer. Radiother Oncol. 2000; 55(3):317–324

[42] Lee NY, Mechalakos JG, Nehmeh S, et al. Fluorine-18-labeled fluoromisonidazole positron emission and computed tomography-guided intensity-modulated radiotherapy for head and neck cancer: a feasibility study. Int J Radiat Oncol Biol Phys. 2008; 70(1):2–13

[43] Lin Z, Mechalakos J, Nehmeh S, et al. The influence of changes in tumor hypoxia on dose-painting treatment plans based on 18F-FMISO positron emission tomography. Int J Radiat Oncol Biol Phys. 2008; 70(4):1219–1228

[44] Grosu AL, Souvatzoglou M, Röper B, et al. Hypoxia imaging with FAZA-PET and theoretical considerations with regard to dose painting for individualization of radiotherapy in patients with head and neck cancer. Int J Radiat Oncol Biol Phys. 2007; 69(2):541–551

[45] Chao KS, Bosch WR, Mutic S, et al. A novel approach to overcome hypoxic tumor resistance: Cu-ATSM-guided intensity-modulated radiation therapy. Int J Radiat Oncol Biol Phys. 2001; 49(4):1171–1182

[46] Søvik A, Malinen E, Olsen DR. Strategies for biologic image-guided dose escalation: a review. Int J Radiat Oncol Biol Phys. 2009; 73(3):650–658

[47] Thorwarth D, Eschmann SM, Paulsen F, Alber M. Hypoxia dose painting by numbers: a planning study. Int J Radiat Oncol Biol Phys. 2007; 68(1):291–300

[48] Geets X, Lee L, Lonneux M, Coche E, Cosnard G, Grégoire V. Re-assessment of HNSCC tumor volume during radiotherapy with anatomic and functional imaging. Radiother Oncol. 2006; 78 Suppl 1:S59

[49] Humm JL, Lee J, O'Donoghue JA, et al. Changes in FDG tumor uptake during and after fractionated radiation therapy in a rodent tumor xenograft. Clin Positron Imaging. 1999; 2(5):289–296

[50] Brahme A. Biologically optimized 3-dimensional in vivo predictive assay-based radiation therapy using positron emission tomography-computerized tomography imaging. Acta Oncol. 2003; 42(2):123–136

[51] Bentzen SM. Theragnostic imaging for radiation oncology: dose-painting by numbers. Lancet Oncol. 2005; 6(2):112–117

[52] Livieratos L, Stegger L, Bloomfield PM, Schafers K, Bailey DL, Camici PG. Rigid-body transformation of list-mode projection data for respiratory motion correction in cardiac PET. Phys Med Biol. 2005; 50(14):3313–3322

[53] Wang Y, Baghaei H, Li H, et al. A simple respiration gating technique and its application in high resolution PET. IEEE Trans Nucl Sci. 2005; 52:125

[54] Guivarc'h O, Turzo A, Visvikis D, et al. Synchronisation of pulmonary scintigraphy by respiratory flow and by impedance plethysmography. Proc SPIE Med Imaging. 2004; 5370:1166–1175

[55] Erdi YE, Nehmeh SA, Pan T, et al. The CT motion quantitation of lung lesions and its impact on PET-measured SUVs. J Nucl Med. 2004; 45(8):1287–1292

[56] Hof H, Rhein B, Haering P, Kopp-Schneider A, Debus J, Herfarth K. 4D-CT-based target volume definition in stereotactic radiotherapy of lung tumours: comparison with a conventional technique using individual margins. Radiother Oncol. 2009; 93(3):419–423

[57] Rietzel E, Liu AK, Doppke KP, et al. Design of 4D treatment planning target volumes. Int J Radiat Oncol Biol Phys. 2006; 66(1):287–295

[58] Park SJ, Ionascu D, Killoran J, et al. Evaluation of the combined effects of target size, respiratory motion and background activity on 3D and 4D PET/CT images. Phys Med Biol. 2008; 53(13):3661–3679

[59] Li G, Citrin D, Camphausen K, et al. Advances in 4D medical imaging and 4D radiation therapy. Technol Cancer Res Treat. 2008; 7(1):67–81

[60] Grégoire V, Haustermans K, Geets X, Roels S, Lonneux M. PET-based treatment planning in radiotherapy: a new standard? J Nucl Med. 2007; 48 Suppl 1:68S–77S

[61] Senan S, De Ruysscher D. Critical review of PET-CT for radiotherapy planning in lung cancer. Crit Rev Oncol Hematol. 2005; 56(3):345–351

31 FDG-PET/CT in the Evaluation of Infection and Inflammation

Sandip Basu, Abass Alavi, and Eugene C. Lin

31.1 Introduction

Although several molecular mechanisms have been proposed as the basis for fluorodeoxyglucose (FDG) uptake in cells, overexpression of glucose transporter protein 1 (GLUT1) subtype in the stimulated macrophages, neutrophils, and lymphocytes is considered the most likely underlying biological phenomenon responsible for this observation (one proposed hypothesis of increased glucose metabolism of activated phagocytes has been related to "respiratory or oxidative burst," increased oxygen uptake by around 50-fold, and increase in glucose metabolism by hexose monophosphate pathway [HMP], though another study reports dissociation between respiratory burst and FDG uptake).[1] The combined PET/CT in the assessment of infection and inflammation undoubtedly proves to be even more effective than PET alone for evaluating certain clinical scenarios where surgical interventions are being considered.

31.2 Comparison of FDG-PET with Other Imaging Modalities for Evaluating Infection and Inflammation

31.2.1 Conventional Nuclear Medicine Techniques

1. Advantages of **FDG-PET:**
   a) Securing results within a short period of time (1.5–2 hours).
   b) High-resolution tomographic images.
   c) High target-to-background contrast ratio.
   d) Sensitive for chronic infections.
   e) Technically not demanding or less labor intensive.
   f) High interobserver agreement.
   g) Radiation dose two to three times lower than that of conventional nuclear medicine techniques.

h) Useful in detecting infection in the axial skeleton, where white blood cell (WBC) scanning is of limited value.
2. Disadvantages of **FDG-PET:**
   a) Relatively high cost.
   b) Differentiation between tumor and infection or inflammation is not possible, but delayed imaging and dual-time-point PET is of help.
   c) Availability (this disadvantage in previous years is now not valid; FDG-PET is now more widely available and an attractive alternative to combined leukocyte–marrow scintigraphy because it requires only one injection and user-friendly procedure).

31.2.2 Anatomical Imaging Modalities (CT/MRI)

1. Advantages of **FDG-PET:**
   a) Whole-body technique.
   b) Not affected by metallic implants.
   c) Assessment of metabolic activity of inflammatory process is more specific in the right setting than hyperperfusion or edema (CT/MRI).
2. Disadvantages of **FDG-PET:**
   a) Not widely available in most of the world (this disadvantage in previous years does not hold true now).
   b) Relatively low spatial resolution compared with structural techniques.

31.3 Potential Clinical Applications

Though there has been regional difference in the stand of its routine clinical use in infection and inflammation, the European Medicines Agency (EMEA) Committee for Medicinal Products for Human Use (CHMP), through a debate, has deemed the use of FDG beneficial in the following series of indications for in infectious or inflammatory diseases[2]:
1. Localization of abnormal foci to guide the etiological diagnosis in the presence of fever of unknown origin (FUO).

2. Diagnosis of infection in suspected chronic infection of bone and/or adjacent structures (osteomyelitis, spondylitis, diskitis, or osteitis including presence of metallic implants), diabetes with suspicion of Charcot's neuroarthropathy, osteomyelitis and/or soft-tissue infection, painful hip prosthesis, vascular prosthesis, and fever in acquired immunodeficiency syndrome (AIDS).

3. Detection of the extent of inflammation in sarcoidosis, inflammatory bowel disease (IBD), and vasculitis involving the great vessels.

4. Therapeutic follow-up of unresectable alveolar echinococcosis, in which it may be used in the search for active localizations of the parasite during medical treatment and after treatment discontinuation.

Based upon the published literature, the 2013 EANM/SNMMI Guideline for ^{18}F-FDG Use in Inflammation and Infection *classifies the different indication into three groups.* Among this, the "major indications" (cumulated reported accuracy [> 85%] and expert opinion) for ^{18}F- FDG-PET/CT in infection and inflammation are as follows[3]:

1. Sarcoidosis.
2. Peripheral bone osteomyelitis (non-postoperative, nondiabetic foot).

3. Suspected spinal infection (spondylodiskitis or vertebral osteomyelitis, non-postoperative).

4. Evaluation of FUO, including true FUO (defined according to the criteria of Durack and Street), postoperative fever and recurrent sepsis, immunodeficiency-related (both induced and acquired) FUO, neutropenic fever, and isolated acute-phase inflammation markers (persistently raised C-reactive protein and/or erythrocyte sedimentation rate).

5. Evaluation of metastatic infection and of high-risk patients with bacteremia.

6. Primary evaluation of vasculitides (e.g., giant cell arteritis).

31.3.1 Chronic Osteomyelitis

Overview

1. Limited added value in the diagnosis of uncomplicated cases of acute osteomyelitis compared with the combination of physical examination, biochemical alterations in combination with three-phase bone scanning, or MRI.

2. Several studies have documented the important role of FDG-PET in diagnosing patients with chronic osteomyelitis (► Fig. 31.1, ► Fig. 31.2, ► Fig. 31.3).

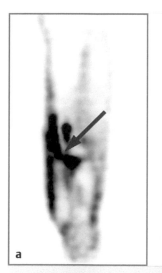
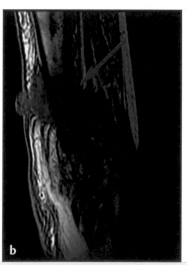
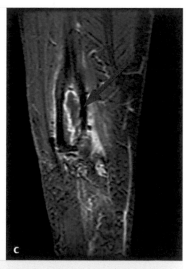

Fig. 31.1 (a) Sagittal fluorodeoxyglucose (FDG) PET. **(b)** Precontrast spoiled gradient (SPGR). **(c)** Postcontrast SPGR. Avid FDG uptake in the sinus tract (*arrow*) connecting soft-tissue abscess with the medullary track of the femur in a patient of proven chronic osteomyelitis. Corresponding MRI abnormalities are also shown in this figure. (From Kumar R, Basu S, Torigian D, Anand V, Zhuang H, Alavi A. Role of modern imaging techniques for diagnosis of infection in the era of ^{18}F-fluorodeoxyglucose positron emission tomography. Clin Microbiol Rev 2008;21(1):209–224. Reproduced with permission.[4])

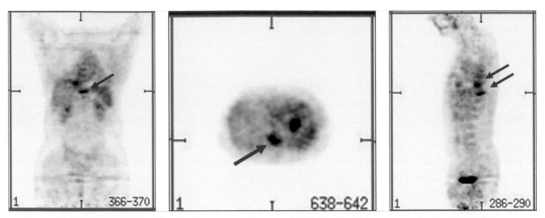

Fig. 31.2 Foci of fluorodeoxyglucose uptake in chronic osteomyelitis of the thoracic spine in two adjacent vertebral bodies (*arrows*). Radiolabeled white blood cell imaging in general has a low yield in this setting. (From Kumar R, Basu S, Torigian D, Anand V, Zhuang H, Alavi A. Role of modern imaging techniques for diagnosis of infection in the era of ^{18}F-fluorodeoxyglucose positron emission tomography. Clin Microbiol Rev 2008;21(1):209–224. Reproduced with permission.[4])

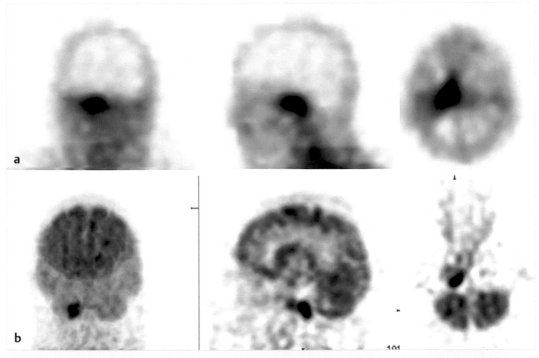

Fig. 31.3 (a) Gallium single-photon emission tomography (SPECT). **(b)** Fluorodeoxyglucose (FDG) PET. Avid FDG uptake in the focus of infection in a patient of proven malignant otitis with corresponding gallium-67 citrate-SPECT images. Note that PET images reveal the site of the disease more precisely than those of SPECT. *(From Kumar R, Basu S, Torigian D, Anand V, Zhuang H, Alavi A. Role of modern imaging techniques for diagnosis of infection in the era of ^{18}F-fluorodeoxyglucose positron emission tomography. Clin Microbiol Rev 2008;21(1):209–224. Reproduced with permission.[4])*

3. In contrast to other nuclear medicine modalities, such as gallium scintigraphy and labeled leukocyte imaging, FDG has high resolution and can distinguish soft-tissue infection from osteomyelitis.
4. It is expected that FDG-PET/CT imaging will be used routinely in the near future to determine the presence or absence of an infectious focus, to monitor response to antimicrobial treatment, and to develop criteria for deciding when the treatment can be safely stopped.

Accuracy

1. Guhlmann et al[5,6] reported a higher accuracy for FDG-PET than antigranulocyte antibody scintigraphy in imaging the central skeleton for infection in patients with suspected chronic osteomyelitis.
2. de Winter et al[7] reported a sensitivity of 100%, a specificity of 86%, and an accuracy of 93% in 60 patients with suspected chronic musculoskeletal infections.
3. Another prospective study by Meller et al[8] on 30 patients with suspected active chronic osteomyelitis concluded that FDG-PET is

superior to indium 111–labeled leukocyte imaging in the diagnosis of chronic osteomyelitis in the central skeleton.
4. FDG-PET accurately detects spinal osteomyelitis (▶ Fig. 31.1) and could potentially replace gallium-67 (^{67}Ga) for this purpose.[9,10,11]
5. A recent meta-analysis showed that FDG-PET not only is the most sensitive imaging modality for detecting chronic osteomyelitis, but also has a greater specificity than radiolabeled WBC scintigraphy, bone scintigraphy, or MRI.[12,13,14]

31.3.2 Complicated Diabetic Foot

Overview

Detection of infection and differentiating it from acute neuropathic osteoarthropathy in the setting of a complicated diabetic foot is a clinical and radiological challenge. The presence of ulceration also complicates the scenario because in this setting infection is strongly considered until proven otherwise. Distinguishing osteomyelitis from Charcot's osteoarthropathy by MRI is a difficult task. Three areas where FDG-PET has been investigated as potential tool of interest are as follows (▶ Fig. 31.4):

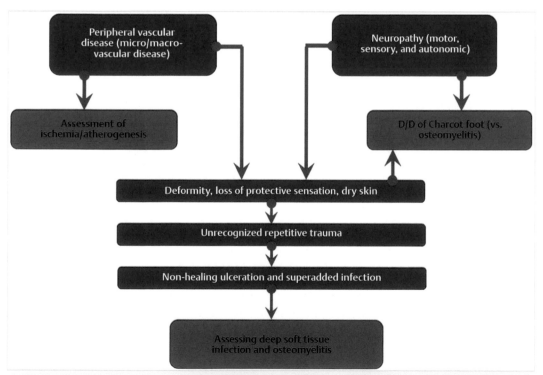

Fig. 31.4 Primary pathogenetic factors (*blue*), the further complicating factors (*brown*) in diabetic foot syndrome, and diagnostic challenges where PET-CT/PET-MRI has a potential role (*green*). (Basu S, Zhuang H, Alavi A. FDG PET and PET/CT Imaging in Complicated Diabetic Foot. PET Clin. 2012 Apr;7(2):151–160. Reproduced with permission.[15])

1. Diagnosis of deep soft-tissue infection and osteomyelitis.
2. Differentiating Charcot's arthropathy from osteomyelitis.
3. Evaluating the ischemia/atherogenesis component in a case of complicated diabetic foot.

Accuracy

1. Preliminary data provide evidence for an important role for FDG-PET imaging in the setting of complicated and uncomplicated diabetic osteoarthropathy.[11,12]
2. FDG-PET/CT was found to be highly accurate in detection of osteomyelitis (▶ Fig. 31.5 and ▶ Fig. 31.6) by Keidar et al.[16]
3. It can differentiate between Charcot's neuroarthropathy and osteomyelitis and also soft-tissue infection (▶ Fig. 31.7).[17,18]

31.3.3 Infected Prosthesis

Overview

1. One particular challenge for orthopaedic surgeons has been differentiating mechanical loosening of prosthesis from superimposed infection and has been the subject of multiple research studies during the past several years.
2. FDG-PET has a great potential for detecting infection in hip prostheses (▶ Fig. 31.8, ▶ Fig. 31.9, ▶ Fig. 31.10) and, to a lesser extent, in knee prostheses.
3. FDG-PET is advantageous over anatomical imaging modalities because it is not affected by the metal implants and provides better resolution images than those of the conventional nuclear medicine techniques, and it is exquisitely sensitive.
4. Noninfectious reactions are common months and even years after surgery, and the recognition of such reactions is important in managing these patients.
5. **Criteria for infection**: Increased FDG uptake around the neck and/or head of the prosthesis is very common and should not be interpreted as a finding suggestive of infection. Most infection is found at the bone–prosthesis interface, and most noninfectious inflammatory reactions are found outside the bone–prosthesis junction. For hip arthroplasty, increased FDG uptake was noted at the bone–prosthesis interface in the middle portion of the shaft of the hip prosthesis, which is considered positive for infection in THAs, whereas FDG uptake was limited to the soft tissues, or adjacent only to the neck of the prosthesis, which is considered negative for infection.
6. Presently, the potential of FDG-PET in the evaluation of prostheses is relatively less defined. More research may further enhance the role of FDG-PET in the evaluation of prostheses.

Accuracy

1. In a prospective study involving 89 patients with 92 painful hip prostheses, our group[21] reported that the respective sensitivity, specificity, positive predictive value (PPV), and negative predictive value (NPV) of FDG-PET for detecting infection was 95.2, 93, 80, and 98.5%, respectively. Similar figures of technetium-99 m sulfur colloid indium 111–labeled WBC

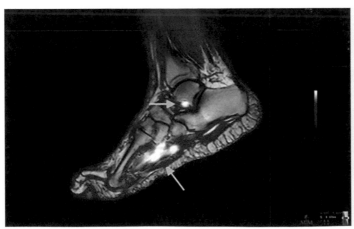

Fig. 31.5 Fused fluorodeoxyglucose (FDG) PET and MR images of a patient with diabetic foot and suspected bone infection. The FDG-PET image shows significant uptake in the soft tissue in the plantar aspect of the foot (suggestive of cellulitis, *longer arrow*); in addition, it reveals a focus of abnormal activity in the talus (consistent with talar bone osteomyelitis, *shorter arrow*). (Reproduced with permission from Diagnostic Imaging.[19])

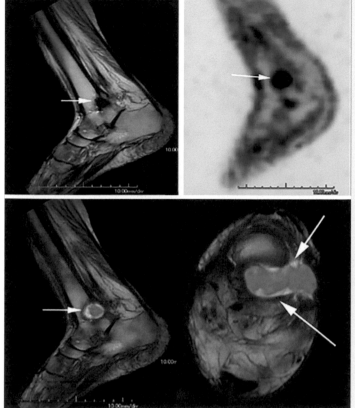

Fig. 31.6 A 70-year-old woman with diabetes with history of resection of the distal fibula, fusion of the tibia–talar joint, and placement of orthopedic hardware. MR image demonstrates chronic sinus tract (*arrows*) extending from the lateral skin margin into the lateral distal tibia likely from prior hardware placement. The findings did not suggest osteomyelitis. PET image demonstrates an abnormally increased focus of fluorodeoxyglucose uptake at the site (*arrows*), consistent with an active osteomyelitis. (Reproduced with permission from Nawaz A, Torigian DA, Siegelman ES, et al. Diagnostic performance of FDG-PET, MRI, and plain film radiography (PFR) for the diagnosis of osteomyelitis in the diabetic foot. Mol Imaging Biol 2010;12:335–42.[20])

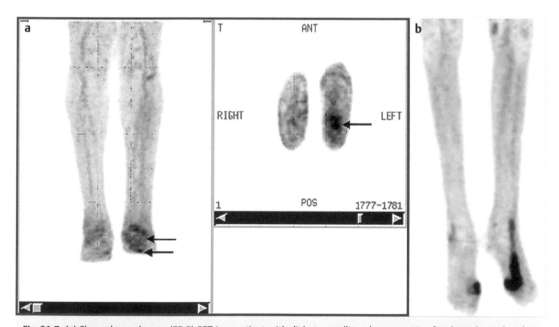

Fig. 31.7 **(a)** Fluorodeoxyglucose (FDG) PET in a patient with diabetes mellitus demonstrating focal uptake in the ulcer (*arrows*) in the transaxial images and the relatively low-grade diffuse uptake in the neuropathic osteoarthropathy (*arrows*) are clearly distinguishable from the uptake observed on the unaffected contralateral limb by visual inspection. **(b)** High-grade FDG uptake clearly distinctive from that of Charcot's neuroarthropathy. (Reproduced with permission from Basu S, Chryssikos T, Houseni M, et al. Potential role of FDG-PET in the setting of diabetic neuro-osteoarthropathy: can it differentiate uncomplicated Charcot's neuropathy from osteomyelitis and soft tissue infection? Nucl Med Commun 2007; 28: 465–72.[17])

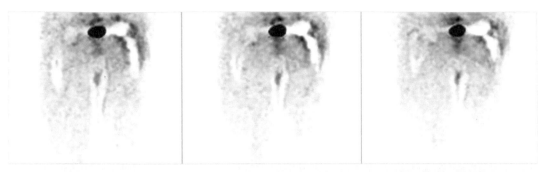

Fig. 31.8 The coronal images shown belong to a patient with a painful left hip following arthroplasty. Although there is some inflammation seen around the neck of the prosthesis and the proximal femur, this is a common reaction in patients after insertion of hip prostheses. The images show no clear evidence of infection due to lack of fluorodeoxyglucose uptake at the bone–prosthesis interface; this aseptic diagnosis was confirmed by surgical intervention in this patient.

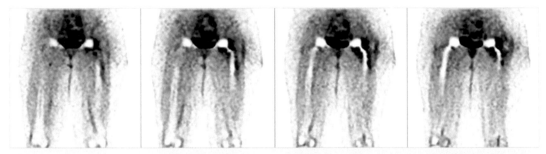

Fig. 31.9 Coronal images of the pelvis and thigh regions show no evidence of infection in the right hip prosthesis. On the left side, however, there is significant uptake of fluorodeoxyglucose at the bone–prosthesis interface surrounding the acetabular component and in the proximal half of the femoral stem. There is also evidence of extension of infection into the proximal soft-tissue structures. The right prosthesis appears aseptic, and the left prosthesis appears infected. This was confirmed by surgical exploration.

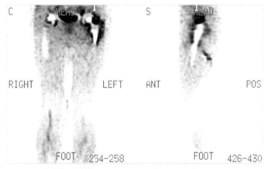

Fig. 31.10 The images shown represent fluorodeoxyglucose PET images of the pelvis and thighs taken in a patient with bilateral hip prostheses complaining of pain in the left hip. A fistula tract leading to the posterior thigh can be clearly seen in the sagittal image. The right prosthesis, meanwhile, appears uncomplicated and free of infection. The infection of the left hip was confirmed by surgical intervention.

scintigraphy (TcSC-Ind BM/WBC) in the diagnosis of periprosthetic infection for hip prostheses were 50, 95.1, 41, and 88.6%, respectively.

2. In a larger population study by Basu et al[22] in 221 prostheses (134 hip and 87 knee prostheses), sensitivity, specificity, PPV, and NPV of FDG-PET in hip prostheses were 81.8, 93.1, 79.4, and 94.0%, respectively, and in knee prostheses were 94.7, 88.2, 69.2, and 98.4%, respectively. For those who underwent both FDG-PET and WBC/BM imaging, there was a trend toward a higher sensitivity for FDG-PET in hip prostheses.

3. A recent systematic review[23] demonstrated a pooled sensitivity of 87% and a pooled specificity of 87% in diagnosing prosthetic joint infection by FDG-PET/CT.

31.3.4 Fever of Unknown Origin

Overview

FUO is a clinical challenge, especially in the elderly, and appears to be an accepted indication for FDG-PET in clinical practice. The nonspecificity of FDG is of great value in evaluating patients with FUO because it accumulates in infections, malignancies, and inflammatory diseases, which are the three major causes of FUO. Being a "catch-all" tracer, it has the potential to replace ^{67}Ga and labeled leukocyte imaging in this setting. However, overall, FDG-PET has had an added value to conventional techniques in 40 to 70% of the patients.

Accuracy

1. In a subgroup of 40 patients who had both PET and a ^{67}Ga study, Blockmans et al[24] found that FDG-PET revealed more abnormalities than the gallium scintigraphy (77 vs. 67%, respectively).
2. Stumpe et al[25] reported 98% sensitivity, 75% specificity, and 91% accuracy for FDG-PET in 39 patients with suspected infections.
3. Meller et al[26] compared FDG and gallium scanning in patients referred for assessment for FUO and reported a sensitivity of 81% and a specificity of 86% for FDG-PET in detecting the cause of the fever and a sensitivity and specificity of 67 and 78%, respectively, for gallium scanning.
4. Bleeker-Rovers et al[27] evaluated 35 patients with FUO and reported that FDG-PET was clinically helpful in 37% of cases, with a sensitivity and specificity of 93 and 90%, respectively, a PPV of 87%, and an NPV of 95%.
5. A pilot study suggests that, in spite of the normal myocardial FDG uptake, FDG-PET accurately helps identify sites of infective endocarditis and is a promising supplement to conventional echocardiography.[28]

31.3.5 Acquired Immunodeficiency Syndrome Patients

Overview

PET has a major role to play in the management of human immunodeficiency virus (HIV) infected patients and is especially valuable in the assessment of diseases affecting the central nervous system (CNS). Quantitative assessment has shown

that the standardized uptake values (SUVs) of toxoplasmosis are significantly lower than those of lymphoma, with virtually no overlap between the uptake values of the two conditions.

Accuracy

1. Hoffman et al[29] studied 11 individuals with AIDS and CNS lesions and found FDG-PET imaging to be more accurate than CT or MRI in differentiating between malignant and nonmalignant etiologies for the CNS lesions.
2. O'Doherty et al[30] showed that PET had an overall sensitivity and specificity of 92 and 94%, respectively, in the detection of infections (▶ Fig. 31.11) or malignancies in patients with AIDS.
3. Using FDG-PET in 47 AIDS patients, Santiago et al[31] found a lesion sensitivity of 82.5% for FDG imaging.

31.3.6 Sarcoidosis

Overview

FDG-PET/CT is of particular advantage in the management of sarcoidosis in the following ways: (1) it is very useful for detecting extrathoracic sarcoidosis or may uncover occult sites that were previously unknown due to whole-body assessment in a single examination and (2) assessment of inflammatory activity and extent helps in treatment response monitoring where it serves as an important sensitive and objective marker. Assessment of disease activity in sarcoidosis is an important parameter during the course of disease to decide upon therapeutic intervention. Additionally, FDG-PET can help in the correct assessment of disease activity in sarcoidosis, which is critical for initiating an optimal management plan because most patients will have a self-limited course, whereas a small percentage may die without treatment soon after diagnosis. FDG uptake patterns in sarcoidosis (▶ Fig. 31.12) can be misinterpreted as malignancy; thus, this test is to be interpreted with other investigations during initial diagnosis.

Accuracy

1. Several groups have reported FDG uptake by sarcoid granulomas,[32,33,34] which appear as typically active lymph nodes in the mediastinum and hilar regions.

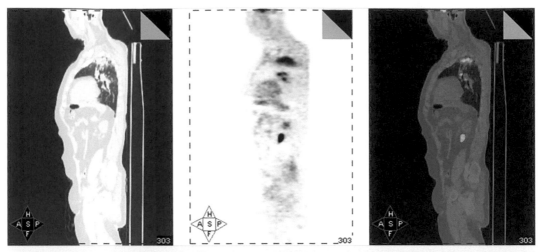

Fig. 31.11 Tubercular inflammatory lesion in the apex of the left lung, which shows intense fluorodeoxyglucose uptake fused with the corresponding CT scan. (From Kumar R, Basu S, Torigian D, Anand V, Zhuang H, Alavi A. Role of modern imaging techniques for diagnosis of infection in the era of ^{18}F-fluorodeoxyglucose positron emission tomography. Clin Microbiol Rev 2008;21(1):209–224. Reproduced with permission.[4])

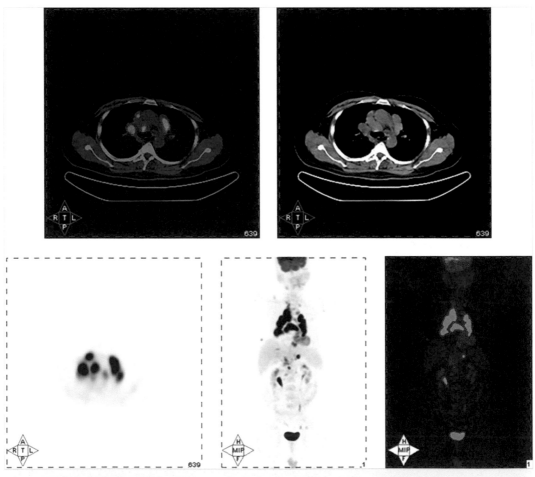

Fig. 31.12 Fluorodeoxyglucose PET images of a case of sarcoidosis where typical uptake is seen in the chest. In patients with active sarcoidosis, significant uptake is seen at the disease sites and can be mistaken for lymphoma or other lymphoproliferative disorders. (Reproduced with permission from Kumar R, Basu S, Torigian D, Anand V, Zhuang H, Alavi A. Role of modern imaging techniques for diagnosis of infection in the era of ^{18}F-fluorodeoxyglucose positron emission tomography. Clin Microbiol Rev 2008;21(1):209–224.[4])

2. By quantifying glucose metabolism in sarcoidosis, Brudin et al[32] have suggested that FDG uptake reflects likely disease activity and its extent at different stages of this unpredictable systemic disorder.

31.3.7 Atherosclerosis

Overview

FDG-PET imaging has the potential to assess atherosclerosis as an inflammatory process at the early stages of the disease, during its natural course, and following therapeutic intervention. The mechanism of this uptake is unclear, and possibilities include high glucose metabolism by macrophages in the atherosclerotic plaque, by smooth muscle in the media, or by proliferating subendothelial muscles.

Accuracy

1. Our group has investigated the frequency of FDG uptake in the large arteries in relation to the atherogenic risk factors.[35] The positive correlation of arterial FDG uptake with the atherogenic risk factors suggested a promising role for FDG-PET imaging in the diagnosis of atherosclerosis and follow-up after treatment intervention.[36,37] In a population of 149 subjects, the mean SUVs of the ascending aorta, aortic arch, descending thoracic aorta, iliac arteries, and femoral arteries increased with age ($p < 0.01$).[38]
2. High correlation is reported between the FDG uptake in the aorta and macrophage content of atherosclerotic lesions.[39]
3. Locally increased concentration of FDG is readily demonstrable in experimental lesions by ex vivo autoradiography. The feasibility of detection of vulnerable atheroma by intravascular catheter and positron-sensitive probe has been explored by various investigators.[40,41]
4. In animal studies, a promising application of FDG-PET for monitoring the therapeutic effect of anti-inflammatory drugs on stabilization of vulnerable atherosclerotic plaques has been demonstrated. FDG-PET was able to image the reduction of inflammation by probucol.[42] FDG-PET, by its ability to image reduction of macrophage infiltration, may be useful for evaluating the therapeutic effect of new drugs clinically that can stabilize vulnerable plaques.

31.3.8 Vasculitis

Overview

Histology is considered the gold standard for the diagnosis of vasculitis, but histopathological confirmation of the diagnosis of vasculitis is not always possible. FDG-PET has the potential to be added to the imaging armamentarium as a functional technique for scanning and detection of metabolically active processes along large- and medium-sized arteries. It has been reported to be useful in the diagnosis and treatment response assessment of patients with vasculitis by several investigators, especially it appears to have great potential in the diagnosis and treatment monitoring of patients with aortitis.

Accuracy

1. In a series of 15 patients with early aortitis, Meller et al[43] compared FDG-PET and MRI for the initial diagnosis and following immunosuppressive therapy. The results of FDG-PET and MRI for the initial diagnosis were comparable, but FDG-PET detected more inflammatory vascular regions and was more reliable in assessing disease activity following therapy than the latter modality.
2. Webb et al[44] found that FDG-PET had a sensitivity of 92%, a specificity of 100%, and NPVs and PPVs of 85 and 100%, respectively, in the initial assessment of active vasculitis in Takayasu's arteritis. Their conclusion was that FDG-PET could be used to evaluate the activity of the disease and to monitor the effectiveness of treatment.
3. In the initial studies of FDG-PET examining CNS involvement in patients with systemic lupus erythematosus (SLE), cerebral blood flow and glucose uptake were found to be reduced during active focal and diffuse CNS lupus.[45] In these and the subsequent studies, FDG-PET was considered to be the most sensitive method for demonstrating reversible deficits and for correlating the functional imaging results with neurologic findings.[46,47,48]

31.3.9 Inflammatory Bowel Disease

FDG-PET has been reported to be useful in detecting disease activity in patients with IBD. Normal FDG uptake in the bowel varies in distribution and intensity due to several factors[49,50,51] and can affect the sensitivity and specificity of this technique in this disorder. FDG-PET can play a major role in the evaluation of IBD in the pediatric age group because this population has low FDG activity in the bowel.

31.3.10 Treatment Response Assessment and Follow-Up with FDG-PET/CT

A potential future use of FDG-PET includes following disease activity after therapeutic interventions.[13] This has been a very useful application that has found use in many of the aforementioned infectious and inflammatory conditions. Further well-designed studies are warranted to investigate whether FDG-PET has an incremental value in this setting when compared with other techniques. Theoretically, it can be argued that imaging-activated inflammatory cells (▶ Fig. 31.13) with FDG is

likely to be more sensitive and specific than changes in perfusion or edema detected by CT/MRI or scintigraphic techniques (▶ Fig. 31.14).

31.3.11 Nonspecific Uptake in the Joints: Potential for Assessing Arthritis

1. FDG accumulation is frequently observed in various joints (particularly inferior glenohumeral joints at the shoulder); this is likely to represent inflammatory reactions.[53,54]
2. The exact location of FDG accumulation at these sites is unclear, but it is likely in the synovial tissue surrounding the joint. These are usually chronic in nature and represent a long-standing process that is detected as an incidental finding on FDG-PET scan.
3. The degree of FDG uptake as an indication of the severity of the inflammatory process may

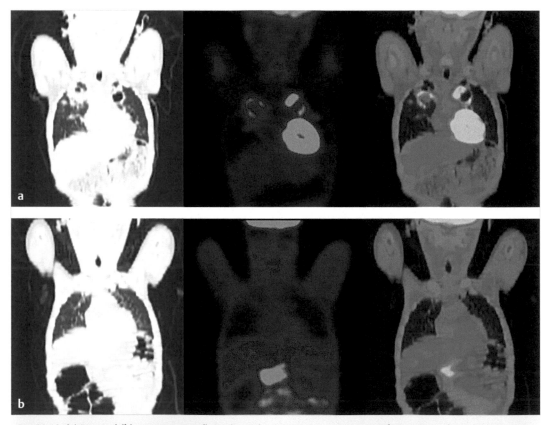

Fig. 31.13 (a) Pre- and **(b)** posttreatment fluorodeoxyglucose PET in a proven case of pneumonia showing therapeutic response. Corresponding CT and fused images are shown in this figure. (Reproduced with permission from Kumar R, Basu S, Torigian D, Anand V, Zhuang H, Alavi A. Role of modern imaging techniques for diagnosis of infection in the era of 18F-fluorodeoxyglucose positron emission tomography. Clin Microbiol Rev 2008;21(1):209–224.[4])

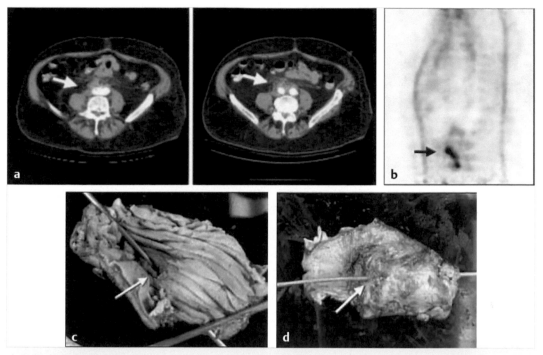

Fig. 31.14 (a) In this patient with suspected graft infection, while the CT scan did show evidence of retroperitoneal stranding (*arrows*), no definite evidence of aortic graft infection such as ectopic air, perigraft abscess, or pseudoaneurysm was noted on the respective images. **(b)** PET scan revealed an abnormal site of fluorodeoxyglucose (FDG) uptake in the area of the aorta corresponding to the graft (*arrow*). A fistulous connection between the jejunum and the aortic graft was evident at laparotomy. *Arrows* point to a probe placed through the fistula as seen from the luminal **(c)** and serosal side **(d)**. (Reproduced with permission from Krupnick AS, Lombardi JV, Engels FH, et al. 18-fluorodeoxyglucose positron emission tomography as a novel imaging tool for the diagnosis of aortoenteric fistula and aortic graft infection-a case report Vasc Endovascular Surg 2003;37(5):363–366.[52])

become an important source of information in rheumatologic conditions like osteoarthritis and rheumatoid arthritis.[55]

4. In patients of rheumatoid arthritis being treated with disease-modifying antirheumatic drugs (DMARD), quantitative metabolic volumetric product on FDG-PET/CT can serve as a valuable adjunct and complementary objective imaging parameter to clinical assessment to American College of Rheumatology/European League against Rheumatism (EULAR) criteria.[56]

References

[1] Jones HA, Cadwallader KA, White JF, Uddin M, Peters AM, Chilvers ER. Dissociation between respiratory burst activity and deoxyglucose uptake in human neutrophil granulocytes: implications for interpretation of (18)F-FDG PET images. J Nucl Med. 2002; 43(5):652–657

[2] Glaudemans AW, Signore A. FDG-PET/CT in infections: the imaging method of choice? Eur J Nucl Med Mol Imaging. 2010; 37(10):1986–1991

[3] Jamar F, Buscombe J, Chiti A, et al. EANM/SNMMI guideline for 18F-FDG use in inflammation and infection. J Nucl Med. 2013; 54(4):647–658

[4] Kumar R, Basu S, Torigian D, Anand V, Zhuang H, Alavi A. Role of modern imaging techniques for diagnosis of infection in the era of 18F-fluorodeoxyglucose positron emission tomography. Clin Microbiol Rev. 2008; 21(1):209–224

[5] Guhlmann A, Brecht-Krauss D, Suger G, et al. Fluorine-18-FDG PET and technetium-99m antigranulocyte antibody scintigraphy in chronic osteomyelitis. J Nucl Med. 1998; 39(12):2145–2152

[6] Guhlmann A, Brecht-Krauss D, Suger G, et al. Chronic osteomyelitis: detection with FDG PET and correlation with histopathologic findings. Radiology. 1998; 206(3):749–754

[7] de Winter F, van de Wiele C, Vogelaers D, de Smet K, Verdonk R, Dierckx RA. Fluorine-18 fluorodeoxyglucose-position emission tomography: a highly accurate imaging modality for the diagnosis of chronic musculoskeletal infections. J Bone Joint Surg Am. 2001; 83-A(5):651–660

[8] Meller J, Köster G, Liersch T, et al. Chronic bacterial osteomyelitis: prospective comparison of (18)F-FDG imaging with a dual-head coincidence camera and (111)In-labelled autologous leucocyte scintigraphy. Eur J Nucl Med Mol Imaging. 2002; 29(1):53–60

[9] Gratz S, Dörner J, Fischer U, et al. 18F-FDG hybrid PET in patients with suspected spondylitis. Eur J Nucl Med Mol Imaging. 2002; 29(4):516–524

[10] Love C, Palestro C. F-18-FDG and (67) GA-SPECT imaging in suspected vertebral osteomyelitis: an intraindividual comparison. J Nucl Med. 2003; 45(suppl):148P

[11] Stumpe KD, Zanetti M, Weishaupt D, Hodler J, Boos N, Von Schulthess GK. FDG positron emission tomography for differentiation of degenerative and infectious endplate abnormalities in the lumbar spine detected on MR imaging. AJR Am J Roentgenol. 2002; 179(5):1151–1157

[12] Crymes WB, Jr, Demos H, Gordon L. Detection of musculoskeletal infection with 18F-FDG PET: review of the current literature. J Nucl Med Technol. 2004; 32(1):12–15

[13] Zhuang H, Alavi A. 18-fluorodeoxyglucose positron emission tomographic imaging in the detection and monitoring of infection and inflammation. Semin Nucl Med. 2002; 32(1):47–59

[14] Alnafisi N, Yun M, Alavi A. F-18 FDG positron emission tomography to differentiate diabetic osteoarthropathy from septic arthritis. Clin Nucl Med. 2001; 26(7):638–639

[15] Basu S, Zhuang H, Alavi A. FDG PET and PET/CT imaging in complicated diabetic foot. PET Clin. 2012; 7(2):151–160

[16] Keidar Z, Militianu D, Melamed E, Bar-Shalom R, Israel O. The diabetic foot: initial experience with 18F-FDG PET/CT. J Nucl Med. 2005; 46(3):444–449

[17] Basu S, Chryssikos T, Houseni M, et al. Potential role of FDG PET in the setting of diabetic neuro-osteoarthropathy: can it differentiate uncomplicated Charcot's neuroarthropathy from osteomyelitis and soft-tissue infection? Nucl Med Commun. 2007; 28(6):465–472

[18] Hopfner S, Krolak C, Kessler S, et al. Preoperative imaging of Charcot neuroarthropathy: does the additional application of (18)F-FDG-PET make sense? Nucl Med (Stuttg). 2006; 45:15–20

[19] Basu S, Alavi A. Nuclear medicine-FDG-PER takes lead role in suspected or proven infection. Diagn Imaging (San Franc). 2007; 29:59–66

[20] Nawaz A, Torigian DA, Siegelman ES, Basu S, Chryssikos T, Alavi A. Diagnostic performance of FDG-PET, MRI, and plain film radiography (PFR) for the diagnosis of osteomyelitis in the diabetic foot. Mol Imaging Biol. 2010; 12(3):335–342

[21] Pill SG, Parvizi J, Tang PH, et al. Comparison of fluorodeoxyglucose positron emission tomography and (111)indium-white blood cell imaging in the diagnosis of periprosthetic infection of the hip. J Arthroplasty. 2006; 21(6) Suppl 2:91–97

[22] Basu S, Kwee TC, Saboury B, et al. FDG PET for diagnosing infection in hip and knee prostheses: prospective study in 221 prostheses and subgroup comparison with combined (111)In-labeled leukocyte/(99m)Tc-sulfur colloid bone marrow imaging in 88 prostheses. Clin Nucl Med. 2014; 39(7):609–615

[23] Hao R, Yuan L, Kan Y, et al. 18F-FDG PET for diagnosing painful arthroplasty/prosthetic joint infection. Clin Transl Imaging. 2017; 5:315–323

[24] Blockmans D, Knockaert D, Maes A, et al. Clinical value of [(18)F]fluoro-deoxyglucose positron emission tomography for patients with fever of unknown origin. Clin Infect Dis. 2001; 32(2):191–196

[25] Stumpe KD, Dazzi H, Schaffner A, von Schulthess GK. Infection imaging using whole-body FDG-PET. Eur J Nucl Med. 2000; 27(7):822–832

[26] Meller J, Altenvoerde G, Munzel U, et al. Fever of unknown origin: prospective comparison of [18F]FDG imaging with a double-head coincidence camera and gallium-67 citrate SPET. Eur J Nucl Med. 2000; 27(11):1617–1625

[27] Bleeker-Rovers CP, de Kleijn EM, Corstens FH, van der Meer JW, Oyen WJ. Clinical value of FDG PET in patients with fever of unknown origin and patients suspected of focal infection or inflammation. Eur J Nucl Med Mol Imaging. 2004; 31(1):29–37

[28] Yen RF, Chen YC, Wu YW, Pan MH, Chang SC. Using 18-fluoro-2-deoxyglucose positron emission tomography in detecting infectious endocarditis/endoarteritis: a preliminary report. Acad Radiol. 2004; 11(3):316–321

[29] Hoffman JM, Waskin HA, Schifter T, et al. FDG-PET in differentiating lymphoma from nonmalignant central nervous system lesions in patients with AIDS. J Nucl Med. 1993; 34(4):567–575

[30] O'Doherty MJ, Barrington SF, Campbell M, Lowe J, Bradbeer CS. PET scanning and the human immunodeficiency virus-positive patient. J Nucl Med. 1997; 38(10):1575–1583

[31] Santiago JF, Jana S, Gilbert HM, et al. Role of fluorine-18-fluorodeoxyglucose in the work-up of febrile AIDS patients. Experience with dual head coincidence imaging. Clin Positron Imaging. 1999; 2(6):301–309

[32] Brudin LH, Valind SO, Rhodes CG, et al. Fluorine-18 deoxyglucose uptake in sarcoidosis measured with positron emission tomography. Eur J Nucl Med. 1994; 21(4):297–305

[33] Lewis PJ, Salama A. Uptake of fluorine-18-fluorodeoxyglucose in sarcoidosis. J Nucl Med. 1994; 35(10):1647–1649

[34] Yasuda S, Shohtsu A, Ide M, et al. High fluorine-18 labeled deoxyglucose uptake in sarcoidosis. Clin Nucl Med. 1996; 21(12):983–984

[35] Yun M, Jang S, Cucchiara A, Newberg AB, Alavi A. 18F FDG uptake in the large arteries: a correlation study with the atherogenic risk factors. Semin Nucl Med. 2002; 32(1):70–76

[36] Lin EC, Quaife RA. FDG uptake in chronic superior vena cava thrombus on positron emission tomographic imaging. Clin Nucl Med. 2001; 26(3):241–242

[37] Zhang Z, Machac J, Helft G, et al. Noninvasive serial monitoring of atherosclerotic progression and regression with FDG-PET in a rabbit model. J Nucl Med. 2000; 41(5):7P

[38] Bural GG, Torigian DA, Chamroonrat W, et al. FDG-PET is an effective imaging modality to detect and quantify age-related atherosclerosis in large arteries. Eur J Nucl Med Mol Imaging. 2008; 35(3):562–569

[39] Vallabhajosula S, Machac J, Knesaurek K, et al. Imaging atherosclerotic macrophage density by positron emission tomography using F-18-fluorodeoxyglucose (FDG). J Nucl Med. 1996; 37:144–144

[40] Lederman RJ, Raylman RR, Fisher SJ, et al. Detection of atherosclerosis using a novel positron-sensitive probe and 18-fluorodeoxyglucose (FDG). Nucl Med Commun. 2001; 22(7):747–753

[41] Strauss HW, Mari C, Patt BE, Ghazarossian V. Intravascular radiation detectors for the detection of vulnerable atheroma. J Am Coll Cardiol. 2006; 47(8) Suppl:C97–C100

[42] Ogawa M, Magata Y, Kato T, et al. Application of 18F-FDG PET for monitoring the therapeutic effect of antiinflammatory drugs on stabilization of vulnerable atherosclerotic plaques. J Nucl Med. 2006; 47(11):1845–1850

[43] Meller J, Strutz F, Siefker U, et al. Early diagnosis and follow-up of aortitis with [(18)F]FDG PET and MRI. Eur J Nucl Med Mol Imaging. 2003; 30(5):730–736

[44] Webb M, Chambers A, AL-Nahhas A, et al. The role of 18F-FDG PET in characterising disease activity in Takayasu arteritis. Eur J Nucl Med Mol Imaging. 2004; 31(5):627–634

[45] van Dam AP. Diagnosis and pathogenesis of CNS lupus. Rheumatol Int. 1991; 11(1):1–11

[46] Sailer M, Burchert W, Ehrenheim C, et al. Positron emission tomography and magnetic resonance imaging for cerebral involvement in patients with systemic lupus erythematosus. J Neurol. 1997; 244(3):186–193

[47] Stoppe G, Wildhagen K, Seidel JW, et al. Positron emission tomography in neuropsychiatric lupus erythematosus. Neurology. 1990; 40(2):304–308

[48] Weiner SM, Otte A, Schumacher M, et al. Diagnosis and monitoring of central nervous system involvement in systemic lupus erythematosus: value of F-18 fluorodeoxyglucose PET. Ann Rheum Dis. 2000; 59(5):377–385

[49] Shreve PD, Anzai Y, Wahl RL. Pitfalls in oncologic diagnosis with FDG PET imaging: physiologic and benign variants. Radiographics. 1999; 19(1):61–77, quiz 150–151

[50] Miraldi F, Vesselle H, Faulhaber PF, Adler LP, Leisure GP. Elimination of artifactual accumulation of FDG in PET imaging of colorectal cancer. Clin Nucl Med. 1998; 23(1):3–7

[51] Pio BS, Byrne FR, Aranda R, et al. Noninvasive quantification of bowel inflammation through positron emission tomography imaging of 2-deoxy-2-[18F]fluoro-D-glucose-labeled white blood cells. Mol Imaging Biol. 2003; 5(4):271–277

[52] Krupnick AS, Lombardi JV, Engels FH, et al. 18-fluorodeoxyglucose positron emission tomography as a novel imaging tool for the diagnosis of aortoenteric fistula and aortic graft infection–a case report. Vasc Endovascular Surg. 2003; 37(5):363–366

[53] von Schulthess GK, Meier N, Stumpe KD. Joint accumulations of FDG in whole body PET scans. Nucl Med (Stuttg). 2001; 40 (6):193–197

[54] Wandler E, Kramer EL, Sherman O, Babb J, Scarola J, Rafii M. Diffuse FDG shoulder uptake on PET is associated with clinical findings of osteoarthritis. AJR Am J Roentgenol. 2005; 185 (3):797–803

[55] Polisson RP, Schoenberg OI, Fischman A, et al. Use of magnetic resonance imaging and positron emission tomography in the assessment of synovial volume and glucose metabolism in patients with rheumatoid arthritis. Arthritis Rheum. 1995; 38(6):819–825

[56] Kumar NS, Shejul Y, Asopa R, Basu S. Quantitative metabolic volumetric product on 18fluorine-2fluoro-2-deoxy-D-glucose-positron emission tomography/computed tomography in assessing treatment response to disease-modifying anti-rheumatic drugs in rheumatoid arthritis: multiparametric analysis integrating American College of Rheumatology/European League Against Rheumatism Criteria. World J Nucl Med. 2017; 16(4):293–302

32 Neurological Applications of Fluorodeoxyglucose PET

Eugene C. Lin

32.1 Seizure Localization[1]

PET is useful in lateralizing epileptogenic foci in patients with equivocal clinical, electroencephalographic (EEG), and MRI examinations, specifically when MRI findings are negative or ictal EEG is discordant with the MRI. Patients with temporal lobe epilepsy, negative MRI studies, and positive PET studies who undergo surgery have good surgical outcomes, comparable to patients with evidence of medial temporal sclerosis on MRI.[2,3] In addition, the pattern of PET findings can aid in predicting surgical outcome. PET does not add value in patients already localized by ictal scalp EEG and MRI.[4]

32.1.1 Accuracy[5,6]

1. **Prognosis**. Ipsilateral PET hypometabolism is an indicator for good postoperative outcome in the presurgical evaluation of drug-resistant temporal lobe epilepsy. Ipsilateral PET hypometabolism has a predictive value of 86% for good outcome (80% in patients with a normal MRI and 72% in patients with a nonlocalized scalp EEG).[4]
2. PET is more accurate for temporal epilepsy.
3. **Interictal PET:**
   a) *Temporal lobe epilepsy*: sensitivity of 84% and specificity of 86%.
   b) *Extratemporal lobe epilepsy*: sensitivity of 33% and specificity of 95%.

32.1.2 Comparison to Other Modalities

1. Interictal PET is more sensitive than interictal single-photon emission computed tomography (SPECT) but less sensitive than ictal SPECT.
2. **SPECT** (temporal epilepsy):
   a) *Ictal SPECT*: sensitivity of 90% and specificity of 73%.
   b) *Interictal SPECT*: sensitivity of 66% and specificity of 68%.

32.1.3 Pearls[7,8]

1. In the interictal state, the involved region will be hypometabolic (▶ Fig. 32.1). The extent of

hypometabolism may be a dynamic process related to the duration, frequency, and severity of seizures.[9,10] During ictus, the involved region is hypermetabolic.

2. Temporal lobe hypometabolism usually involves the entire temporal lobe:
   a) Lateral hypometabolism may be more pronounced.
   b) Even if a focal lesion is present on anatomic images, the temporal lobe hypometabolism is usually diffuse.
3. **MRI negative.** PET is accurate even when there is no MRI evidence of mesial temporal sclerosis.[11] In patients with a negative MRI, the hypometabolism tends to involve the inferolateral temporal lobe rather than the mesial temporal lobe.[12]
4. **Contralateral temporal lobe.** Rarely, the temporal lobe contralateral to the seizure focus may appear mildly hypermetabolic.
5. **Interpretation criteria.** In patients with suspected temporal lobe epilepsy, any degree of hypometabolism on visual inspection should be considered significant. A quantitative difference

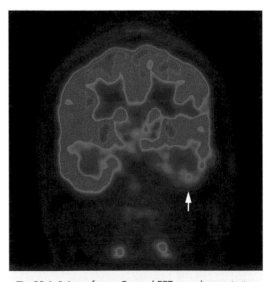

Fig. 32.1 Seizure focus. Coronal PET scan demonstrates decreased left temporal lobe activity (*arrow*) consistent with an interictal seizure focus.

of 15% or more between the temporal lobes is usually significant.[13]

6. **Extratemporal hypometabolism.** Ipsilateral extratemporal hypometabolism in combination with temporal hypometabolism is relatively common:

a) Extratemporal hypometabolism can be seen in the ipsilateral thalamus (most common), the frontal and parietal lobes, and very uncommonly in the occipital lobes and basal ganglia. The greatest degree of hypometabolism is usually seen in the ipsilateral frontal lobe.[14]

b) Bilateral cerebellar hypometabolism is common, which is likely related to chronic use of anti-epilepsy drugs. Crossed cerebellar diaschisis contralateral to the seizure focus can also be seen, more commonly in frontal or parietal lobe seizures.[15]

c) Extratemporal areas of cortical hypometabolism are usually contiguous with each other and the main site in the temporal lobe.

d) Extratemporal hypometabolism is less severe than the temporal hypometabolism. However, frontal lobe hypometabolism can occasionally be greater than hypometabolism in the temporal seizure focus.

e) Hypometabolism can rarely be seen in a contralateral mirror region, likely secondary to functional suppression of these regions through callosal fibers or the fornix.[9]

7. Thalamic hypometabolism[1]:

a) Ipsilateral thalamic hypometabolism is associated with long-standing epilepsy and secondary generalization of seizures.

b) Contralateral thalamic hypometabolism is a predictor of poor surgical outcome (higher risk of postoperative seizures) compared to ipsilateral or no thalamic hypometabolism.

8. **Prognosis.** Unilateral focal temporal hypometabolism is associated with a good surgical outcome. Symmetric bilateral temporal, extratemporal, or thalamic hypometabolism is associated with a higher incidence of postoperative seizures.[16]

9. **Pediatric patients**. PET is useful in the pediatric population in which cortical dysplasia is a major etiology for epilepsy, unlike adult epilepsy in which hippocampal sclerosis is a common etiology. Fluorodeoxyglucose (FDG) PET is positive in 75 to 90% of patients with cortical dysplasia.[17]

32.1.4 Pitfalls[8]

1. **Localization.** PET is primarily useful in lateralizing the epileptogenic focus rather than in exact localization. As hypometabolism often diffusely involves the temporal lobe and extends into extratemporal regions, hypometabolism on PET should not guide the extent of surgical resection without further supportive evidence.[11]

2. **Intracranial electrodes.** Intracranial electrode insertion can cause areas of hypometabolism. PET should be performed before intracranial electroencephalogram.

3. **Subclinical seizures.** Unrecognized subclinical seizure activity during the administration of FDG can result in false-positive apparent hypometabolism in the contralateral temporal lobe (relative to the ictal hypermetabolism in the involved temporal lobe). Therefore, patients should be monitored if possible before the dose is injected.

4. **Children.** Interictal hypermetabolism in the seizure focus can occur in children but rarely in adults.

5. **Focal cortical malformations.** Focal cortical malformations can be associated with decreased, normal, or increased uptake. Focal subcortical heterotopia and lobar dysplasia can be associated with increased uptake on interictal PET.[18]

32.2 Dementia: Alzheimer's Disease[19,20]

Diagnostic guidelines from the National Institute on Aging and the Alzheimer's association[21] incorporate FDG-PET as a biomarker of neuronal injury (along with cerebrospinal fluid tau and structural MRI) and PET amyloid imaging agents are incorporated as biomarkers of brain amyloidosis. In patients with mild cognitive impairment (MCI), neuronal injury biomarkers such as FDG-PET have a more significant role in predicting disease progression than amyloid biomarkers.[22] Amyloid biomarkers are elevated in the initial asymptomatic phase of Alzheimer's disease (AD) and close to a plateau at the MCI phase, and thus provide little predictive information concerning disease progression at the MCI phase. Neuronal injury biomarkers are more associated with future cognitive deterioration.

Compared to another biomarker of neuronal injury, structural MRI, MRI may be more related to the current cognitive state at the MCI phase, while FDG-PET may be a more sensitive biomarker for disease progression.

FDG-PET is a valuable imaging study in patients with suspected AD with mild to moderate cognitive impairment who (1) meet standard criteria for dementia without identifiable cause after full workup or (2) exhibit progressive cognitive dysfunction during a period of observation. FDG-PET is a biomarker of neurodegeneration in which hypometabolism can precede the appearance of cognitive symptoms, and predicts the rate of cognitive decline in individuals who later progress to AD. In addition, FDG-PET has clinical utility when confounding diagnoses such as frontotemporal dementia (FTD) and dementia with Lewy bodies (DLB) are also possible. A negative FDG-PET scan in the setting of suspected dementia makes a dementia diagnosis very unlikely. Although the diagnostic accuracy of FDG-PET is highest in moderate to severe disease, the accuracy is also fairly high in patients with mild disease who may present the most challenging differential diagnoses. The sensitivity and specificity of FDG-PET near the time of initial AD diagnosis is similar to longitudinal clinical diagnosis over 3 to 4 years.[23]

Non-FDG tracers for the evaluation of patients with dementia will be discussed in Chapter 33.

32.3 Accuracy/Comparison to Other Modalities

1. Diagnostic accuracy for AD with clinical and autopsy standard (meta-analysis; ▶ Table 32.1).[24]

Table 32.1 Diagnostic accuracy for AD with clinical and autopsy standard

	Sensitivity %	Specificity %
FDG PET	91	86
SPECT	79	84
MRI	83	85

Abbreviations: FDG, fluorodeoxyglucose; SPECT, single-photon emission computed tomography.

2. Diagnostic accuracy for AD with autopsy standard (meta-analysis; ▶ Table 32.2).[25]

3. FDG-PET has a high sensitivity but variable specificity for the diagnosis of AD. Compared to nondemented controls, the specificity is as high as 89%, but the specificity can decrease to as low as 78% versus non-AD dementia with MCI, and 70% versus non-AD dementia without MCI.[24]

Table 32.2 Diagnostic accuracy for AD with autopsy standard

	Sensitivity %	Specificity %
FDG PET	93	73
SPECT	86	85
MRI	81	84

Abbreviations: FDG, fluorodeoxyglucose; SPECT, single-photon emission computed tomography.

4. Diagnostic accuracy and prognostic accuracy. In a meta-analysis,[26] the diagnostic accuracy was highest for PET amyloid, followed by FDG-PET, SPECT, and structural MRI. The prognostic accuracy to predict progression was highest for FDG-PET, followed by structural MRI, SPECT, and PET amyloid.

5. FDG-PET versus structural MRI. There are conflicting results as to which neuronal injury biomarker (FDG-PET or structural MRI) is superior.[22] FDG-PET may perform better in rapidly converting younger MCI patients, while structural MRI may be superior in older MCI patients.

32.3.1 Pearls/Pitfalls

1. Interpretation criteria for a positive study[27]:
   a) Bilateral symmetric temporoparietal hypometabolism (▶ Fig. 32.2):
      • Parietal activity is usually decreased more than temporal activity.
      • Temporoparietal hypometabolism tends to increase during disease progression.[28]
   b) Posterior cingulate cortex (PCC) hypometabolism:
      • PCC hypometabolism is the most sensitive marker for predicting conversion of MCI to AD.[29]
      • PCC hypometabolism is most easily identified on parasagittal images.
      • PCC hypometabolism usually extends into the precuneus.[30]
      • In contrast to the PCC hypometabolism in amnestic MCI, PCC hypometabolism in wider in AD and extends to the precuneus and lateral parietal cortex.[31]
   c) Hypometabolism may be asymmetric or unilateral early during the disease (▶ Fig. 32.3). If asymmetric hypometabolism is present, this tends to be preserved during disease progression.[28]
   d) Hypometabolism can involve frontal lobes in advanced disease (▶ Fig. 32.4). Increasing

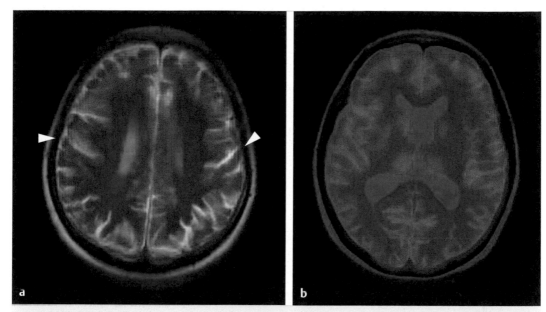

Fig. 32.2 Alzheimer's disease. **(a)** Fused axial PET/MR demonstrates bilateral parietal hypometabolism consistent with Alzheimer's disease. Preserved activity in the motor-sensory cortex (*arrowheads*) around the central sulcus is characteristic in Alzheimer's disease. **(b)** Fused axial PET/MR in the same patient demonstrates preservation of activity in the visual cortex.

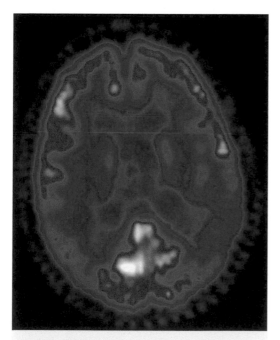

Fig. 32.3 Alzheimer's disease. Axial PET scan demonstrates bilateral parietal hypometabolism in a patient with Alzheimer's disease. The hypometabolism is greater in the left parietal region.

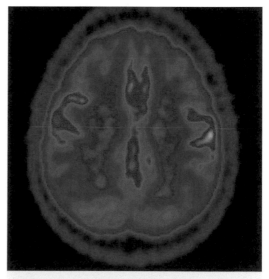

Fig. 32.4 Late-stage Alzheimer's disease. Axial PET scan demonstrates bilateral frontal and parietal hypometabolism. The frontal lobe hypometabolism is seen in the later stages of Alzheimer's disease.

frontal hypometabolism is often the main finding during progression from MCI to AD[28]:

- Frontal lobe abnormalities are not seen without temporoparietal disease.

e) Preserved metabolism in the sensorimotor and visual cortices (▶ Fig. 32.2), cerebellum, basal ganglia, and thalamus.

f) Cerebellar activity remains constant throughout the stages of the disease and therefore it can be used as a reference point for generating semiquantitative indices for affected sites.

g) Glucose metabolism is lower throughout the cortex in patients with AD compared to normals.[32]

2. **Differentiation from other dementias:** AD can usually be differentiated from the following:

a) *FTD (Pick's disease).*[19] Frontal and temporal hypometabolism is the dominant pattern (▶ Fig. 32.5):

- Reduced activity in the PCC seen in AD is not noted in FTD.[33] Anterior cingulate hypometabolism is often seen in FTD.[34]
- FTD primarily affects the anterior and medial temporal cortices. The anterior temporal involvement in particular would be atypical for AD. AD typically involves the posterolateral temporal cortices.

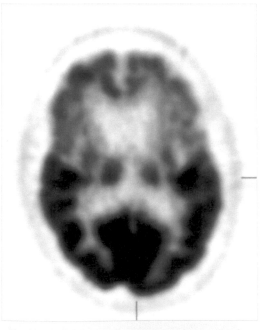

Fig. 32.5 Pick's disease. Axial PET scan demonstrates frontal hypometabolism characteristic for Pick's disease.

- The greatest decrease is often in the medial frontal cortices.
- As FTD progresses, hypometabolism spreads from the frontal lobe to the parietal and temporal lobes.[35]
- Hemispheric asymmetry of hypometabolism is common in FTD.[35]
- There is relative sparing of parietal lobes in FTD. However, some patients present with frontal and temporoparietal hypometabolism to a similar degree, which can make the differentiation between AD and FTD difficult. In one report,[36] temporoparietal hypometabolism was relatively common in patients with FTD. In these cases, hypometabolism of the anterior cingulate and anterior temporal regions is helpful in diagnosing FTD.
- Depression, schizophrenia, alcohol, and substance abuse can also result in mild decreases in frontal metabolism and should be considered in the differential diagnosis.[28]

b) *Vascular dementia (multi-infarct dementia).* Multiple focal cortical and subcortical defects are seen in this type of dementia:

- Areas of decreased metabolism differentiating vascular dementia from AD are the deep gray nuclei, cerebellum, primary cortices, middle temporal gyrus, and anterior cingulate gyrus.[37]
- Note that these defects should be accounted for by areas of abnormal signal on MRI. If these defects have no MRI correlate, this pattern could suggest a primary neurodegenerative disorder rather than vascular dementia.[19]
- However, frontal lobe metabolism is usually decreased in patients with white matter signal abnormalities on MRI secondary to subcortical ischemic vascular disease, regardless of the location of the signal abnormalities.[38]

c) *DLB:*

- DLB not only has bilateral temporoparietal hypometabolism like AD but also involves the occipital lobes (▶ Fig. 32.6).
- The most prominent difference between DLB and AD is reduction in visual cortex activity in DLB.[39]
- In DLB, PCC metabolism is typically preserved relative to the cuneus and precuneus. This has been termed the

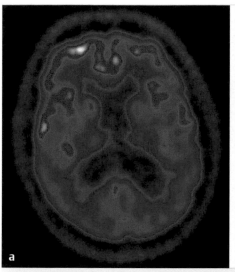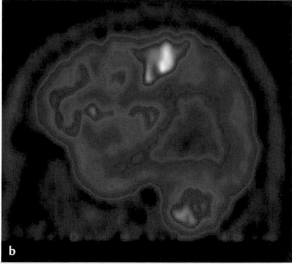

Fig. 32.6 Lewy body dementia. Axial (**a**) and sagittal (**b**) PET scans demonstrate hypometabolism involving the bilateral parietal, temporal, and occipital lobes. The occipital and visual cortex involvement distinguishes Lewy body dementia from Alzheimer's disease.

"cingulate island" sign.[40] In contrast, posterior cingulate metabolism is typically severely reduced early in AD.

- In mild DLB, hypometabolism usually involves substantially larger portions of the cortex than in mild AD. In mild AD, there is often hypometabolism in the medial temporal lobe (hippocampus), which is not present in mild DLB.[41]
- In practice, DLB may be difficult to distinguish from AD with PET; the accuracy is around 70% for this purpose.[42]

d) *Parkinson's dementia:*

- Parkinson's disease with dementia can have the same pattern of hypometabolism as AD and DLB.
- However, compared to AD, Parkinson's dementia tends to have greater reduction in the visual cortex and less reduction in the medial temporal lobe.[43]
- Compared to DLB, there is less reduction in the anterior cingulate cortex in Parkinson's dementia.[44]

3. **Early- versus late-onset AD.** The diagnostic sensitivity for late-onset AD is lower than in early-onset AD.[45] Glucose metabolism is most severely affected in the parietal, frontal, posterior cingulate cortices, and subcortical area in early-onset AD and in the limbic system and medial frontal lobe in late-onset AD.[46,47]

The overall hypometabolism in early-onset AD is greater in magnitude and extent.[47]

4. **Aging.** Aging is associated with a tendency for global reduction in cerebral glucose metabolism, most prominent in the frontal lobes, particularly in the anterior cingulate and frontomesial cortex. This can typically be differentiated from the posterior association cortex reduction seen in AD. However, patients with late-onset AD tend to have a lesser degree of hypometabolism in the temporoparietal cortex, PCC, and precuneus compared to patients with early-onset AD. This may result in a lesser degree of contrast between the hypometabolic posterior association areas secondary to AD, and the frontal hypometabolism secondary to aging.

5. **Depression and hypothyroidism.** Decreased activity due to depression or hypometabolism from thyroid disease may be a confounding factor. In particular, coexisting depression or thyroid disease may be problematic if the degree of decreased uptake on an initial PET scan is used as a prognostic factor.

6. **Plasma glucose levels.** Increased plasma glucose levels in both fasting and glucose-loading conditions can reduce glucose uptake, especially in the precuneus.[48] This can result in an AD-like pattern in cognitively normal subjects. This can appear even with mildly elevated levels of fasting

plasma glucose (100–110 mg/dL), although higher levels typically would be needed to be easily detected by visual inspection. This AD-like pattern can disappear with decreasing plasma glucose levels.[49] While greater insulin resistance can result in an AD-like pattern in cognitively normal patients with prediabetes or early type 2 diabetes,[50] this pattern can also occur without insulin resistance.[51]

References

[1] Newberg AB, Alavi A. PET in seizure disorders. Radiol Clin North Am. 2005; 43(1):79–92

[2] LoPinto-Khoury C, Sperling MR, Skidmore C, et al. Surgical outcome in PET-positive, MRI-negative patients with temporal lobe epilepsy. Epilepsia. 2012; 53(2):342–348

[3] Yang PF, Pei JS, Zhang HJ, et al. Long-term epilepsy surgery outcomes in patients with PET-positive, MRI-negative temporal lobe epilepsy. Epilepsy Behav. 2014; 41:91–97

[4] Willmann O, Wennberg R, May T, Woermann FG, Pohlmann-Eden B. The contribution of 18F-FDG PET in preoperative epilepsy surgery evaluation for patients with temporal lobe epilepsy. A meta-analysis. Seizure. 2007; 16(6):509–520

[5] Bernal B, Altman NR. Evidence-based medicine: neuroimaging of seizures. Neuroimaging Clin N Am. 2003; 13(2):211–224

[6] Spencer SS. The relative contributions of MRI, SPECT, and PET imaging in epilepsy. Epilepsia. 1994; 35 Suppl 6:S72–S89

[7] Bohnen N. Neurological Applications. In: Wahl R ed. Principles and Practice of Positron Emission Tomography. Philadelphia, PA: Lippincott Williams & Wilkins; 2002:276–297

[8] Henry TR, Van Heertum RL. Positron emission tomography and single photon emission computed tomography in epilepsy care. Semin Nucl Med. 2003; 33(2):88–104

[9] Kumar A, Chugani HT. The role of radionuclide imaging in epilepsy, part 1: sporadic temporal and extratemporal lobe epilepsy. J Nucl Med. 2013; 54(10):1775–1781

[10] Van Paesschen W, Dupont P, Sunaert S, Goffin K, Van Laere K. The use of SPECT and PET in routine clinical practice in epilepsy. Curr Opin Neurol. 2007; 20(2):194–202

[11] Knowlton RC. The role of FDG-PET, ictal SPECT, and MEG in the epilepsy surgery evaluation. Epilepsy Behav. 2006; 8(1):91–101

[12] Carne RP, Cook MJ, MacGregor LR, Kilpatrick CJ, Hicks RJ, O'Brien TJ. "Magnetic resonance imaging negative positron emission tomography positive" temporal lobe epilepsy: FDG-PET pattern differs from mesial temporal lobe epilepsy. Mol Imaging Biol. 2007; 9(1):32–42

[13] Delbeke D, Lawrence SK, Abou-Khalil BW, Blumenkopf B, Kessler RM. Postsurgical outcome of patients with uncontrolled complex partial seizures and temporal lobe hypometabolism on 18FDG-positron emission tomography. Invest Radiol. 1996; 31(5):261–266

[14] Nelissen N, Van Paesschen W, Baete K, et al. Correlations of interictal FDG-PET metabolism and ictal SPECT perfusion changes in human temporal lobe epilepsy with hippocampal sclerosis. Neuroimage. 2006; 32(2):684–695

[15] Kawai N, Kawanishi M, Tamiya T, Nagao S. Crossed cerebellar glucose hypermetabolism demonstrated using PET in symptomatic epilepsy: case report. Ann Nucl Med. 2005; 19(3):231–234

[16] Salmenpera TM, Duncan JS. Imaging in epilepsy. J Neurol Neurosurg Psychiatry. 2005; 76 Suppl 3:iii2–iii10

[17] Alavi A, Yakir S, Newberg AB. Positron emission tomography in seizure disorders. Ann N Y Acad Sci. 2011; 1228:E1–E12

[18] Poduri A, Golja A, Takeoka M, Bourgeois BF, Connolly L, Riviello JJ, Jr. Focal cortical malformations can show asymmetrically higher uptake on interictal fluorine-18 fluorodeoxyglucose positron emission tomography (PET). J Child Neurol. 2007; 22(2):232–237

[19] Silverman DH. Brain 18F-FDG PET in the diagnosis of neurodegenerative dementias: comparison with perfusion SPECT and with clinical evaluations lacking nuclear imaging. J Nucl Med. 2004; 45(4):594–607

[20] Van Heertum RL, Greenstein EA, Tikofsky RS. 2-deoxy-fluorglucose-positron emission tomography imaging of the brain: current clinical applications with emphasis on the dementias. Semin Nucl Med. 2004; 34(4):300–312

[21] McKhann GM, Knopman DS, Chertkow H, et al. The diagnosis of dementia due to Alzheimer's disease: recommendations from the National Institute on Aging-Alzheimer's Association workgroups on diagnostic guidelines for Alzheimer's disease. Alzheimers Dement. 2011; 7(3):263–269

[22] Sanchez-Catasus CA, Stormezand GN, van Laar PJ, De Deyn PP, Sanchez MA, Dierckx RA. FDG-PET for prediction of AD dementia in mild cognitive impairment. A review of the state of the art with particular emphasis on the comparison with other neuroimaging modalities (MRI and perfusion SPECT). Curr Alzheimer Res. 2017; 14(2):127–142

[23] Bohnen NI, Djang DS, Herholz K, Anzai Y, Minoshima S. Effectiveness and safety of 18F-FDG PET in the evaluation of dementia: a review of the recent literature. J Nucl Med. 2012; 53(1):59–71

[24] Bloudek LM, Spackman DE, Blankenburg M, Sullivan SD. Review and meta-analysis of biomarkers and diagnostic imaging in Alzheimer's disease. J Alzheimers Dis. 2011; 26(4):627–645

[25] Cure S, Abrams K, Belger M, Dell'agnello G, Happich M. Systematic literature review and meta-analysis of diagnostic test accuracy in Alzheimer's disease and other dementia using autopsy as standard of truth. J Alzheimers Dis. 2014; 42(1):169–182

[26] Frisoni GB, Bocchetta M, Chételat G, et al. ISTAART's Neuroimaging Professional Interest Area. Imaging markers for Alzheimer disease: which vs how. Neurology. 2013; 81(5):487–500

[27] Van Heertum RL, Tikofsky RS. Positron emission tomography and single-photon emission computed tomography brain imaging in the evaluation of dementia. Semin Nucl Med. 2003; 33(1):77–85

[28] Herholz K. Cerebral glucose metabolism in preclinical and prodromal Alzheimer's disease. Expert Rev Neurother. 2010; 10(11):1667–1673

[29] Nordberg A, Rinne JO, Kadir A, Långström B. The use of PET in Alzheimer disease. Nat Rev Neurol. 2010; 6(2):78–87

[30] Herholz K. Guidance for reading FDG PET scans in dementia patients. Q J Nucl Med Mol Imaging. 2014; 58(4):332–343

[31] Shivamurthy VK, Tahari AK, Marcus C, Subramaniam RM. Brain FDG PET and the diagnosis of dementia. AJR Am J Roentgenol. 2015; 204(1):W76–W85

[32] Coleman RE. Positron emission tomography diagnosis of Alzheimer's disease. Neuroimaging Clin N Am. 2005; 15(4):837–846, x

[33] Bonte FJ, Harris TS, Roney CA, Hynan LS. Differential diagnosis between Alzheimer's and frontotemporal disease by the posterior cingulate sign. J Nucl Med. 2004; 45(5):771–774

[34] Foster NL, Heidebrink JL, Clark CM, et al. FDG-PET improves accuracy in distinguishing frontotemporal dementia and Alzheimer's disease. Brain. 2007; 130(Pt 10):2616–2635

[35] Kato T, Inui Y, Nakamura A, Ito K. Brain fluorodeoxyglucose (FDG) PET in dementia. Ageing Res Rev. 2016; 30:73–84

[36] Womack KB, Diaz-Arrastia R, Aizenstein HJ, et al. Temporoparietal hypometabolism in frontotemporal lobar degeneration and associated imaging diagnostic errors. Arch Neurol. 2011; 68(3):329–337

[37] Kerrouche N, Herholz K, Mielke R, Holthoff V, Baron JC. 18FDG PET in vascular dementia: differentiation from Alzheimer's disease using voxel-based multivariate analysis. J Cereb Blood Flow Metab. 2006; 26(9):1213–1221

[38] Tullberg M, Fletcher E, DeCarli C, et al. White matter lesions impair frontal lobe function regardless of their location. Neurology. 2004; 63(2):246–253

[39] Gilman S, Koeppe RA, Little R, et al. Differentiation of Alzheimer's disease from dementia with Lewy bodies utilizing positron emission tomography with [18F]fluorodeoxyglucose and neuropsychological testing. Exp Neurol. 2005; 191 Suppl 1:S95–S103

[40] Graff-Radford J, Murray ME, Lowe VJ, et al. Dementia with Lewy bodies: basis of cingulate island sign. Neurology. 2014; 83(9):801–809

[41] Ishii K, Soma T, Kono AK, et al. Comparison of regional brain volume and glucose metabolism between patients with mild dementia with Lewy bodies and those with mild Alzheimer's disease. J Nucl Med. 2007; 48(5):704–711

[42] Koeppe RA, Gilman S, Joshi A, et al. 11C-DTBZ and 18F-FDG PET measures in differentiating dementias. J Nucl Med. 2005; 46(6):936–944

[43] Vander Borght T, Minoshima S, Giordani B, et al. Cerebral metabolic differences in Parkinson's and Alzheimer's diseases matched for dementia severity. J Nucl Med. 1997; 38(5):797–802

[44] Yong SW, Yoon JK, An YS, Lee PH. A comparison of cerebral glucose metabolism in Parkinson's disease, Parkinson's disease dementia and dementia with Lewy bodies. Eur J Neurol. 2007; 14(12):1357–1362

[45] Haense C, Herholz K, Jagust WJ, Heiss WD. Performance of FDG PET for detection of Alzheimer's disease in two independent multicentre samples (NEST-DD and ADNI). Dement Geriatr Cogn Disord. 2009; 28(3):259–266

[46] Ishii K, Minoshima S. PET is better than perfusion SPECT for early diagnosis of Alzheimer's disease: for. Eur J Nucl Med Mol Imaging. 2005; 32(12):1463–1465

[47] Kim EJ, Cho SS, Jeong Y, et al. Glucose metabolism in early onset versus late onset Alzheimer's disease: an SPM analysis of 120 patients. Brain. 2005; 128(Pt 8):1790–1801

[48] Ishibashi K, Onishi A, Fujiwara Y, Ishiwata K, Ishii K. Relationship between Alzheimer disease-like pattern of 18F-FDG and fasting plasma glucose levels in cognitively normal volunteers. J Nucl Med. 2015; 56(2):229–233

[49] Ishibashi K, Onishi A, Fujiwara Y, Ishiwata K, Ishii K. Plasma glucose levels affect cerebral 18F-FDG distribution in cognitively normal subjects with diabetes. Clin Nucl Med. 2016; 41(6):e274–e280

[50] Baker LD, Cross DJ, Minoshima S, Belongia D, Watson GS, Craft S. Insulin resistance and Alzheimer-like reductions in regional cerebral glucose metabolism for cognitively normal adults with prediabetes or early type 2 diabetes. Arch Neurol. 2011; 68(1):51–57

[51] Ishibashi K, Kawasaki K, Ishiwata K, Ishii K. Reduced uptake of 18F-FDG and 15O-H2O in Alzheimer's disease-related regions after glucose loading. J Cereb Blood Flow Metab. 2015; 35(8):1380–1385

33 Neurological Applications of Nonfluorodeoxyglucose Tracers

Mohsen Khosravi, Andrew B. Newberg, and Abass Alavi

33.1 Introduction

1. Since its introduction into clinical neurology practice, PET has been associated with the use of ^{18}F-fluorodeoxyglucose (FDG).[1]
2. FDG has been widely used in the identification of several types of dementia like Alzheimer's disease, epilepsy, movement disorders like Parkinsonism, and many other neurologic disorders.[2,3,4]
3. Despite the large field of application for FDG, unavoidably there are some drawbacks and limitations associated with the use of FDG in clinical neurology. For these reasons, expansion of the pool of non-FDG PET tracers available for use in neurology was considered of primary importance.[1]
4. Significant improvements and an increase in the growing number of available PET non-FDG and receptor-specific tracers have led to an increase in neurological applications of PET over the past decade.[1]
5. Non-FDG tracers currently available include amyloid tracers, fluorodopa, cerebral blood flow tracers, tumor tracers, and neurotransmitter-associated tracers.
6. Neurological disorders for which non-FDG PET tracers may be useful for include Alzheimer's disease and other dementias, Parkinson's disease and other movement disorders, seizures and epilepsy, brain tumors, and cerebrovascular disease.[2,3,4,5]
7. The basic requirements for neurological tracers are the ability to cross the blood–brain barrier (BBB; neutral; molecular weight [MW] < 700; log-*P*: 1.0–3.0) whether by free diffusion or by specific transport mechanisms, in vivo stability, high and selective binding affinity for the target receptor (IC50 < 10 nM), and high uptake in the brain.[5,6]
8. Of the numerous available PET tracers, a few have been selected that have been extensively studied and used in common neurologic disorders. ▶ Table 33.1 lists the most common PET radiotracers/ligands and their intended applications in clinical neurology.

The aim of this chapter is to provide a brief overview of the neurological application of the most commonly used non-FDG tracers and review the most promising developments in the field.

33.2 Indications

33.2.1 Alzheimer's Disease and Other Dementias

Accuracy/Comparison to Other Modalities

(^{11}C) Pittsburgh Compound B

1. A radiolabeled analog of thioflavin dye, which has been established as an effective biomarker for fibrillar β-amyloid in the human brain.[7]
2. The regional brain binding of [11]C Pittsburgh compound B (PiB) is highest in the frontal cortex, cingulate gyrus, precuneus, striatum, parietal cortex, and lateral temporal cortex studied in AD patients.[8]
3. Significant ^{11}C-PiB retention was reported in approximately 50 to 60% of individuals with mild cognitive impairment (MCI).[9]
4. The occipital cortex, sensorimotor cortex, and medial temporal cortex are usually spared.[8]
5. Sensitivity and specificity of ^{11}C-PiB for predicting progression from MCI to AD ranged from 83.3 to 100% and from 41.1 to 100%, with pooled estimates of 94.7 and 57.2%, respectively.
6. ^{11}C-PiB is strongly correlated with postmortem pathological results.[10]
7. PiB negativity indicated a 100% negative predictive value for progression to AD.[11]

[18]F-Florbetapir (Amyvid), ^{18}F-Flutemetamol (Vizamyl), and ^{18}F-Florbetaben (NeuraCeq)

1. All three ^{18}F-labeled amyloid-binding PET radiopharmaceuticals have been approved by the U.S. Food and Drug Administration (FDA) for clinical use.[12,13,14]
2. A positive amyloid PET shows uptake of radiotracer in the cortical gray matter and the

Table 33.1 Common non-FDG PET tracers used to study neurological disorders

Neurologic disorder	Tracer	Application area
Alzheimer's disease and other dementia	^{11}C-Pittsburgh compound B (PiB) ^{18}F-florbetapir (Amyvid) ^{18}F-flutemetamol (Vizamyl) ^{18}F-florbetaben (NeuraCeq)	Amyloid detection Amyloid detection Amyloid detection Amyloid detection
Parkinson's disease and other movement diseases	^{18}F-fluorodopa (FDOPA) ^{11}C-dihydrotetrabenazine (DTBZ) ^{18}F-dihydrotetrabenazine (DTBZ) ^{11}C-fluoropropyl (FP) ^{18}F-fluoropropyl (FP) ^{11}C-raclopride ^{11}C-SCH 23390 ^{11}C-NNC 756 N-[11C] methyl-4-piperidinyl propionate (^{11}C-PMP) N-[11C] methylpiperidin-4-yl acetate (^{11}C-MP4A) Carbon-11 WAY 100635	Presynaptic dopaminergic system Presynaptic dopaminergic system Presynaptic dopaminergic system Presynaptic dopaminergic system Presynaptic dopaminergic system D2 dopamine receptor activity D1 dopamine receptor activity D1 dopamine receptor activity Acetylcholinesterase activity Acetylcholinesterase activity Serotonin 5-HT1A receptor activity
Seizure and epilepsy	^{11}C-flumazenil (FMZ) ^{18}F-flumazenil (FMZ) ^{11}C-a-methyl tryptophan (AMT)	Benzodiazepine receptor activity Benzodiazepine receptor activity Serotonin synthesis
Brain tumors	[11C] L-methionine (MET) O-(2-[18F] fluoroethyl)-L-tyrosine (FET) 6-[18F] fluoro-3,4-dihydroxy-L-phenylalanine (FDOPA) 3'-deoxy-3'-fluorothymidine (^{18}F-FLT)	Amino acid metabolism Amino acid metabolism Amino acid metabolism DNA synthesis
Cerebrovascular disease	^{15}O-H$_2$O	Blood flow

negative image shows nonspecific uptake only in the white matter.[15]

3. Cortical retention of ^{18}F-labeled tracers was strongly correlated with that of ^{11}C-PiB.[16]

4. ^{18}F-flutemetamol had higher white matter retention, whereas ^{18}F-florbetapir had lower cortical retention compared to PiB.[16]

5. A positive amyloid PET raises confidence in the AD diagnosis and allows early and appropriate symptomatic treatment, yet negative amyloid PET reduces the probability of AD and helps prevent inappropriate treatment.[9]

6. The appropriate clinical indications of PET amyloid imaging by the Society of Nuclear Medicine, Amyloid Imaging Task Force and Molecular Imaging and the Alzheimer Association involve patients with persistent or progressive unexplained MCI, patients satisfying core clinical criteria for possible AD (atypical clinical course or etiologically mixed presentation), and patients with atypically young-onset dementia.[17]

7. Amyloid imaging also has a role in evaluation of patients with MCI: 70% chance of progression to AD over a 3-year period for positive amyloid scan and only a 10% chance in negative scans.[8]

8. Overall accuracy of amyloid imaging for AD is estimated to be more than 90% for patients younger than 70 years, about 85% for patients in their 70 s, and 75 to 80% for those older than 80 years.[8]

9. The sensitivity and specificity, compared with the clinical diagnosis of AD, for the ^{18}F-florbetapir scans were 95% for both.[18]

10. Amyloid imaging can be useful in differentiating AD from frontotemporal dementia that does not show significant amyloid deposition.[8]

11. Amyloid PET imaging may predict future hemorrhages, since cerebral amyloid angiopathy (CAA) related hemorrhages occur preferentially at sites of increased amyloid deposition.[19]

12. Amyloid PET is often positive in diffuse Lewy body disease (DLBD) patients with an uptake pattern similar to Alzheimer's disease.[20]

13. While FDG-PET is a marker of neurodegeneration, amyloid agents mark neuropathology; to date, no single diagnostic imaging is considered sufficient; maybe their combined interpretation may help the diagnosis of AD in a right clinical background.[21]

14. Neurodegeneration targeted by ^{18}F-FDG-PET as hypometabolism has been used extensively to study dementia and it may be an effective tool for early diagnosis and differentiation of various types of dementia.[22]

15. Temporoparietal glucose hypometabolism with frontal involvement in progressed disease has shown to be characteristic for Alzheimer's disease.[23]

16. The degree of hypometabolism may correlate with the severity of dementia.[24]

17. There has always been a controversy about the overall and relative efficacy of these PET agents with respect to FDG-PET in AD diagnosis (▶ Fig. 33.1).[25,26,27,28]

Pearls/Pitfalls

1. High-affinity and high-specificity binding to fibrillar amyloid.

2. Short half-life of [11]C (20 minutes) limits the use of ^{11}C-PiB to centers with an onsite cyclotron.[15]

3. Longer half-life (110 minutes) of ^{18}F-labeled tracers makes them commercially and widely available.[15]

4. Higher normal white matter uptake than ^{11}C-PiB.[15]

5. Significant ^{11}C-PiB retention was reported in approximately 30% of normal healthy older people, 18% of persons aged 60 to 69 years and in 65% of those older than 80 years, and the mean cortical binding potential for PiB rose in an age-dependent manner.[9,29]

6. A positive PET can also be seen in normal older individuals as well as in other medical conditions, such as DLBD and CAA.[9,29]

7. Some clinically diagnosed patients with AD were reported negative by ^{18}F-florbetapir PET

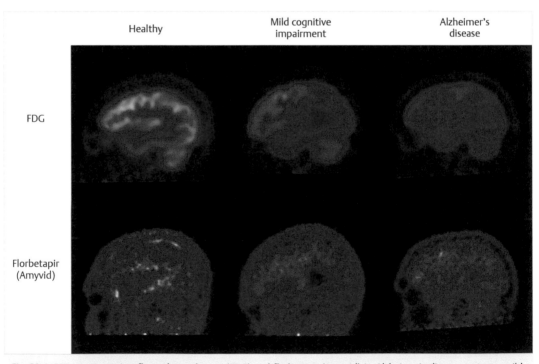

Fig. 33.1 PET imaging using fluorodeoxyglucose (FDG) and florbetapir (Amyvid) in Alzheimer's disease patients, mild cognitive impairment subjects, and health controls. FDG shows temporoparietal glucose hypometabolism, which has shown to be characteristic for Alzheimer's disease, while amyloid imaging with florbetapir (Amyvid) shows diffuse uptake pattern mostly denoted in the frontal lobe.

and 10 to 20% of clinically diagnosed patients with AD do not have amyloid disease at autopsy.[30]

8. False-positive results may be achieved in apparently healthy subjects and are found in 12% of those in their 60 s, 30% of those in their 70 s, and approximately 50% of those older than 80 years.[8]

33.2.2 Parkinson's Disease and Other Movement Disorders

Accuracy/Comparison to Other Modalities

Presynaptic

1. Dopamine is the key neurotransmitter in the nigrostriatal-pallidal-thalamo-cortical circuit. ^{18}F-fluorodopa (FDOPA) PET has been extensively used to study the integrity of nigrostriatal projections, as a marker for dopamine synthesis and storage in the presynaptic terminals.[31]

2. FDOPA uptake is reduced in idiopathic Parkinson's disease, which is most prominent in posterior putamen, which correlates with severity of symptoms, particularly rigidity and bradykinesia.[32]

3. Parkinson's disease is typically characterized by an asymmetric reduction in tracer uptake with a caudal to rostral gradient in which the posterior striatum is maximally affected (▶ Fig. 33.2).[33]

4. Extrastriatal FDOPA uptake increase in the dorsolateral prefrontal cortex, anterior cingulate, and pallidum has been shown at disease onset, but not in more advanced disease.[34]

5. There is progressive decline in FDOPA uptake in the striatum (posterior putamen) contralateral to the clinically most affected side as PD progresses and the caudate nucleus is also affected later.[35,36]

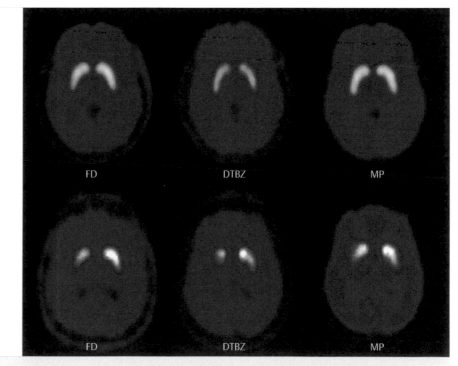

Fig. 33.2 PET images using presynaptic from a healthy control individual and a patient with Parkinson's disease. Parkinson's disease is typically characterized by an asymmetric reduction in tracer uptake with a caudal to rostral gradient in which the posterior striatum is maximally affected. FD, 6–18F-fluoro-levodopa; DTBZ, ^{11}C-dihydrotetrabenazine; MP, ^{11}C-d-threo-methylphenidate. (Reproduced with permission from The Lancet. Stoessl AJ, Lehericy S, Strafella AP. Imaging insights into basal ganglia function, Parkinson's disease, and dystonia. Lancet. 2014;384 (9942):532–544.)

6. Striatal FDOPA Ki is indicated to correlate with postmortem dopaminergic cell density in the substantia nigra.[37]

7. Diffuse loss of nigrostriatal dopaminergic projection is seen in multiple system atrophy (MSA) and progressive supranuclear palsy (PSP), as reflected by the symmetrical loss of FDOPA signal in the entire striatum.[38]

8. ^{11}C-dihydrotetrabenazine (DTBZ) and ^{18}F-DTBZ are used to image vesicular monoamine transporter 2 (VMAT2) and is considered a marker of nigrostriatal terminal density.

9. PET studies were utilized to assess the effects of therapeutic agents in PD. ^{18}F-DOPA was used to compare the therapeutic effect of ropinirole and L-DOPA on the rate of progression.

10. DTBZ shows decreased binding in caudate nucleus and anterior and posterior putamen in Parkinson's disease and DLBD compared with the healthy subjects and AD patients.[39]

11. ^{18}F-DTBZ PET images demonstrated that the reduction of VMAT2 availability was obviously correlated with the severity of disease in PD.[40]

12. 11C-fluoropropyl (FP), ^{18}F-FP and [11]C-2β-carbomethoxy-3β-(4-fluorophenyl)tropane, used to assess the availability of presynaptic dopamine transporters (DATs).

13. Presynaptic dopaminergic imaging can be useful in distinguishing psychogenic movement disorders from early idiopathic Parkinson's disease (PD and also for confirming the diagnosis of Parkinson's disease in a patient with atypical clinical features such as an early age of onset or to enable distinction from essential tremors.[31,41,42,43]

Postsynaptic

1. ^{11}C-raclopride studied for postsynaptic changes in basal ganglia, and binds to D2 receptors, while ^{11}C-SCH 23390 and ^{11}C-NNC 756 bind to D1 receptor.

2. While the uptake for ^{11}C-raclopride is preserved or increased in early PD, it is decreased in patients with atypical parkinsonism (MSA or PSP).[44]

3. ^{11}C-SCH 23390 (D1 receptor binding) uptake in the putamen was reported to be normal in early PD.[45]

4. ^{11}C-raclopride PET studies were helpful to assess motor fluctuations as a major disabling complication in the treatment of PD and to evaluate the effects of deep brain stimulation of the subthalamic nucleus.[46,47]

5. ^{11}C-raclopride PET was reported to be useful for assessing the therapeutic value and/or placebo effect of repetitive transcranial magnetic stimulation in patients with PD.[48]

6. Striatal D2 receptor binding decreases by approximately 5% per year in Huntington's disease, and the reduction correlates with the duration and clinical severity of the disease.[49]

Pearls/Pitfalls

1. In early Parkinson's disease, FDOPA may underestimate the degree of neuronal degeneration owing to compensatory upregulation of amino acid decarboxylase enzyme.[32]

2. Radiolabeled DATs are more sensitive than FDOPA in the early detection of PD, as decarboxylating enzyme upregulates as a compensatory phenomenon and the DAT is downregulated in the striatum.[50,51]

3. FDOPA PET is indicated to discriminate PD from the striatonigral degeneration form of MSA in 70% of cases and from PSP in 90% of cases; however, it is less effective in discriminating between the atypical Parkinsonian syndromes.[38]

33.2.3 Seizure and Epilepsy

Accuracy/Comparison to Other Modalities

1. ^{11}C-flumazenil (FMZ) PET, ^{18}F-FMZ PET, and ^{11}C-a-methyl tryptophan (AMT) PET have been mostly introduced as tracers to be studied in epilepsy.

2. One of the main clinical uses of PET in epilepsy is localization of epileptogenic foci in potential surgical candidates with partial seizures and corroborating findings from other investigational modalities such as electroencephalography (EEG) and MRI.[22]

3. Functional information delivered by PET and the morphologic information delivered by CT or MR are essential in presurgical evaluation of epilepsy.[52]

4. Flumazenil is a specific benzodiazepine antagonist, which is reversibly bound at the benzodiazepine binding sites of γ-aminobutyric acid (GABA)-A receptors.

5. In focal epilepsies, an average reduction of 30% has been reported in the GABA-A receptor density in the epileptogenic focus using ^{11}C-FMZ.[53]

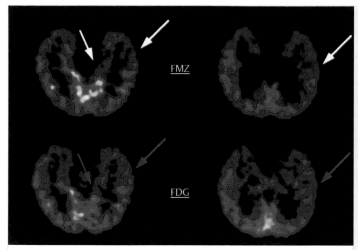

Fig. 33.3 Decreased ^{18}F-flumazenil (FMZ) binding extending outside the mesial temporal structure in a patient with temporal lobe epilepsy with MRI signs of mesial temporal sclerosis, left mesial and lateral temporal FMZ binding (*white arrows*) and a coextensive hypometabolism on FDG-PET (*green arrows*) which closely correspond with ictal onset zone. (Reproduced with permission from The Journal of Brain. Ryvlin P, Bouvard S, Le Bars D, et al. Clinical utility of flumazenil-PET versus [18F] fluorodeoxyglucose-PET and MRI in refractory partial epilepsy. A prospective study in 100 patients. Brain. 1998;121(11):2067–2081.)

6. The degree of decreased ^{11}C-FMZ binding has been indicated to correlate with seizure frequency (▶ Fig. 33.3).[54,55]

7. Increased uptake of ^{11}C-AMT is seen in epileptic foci, unlike FDG or FMZ, particularly in patients with tuberous sclerosis and cortical developmental malformations.[56]

8. The focus localizing abilities of ^{11}C-FMZ and ^{18}F-FDG PET were studied using extra- and intracranial EEG recordings as reference. ^{11}C-FMZ indicated to be more sensitive and accurate.[57]

9. PET may reduce the need for invasive EEG as part of the preoperative localization of surgical targets.[22]

10. PET is less useful clinically for primary generalized seizures.[22]

Pearls/Pitfalls

1. Correction for partial volume effects is considered mandatory when structural changes are present.[53,58]

2. Epileptogenic foci identified by FMZ-PET tend to be smaller than the areas of hypometabolism on FDG-PET.[59]

3. ^{18}F-FMZ may be recognized as one of the tracers of choice for patients with refractory epilepsy because of better sensitivity and anatomical resolution than FDG.[52]

4. Benzodiazepine-receptor scans appear "sharper" in comparison to FDG PET/CT scans.[52]

5. Patients with coma and vegetative state, motor neuron disease, and cerebral ischemia may have decreased FMZ binding.[60,61]

6. After a seizure, false lateralization may be seen in contralateral temporal lobe, reflecting rapid neuronal plasticity of GABA-A receptors.[62]

33.2.4 Brain Tumors

Accuracy/Comparison to Other Modalities

1. While the most widely used PET tracers for this application is still ^{18}F-FDG, radiolabeled amino acids (AAs) such as [11C] L-methionine (11C-MET); O-(2-[18F] fluoroethyl)-L-tyrosine (18F-FET); 6-[18F] fluoro-3,4-dihydroxy-L-phenylalanine (18F-FDOPA); and the nucleoside analogue 3′-deoxy-3′-fluorothymidine (18F-FLT) have the largest amount of supporting data for their efficacy, (methyl-11C)-L-methionine (11C-MET) is the most commonly used amino radiolabel.[63]

2. AAs may be the best suited for estimating gross tumor volumes and margins.[63]

3. AAs are more tumor specific as their uptake is less influenced by inflammation.[63]

4. Increased uptake of ^{11}C-MET, which reflects cellular amino acid uptake, is indicative of high-grade glioma and poorer survival.[64]

5. ^{11}C-MET indicated 89% sensitivity and 100% specificity in detecting malignant brain tumors and 92% sensitivity and 100% specificity for glioma.

6. 11C-MET is useful for discriminating between recurrences of local or metastatic tumors and radiation-induced changes with a sensitivity of 77.8% and specificity of 100% for differentiating

recurrence of metastatic brain tumors from postradiotherapy changes.

7. Brain lesions that show hypo- or isometabolism on FDG PET can be detected and differentiated with high sensitivity and good contrast using ^{11}C-methionine PET.[65]

8. An initial study demonstrated that uptake of ^{18}F-FET in brain tumors is similar to that of ^{11}C-methionine.[66]

9. In a study, both MET and FET differentiated tumor tissue and treatment-related changes with a sensitivity of 91% and a specificity of 100%. They provide comparable diagnostic information on gliomas and brain metastases.[67]

10. FET-PET can be used for differentiation of residual or recurrent tumor from treatment-related changes/pseudoprogression, as well as for delineation of gliomas.[67]

11. Combined use of ^{11}C-MET and ^{18}F-FDG-PET improves the accuracy of discrimination between recurrent tumor and postradiotherapy changes.[68]

12. ^{18}F-FET was able to distinguish between recurrent tumor and therapy-induced benign changes with 100% accuracy.[69]

13. ^{18}F-FDOPA indicated to be more sensitive and specific for evaluating recurrent tumors than was ^{18}F-FDG PET, particularly recurrent low-grade gliomas, as these tumors are difficult to evaluate by MRI and are usually not visible on ^{18}F-FDG PET scans (▶ Fig. 33.4a, b).[70]

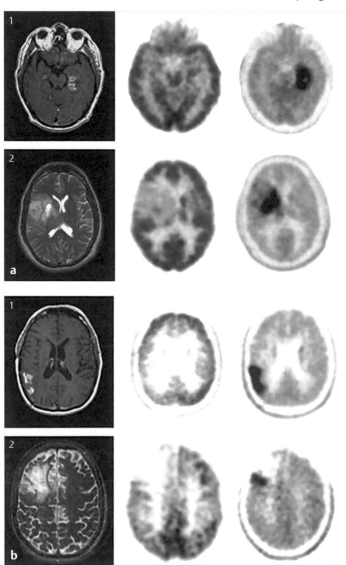

Fig. 33.4 (a) MRI (left), ^{18}F-fluorodeoxyglucose (FDG) PET (middle), and ^{18}F-fluorodopa (FDOPA) PET (right) of newly diagnosed tumors. (1) Glioblastoma. (2) Grade II oligodendroglioma. **(b)** MRI (left), ^{18}F-FDG PET (middle), and ^{18}F-FDOPA PET (right) for evaluating recurrent tumors. (1) Recurrent glioblastoma. (2) Recurrent grade II oligodendroglioma. (This figure was originally published in JNM. Chen W, Silverman DH, Delaloye S, et al. 18F-FDOPA PET imaging of brain tumors: comparison study with 18F-FDG PET and evaluation of diagnostic accuracy. J Nucl Med. 2006;47(6):904–911. © 2018 by the Society of Nuclear Medicine and Molecular Imaging, Inc.)

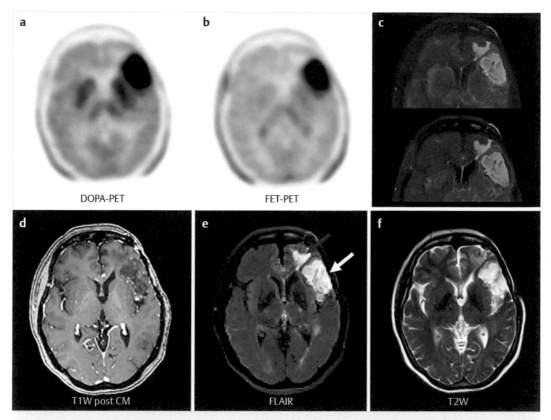

Fig. 33.5 A participant with low-grade glioma, which is rarely delineable in contrast-enhanced T1-weighted images **(d)**. The fluid-attenuated inversion recovery **(e)** and T2-weighted **(f)** sequences demonstrate elevated signal intensity in the anterior temporal **(e,** *white arrow*) and the lateral frontal lobe **(e,** *red arrow*) but cannot differentiate between tumor and edema. With both DOPA **(a)** and FET **(b)** PET, the malignant tissue was equally demarcated as presented in the fusion images **(c)**. (Adapted from Kratochwil et al.[74])

14. No significant difference in uptake between ^{18}F-FDOPA and ^{11}C-METwas found in either low- or high-grade tumors.[71]
15. ^{18}F-FDOPA had a sensitivity of 96% and a specificity of 43%, with an overall accuracy of 83% (95% confidence interval [CI]: 70–97%); it indicated to be more sensitive overall than ^{18}F-FDG in identifying tumors.
16. The increasing use of advanced MRI techniques and the introduction of integrated PET/MRI systems will facilitate the optimal use of both modalities for neuro-oncologic imaging, and multiparametric analysis of combined PET and MRI data may improve diagnostic accuracy in the evaluation of brain tumors before and after therapy.[72,73]
17. Patients with low-grade gliomas without striatum involvement may benefit from the higher contrast of FDOPA, whereas patients

with possible basal ganglia involvement should be examined with ^{18}F-FET irrespective of tumor grade. FDOPA-PET demonstrates superior contrast ratios for lesions outside the striatum, but FET-PET can provide additional information on tumor grading (▶ Fig. 33.5).[74]

Pearls/Pitfalls

1. Because of the short half-life of ^{11}C, in ^{11}C-MET the applicability of this tracer is limited to facilities with onsite cyclotrons.[75]
2. Superior contrast of AAs to that of ^{18}F-FDG because of the low uptake in normal brain tissue. This higher contrast proved useful in detecting low-grade and recurrent tumors.[76]
3. There are data supporting the superiority of radiolabeled AAs and ^{11}C-CHO over ^{18}F-FDG in distinguishing radiation necrosis from

recurrence in patients with primary and metastatic brain tumors.[63]

4. 11C-MET uptake may also be elevated in other conditions like cerebral hematoma or necrotic areas caused by radiotherapy.[77]

5. Tumor-to-background ratio (TBR) values on FET-PET are better in distinguishing between tumoral and nontumoral lesions, confirming the potential advantage of FET-PET over FDG-PET for brain lesion characterization.[78]

6. Generally, ^{18}F-FET PET has not been indicated to be useful in discriminating low- from high-grade tumors.[79]

33.2.5 Cerebrovascular Disease and Other Blood Flow Measurement Applications

Accuracy/Comparison to Other Modalities

1. ^{15}O-H$_2$O is helpful for quantification of regional cerebral blood flow (rCBF), which may be useful to characterize the altered brain perfusion in patients with cerebrovascular disease.

2. ^{15}O-H$_2$O PET and subsequently MR perfusion weighted imaging (PWI) have been used to study cerebral blood flow in reversible cerebral ischemia.[80]

3. ^{15}O-H$_2$O is useful for quantification of rCBF changes to detect network dysfunction in the brain.[81]

4. ^{15}O-H$_2$O PET has been able to detect perfusion changes in the prefrontal and parietal cortices of behavioral performance deficit in schizophrenia.[81,82]

5. Simultaneous ^{15}O-H$_2$O-PET/MRI is feasible in an acute-stroke setting without significantly delaying clinical pathways and without compromising the diagnostic quality of the MR data.[83]

6. ^{15}O-H$_2$O PET helps localizing the region of the epileptogenic focus, which shows an increase blood flow during the ictal period of partial seizures.[22]

7. fMRI requires one to measure the difference between an activated state and baseline. If this comparison must take place in a single scan, fMRI is impracticable for longitudinal studies, such as studying a patient before and after the treatment. With PET, images of changes in blood flow or regional cerebral glucose metabolism at different points in time can be compared. However, this is also now possible with perfusion MRI.[84]

8. rCBF measured with perfusion CT does contain perfusion information, but neither quantitative nor relative values can substitute rCBF measured by water PET.[85]

9. The practical application of ^{15}O-H$_2$O PET for stroke is challenging, because of problems in supplying a radiotracer with a short half-life within the right time frame to study cerebral hemodynamics throughout an acute stroke.[86]

Pearls/Pitfalls

1. The relative simplicity of producing both ^{15}O-H$_2$O and [15]C-O$_2$.[87]

2. The short half-life of [15]O (2.05 minutes), allowing for repeat measurements during one scanning session and/or combination of rCBF measurements with any other study.[87]

3. The partition coefficient of water being less dependent on pathology than that of most other tracers.[87]

4. The possibility to combine rCBF measurements with oxygen utilization measurements using [15]O$_2$, resulting in the same tracer characteristics for both measurements-circulating H$_2$[15]O for flow and H$_2$[15]O of metabolism for oxygen utilization, respectively.[87]

5. A potential drawback of H$_2$[15]O is the fact that water is not strictly freely diffusible. This might lead to underestimation of rCBF at high flow rates.[87]

6. Compared to fMRI (arterial spin labeling or blood oxygen level dependent), water PET is preferable in cases where movement, such as mastication, is unavoidable.[84,88]

7. Water PET has the advantage that the attenuation of annihilation radiation is less for the surface than central parts, while MRI has the relative disadvantage that the parts in contact with the air have a large susceptibility artifact.[84]

8. Also, if the action, thought, or experience being studied is not reliably replicable, it may be best captured by PET, which has a good signal-to-noise ratio (SNR) for a single trial.[84]

33.3 Conclusion

Overall, PET imaging has been utilized to assess a wide variety of neurologic and psychiatric disorders. Most of these imaging results still lie in the realm of research, helping understand the pathophysiology of different disorders, explore diagnostic criteria, and evaluate the effects of treatment.

Future studies will be needed to determine how the growing number of neurotransmitter ligands can be utilized in the study of neurologic disorders. Ultimately, identifying and validating clinical applications will be necessary so that PET imaging continues to play a key role in the management of neurologic disorders.

References

[1] Nanni C, Fantini L, Nicolini S, Fanti S. Non FDG PET. 2010; 65: 536–548

[2] Noble JM, Scarmeas N. Application of pet imaging to diagnosis of Alzheimer's disease and mild cognitive impairment. Int Rev Neurobiol. 2009; 84(9):133–149

[3] Peter J, Houshmand S, Werner TJ, Rubello D, Alavi A. Applications of global quantitative 18F-FDG-PET analysis in temporal lobe epilepsy. Nucl Med Commun. 2016; 37(3):223–230

[4] Meles SK, Teune LK, de Jong BM, Dierckx RA, Leenders KL. Metabolic imaging in Parkinson disease. J Nucl Med. 2017; 58 (1):23–28

[5] Pike VW. PET radiotracers: crossing the blood-brain barrier and surviving metabolism. Trends Pharmacol Sci. 2009; 30 (8):431–440

[6] Pimlott SL, Sutherland A. Molecular tracers for the PET and SPECT imaging of disease. Chem Soc Rev. 2011; 40(1):149–162

[7] Klunk WE, Engler H, Nordberg A, et al. Imaging brain amyloid in Alzheimer's disease with Pittsburgh Compound-B. Ann Neurol. 2004; 55(3):306–319

[8] Rowe CC, Villemagne VL. Brain amyloid imaging. J Nucl Med Technol. 2013; 41(1):11–18

[9] Fodero-Tavoletti MT, Cappai R, McLean CA, et al. Amyloid imaging in Alzheimer's disease and other dementias. Brain Imaging Behav. 2009; 3(3):246–261

[10] Ikonomovic MD, Abrahamson EE, Price JC, et al. Early AD pathology in a [C-11]PiB-negative case: a PiB-amyloid imaging, biochemical, and immunohistochemical study. Acta Neuropathol. 2012; 123(3):433–447

[11] Nordberg A, Carter SF, Rinne J, et al. A European multicentre PET study of fibrillar amyloid in Alzheimer's disease. Eur J Nucl Med Mol Imaging. 2013; 40(1):104–114

[12] Yang L, Rieves D, Ganley C. Brain amyloid imaging–FDA approval of florbetapir F18 injection. N Engl J Med. 2012; 367 (10):885–887

[13] World Molecular Imaging Society. FDA Approves Piramal Imaging's NeuraceqTM (florbetaben F18 injection) for PET Imaging of Beta-Amyloid Neuritic Plaques in the Brain. Available at: http://www.wmis.org/fda-approves-piramal-imagings-neuraceqtm-florbetaben-f18-injection-for-pet-imaging-of-beta-amyloid-neuritic-plaques-in-the-brain/. Accessed July 29, 2017

[14] Garber K. First FDA-approved beta-amyloid diagnostic hits the market. Nat Biotechnol. 2012; 30(7):575–575

[15] Sarikaya I. PET imaging in neurology: Alzheimer's and Parkinson's diseases. Nucl Med Commun. 2015; 36(8):775–781

[16] Landau SM, Thomas BA, Thurfjell L, et al. Alzheimer's Disease Neuroimaging Initiative. Amyloid PET imaging in Alzheimer's disease: a comparison of three radiotracers. Eur J Nucl Med Mol Imaging. 2014; 41(7):1398–1407

[17] Johnson KA, Minoshima S, Bohnen NI, et al. Guidelines for brain amyloid imaging published. J Nucl Med. 2013; 54(3):476–490

[18] Newberg AB, Arnold SE, Wintering N, Rovner BW, Alavi A. Initial clinical comparison of 18F-florbetapir and 18F-FDG PET in patients with Alzheimer disease and controls. J Nucl Med. 2012; 53(6):902–907

[19] Gurol ME, Dierksen G, Betensky R, et al. Predicting sites of new hemorrhage with amyloid imaging in cerebral amyloid angiopathy. Neurology. 2012; 79(4):320–326

[20] Gomperts SN, Rentz DM, Moran E, et al. Imaging amyloid deposition in Lewy body diseases. Neurology. 2008; 71(12): 903–910

[21] McKhann GM, Knopman DS, Chertkow H, et al. The diagnosis of dementia due to Alzheimer's disease: recommendations from the National Institute on Aging-Alzheimer's Association workgroups on diagnostic guidelines for Alzheimer's disease. Alzheimers Dement. 2011; 7(3):263–269

[22] Tai YF, Piccini P. Applications of positron emission tomography (PET) in neurology. J Neurol Neurosurg Psychiatry. 2004; 75(5):669–676

[23] Salmon E. Functional brain imaging applications to differential diagnosis in the dementias. Curr Opin Neurol. 2002; 15 (4):439–444

[24] Mazziotta JC, Frackowiak RSJ, Phelps ME. The use of positron emission tomography in the clinical assessment of dementia. Semin Nucl Med. 1992; 22(4):233–246

[25] Kepe V, Moghbel MC, Långström B, et al. Amyloid-β positron emission tomography imaging probes: a critical review. J Alzheimers Dis. 2013; 36(4):613–631

[26] Moghbel MC, Saboury B, Basu S, et al. Amyloid-β imaging with PET in Alzheimer's disease: is it feasible with current radiotracers and technologies? Eur J Nucl Med Mol Imaging. 2012; 39(2):202–208

[27] Villemagne VL, Doré V, Bourgeat P, et al. Aβ-amyloid and tau imaging in dementia. Semin Nucl Med. 2017; 47(1):75–88

[28] Villemagne VL, Klunk WE, Mathis CA, et al. Aβ Imaging: feasible, pertinent, and vital to progress in Alzheimer's disease. Eur J Nucl Med Mol Imaging. 2012; 39(2):209–219

[29] Rowe CC, Ellis KA, Rimajova M, et al. Amyloid imaging results from the Australian Imaging, Biomarkers and Lifestyle (AIBL) study of aging. Neurobiol Aging. 2010; 31(8):1275–1283

[30] Lim A, Tsuang D, Kukull W, et al. Clinico-neuropathological correlation of Alzheimer's disease in a community-based case series. J Am Geriatr Soc. 1999; 47(5):564–569

[31] Brooks DJ, Pavese N. Imaging biomarkers in Parkinson's disease. Prog Neurobiol. 2011; 95(4):614–628

[32] Ishikawa T, Dhawan V, Chaly T, et al. Clinical significance of striatal DOPA decarboxylase activity in Parkinson's disease. J Nucl Med. 1996; 37(2):216–222

[33] Stoessl AJ, Lehericy S, Strafella AP. Imaging insights into basal ganglia function, Parkinson's disease, and dystonia. Lancet. 2014; 384(9942):532–544

[34] Kaasinen V, Någren K, Hietala J, et al. Extrastriatal dopamine D2 and D3 receptors in early and advanced Parkinson's disease. Neurology. 2000; 54(7):1482–1487

[35] Brooks DJ, Ibanez V, Sawle GV, et al. Differing patterns of striatal 18F-dopa uptake in Parkinson's disease, multiple system atrophy, and progressive supranuclear palsy. Ann Neurol. 1990; 28(4):547–555

[36] Brooks DJ. PET studies on the early and differential diagnosis of Parkinson's disease. Neurology. 1993; 43(12) Suppl 6:S6–S16

[37] Snow BJ, Tooyama I, McGeer EG, et al. Human positron emission tomographic [18F]fluorodopa studies correlate with dopamine cell counts and levels. Ann Neurol. 1993; 34(3): 324–330

[38] Burn DJ, Sawle GV, Brooks DJ. Differential diagnosis of Parkinson's disease, multiple system atrophy, and Steele-Richardson-

Olszewski syndrome: discriminant analysis of striatal 18F-dopa PET data. J Neurol Neurosurg Psychiatry. 1994; 57(3):278–284

[39] Koeppe RA, Gilman S, Junck L, Wernette K, Frey KA. Differentiating Alzheimer's disease from dementia with Lewy bodies and Parkinson's disease with (+)-[11C]dihydrotetrabenazine positron emission tomography. Alzheimers Dement. 2008; 4 (1) Suppl 1:S67–S76

[40] Hsiao I-T, Weng Y-H, Hsieh C-J, et al. Correlation of Parkinson disease severity and 18F-DTBZ positron emission tomography. JAMA Neurol. 2014; 71(6):758–766

[41] Stoessl AJ, Martin WW, McKeown MJ, Sossi V. Advances in imaging in Parkinson's disease. Lancet Neurol. 2011; 10(11):987–1001

[42] Burn DJ, Mark MH, Playford ED, et al. Parkinson's disease in twins studied with 18F-dopa and positron emission tomography. Neurology. 1992; 42(10):1894–1900

[43] Piccini P, Morrish PK, Turjanski N, et al. Dopaminergic function in familial Parkinson's disease: a clinical and 18F-dopa positron emission tomography study. Ann Neurol. 1997; 41 (2):222–229

[44] Brooks DJ, Ibanez V, Sawle GV, et al. Striatal D2 receptor status in patients with Parkinson's disease, striatonigral degeneration, and progressive supranuclear palsy, measured with 11C-raclopride and positron emission tomography. Ann Neurol. 1992; 31(2):184–192

[45] Shinotoh H, Inoue O, Hirayama K, Aotsuka A. Dopamine D1 receptors in Parkinson's disease and striatonigral degeneration: a positron emission tomography study. J Neurol Neurosurg Psychiatry. 1993; 56(5):467–472

[46] La Fuente-Fernández D, Lu J, Sossi V. Biochemical variations in the synaptic level of dopamine precede motor fluctuations in Parkinson's disease: PET evidence of increased dopamine turnover. Ann Neurol. 2001; 49:298–303

[47] Nimura T, Yamaguchi K, Ando T, Shibuya S. Attenuation of fluctuating striatal synaptic dopamine levels in patients with Parkinson disease in response to subthalamic nucleus stimulation: a positron emission. J Neurol Neurosurg. 2005; 117 (1):1968–1973

[48] Kim J, Chung E, Lee W, Shin H. Therapeutic effect of repetitive transcranial magnetic stimulation in Parkinson's disease: analysis of raclopride PET study. Mov Disord. 2008; 23(2):207–211

[49] Pavese N, Andrews TC, Brooks DJ, et al. Progressive striatal and cortical dopamine receptor dysfunction in Huntington's disease: a PET study. Brain. 2003; 126(Pt 5):1127–1135

[50] Lee CS, Samii A, Sossi V, et al. In vivo positron emission tomographic evidence for compensatory changes in presynaptic dopaminergic nerve terminals in Parkinson's disease. Ann Neurol. 2000; 47(4):493–503

[51] Brooks DJ, Frey KA, Marek KL, et al. Assessment of neuroimaging techniques as biomarkers of the progression of Parkinson's disease. Exp Neurol. 2003; 184 Suppl 1:S68–S79

[52] Hodolic M, Topakian R, Pichler R. (18)F-fluorodeoxyglucose and (18)F-flumazenil positron emission tomography in patients with refractory epilepsy. Radiol Oncol. 2016; 50(3):247–253

[53] Hammers A. Flumazenil positron emission tomography and other ligands for functional imaging. Neuroimaging Clin N Am. 2004; 14(3):537–551

[54] Savic I, Svanborg E, Thorell JO. Cortical benzodiazepine receptor changes are related to frequency of partial seizures: a positron emission tomography study. Epilepsia. 1996; 37(3):236–244

[55] Ryvlin P, Bouvard S, Le Bars D, et al. Clinical utility of flumazenil-PET versus [18F]fluorodeoxyglucose-PET and MRI in refractory partial epilepsy. A prospective study in 100 patients. Brain. 1998; 121(Pt 11):2067–2081

[56] Rubí S, Costes N, Heckemann RA, et al. Positron emission tomography with α-[11C]methyl-L-tryptophan in tuberous sclerosis complex-related epilepsy. Epilepsia. 2013; 54(12):2143–2150

[57] Savic I, Ingvar M, Stone-Elander S. Comparison of [11C]flumazenil and [18F]FDG as PET markers of epileptic foci. J Neurol Neurosurg Psychiatry. 1993; 56(6):615–621

[58] Koepp MJ, Hand KSP, Labbé C, et al. In vivo [11C]flumazenil-PET correlates with ex vivo [3H]flumazenil autoradiography in hippocampal sclerosis. Ann Neurol. 1998; 43(5):618–626

[59] Muzik O, da Silva EA, Juhasz C, et al. Intracranial EEG versus flumazenil and glucose PET in children with extratemporal lobe epilepsy. Neurology. 2000; 54(1):171–179

[60] Heiss W-D. PET in coma and in vegetative state. Eur J Neurol. 2012; 19(2):207–211

[61] Heiss WD. The ischemic penumbra: how does tissue injury evolve? Ann N Y Acad Sci. 2012; 1268(1):26–34

[62] Ryvlin P, Bouvard S, Le Bars D, Mauguière F. Transient and falsely lateralizing flumazenil-PET asymmetries in temporal lobe epilepsy. Neurology. 1999; 53(8):1882–1885

[63] Sharma A, McConathy J. Overview of PET tracers for brain tumor imaging. PET Clin. 2013; 8(2):129–146

[64] De Witte O, Goldberg I, Wikler D, et al. Positron emission tomography with injection of methionine as a prognostic factor in glioma. J Neurosurg. 2001; 95(5):746–750

[65] Chung J-K, Kim YK, Kim SK, et al. Usefulness of 11C-methionine PET in the evaluation of brain lesions that are hypo- or isometabolic on 18F-FDG PET. Eur J Nucl Med Mol Imaging. 2002; 29(2):176–182

[66] Weber WA, Wester H-J, Grosu AL, et al. O-(2-[18F]fluoroethyl)-L-tyrosine and L-[methyl-11C]methionine uptake in brain tumours: initial results of a comparative study. Eur J Nucl Med. 2000; 27(5):542–549

[67] Grosu AL, Astner ST, Riedel E, et al. An interindividual comparison of O-(2-[18F]fluoroethyl)-L-tyrosine (FET)- and L-[methyl-11C]methionine (MET)-PET in patients with brain gliomas and metastases. Int J Radiat Oncol Biol Phys. 2011; 81(4):1049–1058

[68] Ogawa T, Kanno I, Shishido F, et al. Clinical value of PET with 18F-fluorodeoxyglucose and L-methyl-11C-methionine for diagnosis of recurrent brain tumor and radiation injury. Acta Radiol. 1991; 32(3):197–202

[69] Pöpperl G, Götz C, Rachinger W, Gildehaus FJ, Tonn JC, Tatsch K. Value of O-(2-[18F]fluoroethyl)- L-tyrosine PET for the diagnosis of recurrent glioma. Eur J Nucl Med Mol Imaging. 2004; 31(11):1464–1470

[70] Chen W, Silverman DH, Delaloye S, et al. 18F-FDOPA PET imaging of brain tumors: comparison study with 18F-FDG PET and evaluation of diagnostic accuracy. J Nucl Med. 2006; 47(6):904–911

[71] Becherer A, Karanikas G, Szabó M, et al. Brain tumour imaging with PET: a comparison between [18F]fluorodopa and [11C]methionine. Eur J Nucl Med Mol Imaging. 2003; 30(11):1561–1567

[72] Neuner I, Kaffanke J, Langen K, Kops E. Multimodal imaging utilising integrated MR-PET for human brain tumour assessment. Eur Radiol. 2012; 22(12):2568–2580

[73] Bisdas S, Ritz R, Bender B, et al. Metabolic mapping of gliomas using hybrid MR-PET imaging: feasibility of the method and spatial distribution of metabolic changes. Invest Radiol. 2013; 48(5):295–301

[74] Kratochwil C, Combs SE, Leotta K, et al. Intra-individual comparison of 18F-FET and 18F-DOPA in PET imaging of recurrent brain tumors. Neuro-oncol. 2014; 16(3):434–440

[75] Ricci PE, Karis JP, Heiserman JE, Fram EK, Bice AN, Drayer BP. Differentiating recurrent tumor from radiation necrosis: time

for re-evaluation of positron emission tomography? AJNR Am J Neuroradiol. 1998; 19(3):407–413

[76] Herholz K, Hölzer T, Bauer B, et al. 11C-methionine PET for differential diagnosis of low-grade gliomas. Neurology. 1998; 50(5):1316–1322

[77] Dethy S, Goldman S, Blecic S, Luxen A, Levivier M, Hildebrand J. Carbon-11-methionine and fluorine-18-FDG PET study in brain hematoma. J Nucl Med. 1994; 35(7):1162–1166

[78] Dunet V, Pomoni A, Hottinger A, Nicod-Lalonde M, Prior JO. Performance of 18F-FET versus 18F-FDG-PET for the diagnosis and grading of brain tumors: systematic review and meta-analysis. Neuro-oncol. 2016; 18(3):426–434

[79] Weckesser M, Langen KJ, Rickert CH, et al. O-(2-[18F]fluorethyl)-L-tyrosine PET in the clinical evaluation of primary brain tumours. Eur J Nucl Med Mol Imaging. 2005; 32(4): 422–429

[80] Barber PA, Consolo HK, Yang Q, et al. Comparison of MRI perfusion imaging and single photon emission computed tomography in chronic stroke. Cerebrovasc Dis. 2001; 11(2):128–136

[81] Seok J-H, Park H-J, Lee J-D, et al. Regional cerebral blood flow changes and performance deficit during a sustained attention task in schizophrenia: (15) O-water positron emission tomography. Psychiatry Clin Neurosci. 2012; 66(7):564–572

[82] Lahti AC, Holcomb HH, Medoff DR, Weiler MA, Tamminga CA, Carpenter WT, Jr. Abnormal patterns of regional cerebral blood flow in schizophrenia with primary negative symptoms during an effortful auditory recognition task. Am J Psychiatry. 2001; 158(11):1797–1808

[83] Werner P, Saur D, Lobsien D, Zeisig V. Feasibility of combined H2O-PET/MRI in patients with acute stroke. J Nucl Med. 2013; 54:87

[84] Kameyama M, Murakami K, Jinzaki M. Comparison of [15O] H2O positron emission tomography and functional magnetic resonance imaging in activation studies. World J Nucl Med. 2016; 15(1):3–6

[85] Grüner JM, Paamand R, Højgaard L, Law I. Brain perfusion CT compared with 15O-H2O-PET in healthy subjects. EJNMMI Res. 2011; 1:28

[86] Werner P, Saur D, Zeisig V, et al. Simultaneous PET/MRI in stroke: a case series. J Cereb Blood Flow Metab. 2015; 35(9): 1421–1425

[87] Lammertsma AA, Frackowiak RS, Hoffman JM, et al. The C15O2 build-up technique to measure regional cerebral blood flow and volume of distribution of water. J Cereb Blood Flow Metab. 1989; 9(4):461–470

[88] Momose T, Nishikawa J, Watanabe T, et al. Effect of mastication on regional cerebral blood flow in humans examined by positron-emission tomography with 15O-labelled water and magnetic resonance imaging. Arch Oral Biol. 1997; 42(1):57–61

34 Cardiac PET and PET/CT

Amol Takalkar, Umesh Sharma, and Eugene C. Lin

34.1 Myocardial Perfusion Assessment

Myocardial perfusion assessment at rest and with stress (exercise or pharmacologic) is important in patients with known or suspected coronary artery disease (CAD). The new SNMMI-ASNC position statement on myocardial perfusion PET imaging[1,2,3] upgrades PET to a "**Preferred**" test for patients who meet criteria for stress imaging but are unable to complete a diagnostic level of exercise. The statement also identifies five distinct clinical situations where cardiac PET is "**Recommended**":

- Poor quality, equivocal, or inconclusive prior stress-imaging study.
- Patients with certain body characteristics that commonly affect image quality.
- Higher-risk patients.
- Younger patients to minimize accumulated lifetime radiation exposure.
- When myocardial blood flow quantification is identified by clinicians to be a needed adjunct to the image findings.

Single-photon emission tomography (SPECT) myocardial perfusion imaging (MPI) with thallium or technetium-99m-labeled agents is routinely practiced. However, SPECT imaging has several limitations and MPI with PET is superior to SPECT,[4] making it a key nuclear cardiology test in the current era of high-value initiatives for appropriate patients, in theory supporting the Center for Medicare and Medicaid Services' (CMS) initiatives to improve the quality and efficiency of health care while controlling costs. In practice, PET MPI is constrained by the need for an onsite cyclotron to perform nitrogen-13 (^{13}N) ammonia imaging. Rubidium-82 (^{82}Rb) chloride imaging can be performed with a generator. Given the cost of the generator and current reimbursements, approximately six studies a day may need to be performed for PET to be cost-effective. An ^{18}F-labeled PET myocardial perfusion agent could potentially circumvent these issues with ^{13}N ammonia (need for onsite cyclotron) and ^{82}Rb chloride (need to lease a generator necessity steady patient volume) by providing single patient ready doses on an as-needed basis, but is still not clinically available.

34.1.1 Tracers

^{13}N ammonia (cyclotron-produced) and ^{82}Rb chloride (generator produced) are Food and Drug Administration (FDA) approved PET radiopharmaceuticals for assessing myocardial blood flow. ^{18}F-flurpiridaz remains an investigational product in phase III trials, still not FDA approved, and is awaiting further development and commercialization. Oxygen-15 (^{15}O) labeled water and ^{62}Cu-pyruvaldehyde bis (N4-methylthiosemicarbazone) (Cu-PTSM) can also be used but are mostly restricted to the research setting.

^{82}Rb can be eluted from a strontium-82 generator, which needs to be replaced approximately every 4 weeks. The half-life of ^{82}Rb is 75 seconds.

^{13}N ammonia has a half-life of approximately 10 minutes.

The advantages of ^{82}Rb are that a cyclotron is not needed, and it is ideal for peak dipyridamole or regadenoson stress gated imaging. ^{82}Rb as imaging typically starts 90 to 120 seconds after injection compared with 3 to 5 minutes with ^{13}N ammonia. The disadvantages are poorer resolution (due to a positron range of 2.6 mm), lower extraction, and more difficulty with quantitation compared with ^{13}N ammonia. It is also very difficult to perform exercise stress testing with ^{82}Rb, given the short half-life of the tracer.

34.1.2 Protocols

Generally, similar protocols (except for dose of radiotracer and imaging time and duration) to those used for SPECT are followed; however, usually pharmacologic stress testing is performed. Exercise stress testing is difficult due to the short half-life of the tracers. With ^{13}N ammonia, exercise stress testing can be done, but it requires meticulous coordination and setup. The images are displayed and reviewed similar to the cardiac SPECT images (▶ Fig. 34.1 and ▶ Fig. 34.2).

34.1.3 Accuracy and Comparison with Other Modalities

PET imaging provides better spatial and temporal resolution and hence is better suited in patients with thick/muscular chest wall, large breast tissue, or overall body habitus that frequently leads to

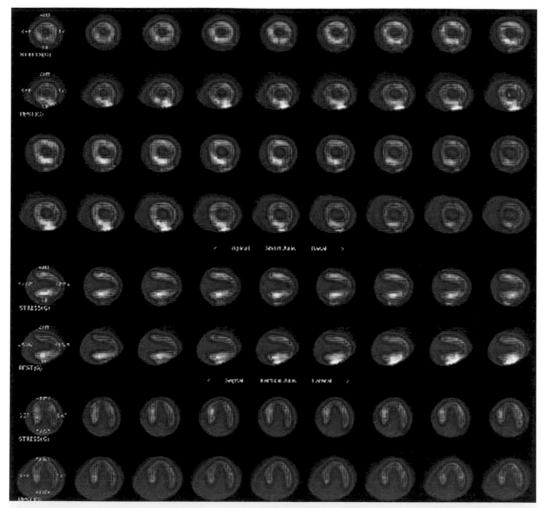

Fig. 34.1 Rest and dipyridamole stress myocardial perfusion PET rubidium-82 images displayed conventionally in the short, vertical, and horizontal long axes, showing normal myocardial perfusion at rest and stress. (This image is provided courtesy of Elias Botvinick, MD, San Francisco, CA.)

indeterminate SPECT myocardial perfusion studies (▶ Fig. 34.3). Due to the short half-life of the PET tracers, pure stress-related images uncontaminated by the prior rest injection can be obtained. Unlike gated SPECT, left ventricular (LV) ejection fraction can be assessed at peak stress, as imaging is performed soon after injection. PET imaging, with absolute quantification of regional radiotracer uptake, is better suited when serial studies are required to assess perfusion in a particular myocardial segment. It also allows better evaluation of endothelial dysfunction and coronary flow reserve as a measure of coronary stenosis. Moreover, PET allows for more efficient imaging protocols, leading to faster studies (around 45 minutes

compared with 3 to 4 hours for SPECT studies) and lower radiation exposure.

Numerous studies have shown that myocardial perfusion PET has higher accuracy,[5] sensitivity,[6] and specificity[7] compared with SPECT.

34.1.4 Pitfalls

1. If ^{13}N ammonia is used for perfusion imaging, there is decreased lateral wall activity (on stress and rest images) in ~10% of normal patients. The etiology of this is unknown.
2. Decreased activity in the apex (on stress and rest) is a normal variant, probably related to partial volume artifact due to

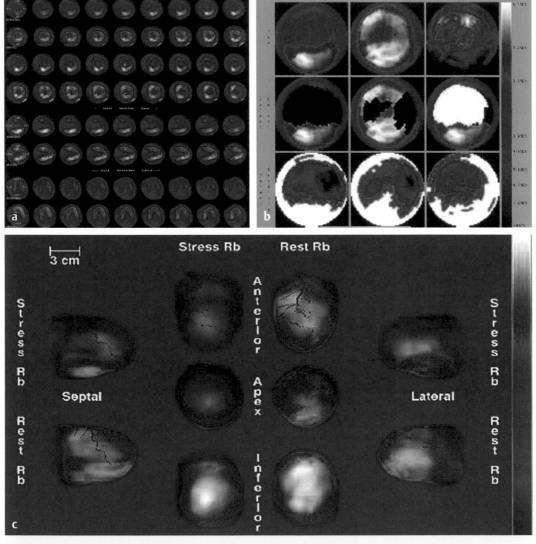

Fig. 34.2 (a) Rest and dipyridamole stress myocardial perfusion PET rubidium-82 images showing a large region of ischemia in the anterior wall, anterior septum, and anterior and midlateral walls and gross stress-induced cavitary dilation by conventional display. (b) The polar map shows the defect distribution and magnitude. (c) A model 3D ventricle fused with a model coronary tree (can be patient's own coronary tree if the patient had undergone a PET study with CT coronary angiography) showing the extent and density of the abnormality. (These images are provided courtesy of Elias Botvinick, MD, San Francisco, CA.)

apical thinning relative to the remainder of the myocardium. It can be seen with ^{82}Rb or ^{13}N ammonia—often more evident with ^{13}N-ammonia and with time-of-flight (TOF) cameras.

3. Misregistration artifact during a cardiac PET/CT scan can result in artifactual defects (see Pitfalls in Myocardial Viability section).

34.2 Myocardial Viability

1. PET imaging with fluorodeoxyglucose (FDG) with MPI is the current gold standard for the assessment of myocardial viability.
2. Demonstration of significant viable myocardium in a patient with chronic ischemic heart disease with left ventricular (LV)

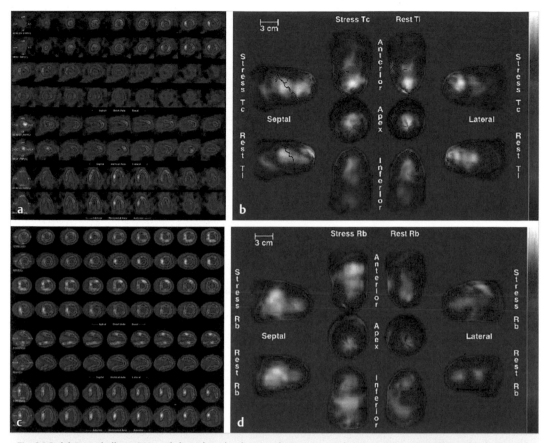

Fig. 34.3 (a) Rest thallium-201 and dipyridamole pharmacologic stress technetium-99 m sestamibi single-photon emission tomography myocardial perfusion images of an obese 63-year-old woman with atypical chest pain showing irregular uptake with an apparent fixed inferior wall defect with possible stress-induced abnormality in the lateral wall, **(b)** also well seen on the model left ventricular display. **(c)** A repeat pharmacologic stress imaging study performed with PET shows normal rest and stress perfusion **(d)** with normal ventricular model of myocardial uptake. (These images are provided courtesy of Elias Botvinick, MD, San Francisco, CA.)

dysfunction indicates a need for prompt revascularization and predicts low perioperative mortality and morbidity, significant improvement in left ventricular ejection fraction (LVEF) and congestive heart failure (CHF) symptoms, and improved survival.

3. Absence of viable myocardium in a patient with chronic ischemic heart disease with LV dysfunction supports the decision for medical management and/or cardiac transplantation.

34.2.1 Clinical Scenario

Patients with severe LV dysfunction and CAD continue to pose a significant management dilemma to clinicians who frequently need to choose between aggressive medical treatment and revascularization therapy.[8] Revascularization therapy results in better long-term survival rates, and several investigators have demonstrated the benefit of revascularization in CAD patients with poor LV function.[9,10,11,12,13,14,15,16,17] However, it is associated with significant periprocedure morbidity and mortality, making identification and selection of only those patients who will benefit maximally from revascularization extremely crucial. Improvement in the LV function after revascularization is mainly dependent on the reversibility of contractile dysfunction. Dysfunctional but "viable" myocardium is said to be reversibly dysfunctional, whereas scar tissue usually results in nonreversibly dysfunctional myocardium. Thus, accurate

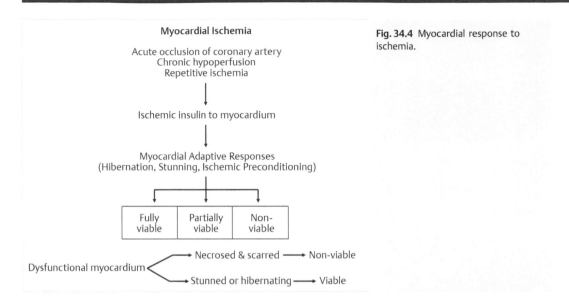

Fig. 34.4 Myocardial response to ischemia.

identification of myocardial viability is a critical component in the diagnostic workup of these patients.

34.2.2 Mechanism of Myocardial Ischemia

Myocardial ischemia may result from acute coronary artery occlusion or from chronic hypoperfusion or repetitive ischemic processes. The severity and duration of myocardial ischemia will determine the myocardial response to the ischemic process. Although the myocardium has several immediate as well as sustained mechanisms of adaptations (e.g., hibernation, stunning, and ischemic preconditioning[18,19,20]) to withstand acute and chronic ischemia, the end result of ischemic injury is a mechanically dysfunctional myocardium. The dysfunctional myocardium may be related to ischemic but viable myocardium, such as stunned or hibernating myocardium or necrosed and scarred myocardium that may be completely nonviable (▶ Fig. 34.4).

34.2.3 Identification of Myocardial Viability by PET

The normal myocardium preferentially uses free fatty acids (FFAs) as energy substrates during normal fasting conditions. During hypoxia and ischemia, FFA oxidation is markedly decreased, and the rate of anaerobic glycolysis is enhanced. Thus, the ischemic myocardium uses glucose in

preference to FFAs as the energy substrate.[21,22,23,24,25,26,27,28,29,30] FDG-PET can reliably and accurately assess the initial steps of glucose metabolism in the ischemic myocardium by evaluating myocardial glucose uptake. The protocol for assessing myocardial viability using PET and ^{13}N ammonia for MPI and FDG for myocardial metabolism imaging is depicted in ▶ Fig. 34.5.

Using the combination of myocardial blood flow and myocardial metabolism, three possible patterns have been described in the dysfunctional myocardium: (1) normal myocardial blood flow and FDG activity; (2) decreased myocardial blood flow with normal or increased FDG activity —"flow-metabolism mismatch" (▶ Fig. 34.6); and (3) decreased myocardial blood flow and FDG activity—"matched defect" (▶ Fig. 34.7).[8,31] The first two patterns represent viable myocardium; the third pattern represents nonviable myocardium. The flow-metabolism mismatch pattern is considered to be the scintigraphic hallmark of dysfunctional, ischemic, but viable myocardium.

34.2.4 Accuracy and Comparison with Other Modalities

Methods to Assess Myocardial Viability

Myocardial viability can be assessed by several imaging modalities that assess different biological characteristics of the myocardium.

N-13 AMMONIA / F-18 FDG IMAGING

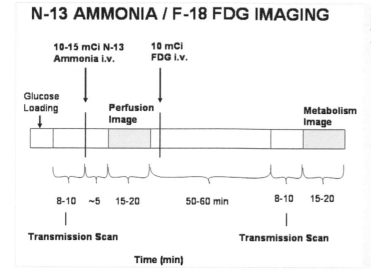

Fig. 34.5 Protocol to assess myocardial viability with PET. FDG, fluorodeoxyglucose.

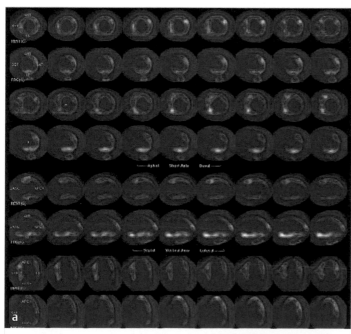

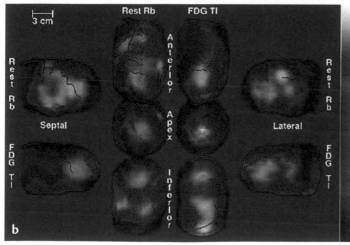

Fig. 34.6 (a) A rest rubidium-82 perfusion image with a rest fluorine-18 fluorodeoxyglucose (FDG) scan in a patient with known coronary artery disease and recent myocardial infarction for viability evaluation showing perfusion in all regions except the left ventricular apex, related anterior wall, and inferolateral wall, which show positive FDG uptake (mismatch), indicating regional viability and a high likelihood of functional improvement after bypass graft surgery. **(b)** The findings are superimposed on a model left ventricle, where defects are shown in blue. (Courtesy of Elias Botvinick, MD, San Francisco, CA.)

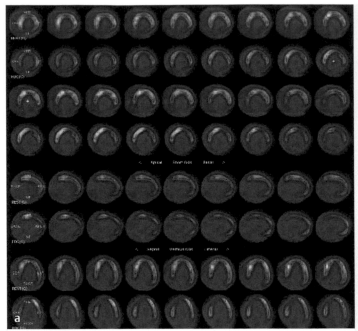

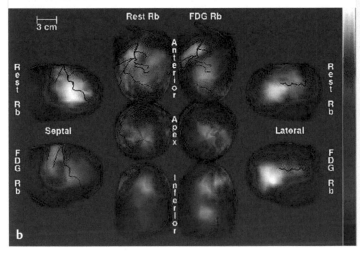

Fig. 34.7 **(a)** Rest rubidium-82 (^{82}Rb) myocardial perfusion images above fluorodeoxyglucose (FDG) PET myocardial metabolic images showing a large, dense, matched defect in the inferior wall, extending into posteroseptal and basal posterolateral regions, that suggests a scar in the right coronary and the basal region of the left circumflex coronary artery territories. There is apparent paradox of ^{82}Rb uptake (indicating viability) with reduced FDG uptake in the distal left ventricular septum (likely a metabolic variation without implications of nonviability). **(b)** A color-coded model of the left ventricle also shows the defects well. (These images are provided courtesy of Elias Botvinick, MD, San Francisco, CA.)

1. *Assessment of contractile reserve.* Stress echocardiography or MRI with low- or high-dose dobutamine.
2. *Assessment of sarcolemma integrity.* Thallium-201 rest-redistribution studies.
3. *Assessment of myocardial perfusion and mitochondrial membrane integrity.* SPECT with technetium-99 m agents such as sestamibi and tetrofosmin, with or without nitrate enhancement.
4. *Assessment of myocardial metabolism.* PET with myocardial perfusion and fluorine-18 [^{18}F]-FDG[32]
5. *Assessment of cell membrane integrity.* Contrast-enhanced MRI.[33,34]

Accuracy of Methods to Assess Myocardial Viability[35]

All techniques have a higher sensitivity than specificity (▶ Table 34.1).[35] However, PET may be the most sensitive technique, and dobutamine stress echo may be the most specific technique. PET has the greatest value relative to other techniques in patients with severe LV dysfunction. Contrast-enhanced MRI is a newer technique for evaluation

Table 34.1 Sensitivity and specificity of various methods to assess myocardial viability

Imaging method	Sensitivity %	Specificity %
PET	93	58
Thallium rest redistribution	86	59
Thallium reinjection	88	50
Technetium tracers	81	66
Dobutamine echo	81	80

Abbreviation: echo, echocardiogram.

of hibernating myocardium. Initial data suggest that the MRI findings correlate well with PET and have high sensitivity and specificity.

34.2.5 Pearls
Clinical Implications of Myocardial Viability

1. *Prediction of postrevascularization functional recovery.* The ability of PET to predict functional recovery in the form of improved global and regional LV function after revascularization by assessing myocardial viability prior to treatment has been well documented by several investigators.[36,37,38,39,40] Studies have demonstrated a linear correlation between the number of viable segments and the changes in LVEF, and a significantly higher functional improvement occurs in patients with large flow-metabolism mismatches compared with those with minimal or no mismatch on PET.

2. *Prediction of improvement in CHF symptoms, exercise capacity, and quality of life.* The preoperative size of myocardial viability as determined by PET correlates directly to the degree of improvement in heart failure symptoms after coronary artery bypass grafting; thus, myocardial viability evaluation also predicts the level of improvement in CHF symptoms after revascularization.

3. *Prediction of cardiac events, remodeling, and long-term survival.* Chronic ischemic heart disease patients with LV dysfunction are at increased risk for future cardiac events, and the presence of dysfunctional but viable myocardium appears to be a risk indicator for recurrent ischemic events. The natural history of disease progression in heart failure patients is significantly affected by LV remodeling, and

measures that halt or reverse ventricular remodeling result in more favorable outcomes in such patients. In chronic ischemic heart disease patients with LV dysfunction, viable myocardium is independently associated with improved long-term survival after revascularization.

4. *Prediction of perioperative complications and short-term survival.* Establishing the presence of a viable myocardium before revascularization in addition to the clinical and angiographic assessment in the decision-making process results in a low perioperative morbidity and mortality (fewer perioperative complications, less need for inotropic drugs, low early mortality, and promising short-term survival).[41,42]

Interpretation[43]

1. *Partial mismatch.* A partial mismatch is seen when FDG uptake is reduced, but not as much as the perfusion deficit. This may be secondary to a combination of scar and hibernating myocardium.

2. *Stunning.* Normal FDG uptake with a focal wall motion abnormality suggests stunning:
   a) If the wall motion abnormality is global with normal FDG uptake, this could be secondary to a cardiomyopathy or three-vessel disease.

3. *Reverse mismatch:*
   a) Reverse mismatch (normal perfusion with decreased FDG uptake) is often artifactual secondary to normalization errors (see Pitfalls).
   b) Also associated with recent myocardial infarction, multivessel disease, diabetes, and left bundle branch block (septal reverse mismatch).

34.2.6 Pitfalls[43]

1. *Reverse mismatch.* As areas of hibernating myocardium can have increased FDG uptake relative to normal myocardium, it is important to normalize the FDG uptake to the area of maximum perfusion. Failure to do so can result in artifactual reverse mismatched defects (normal perfusion and decreased FDG uptake) in the normal myocardium.

2. *Recent myocardial infarction.* FDG uptake can be seen in recently infarcted myocardium, secondary to leukocytes in the infarct region.

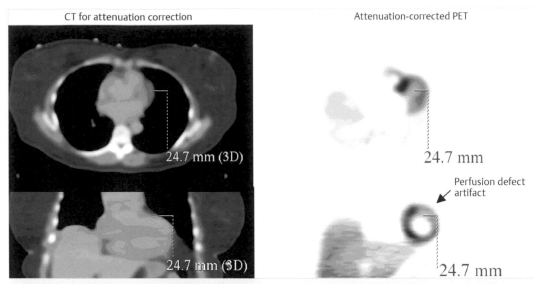

Fig. 34.8 Axial and coronal slices from a ¹³NH₃ stress study performed on a PET/CT scanner. This is an example of attenuation and emission scan mismatch in cardiac PET/CT, which often occurs along the lateral free wall or right diaphragm. The left column shows images from a helical CT scan used for attenuation correction of the PET images in the second column. The same line in 3D space is drawn from the edge of the cardiac lateral wall in the CT to the edge of the wall on the PET, marking the 2.5-cm mismatch at the lateral wall between the attenuation and emission images. This mismatch leads to the artifactual defect highlighted on the same PET slices. (Courtesy of Adam Alessio, PhD, Seattle, WA.)

3. ***Perfusion imaging:***

   a) If PET tracers are not available to assess perfusion, SPECT imaging with standard tracers such as technetium sestamibi can be substituted. However, correlation between PET and SPECT images will be inexact due to attenuation on the SPECT images. Transmission-based attenuation-corrected SPECT imaging may be more accurate for correlation with PET.

   b) ¹³*N ammonia.* If ¹³N ammonia is used as the perfusion tracer, there is decreased lateral wall activity in approximately 10% of normal patients. The etiology of this is unknown.

   c) ***Artifacts.***[44,45,46,47,48,49] One limitation of cardiac PET imaging on a PET/CT system is that misalignment between emission and attenuation image can lead to global and regional perfusion errors. The PET attenuation correction is often formed from a helical CT acquisition, representing a snapshot of the respiratory cycle, whereas the PET image is acquired over multiple respirations. Misalignment of these temporally different scans is common and often occurs in the diagnostic region of interest (along the lateral wall of the myocardium), leading to moderate to severe perfusion artifacts in 40% of cardiac PET–helical CT acquisitions. These misalignment artifacts are well appreciated in cardiac PET/CT (▶ Fig. 34.8) and have been shown to cause errors up to ± 35% over conventional cardiac PET imaging in which attenuation maps are formed over multiple respirations with a transmission rod source.

Several approaches have been proposed to minimize these artifacts. Groups have explored the option of performing the CT scan at an optimal time during respiration, such as at midexpiration, to minimize potential mismatches. Our clinical experience has found that asking a patient to hold his or her breath at a certain point in the respiratory cycle causes highly variable results. Another approach is to acquire the attenuation map with a cine CT acquisition, which acquires multiple low-dose CT scans over a period of time at each slice in the patient. The average or intensity maximum of these cine images can be used to reduce the potential of artifact-forming mismatches. If a mismatch is evident, most vendors offer a realignment tool to manually fix major errors.

34.2.7 Cost-Effectiveness of Cardiac PET versus Other Imaging Modalities

CMS value-based purchasing move is aimed at revolutionizing the business of health care delivery, with many health care stakeholders now focusing on resource utilization to get the most of their spent health care dollars. CMS is now using alternative payment models to reward value and quality with increase of fee-for-service payments from 30% in 2016 to 50% by 2018. Bundling of payments for linked services creates an opportunity and need for clinicians and organizations to provide high-quality, cost-effective care.[50]

There has also been a gradual decline in CMS reimbursement for cardiac imaging services provided by physicians and hospitals alike. Per CMS 2016 Medicare Physician Fee schedule, Medicare reimbursement was $571.02 for cardiac SPECT, $583.54 for cardiac MRI with stress testing, and $93.43 for cardiac PET.[51]

Also, the 2016 Medicare hospital payment $1108.46 for cardiac SPECT stress test, $1108.46 for cardiac MRI with stress imaging, and $1285.17 for cardiac PET.[52]

Many clinicians may not be aware of the financial realities around reimbursement of these tests, especially when it relates to the realities of current health care economics.

Cardiac PET, with its highest sensitivity lends itself for being the most cost-effective single test for evaluation of cardiac viability and can reduce downstream utilization of diagnostic arteriography, compared to SPECT MPI.[53] Tracking of physician resource utilization, variances in utilization, understanding the reasons for the variance, physician education, and collaboration with physicians are needed to achieve equitable utilization of cardiac PET scans.

34.3 Cardiac Sarcoidosis

The Heart Rhythm Society expert consensus statement[54] states that cardiac MRI or FDG-PET can be useful in patients with extracardiac sarcoidosis and one or more abnormalities on initial screening with symptoms/electrocardiogram/echocardiogram. If no abnormalities are present on initial screening, cardiac MRI or FDG-PET is not recommended.

Patient preparation for cardiac sarcoidosis studies is discussed in Chapter 4.

34.3.1 Accuracy/Comparison to Other Modalities

1. PET (meta-analysis)[55]: sensitivity of 89% and specificity of 78%.
2. PET/CT (meta-analysis)[56]: sensitivity of 81% and specificity of 82%.
3. FDG-PET is more sensitive than ^{67}Ga, ^{201}Th, and ^{99m}Tc imaging for the diagnosis of cardiac sarcoidosis.[57]
4. FDG-PET and cardiac MRI identify different pathologies in patients with cardiac sarcoidosis. FDG-PET identifies active inflammation, while late gadolinium enhancement MRI identifies fibrosis. One advantage of PET is that whole-body PET images can evaluate systemic disease outside the myocardium. However, one advantage of MRI is that it does not utilize ionizing radiation. Several authors[57,58] have suggested cardiac MRI as the initial test in patients with suspected cardiac sarcoidosis, with FDG-PET used in patients with contraindications to MRI (not uncommon in this population), such as indwelling cardiac devices. If MRI is negative, PET is not necessary. If MRI is positive, FDG-PET could be performed to assess baseline disease activity and used to monitor response over time (▶ Fig. 34.9).

34.3.2 Pearls

1. **Perfusion imaging**. If possible, resting myocardial perfusion should also be assessed with PET (^{82}Rb or ^{13}N ammonia) or ^{99m}Tc tracers with SPECT. Normal studies have normal rest perfusion and no myocardial FDG uptake. In the early stage of sarcoidosis, focal areas of FDG uptake will be seen without perfusion defects. In more advanced stages, both abnormal FDG uptake and a perfusion defect will be seen. The perfusion defect is usually secondary to scar, but is occasionally secondary to microvascular compression from inflammation. It is important to be aware that FDG uptake with a perfusion defect (perfusion metabolism mismatch) is also a sign of hibernating myocardium, and obstructive coronary disease in the involved territory should be ruled out. In end-stage disease, there is mostly scar, which results in a perfusion defect without FDG uptake.[59]
2. **Diagnostic criteria**. One proposed classification has four types of patterns of FDG uptake: none, diffuse, focal, and focal and diffuse.[60] Focal and focal and diffuse patterns are considered to be

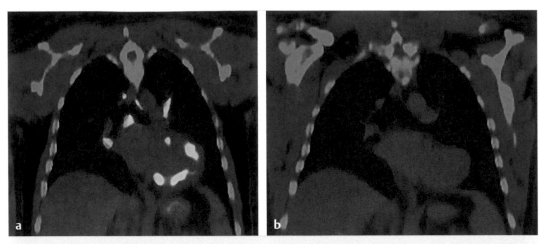

Fig. 34.9 Sarcoidosis. **(a)** Coronal PET/CT fused images demonstrated fluorodeoxyglucose-avid nodes in the mediastinal and bilateral hilar regions, representing sarcoidosis. Foci of uptake are also seen in the left ventricular wall representing cardiac sarcoidosis. **(b)** Post–steroid treatment, with resolution of the foci of uptake. (These images are provided courtesy of Wengen Chen, MD, Baltimore, MD.)

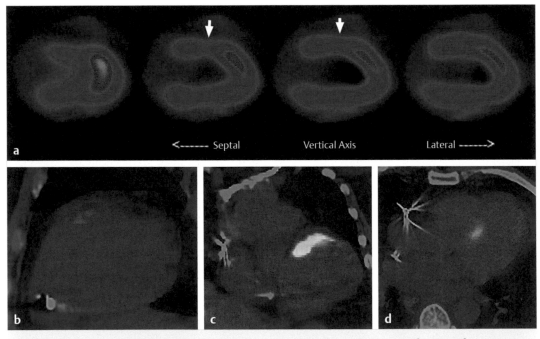

Fig. 34.10 Patterns of cardiac sarcoidosis. **(a)** Vertical long-axis images from a Tc-99 m tetrofosmin perfusion scan in a patient with suspected sarcoidosis demonstrates a perfusion defect at the base of the anterior wall (*arrows*). **(b)** Sagittal PET/CT demonstrates increased FDG uptake in the region of the perfusion defect. The associated perfusion defect could be secondary to scar, or microvascular obstruction from inflammation, and indicates a later stage of cardiac sarcoidosis. However, hibernating myocardium could give a similar perfusion-metabolism mismatch, and obstructive coronary disease in this territory should be ruled out. **(c)** Coronal PET/CT in a different patient with suspected cardiac sarcoidosis demonstrates uptake in the left ventricular free wall. **(d)** Axial PET/CT in a different patient with suspected cardiac sarcoidosis demonstrates uptake in the base of the septum. Both the base of the septum and the free wall are common locations for cardiac sarcoidosis involvement.

positive for cardiac sarcoidosis, with localized uptake only in the lateral wall excluded.[61]

3. *Sites of cardiac sarcoidosis* (▶ Fig. 34.10):

   a) The most frequently involved area in cardiac sarcoidosis is the septum (31.5%), followed by the inferior wall, anterior left ventricle, right ventricle, and lateral left ventricle.[59]

   b) In particular, the base of the ventricular septum is a common site for cardiac sarcoidosis. This may result in second- or third-degree atrioventricular block.

   Thus, localized FDG uptake in the base of the septum in patients with atrioventricular block is likely secondary to sarcoidosis.[60]

   c) The left ventricular free wall is a common site of cardiac sarcoidosis. If the onset site of monomorphic ventricular tachycardia corresponds to the site of FDG uptake, this is more likely to be a sarcoidosis lesion.[60]

   d) Apical involvement is rare.[62]

References

[1] Bateman TM, Dilsizian V, Beanlands RS, et al. American Society of Nuclear Cardiology and Society of Nuclear Medicine and Molecular Imaging Joint Position Statement on the Clinical Indications for Myocardial Perfusion PET. J Nucl Cardiol. 2016; 23(5):1227–1231

[2] Bateman TM, Dilsizian V, Beanlands RS, DePuey EG, Heller GV, Wolinsky DA. American Society of Nuclear Cardiology and Society of Nuclear Medicine and Molecular Imaging Joint Position Statement on the Clinical Indications for Myocardial Perfusion PET. J Nucl Med. 2016; 57(10):1654–1656

[3] Dilsizian V, Bacharach SL, Beanlands RS, et al. ASNC imaging guidelines/SNMMI procedure standard for positron emission tomography (PET) nuclear cardiology procedures. J Nucl Cardiol. 2016; 23(5):1187–1226

[4] Di Carli MF, Dorbala S, Meserve J, El Fakhri G, Sitek A, Moore SC. Clinical myocardial perfusion PET/CT. J Nucl Med. 2007; 48(5):783–793

[5] Bateman TM, Heller GV, McGhie AI, et al. Diagnostic accuracy of rest/stress ECG-gated Rb-82 myocardial perfusion PET: comparison with ECG-gated Tc-99 m sestamibi SPECT. J Nucl Cardiol. 2006; 13(1):24–33

[6] Go RT, Marwick TH, MacIntyre WJ, et al. A prospective comparison of rubidium-82 PET and thallium-201 SPECT myocardial perfusion imaging utilizing a single dipyridamole stress in the diagnosis of coronary artery disease. J Nucl Med. 1990; 31(12):1899–1905

[7] Stewart RE, Schwaiger M, Molina E, et al. Comparison of rubidium-82 positron emission tomography and thallium-201 SPECT imaging for detection of coronary artery disease. Am J Cardiol. 1991; 67(16):1303–1310

[8] Schelbert HR. 18F-deoxyglucose and the assessment of myocardial viability. Semin Nucl Med. 2002; 32(1):60–69

[9] Alderman EL, Fisher LD, Litwin P, et al. Results of coronary artery surgery in patients with poor left ventricular function (CASS). Circulation. 1983; 68(4):785–795

[10] Emond M, Mock MB, Davis KB, et al. Long-term survival of medically treated patients in the Coronary Artery Surgery Study (CASS) Registry. Circulation. 1994; 90(6):2645–2657

[11] Passamani E, Davis KB, Gillespie MJ, Killip T. A randomized trial of coronary artery bypass surgery. Survival of patients with a low ejection fraction. N Engl J Med. 1985; 312(26):1665–1671

[12] Alderman EL, Corley SD, Fisher LD, et al. CASS Participating Investigators and Staff. Five-year angiographic follow-up of factors associated with progression of coronary artery disease in the Coronary Artery Surgery Study (CASS). J Am Coll Cardiol. 1993; 22(4):1141–1154

[13] Mickleborough LL, Maruyama H, Takagi Y, Mohamed S, Sun Z, Ebisuzaki L. Results of revascularization in patients with severe left ventricular dysfunction. Circulation. 1995; 92(9) Suppl:II73–II79

[14] Kaul TK, Agnihotri AK, Fields BL, Riggins LS, Wyatt DA, Jones CR. Coronary artery bypass grafting in patients with an ejection fraction of twenty percent or less. J Thorac Cardiovasc Surg. 1996; 111(5):1001–1012

[15] Miller DC, Stinson EB, Alderman EL. Surgical treatment of ischemic cardiomyopathy; is it ever too late? Am J Surg. 1981; 141(6):688–693

[16] Luciani GB, Faggian G, Razzolini R, Livi U, Bortolotti U, Mazzucco A. Severe ischemic left ventricular failure: coronary operation or heart transplantation? Ann Thorac Surg. 1993; 55(3):719–723

[17] Ellis SG, Fisher L, Dushman-Ellis S, et al. Comparison of coronary angioplasty with medical treatment for single- and double-vessel coronary disease with left anterior descending coronary involvement: long-term outcome based on an Emory-CASS registry study. Am Heart J. 1989; 118(2):208–220

[18] Bengel FM, Schwaiger M. Assessment of myocardial viability by PET. In: Valk P, ed. Positron Emission Tomography: Principles and Clinical Practice. London, UK: Springer Verlag; 2003:447–463

[19] Kloner RA, Bolli R, Marban E, Reinlib L, Braunwald E. Medical and cellular implications of stunning, hibernation, and preconditioning: an NHLBI workshop. Circulation. 1998; 97(18):1848–1867

[20] Wijns W, Vatner SF, Camici PG. Hibernating myocardium. N Engl J Med. 1998; 339(3):173–181

[21] Taegtmeyer H. Myocardial metabolism. In: Phelps ME, Mazziotta JC, Schelbert HR, eds. Positron Emission Tomography and Autoradiography: Principles and Applications for the Brain and Heart. New York, NY: Raven; 1986:149–195

[22] Liedtke AJ. Alterations of carbohydrate and lipid metabolism in the acutely ischemic heart. Prog Cardiovasc Dis. 1981; 23 (5):321–336

[23] Liedtke AJ. The origins of myocardial substrate utilization from an evolutionary perspective: the enduring role of glucose in energy metabolism. J Mol Cell Cardiol. 1997; 29(4):1073–1086

[24] Liedtke AJ, Renstrom B, Hacker TA, Nellis SH. Effects of moderate repetitive ischemia on myocardial substrate utilization. Am J Physiol. 1995; 269(1, Pt 2):H246–H253

[25] Liedtke AJ, Renstrom B, Nellis SH, Hall JL, Stanley WC. Mechanical and metabolic functions in pig hearts after 4 days of chronic coronary stenosis. J Am Coll Cardiol. 1995; 26(3):815–825

[26] Vanoverschelde JL, Wijns W, Depré C, et al. Mechanisms of chronic regional postischemic dysfunction in humans. New insights from the study of noninfarcted collateral-dependent myocardium. Circulation. 1993; 87(5):1513–1523

[27] Schelbert HR, Henze E, Phelps ME, Kuhl DE. Assessment of regional myocardial ischemia by positron-emission computed tomography. Am Heart J. 1982; 103(4)(,)(Pt 2):588–597

[28] Schwaiger M, Fishbein MC, Block M, et al. Metabolic and ultrastructural abnormalities during ischemia in canine myocardium: noninvasive assessment by positron emission tomography. J Mol Cell Cardiol. 1987; 19(3):259–269

[29] Kalff V, Schwaiger M, Nguyen N, McClanahan TB, Gallagher KP. The relationship between myocardial blood flow and glucose uptake in ischemic canine myocardium determined with fluorine-18-deoxyglucose. J Nucl Med. 1992; 33(7):1346–1353

[30] Marwick TH, Nemec JJ, Lafont A, Salcedo EE, MacIntyre WJ. Prediction by postexercise fluoro-18 deoxyglucose positron emission tomography of improvement in exercise capacity after revascularization. Am J Cardiol. 1992; 69(9):854–859

[31] Keng FY. Clinical applications of positron emission tomography in cardiology: a review. Ann Acad Med Singapore. 2004; 33(2):175–182

[32] Bax JJ, Wijns W, Cornel JH, Visser FC, Boersma E, Fioretti PM. Accuracy of currently available techniques for prediction of functional recovery after revascularization in patients with left ventricular dysfunction due to chronic coronary artery disease: comparison of pooled data. J Am Coll Cardiol. 1997; 30(6):1451–1460

[33] Lekx KS, Pereira RS, Prato FS, Sykes J, Wisenberg G. Determining myocardial viability in a chronic occlusion canine model using MRI with a constant infusion of Gd-DTPA. 18th Meeting of International Society for Magnetic Resonance in Medicine (ISMRM). Berkeley, CA; 2000

[34] Shan K, Constantine G, Sivananthan M, Flamm SD. Role of cardiac magnetic resonance imaging in the assessment of myocardial viability. Circulation. 2004; 109(11):1328–1334

[35] Bax JJ, Poldermans D, Elhendy A, Boersma E, Rahimtoola SH. Sensitivity, specificity, and predictive accuracies of various noninvasive techniques for detecting hibernating myocardium. Curr Probl Cardiol. 2001; 26(2):147–186

[36] Baer FM, Voth E, Deutsch HJ, et al. Predictive value of low dose dobutamine transesophageal echocardiography and fluorine-18 fluorodeoxyglucose positron emission tomography for recovery of regional left ventricular function after successful revascularization. J Am Coll Cardiol. 1996; 28(1):60–69

[37] Bax JJ, Cornel JH, Visser FC, et al. F18-fluorodeoxyglucose single-photon emission computed tomography predicts functional outcome of dyssynergic myocardium after surgical revascularization. J Nucl Cardiol. 1997; 4(4):302–308

[38] Knuuti MJ, Saraste M, Nuutila P, et al. Myocardial viability: fluorine-18-deoxyglucose positron emission tomography in prediction of wall motion recovery after revascularization. Am Heart J. 1994; 127(4)(,)(Pt 1):785–796

[39] Schöder H, Campisi R, Ohtake T, et al. Blood flow-metabolism imaging with positron emission tomography in patients with diabetes mellitus for the assessment of reversible left ventricular contractile dysfunction. J Am Coll Cardiol. 1999; 33(5):1328–1337

[40] Tillisch J, Brunken R, Marshall R, et al. Reversibility of cardiac wall-motion abnormalities predicted by positron tomography. N Engl J Med. 1986; 314(14):884–888

[41] Landoni C, Lucignani G, Paolini G, et al. Assessment of CABG-related risk in patients with CAD and LVD. Contribution of PET with [18F]FDG to the assessment of myocardial viability. J Cardiovasc Surg (Torino). 1999; 40(3):363–372

[42] Haas F, Haehnel CJ, Picker W, et al. Preoperative positron emission tomographic viability assessment and perioperative and postoperative risk in patients with advanced ischemic heart disease. J Am Coll Cardiol. 1997; 30(7):1693–1700

[43] Beanlands RSB, Ruddy TD, Mahhadis J. Myocardial viability. In: Wahl RL, Buchanan JW, eds. Principles and Practice of Positron Emission Tomography. Philadelphia, PA: Lippincott Williams & Wilkins; 2002:1334–1350

[44] Alessio AM, Kohlmyer S, Branch K, Chen G, Caldwell J, Kinahan P. Cine CT for attenuation correction in cardiac PET/CT. J Nucl Med. 2007; 48(5):794–801

[45] Goerres GW, Kamel E, Heidelberg TN, Schwitter MR, Burger C, von Schulthess GK. PET-CT image co-registration in the thorax: influence of respiration. Eur J Nucl Med Mol Imaging. 2002; 29(3):351–360

[46] Goerres GW, Burger C, Kamel E, et al. Respiration-induced attenuation artifact at PET/CT: technical considerations. Radiology. 2003; 226(3):906–910

[47] Gould KL, Pan T, Loghin C, Johnson NP, Guha A, Sdringola S. Frequent diagnostic errors in cardiac PET/CT due to misregistration of CT attenuation and emission PET images: a definitive analysis of causes, consequences, and corrections. J Nucl Med. 2007; 48(7):1112–1121

[48] Nakamoto Y, Osman M, Cohade C, et al. PET/CT: comparison of quantitative tracer uptake between germanium and CT transmission attenuation-corrected images. J Nucl Med. 2002; 43(9):1137–1143

[49] Pan T, Mawlawi O, Nehmeh SA, et al. Attenuation correction of PET images with respiration-averaged CT images in PET/CT. J Nucl Med. 2005; 46(9):1481–1487

[50] Press MJ, Rajkumar R, Conway PH. Medicare's New Bundled Payments: Design, Strategy, and Evolution. JAMA. 2016; 315 (2):131–132

[51] American Society of Nuclear Cardiology. Final 2016 Payment Rates Compared to 4Q 2015 Final Rates Medicare Hospital Outpatient Prospective Payment System HOPPS (APC) Nuclear Cardiology Procedures, Radiopharmaceuticals, and Drugs. Revised October 2015. Available at: http://www.asnc. org/Files/Advocacy/ASNC%20HOPPS%20Final%20payment% 20chart%202016%2011_02_2015.pdf. Accessed: July 1, 2017

[52] Karin R. Cardinal Health: 2016 Medicare update. Presented by Rudy Karin, Director, Reimbursement Strategy, NMB Healthcare Consulting. Available at: http://docplayer.net/ 21417293–2016-medicare-update-nmd-healthcare-consulting.html. Accessed: July 1, 2017

[53] Merhige ME, Breen WJ, Shelton V, Houston T, D'Arcy BJ, Perna AF. Impact of myocardial perfusion imaging with PET and (82)Rb on downstream invasive procedure utilization, costs, and outcomes in coronary disease management. J Nucl Med. 2007; 48(7):1069–1076

[54] Birnie DH, Sauer WH, Bogun F, et al. HRS expert consensus statement on the diagnosis and management of arrhythmias associated with cardiac sarcoidosis. Heart Rhythm. 2014; 11 (7):1305–1323

[55] Youssef G, Leung E, Mylonas I, et al. The use of 18F-FDG PET in the diagnosis of cardiac sarcoidosis: a systematic review and metaanalysis including the Ontario experience. J Nucl Med. 2012; 53(2):241–248

[56] Tang R, Wang JT, Wang L, et al. Impact of patient preparation on the diagnostic performance of 18F-FDG PET in cardiac sarcoidosis: a systematic review and meta-analysis. Clin Nucl Med. 2016; 41(7):e327–e339

[57] Hulten E, Aslam S, Osborne M, Abbasi S, Bittencourt MS, Blankstein R. Cardiac sarcoidosis-state of the art review. Cardiovasc Diagn Ther. 2016; 6(1):50–63

[58] Skali H, Schulman AR, Dorbala S. (18)F-FDG PET/CT for the assessment of myocardial sarcoidosis. Curr Cardiol Rep. 2013; 15(5):352

[59] Orii M, Imanishi T, Akasaka T. Assessment of cardiac sarcoidosis with advanced imaging modalities. BioMed Res Int. 2014; 2014:897956

[60] Ishida Y, Yoshinaga K, Miyagawa M, et al. Recommendations for (18)F-fluorodeoxyglucose positron emission tomography imaging for cardiac sarcoidosis: Japanese Society of Nuclear Cardiology recommendations. Ann Nucl Med. 2014; 28(4): 393–403

[61] Ishimaru S, Tsujino I, Takei T, et al. Focal uptake on 18F-fluoro-2-deoxyglucose positron emission tomography images indicates cardiac involvement of sarcoidosis. Eur Heart J. 2005; 26(15):1538–1543

[62] Lynch JP, III, Hwang J, Bradfield J, Fishbein M, Shivkumar K, Tung R. Cardiac involvement in sarcoidosis: evolving concepts in diagnosis and treatment. Semin Respir Crit Care Med. 2014; 35(3):372–390

Index

Note: Page numbers set **bold** or *italic* indicate headings or figures, respectively.

4

4DPET/CT **334**

1

11C Pittsburgh compound B
  (PiB) **360**, 362
11C-DTBZ 364
11C-flumazenil 364, *365*
11C-MET 365, 368
11C-raclopride 364
13N ammonia 372–373, 380–381
18F NaF
– accuracy **304**, *306*, **306**,
  307
– back pain, failed back
  surgery 308
– bisphosphonates
  effects 307
– bone graft evaluation 308
– characterization 303, *303*
– degenerative joint
  disease 308
– enchondroma 308
– false negatives 306
– false positives 304, *305*
– G-CSF effects 307
– inborn source of error 307
– indications **303**
– inflammatory bone
  disease 308
– mandibular condylar
  hyperplasia 308
– metabolic bone disease **309**
– modality comparison **304**,
  306, **306**, *307*
– osseous disease, benign **308**
– osseous disease,
  malignant **303**, *304*
– osteoid osteoma 308
– osteonecrosis
  evaluation 308
– pediatric bone
  scanning **308**
– prosthetic joint
  assessment 308
– quantitative **309**
– rheumatologic bone
  disease 308
– septic loosening 308
– skeletal metastases
  SUV 306
– therapy response **306**, 307
– trauma 308
18F-DTBZ 364
18F-FET 365, 368
18F-florbetaben
  (NeuraCeq) **360**, *362*

18F-florbetapir (Amyvid) **360**,
  362
18F-fluorodopa (FDOPA) 363,
  365, *366–367*
18F-flurpiridaz 372
18F-flutemetamol
  (Vizamyl) **360**, *362*

6

68Ga-based imaging, *see*
  68Ga-SA, PSMA
68Ga-exendin **319**
68Ga-SA
– 18F-FDG combined use **316**
– accuracy **315**
– false negatives 317–318
– false positives 317–318
– image acquisition **316**
– image interpretation *317*,
  317, *318*
– indications **314**, *315*
– management impact **316**
– mimics 318
– modality comparison **315**
– overview 314
– synthesis **316**
68Ga-somatostatin
  antagonists **319**

8

82Rb chloride 372, 381

A

ABVD regimen studies 225
AC images interpretation 90,
  90, 91, *91–92*
acipimox 33
adenocarcinomas
– esophageal cancer 210, 214
– gastric cancer, intestinal/
  diffuse-type 208
– gastric cancer, lepidic
  predominant 180
– lung, FDG avidity 180
– mucinous, differential
  diagnosis 242
– ovarian cancer 256
– pancreatic cancer 28, **245**
– thoracic neoplasms 179,
  184
adrenals
– bilateral uptake 70, *71*
– false negatives 140
– hyperplasia 70, *71*, 186
– metastasis, PET **138**, *139*
– normal variants, benign
  findings **69**

– PET diagnostic
  accuracy **138**
– SUV and visual analysis 139
– thoracic neoplasm
  metastases, PET/CT
  accuracy 182, *183*
– uptake, nonmetastatic
  causes of *71*, 140
aerobic glycolysis **23**, 24
AIDS **345**, *346*
Alzheimer's disease **353**, *354*,
  354, *355*, **360**, *361*
American Association of
  Physicists in Medicine
  (AAPM) 44
amino acids in imaging 365,
  368
amyloid imaging 360–362
Amyvid (18F-florbetapir) **360**,
  362
androgen deprivation
  therapy 313
angiomyolipomas 70, 265
anticonvulsants 151
arterial phase imaging 104
arthritis **348**
atelectasis 64, *64–65*
atherosclerosis **48**, 78, *81*, **347**
autoimmune pancreatitis 246,
  246
axilla
– dose extravasation 60, *61*
– glenohumeral joint 60, *61*
– normal variants, benign
  findings **60**

B

Baastrup's disease (kissing
  spine) 76, *78*
barium artifact *105*
basal ganglia 51, 364
benzodiazepines, myocardial
  uptake 52
bezafibrate, myocardial
  uptake 52
biological target volumes
  (BTV) 332
bladder cancer
– accuracy **269**
– lymph node metastases *270*
– metastatic 269, *269*
– metastatic, urinary
  activity 31, *269*
– PET applications 269, *269*
– PET/MRI **117**, *119*
– prognosis 269
bladder catheterization 31
bleomycin lung toxicity 63, *63*
bone, bone marrow

– 18FNaF, *see* 18FNaF
– accuracy **291**
– arthritis 76
– benign fractures 73, *74*
– benign vs. malignant
  tumors **291**, **291**, 292
– breast cancer
  metastases 199, *199–200*
– chemotherapy 74
– chondrosarcoma 291, *291*
– cortical lesions therapy
  response 148
– degenerative spurring 76,
  76
– enchondroma 291
– erythropoietin 76
– esophageal cancer
  metastases 212, *212*
– false negatives 292
– false positives 292, *292–293*
– FDG accumulation 292
– focal uptake 76
– G-CSF treatment *70*, 73, *75–
  76*
– gastric cancer
  metastases 209, *209*
– giant cell tumor 292, *292*
– hepatocellular carcinoma
  metastases 240
– insufficiency fractures 73,
  75
– intraspinous bursa
  uptake 76, *78*
– lesion detection 91, *91*
– lytic vs. sclerotic
  metastasis 136, *136–139*
– metastases 292
– metastases, PET **136**
– metastases, PET/MRI **119**
– metastases, global disease
  assessment **48**
– normal variants, benign
  findings **73**
– osteosarcoma
  metastases 297
– pediatric PET/CT **324**, *325*
– PET vs. bone scan 136
– prostate cancer
  metastases *272*, *273*, *275*,
  276
– radiation effects 76, *77*
– subchondral cysts 76, *77*
– thoracic neoplasm
  metastases 182, *182–183*
– thyroid cancer
  metastases 172
bowel activity
– cecal uptake 67, *67*
– colon cancer, primary
  metastatic 67, *281*
– colon polyps 67, *280*

- focal and segmental uptake 67, 68, 280–281
- gastrointestinal tract pathology 67
- large 67, 67–68
- normal variants, benign findings 67
- oral contrast 67
- patient preparation 31
- segmental uptake 67, 68
- small 67
- SUV 68, 102

brain
- active small lesion detection 154
- age-related changes 51
- basal ganglia/thalamus lesions 154
- biopsy site determination 150
- crossed cerebellar diaschisis 51, 52
- deep white matter lesions 154
- false negatives 151
- false positives 151, 151–152, 154
- FDG PET accuracy 151
- FDG uptake, factors affecting 150–151
- imaging correlation 152
- melanoma, metastatic 234, 235
- metabolic grading of 150, 150
- non-FDG PET tracers 361
- normal variants, benign findings 51, 355
- oncological PET 138, 139
- postsurgical changes 152
- primary tumors 150
- radiation effects 152
- radiation therapy planning 333
- renal function 51
- seizures 154
- SPECT comparison 51
- SUV 151, 153
- thoracic neoplasm metastases, PET/CT accuracy 182
- transformation evaluation 150
- tumor recurrence 152–153, 154
- tumor vs. radiation necrosis 151, 152–153
- tumors, FDG PET imaging 365, 366–367, 368
- uptake symmetry 51
- uptake, normal pattern of 51
- visual interpretation criteria 152, 153, 153

breast cancer
- accuracy 195, 197, 197, 199, 201, 203, 203
- antiaromatase therapy 204
- axillary nodal metastasis 197–198
- axillary staging 201
- bone marrow metastases 199, 199–200
- brachial plexus metastases 201, 202
- chest wall metastases 201, 202
- contrast-enhanced MRI 195
- degree of FDG uptake 196
- delayed/dual time point imaging 196
- dense breasts 196
- distant metastases 198, 199
- distant recurrence 201
- elevated tumor markers 201
- extra-axillary nodes 198, 198–199
- false negatives 196, 196
- false positives 196, 197
- histology 197, 200
- incidental uptake 195
- interim PET 202
- invasive ductal carcinoma 197
- invasive lobular carcinoma 196
- locoregional recurrence 201, 202
- low FDG uptake tumors 204
- lytic/blastic metastases 200
- malignancy detection 195
- masses 195
- metabolic flare 204
- metastatic 197, 199, 201, 202
- modality comparison 195, 197, 197, 201, 203, 203
- multifocal disease 197, 198
- PET vs. bone scan 137, 138–139
- PET/MRI 117, 204
- prognosis 202
- receptor expression 204
- recurrence 201, 201, 202
- seroma 197
- staging 196
- SUV 195, 204
- therapy response 202, 203
- timing of PET/CT 204

breastfeeding 32, 32

breasts
- focal uptake 60
- implants 60
- lactation 60
- mislocalization 101, 102
- nipple uptake 60
- normal variants, benign findings 60
- postmenopausal 60
- premenopausal 60, 61

bronchoalveolar carcinoma 179, 180

brown fat
- differential diagnosis 79, 82–83, 86
- follow-up 95, 96
- glucose/FDG metabolism 22, 23
- infradiaphragmatic uptake 83
- locations 81, 85
- neck/supraclavicular uptake 82–83, 86
- normal variants, benign findings 81
- suprarenal uptake 83
- thoracic uptake 83
- thyroid cancer 58, 173, 174
- uptake minimization 30

C

caffeine 28

carcinoids vs. hamartomas 179

cardiac PET
- accuracy 372, 375, 376, 378, 379, 381, 382
- activity variations 373
- activity, glucose/FDG metabolism 21, 22
- artifacts 380, 380
- cardiac events prediction 379
- cell membrane integrity assessment 378
- CHF symptoms improvement prediction 379
- clinical scenario 375
- complications prediction 379
- contractile reserve assessment 379
- cost-effectiveness 381
- diagnostic criteria 381
- exercise capacity improvement prediction 379
- functional recovery prediction 379
- interpretation 379
- misregistration artifact 374
- mitochondrial membrane integrity assessment 378
- modality comparison 372, 375, 376, 381, 382
- myocardial infarction, recent 379
- myocardial ischemia mechanism 376, 376
- myocardial metabolism assessment 378
- myocardial perfusion assessment 372, 378

- myocardial viability 374, 376, 377–378, 378, 379
- non-FDG PET tracers 361
- partial mismatch 379
- patient preparation 33
- perfusion imaging 380–381
- protocols 372, 373–374
- quality of life improvement prediction 379
- remodeling prediction 379
- reverse mismatch 379
- sarcolemma integrity assessment 378
- stunning 379
- survival prediction 379
- tracers 372, 372, 380–381

cardiovascular disease 122

cerebrovascular disease 368

cervical cancer
- accuracy 254, 254–255
- dual-time imaging 254
- early-stage 254, 254
- false negatives 254
- false positives 254
- lymph node metastases 254
- metastatic 253
- modality comparison 254, 254–255
- neoadjuvant chemotherapy 255
- pattern of spread 254
- pelvic nodal metastases 253
- PET application 253
- primary tumor 253, 253
- prognosis 254, 255
- radiotherapy effect 255
- recurrence 255
- staging 253, 253
- therapy response 255
- urinary activity 253, 254

Charcot's osteoarthropathy 341, 341, 342, 342, 343

chemoradiotherapy 163

cholangiocarcinoma
- accuracy 242, 242
- extrahepatic 242
- false negatives 242
- false positives 242
- hilar 241–242
- intrahepatic 242
- metastatic 240, 241, 241, 242
- modality comparison 242
- PET/CT imaging 100, 240, 240–241
- primary sclerosing cholangitis 241, 242
- primary tumor detection 241–242
- staging 241
- SUVs 242

cholecystitis 242, 243

chondrosarcoma 291, 291

clinical target volume (CTV) 332

CNS tumors **115**, *116*
cold exposure
  minimization 31
colon cancer
– bowel activity, primary
  metastatic 67, *281*
– lesion detection 92, *92–93*
– metastatic *281*
– peritoneal metastasis 93,
  129
– staging, initial *281*, **282**
– synchronous 159, *160*
colon polyps 67, 243, *280*
colorectal cancer
– accuracy **280**, 282, **282**, **284**
– CEA, elevated 282–283, *283*,
  284
– CEA, normal 286
– colonoscopy, FDG uptake
  and 281
– degree of uptake 280, *280–*
  281
– differential diagnosis *281*
– end of therapy PET 286
– extrahepatic
  metastases 285
– false positives 286
– hepatic resection 285
– interim PET 286
– KRAS mutations 282
– liver metastases 282, 284–
  285, *285*
– lymph node staging 282
– metastatic *281*, 285
– modality comparison **280**,
  282, **282**, **285**
– mucinous tumors 286
– neoadjuvant
  chemotherapy 286
– PET/CT colonography 282
– PET/MRI 116
– polyps 280, *280*
– posttreatment
  differentiation 284, *284*
– primary tumors 280, **280**
– prognosis 286
– recurrence/restaging **282**,
  283, 284, *284*, 285
– staging, initial **282**
– therapy response **286**
– uptake location 281
– uptake pattern 281
– uptake, nonmalignant
  causes 280–281
corticosteroids 150
costovertebral joints 76
Crohn's disease **48**, 123
crossed cerebellar
  diaschisis 51, *52*
Cushing's disease 150
cystic neck masses 165

D

degenerative joint disease 308
delayed imaging

– FDG uptake effects 151
– hepatocellular
  carcinoma 240
– musculoskeletal
  tumors 293
– pancreatic cancer 246
dementia **353**, *354*, **354**, *355*,
  360, *361*
depression 357
diabetic patients
– foot **341**, **341**, *342*, **342**, *343*
– myocardial uptake 52
– patient preparation 29, 33
diazepam 30
diet, fasting **28**
diffuse large B-cell
  lymphoma 220, 223, **226**,
  228
diffuse peritoneal
  carcinomatosis 133, *133*,
  258, *259*
diuretics 31
diverticulitis *281*
dopamine 363
dopamine transporters
  (DATs) 364
dose extravasation 60, *61*
dose painting
– by contours 334, *334*
– by numbers **334**
– characterization **334**
– methodologies **334**
drug-associated lung
  toxicity 63, *63*
DTP PET/CT **40**
ductal carcinoma in-situ
  195

E

electrodes, intracranial 353
enchondroma 291, 308
endometrial cancer **258**, *259*
endometriomas 256
ephedrine 31
epilepsy, *see* seizure, epilepsy
esophageal cancer
– accuracy 212, *212*, **212–214**
– adenocarcinomas 210, 214
– bone metastases 212, *212*
– differential diagnosis 212
– distant metastases *212*
– distant nodes 212, *212*
– end of treatment PET 214
– esophageal ulceration 215
– false negatives 212–213
– false positives 213
– gastroesophageal junction
  uptake *65*, 211
– gastrohepatic vs. celiac
  nodes 212
– hiatal hernias 211
– hilar uptake
  interpretation 212
– interim PET 213

– interval metastases 214,
  214
– level of uptake 210
– locoregional nodes 212, *212*
– metastatic 211, *211–212*,
  214, *214*
– modality comparison *212*,
  212, **214**
– neoadjuvant therapy 213–
  214
– nodal staging 212
– PET/MRI 115
– primary tumor
  detection **210**, 212–213
– prognosis 211
– radiation esophagitis 215
– radiation therapy
  planning **215**
– recurrence 213, **213**
– respiratory
  misregistration 211
– squamous cell
  carcinomas 210
– staging *211*, **211**, 212
– SUV 215
– synchronous
  neoplasms 213
– therapy response **213**
esophagus 65, *65*, **65**, 66
Ewing's sarcoma 294, **296**
exendin **319**
extratemporal lobe
  epilepsy 352

F

[F-18] FDG
– basic modeling/biology *15*,
  15
– design of 12, *12*
– development of 13, **13**
– electrophilic radiosynthetic
  scheme 13, *13*
– first synthesis **12**, *13*
– Julich method *13*, 14
– nucleophilic radiosynthetic
  scheme 13, *13*
– one-pot syntheses 14
– overview 12
– phase-transfer agents 14
– quality control 15
– residual volatile organic
  solvents 15
– solid-phase hydrolysis 14
false negatives
– 18FNaF 306
– 68Ga-SA 317–318
– adrenals 140
– bone, bone marrow 292
– brain 151
– breast cancer 196, *196*
– cervical cancer 254
– cholangiocarcinoma 242
– esophageal cancer 212–213
– head and neck 158, 162

– hepatocellular
  carcinoma 129, *238*
– interpretation 93
– liver 129, *238*
– lymphoma 155
– multiple myeloma 300
– musculoskeletal
  tumors 293
– ovarian cancer 256, 258
– pancreatic cancer 246
– renal cell carcinoma 265,
  265
– therapy response 145
– thoracic neoplasms 177,
  179, *180*
false positives
– 18FNaF 304, *305*
– 68Ga-SA 317–318
– bone, bone marrow 292,
  292–293
– brain 151, *151–152*, 154
– breast cancer 196, *197*
– cervical cancer 254
– cholangiocarcinoma 242
– colorectal cancer 286
– esophageal cancer 213
– flare phenomenon 145
– gallbladder cancer 242
– head and neck 157–158,
  164
– interpretation 93, *94*
– liver 69, *69*, 129, *238*
– lungs 64, 96
– lymphoma 155, 229
– melanoma 232
– musculoskeletal
  tumors 293, *294*
– ovarian cancer *135*, 256
– pancreatic cancer 246, 250
– PET/CT 98, *100*
– renal 70, *265*
– renal cell carcinoma 265
– therapy response 145
– thoracic neoplasms 179,
  186
– ureteral 70
fasting state uptake 52, *52–53*
fatty acids, glucose/FDG
  metabolism 22, *23*
FDG tracers, *see* neurological
  tracers
fever of unknown origin **345**
fibromas 256
fibrous dysplasia 292, *292*
flare phenomenon 145
fluciclovine
– inflammatory uptake **273**
– interpretation **272**
– physiologic uptake **272**
– prostate cancer **270**, 271–
  272, *273*
flumazenil 364, *365*
focal cortical
  malformations 353
follicular lymphoma 222, 227,
  227

follicular neoplasms 170
free fatty acid metabolism, decreasing 33
frontotemporal dementia 356, *356*
furosemide 31

G

gallbladder cancer
- false positives 242
- metastatic 241–242
- PET/CT imaging 240
- polyps 243
- primary tumor detection 241, *241*, 242
- regional lymph nodes 242, *242*
- staging 241
gallbladder/biliary tree
- delayed resolution 94, *95*
- inflammation 69, *95*
- normal variants, benign findings 69, **69**, *95*
- stent placement 69, *69*
gastric cancer
- accuracy 208, **208**
- adenocarcinoma, intestinal/diffuse-type 208
- asymptomatic 209
- comorbid pathologies 209
- gastric remnant 210
- histology 209
- lymph node staging 208
- metastatic *208*, 209, *209*
- modality comparison **208**
- morphology 209
- NCCN guidelines 208
- nodal metastases 208, *208*
- perigastric nodes 210
- PET/MRI 116
- primary tumor 208
- prognosis 208
- recurrent 209
- therapy response 208
gastrointestinal disorders **123**
gastrointestinal stromal tumors
- accuracy **216**
- flare phenomenon 216
- global disease assessment **47**
- imaging, imatinib effects 215
- imatinib refractory 216
- metastatic 216
- morphologic criteria 215
- PET/CT imaging 100, 215, *215*, 216, *216*
- PET/MRI **115**
- prognosis 216
- pseudoprogression 216
- recurrence 216
- therapy response 216
genitourinary tract
- normal variants, benign findings **70**
- renal false positives 70, *265*
- retroperitoneal nodal uptake 70, *71–72*
glenohumeral joint variants, benign findings 60, *61*, 76
glioma
- FDG PET accuracy **151**, *366–367*, 368
- lymphoma vs. *154*, **154**
- metabolic grading of 150, *150*
- transformation evaluation 150
glucose loading, oral 33
glucose-6-phosphatase activity (G-6-Pase) 19–20
glucose/FDG metabolism
- aerobic glycolysis **23**, 24
- aging effects on 357
- altered biological pathways 22
- analogs, chemical structures 12
- cellular level **19**
- glucose/FDG similarities **19**, *20*
- glycolytic metabolism-based therapies **24**
- hypoxic environment **23**
- imaging biology **18**, *20*
- insulin administration 29, *29*
- organ level *21*, **21**
- overview 18
- plasma level, FDG uptake effects 151, 357
- tissue level **20**
- whole-body level **21**, *22–23*
GLUT1 19, 338
GLUT4 19
granulocyte colony stimulating factor (G-CSF) 69, *70*, 73, *75–76*, 307
Graves' disease 60, 62, 77
gray matter, FDG uptake effects 151
gross tumor volume (GTV) 332
gynecologic cancer, PET/MRI **117**
- *See also* specific cancers by anatomic region

H

head and neck
- bone invasion 160
- cervical metastasis, unknown primary *157*, **157**, *158*
- clinical N0 neck **158**
- cystic neck masses 165
- dedicated protocol 161
- distant metastases detection *159*, **159**
- false negatives 158, 162
- false positives 157–158, 164
- hardware artifacts 161
- laryngeal uptake 58, *58*, 162
- length of surveillance 162
- malignancies, global disease assessment **47**
- mislocalization 101, *101–102*
- muscle uptake 59, *59–60*
- mylohyoid muscles, sublingual glands (axial) 53, *56*
- nasopharyngeal uptake 56, *56–57*, 58
- nodal staging **158**
- normal uptake (sagittal) 53, *56*
- normal variants, benign findings **53**
- osteoradionecrosis 164
- parotid lesions 164, *164–165*
- PET limitations 164
- PET scan interpretation 160, *161*
- PET vs. bone scan 137
- PET vs. CT/MRI *160*
- PET vs. MRI *162*
- PET vs. radionuclides 162, *162*
- PET/CT accuracy **157**, **160–161**, *163*, **163**
- PET/CT applications **166**
- PET/CT for bone metastases 160
- PET/CT for M staging 160
- PET/CT timing 158, 164
- PET/MRI **114**, *114*
- postoperative PET/CT 162
- prognosis **160**, **163**
- radiation effects 162
- radiation therapy planning **333**
- reactive lymphadenopathy 160
- regional nodal metastases 160
- salivary glands 55, *57*
- scan volume 160
- soft palate (axial) 53, *57*
- staging **158**
- submandibular gland *57*
- SUV 160, 162
- synchronous lesions detection *159*, **159**, *160*
- therapy response **163**
- tongue uptake 58
- tonsils (coronal) 53, *56–57*
- tumor characterization **164**
- tumor recurrence **161**
- tumor stunning 162
- visual grading criteria 164
heart
- atrial uptake 53, *55–56*
- fasting state uptake 52, *52–53*
- insulin effect *29*, 53
- misregistration *101*
- normal variants, benign findings **52**
- papillary muscle uptake 53, *54*
- perfusion imaging 53
- right ventricular uptake 53
hemangiomas 293
hepatocellular carcinoma
- accuracy **239**
- bone metastases, detection 240
- cirrhosis 240
- delayed imaging 240
- false negatives 129, *238*
- fibrolamellar 240
- hepatitis 240
- metastatic, detection 239
- modality comparison **239**
- monitoring therapy 238, *239*
- PET applications 238, *238*
- post-TACE 240
- primary lesion detection *238*, 239
- prognosis 239
- recurrent, detection 240
- SUV 240
- timing of PET/CT 240
- transplant recipients 239
hexokinase II (HK II) 19–20
hiatal hernias 67, 211
hibernoma 293, *294*
hila
- adenopathy, differential diagnosis 64
- bilateral hilar uptake 64, *65*
- normal variants, benign findings **64**
hip osteonecrosis 308
histiocytosis X 151
Hodgkin's disease 220, *220*, 223, **224**, *226*, 324
Hürthle's cell neoplasms 170
hydration 28–29, 31
hydroxylapatite, FDG uptake and 59
hyperglycemia 28, 151
hyperinsulinemic-euglycemic clamp 33
hypometabolism
- dementia 362, *362*
- temporal lobe epilepsy 352, *352*, 353–354, *355*
hypothyroidism 357
hypoxia induction factor 1 (HIF-1) 23

I

immune checkpoint inhibitors 228, *228*

infection, inflammation
- AIDS **345**, *346*
- atherosclerosis **347**
- bone disease, 18FNaF imaging 308
- diabetic foot *341*, **341**, *342*, **342**, *343*
- FDG-PET/CT applications 338–339
- fever of unknown origin 345
- gallbladder/biliary tree 69, *95*
- inflammatory bowel disease 347
- joints, FDG uptake in **348**
- lungs, global disease assessment **48**
- modality comparison 338
- osteomyelitis, chronic *339*, **339**, *340*, 341
- prostheses *342*, *344*
- quantitative whole-body imaging 48
- sarcoidosis **34**, *135*, **345**, *346*, **381**, *382*, 383
- therapy response 147, *348*, **348**, *349*
- vasculitis **347**
inflammatory bowel disease **347**
injected clot *64*, 180
insulin administration 29, *29*
insulin sensitizers 30
interpretation
- AC images 90, *90*, 91, *91–92*
- accuracy 89
- anatomic correlation **92**
- appropriate indication **89**
- clinical data **90**
- confidence 93
- confirmation of findings 93, *93*
- cost-effectiveness 89
- data correlation **90**, 94, *94*
- delayed resolution 94, *95*
- evidence 89
- false negatives 93
- false positives 93, *94*
- follow-up **95**, *96*
- large lesions 93
- lesion localization *74*, *92*, 93–94, *178*
- lesion size 93, *281*
- management effect 89
- MIP images 90
- motion 94
- NAC images 90, *90*, 91, *91–92*
- patient limitations 89
- PET/CT **106**
- PET/MRI **111**
- reporting **95**
- sensitivity, specificity 89, *92*, **92**
- SUVs in small lesions 93

- technical limitations 89
intracranial electrodes 353
intraductal papillary mucinous tumor 247, *247*
IV fluids 28

J

jaw osteonecrosis 308
joints, FDG uptake in **348**

K

kidneys 103
KRAS mutations 282
Kryptofix 14–15

L

Langerhans cell histiocytosis **326**, *329*
laryngeal tumors metastases 160
leiomyomas 70, *72–73*
lepidic predominant adenocarcinoma 180
lesion localization, *see* localization
levothyroxine, myocardial uptake 52
Lewy body dementia 356, *357*, 361, 363
lipoma 292–293
liposarcomas 292, *293*
liver
- artifacts 130, *131*
- benign vs. malignant, differentiation 129
- colorectal cancer metastases 282, 284–285, *285*
- data correlation 130, *130–131*
- false negatives 129, *238*
- false positives 69, *69*, 129, *238*
- gastric cancer metastases 209, *209*
- hepatic adenomas 129, *129*
- insulin 69
- intravenous contrast 105
- metastases, PET 129, *130–131*
- metastases, PET/MRI 116
- mislocalizations 102, *104*
- NAC images 130
- noise artifact 68
- normal variants, benign findings **68**
- oncological PET **129**
- pancreatic cancer metastasis *249*, 250
- PET/CT differences 103
- small lesion evaluation 129, *130*

- subtle foci of uptake interpretation 130
- SUV 68
- therapy response 148
localization
- interpretation *74*, *92*, 93–94, *178*
- lymph nodes 134, *134–135*
- mislocalizations 102, *104*
- oncological PET 128
- PET/CT 98–99, *99*
- seizure *352*, **352**, 353
lung cancer, *see* non-small cell lung cancer (NSCLC), small cell lung cancer, thoracic neoplasms
- global disease assessment **46**
- PET vs. bone scan 137
- PET/MRI **115**
- prognostic predictors 46
- radiation therapy planning 331, *332*, **333**
- recurrent 187
- synchronous 159, *159*
lungs
- activity, normal gradient of 63
- atelectasis 64, *64–65*
- bases, PET/CT detection 106
- diffuse uptake 63, *63*
- false positives 64, 96
- focal uptake, no CT correlate 63, *64*
- inflammation, global disease assessment **48**
- lesion detection 91, *91*
- metastases, PET 135
- nodular uptake 63
- nodules, PET/CT detection 106
- normal variants, benign findings **63**
- oncological PET **135**
- osteosarcoma metastases 296–297
- PET/CT 106
- PET/CT vs. CT 136
- pulmonary nodules **115**
- radiation pneumonitis 63, *64*
- small nodules 136
- SUV 102
lymph nodes, *see* retroperitoneal nodes
- bladder cancer metastases *270*
- cervical cancer metastases 254
- CT correlation *128*, 134, *134*
- density 135
- endometrial cancer metastases 259
- Inflammatory vs. malignant 133

- location, pattern 134, *134–135*
- oncological PET **133**
- osteosarcoma metastases 297
- ovarian cancer metastases 257–258
- pancreatic cancer metastases 250
- pelvic 135, *135*
- prostate cancer metastases **273**, **312**, *313*
- PSMA staging **312**
- size 133
- SUV 133
- testicular cancer metastases 267, **268**
lymphangitic carcinomatosis 63, *63*
lymphoma
- accuracy **220**, **227**, **229**
- AIDS related B-cell 220
- baseline pretreatment scan 228
- bone marrow activity 224
- bone marrow involvement 223
- Burkitt 222
- Deauville criteria 227
- diffuse large B-cell 220, 223, **226**, 228
- end of therapy PET 227
- extensive **221**
- extranodal disease detection 224
- false negatives 155
- false positives 155, 229
- FDG PET applications 154
- follicular 222, 227, **227**
- gastric 209, *210*
- glioma vs. *154*, **154**
- global disease assessment *46*
- histological subtype 220
- Hodgkin's disease 220, *220*, 223, **224**, *226*, 324
- immunomodulatory agents 228, *228*
- interim PET 227
- liver activity in interpretation 228
- Lugano classification 223, 227
- MALT 222
- mantle cell 222
- marginal zone 222
- modality comparison **223**, **227**
- nodal disease detection 223
- non-Hodgkin's 220, *221–222*, 223
- peripheral T-cell 222
- PET prognostic value 229
- PET/MRI *120*, **120**, *121*
- postradiotherapy imaging 229

- pretransplantation **229**
- primary CNS 155
- relapse **229**
- retroperitoneal nodal
  uptake 70, *72*
- salvage chemotherapy 229
- spectrum of disease *221*
- splenic disease *70,* 223–224
- staging 220, **220,** *221–222*
- steroids and 155
- therapy response **224,** 225,
  226, 227, *228*
- thymic hyperplasia *61–62,*
  224
- toxoplasmosis vs. **154**

M

mandibular condylar
  hyperplasia 308
mediastinum 105
Medicare 381
melanoma
- accuracy 233, 234, **234,** *235*
- asymptomatic, high risk
  patients 234
- bowel, metastatic *233*
- brain, metastatic 234, *235*
- distant disease
  detection 232
- false positives 232
- immunomodulation 235,
  236
- interpretation 235
- isolated limb infusion 233
- melanin content 234
- metastatic *232–233,* 234
- modality comparison **234**
- noncutaneous 233
- peripheral lesions 234
- primary *232*
- prognosis **234**
- recurrence **232,** 234
- scan volume 235
- staging 232, **232,** *233*
- tumor markers 235
- uveal 233
meningioma 151, *151*
mental state, glucose/FDG
  metabolism 22
mesothelioma *47,* 189, *190*
metformin 29, *30*
MIP images 90
monoclonal gammopathy of
  undetermined significance
  (MGUS) **297**
MR enterography 110
MR spectroscopy 151
multi-infarct dementia 356
multiple myeloma
- accuracy **298,** *299,* 300
- extramedullary
  disease 298, *299*
- false negatives 300
- MGUS **297**

- modality comparison **298,**
  299
- MRI 298, *299*
- pathologic fractures **298**
- PET applications 297
- prognosis **297**
- radiographs 298, *299*
- sestamibi 300
- therapy response **297,** *298*
muscle uptake
  minimization 30
musculoskeletal tumors, *see*
  skeletal muscle
- 18FNaF, skeletal metastases
  SUV 306
- accuracy 292
- benign vs. malignant **291**
- bone, benign vs. malignant,
  see bone, bone marrow
- delayed imaging 293
- evaluation of **293**
- false negatives 293
- false positives 293, *294*
- PET/MRI **122**
- prostate cancer
  metastases **274**
- soft tissue, benign vs.
  malignant **292,** 293, *293*
- tumor grade 292
MYC oncogene 23
myocardial perfusion imaging
  (MPI) 372

N

NAC images
- interpretation 90, *90,* 91,
  91–92
- liver 130
- PET/CT 106
nasopharyngeal tumors
  metastases 160, *161*
NeuraCeq (18F-
  florbetaben) **360,** *362*
neuroendocrine tumors
- differential diagnosis 248
- pancreatic *248,* **248,** *249*
- PET/MRI **117**
neurologic diseases PET/
  MRI **122**
neurological tracers 360,
  361
- *See also* specific tracers
niacin 33
nicotine 31
non-FDG PET tracers *361*
non-Hodgkin's
  lymphoma 220, *221–222,*
  223
non-small cell lung cancer
  (NSCLC)
- distant staging 181
- end-of-treatment PET 187,
  187, 188
- interim PET 187

- mediastinal staging 181,
  182
- PET/CT accuracy **182**
- prognosis **186**
- radiation therapy
  planning **188**
- radiofrequency
  ablation **189**
- recurrent 187, *188,* **188**
- restaging 187, *187,* 188
- staging **181**
- therapy response **186**
nonseminomatous germ cell
  tumors **268**

O

oncocytomas 70, 265
oncological PET
- adrenals **138,** *139*
- advantages 128
- bone marrow
  metastases **136**
- brain **138,** *139*
- contrast-tonoise ratio 128,
  129
- disadvantages 128
- early detection 128, *128*
- false positives 128
- liver **129**
- localization 128
- lungs **135**
- lymph nodes **133**
- patient management 128
- peritoneum **131,** *132*
- principles **128**
- sensitivity, specificity 128
- spleen **131**
oral cavity metastases 160
oral glucose loading 33
osteoid osteoma 308
osteomyelitis *341,* **341,** *342,*
  342, *343*
osteomyelitis, chronic *339,*
  339, *340,* **341**
osteoradionecrosis 164
osteosarcoma
- accuracy 295, *296,* **297**
- bone metastases 297
- evaluation of **294**
- Ewing's sarcoma vs. 294
- guiding biopsy *293,* 294
- lung metastases 296–297
- lymph node metastases 297
- metastatic *295*
- modality comparison **295,**
  296, **297**
- postamputation
  evaluation 296
- prognosis 295, **297**
- recurrence 295, *296,* **296–**
  297
- staging 294, *295,* **295**
- therapy monitoring 294,
  295

- therapy response 296, **297**
- tumor grade *293,* 294
ovarian cancer
- accuracy 256, **256–257**
- adenocarcinomas 256
- CA-125 257
- chemotherapy 72
- cost-effectiveness 257
- diffuse peritoneal
  carcinomatosis 258, *259*
- endometriomas 256
- false negatives 256, 258
- false positives *135,* 256
- fibromas 256
- lymph node
  metastases 257–258
- masses **256**
- metastatic *258–259*
- modality comparison *256,*
  256–257
- normal variants, benign
  findings **72,** *73,* 135
- pelvic uptake spectrum *73*
- peritoneal metastases 257–
  258, *258–259*
- postmenopausal uptake 72,
  256
- premenopausal uptake 72
- prognosis 257
- recurrence **257**
- retroperitoneal node
  metastases 257
- second-look
  laparotomy 257
- SUV 256
- teratomas 256
- therapy response **258**
- visual threshold 256

P

Paget's disease *293,* 304
pancreas variants, benign
  findings **69**
pancreatic cancer
- accuracy 245, **245,** *247,*
  250
- adenocarcinoma 28, **245**
- autoimmune pancreatitis
  vs. 246, *246*
- biliary stents 250, *250*
- cholestasis 250
- clinical history 245
- cystic tumors *247,* **247**
- delayed imaging 246
- false negatives 246
- false positives 246, 250
- hyperglycemia 246
- intraductal papillary
  mucinous tumor 247, *247*
- liver metastasis *249,* 250
- lymph node metastases 250
- malignant vs. inflammatory
  masses 245, *245*
- metastatic *245, 249*

- modality comparison *245*, **245**, *247*, **250**
- neoadjuvant therapy 250
- neuroendocrine tumors 248, *248*, **248**, *249*
- peritoneal metastases 250
- prognosis **250**
- pseudocyst *247*
- recurrence 250, *250*
- solid pseudopapillary tumors 248
- staging **248**, *249*
- SUV 246
- therapy response **250**
parametric quantitative whole-body imaging 43, **44**, *45*
parenteral nutrition 28
Parkinson's disease 357, *361*, *363*, **363–364**
parotid lesions 164, *164–165*
pathologic tissues, IV contrast 104
patient preparation
- bladder catheterization 31
- blood glucose levels **28**
- bowel activity 31
- brain uptake 28
- breastfeeding *32*, **32**
- caffeine 28
- cardiac FDG PET **33**
- cold exposure minimization 31
- diabetic patients 29, 33
- diet, fasting **28**
- diuretics 31
- drugs to avoid 31
- FDG administration route *33*, **33**
- FDG uptake in pancreatic adenocarcinoma 28
- free fatty acid metabolism, decreasing 33
- glucose/FDG metabolism effects 21, *22*
- hydration 28–29, 31
- hyperglycemia, acute vs. chronic 28
- hyperinsulinemic-euglycemic clamp 33
- insulin administration 29, *29*
- insulin sensitizers 30
- IV fluids 28
- metformin 29, *30*
- myocardial viability **33**
- oral glucose loading 33
- parenteral nutrition 28
- PET scan timing **31**, *32*
- PET/CT **106**
- pharmacologic interventions 30
- physiologic uptake minimization **30**
- sarcoidosis **34**
- sulfonylureas 30
- urinary activity 31, *253*, *265*, *269*
pediatric PET/CT
- 18FNaF bone scanning **308**
- applications 324, *324*
- bone tumors 324, *325*
- Langerhans cell histiocytosis **326**, *329*
- PET/MRI **121**, *122*
- pregnancy, contraindications 324
- seizures 353
- soft-tissue malignancies **325**, *326–328*
peritoneum
- diffuse peritoneal carcinomatosis 133, *133*
- gastric cancer metastases 209, *209*
- implant *132*
- liver border 133
- medial to cecum 132, *132*
- metastases *132*
- metastases, bowel activity vs. *129*, 133
- oncological PET **131**, *132*
- ovarian cancer metastases 257–258, *258–259*
- pancreatic cancer metastases 250
- pelvis 132, *132*
- seeding patterns 131, *132*
- straight line sign 133
perivascular tumor infiltration 78, *85*
PET image segmentation **43**
PET/CT
- accuracy 98
- advantages **98**
- calcified lesions 105, *295*
- contemporaneous correlation 98
- CT-based attenuation correction 98
- degree of certainty 98, *100*
- dense material, attenuation artifacts secondary to **103**
- differences 102
- disadvantages **98**
- false positives 98, *100*
- free breathing 99
- inspiration 99, *101*
- interpretation **106**
- intravenous contrast 103, *105*, 106–107
- lesion localization 98–99, *99*
- lung 106
- metallic/dense material artifact 105
- mislocalizations 102, *104*
- misregistration **98**
- NAC images 106
- nonrespiratory motion 101, *101–102*
- normal expiration 99
- oral contrast 103, *105*, 106
- patient preparation **106**
- registration 106
- respiration type 99, *101*
- respiratory averaged low-dose CT scanning 100
- respiratory gating 100
- SUV 102, 106
- true whole-body **107**
- truncation artifact 106
- uptake levels, incorrect 99
PET/MRI
- ADC images, interpretation 111
- advantages **109**
- attenuation correction **112**, *113*
- basic sequences, interpretation **111**
- bladder cancer 117, *119*
- breast cancer **117**
- cardiovascular diseases **122**
- CNS tumors 115, *116*
- contraindications 109–110
- contrast materials 110
- disadvantages **109**
- DW images, interpretation 111
- ear protection 110
- examination times 109
- functional imaging capability 109
- GI disease **123**
- GI tract malignancies **115**
- gynecologic cancer **117**
- head and neck 114, *114*
- image acquisition 110
- image registration 112
- infrastructure requirements 109
- interpretation **111**
- lymphoma 120, **120**, *121*
- musculoskeletal disorders **122**
- neuroendocrine tumors **117**
- neurologic diseases **122**
- nononcologic applications **121**
- oncologic applications **114**
- osseous metastases **119**
- overview 109
- patient preparation **110**
- pediatric malignancies **121**, *122*
- precontrast/postcontrast T1-weighted, interpretation 111
- prostate cancer 117, *118*
- quantification **112**
- radiation exposure 109
- sensitivity, specificity 109, 119
- signal intensity 112
- soft-tissue contrast 109
- T1-weighted GRE, interpretation 111
- T2-weighted RARE, interpretation 111
- thoracic malignancies **115**
physics principles
- 2D vs. 3D acquisition **6**, 7
- AC corrections 7, 8
- annihilation **3**
- block detectors 4, *4*
- coincident photon events **4**, *5*
- collimation effects 6, *7*
- Compton scatter 3
- corrections **7**, 8
- CT-based attenuation correction **9**, *11*
- data acquisition **3**
- decay constant 3
- energy resolution 3
- expectation maximization (EM) algorithm 8, *9*
- filtered back-projection (FBP) 7–8, *8*
- image quality 9, **9**
- image reconstruction **7**, 8
- imaging field of view (FOV) 4, *5*
- light output 3
- noise/resolution trade-offs 9, **9**
- ordered-subsets expectation maximization (OSEM) 7–8, *8*
- overview 2, *2*
- photomultiplier tubes (PMTs) 4
- photon detection **3**
- radioactive decay **2**
- scanner components, function **9**, *10–11*
- scintillation detectors **3**, *4*
- sinograms 6, **6**
- stopping power 3
- time-of-flight 6, **6**
Pick's disease 356, *356*
pioglitazone 30
pituitary adenoma 151, *152*
planning target volume (PTV) 332
positron emission mammography (PEM) 195
posterior cingulate cortex hypometabolism 354
primary sclerosing cholangitis 241, *242*
progressive multifocal leukoencephalopathy 155
propranolol 30
prostate cancer
- 18FNaF 304, *305–307*
- accuracy **275**
- biochemical recurrence 271, *272*
- bone metastases **272**, *273*, 275, *276*

- calcification 270
- FDG uptake, incidental **270**
- fluciclovine **270**, 271–272, *273*
- fluciclovine, interpretation **272**
- global disease assessment **47**
- inflammatory uptake **273**
- lymph node metastases **273**, *313*
- metastatic *272*, *275–276*
- modality comparison **275**
- non-prostatectomy **273**
- PET/MRI **117**, *118*
- physiologic uptake **272**
- primary staging **271**
- prognosis 275
- prostatectomy bed **273**
- PSMA, *see* PSMA
- recurrence 275, *312*, *314*
- skeletal metastases **274**
- staging/restaging 270, *271*, *274*, **274**
- therapy response 275
prostate specific membrane antigen, *see* PSMA
prostheses 84, *99*, **342**, *344*
PSMA
- accuracy 312
- intraprostatic diagnosis **312**
- lymph nodal staging **312**, *313*
- prostate cancer 270, 271–272, 311, *311*
- recurrence **312**, *314*
- staging 312
- technical aspects **311**

Q

quantitative whole-body imaging
- dynamic **42**, *43*
- global disease assessment, cancer *46*, **46**
- global disease assessment, inflammatory diseases **48**
- global metabolic activity **46**
- overview 42
- parametric 43, **44**, *45*
- peer-reviewed publications 42, *42*
- PET image segmentation **43**
- qualitative visual assessment 42
- radiomics **44**
- semiquantitative metrics **42**
- single-bed FOV imaging 44
- standardized uptake value **43**
- static vs. dynamic **43**
- texture analysis **44**
- tracer kinetic analysis 43

R

R-CHOP studies 226, 228, *228*
radiation esophagitis 215
radiation pneumonitis 63, *64*, 188
radiation therapy planning
- ABVD regimen studies 225
- automated segmentation methods **332**
- brain tumors **333**
- clinical applications **333**
- clustering methods 332
- delineation by visual assessment **332**
- dose painting **334**
- esophageal cancer **215**
- hard thresholding 332
- head and neck **164**, **333**
- lung cancer 331, *332*, **333**
- non-small cell lung cancer (NSCLC) **188**
- PET-CT in **331**
- residual disease evaluation 163
- respiratory gating of PET/CT **334**
- semiautomated segmentation methods **332**
- soft thresholding 332
- staging and **331**
- target volumes in **332**
- theragnostic imaging **334**
- thresholding 331, **332**
- tumor volume delineation **331**
radiofrequency ablation **189**, 286
radiomics **44**
rectal cancer **282**, 287
renal cell carcinoma
- accuracy *264*, **264**, **266**
- adjacent lesions *92*, 265
- angiomyolipomas 265
- bone metastases 266
- degree of uptake 265, *265*
- false negatives 265, *265*
- false positives 265
- indeterminate renal cysts *264*, **264**
- inflammatory lesions 265
- masses *264*, **264**
- metastases 264
- metastatic 265, *266*
- modality comparison *264*, **264**, **266**
- oncocytomas 265
- prognosis 265–266
- staging/restaging **265**, 266, *266*
- therapy response **266**
- urinary activity *265*
resperine 30
respiratory gating of PET/CT **334**

retroperitoneal nodes, *see* lymph nodes
- evaluation of 31, *253*
- genitourinary tract 70, *71–72*
- lymphoma 70, *72*
- ovarian cancer metastases 257
- testicular cancer metastases 267, **268**
rosiglitazone 30
Rotter's node metastases *198*

S

sacroiliitis 308
sarcoidosis **34**, *135*, **345**, *346*, **381**, *382*, 383
sedatives, FDG uptake effects 151
seizure, epilepsy, *see* temporal lobe epilepsy
- accuracy **364**, *365*
- benzodiazepine-receptor scans 365
- decreased FMZ binding 365
- epileptogenic foci size 365
- false lateralization 365
- localization *352*, **352**, 353
- modality comparison **364**
- partial volume effects 365
- refractory 365
seizures, subclinical 353
seminoma 267, **267**, *268*, 269, *269*
SEMPET trial 268
skeletal muscle, *see* musculoskeletal tumors
- anxiety 77
- brown fat uptake 78, *79*
- diaphragmatic crus uptake 78, *80–81*
- exercise 77
- insulin **29**, 77
- intercostal muscle uptake 78
- longus colli muscles *59*, 78
- mimics 77
- nodal uptake 77, *79*
- normal variants, benign findings **77**
- retrocrural node 78, *81*
- teres minor uptake 78
small cell lung cancer **189**
soft tissue sarcomas
- accuracy **295**, *296*
- evaluation of **294**
- lung metastases 296
- modality comparison **295**, *296*
- pediatric PET/CT **325**, *326–327*
- postamputation evaluation 296
- recurrence **296**

- staging **295**
- therapy response 296
- tumor grade *293*, 294
soft tissue variants, benign findings **78**
solid pseudopapillary tumors 248
somatostatin analogs, *see* 68Ga-SA
somatostatin antagonists **319**
SPECT
- accuracy 119, 152, 160, 315, *340*, 354, *354*
- bone metastases 160, 172
- cardiac imaging 372–373, 378, 380–381
- dementia 354, *354*
- FDG uptake and 51
- head and neck metastases 160
- hip osteonecrosis 308
- hypoperfusion 51
- infection, inflammation *340*
- limitations of 4, 372
- Medicare reimbursement 381
- perfusion imaging 381
- temporal lobe epilepsy 352
- thallium, accuracy 152
- thoracic neoplasms 177
spinal cord variants, benign findings **52**
spleen
- G-CSF treatment 69, *70*
- normal variants, benign findings **69**
- oncological PET **131**
- PET/CT differences 103
- therapy response 148
spondylodiscitis *123*, **123**
squamous cell carcinomas 179, 210
standardized uptake value (SUV)
- acronyms 36
- attenuation correction method 38
- background activity 37
- brain 151, 153
- breast cancer 195, 204
- calculation **36**
- cholangiocarcinoma 242
- CT-based attenuation correction 38
- delayed time point imaging 40
- dose extravasation 37
- dual time point imaging **40**
- EORTC guidelines 39
- esophageal cancer 215
- filtered back vs. interactive reconstruction 37
- head and neck 160, 162
- hepatocellular carcinoma 240
- interpretation 38

– intraductal papillary
mucinous tumor 247
– lean body mass
calculation 36
– lymph nodes 133
– maximum SUV
(SUVmax) 38
– mean SUV (SUVmean) 39
– measurement methods **38**
– number of iterations 37
– ovarian cancer 256
– overview 36
– pancreatic cancer 246
– partial volume
correction 37
– partial volume effects 37
– patient size 36
– peak SUV (SUVpeak) 39
– pearls/pitfalls **40**
– PERCIST criteria 36–37, 39
– PET/CT 102, 106
– pitfalls **36**
– plasma glucose levels 37
– reconstruction
parameters 37
– region of interest **38**
– repeatability **39**
– reporting **95**
– reproducibility **39**
– testicular cancer 269
– time of measurement 37
– truncation artifact 38
sternoclavicular joints 76
stomach
– hiatal hernia 67
– normal variants, benign
findings **66**
– uptake patterns 66, *66*
subclinical seizures 353
sulfonylureas 30
supraglottic larynx
metastases 160, *161*
SUV, *see* standardized uptake
value (SUV)

T

talc pleurodesis 186,
186
Teflon, FDG uptake and 59
temporal lobe epilepsy 352,
352, 353–354
– *See also* seizure, epilepsy
teratomas 256, 267, 269
testes variants, benign
findings **73**, *90*
testicular cancer
– accuracy **267–268**, *269*
– metastatic 267, *267*
– modality comparison **267–
268**, *269*
– nonseminomatous germ cell
tumors **268**
– PET applications 266
– recurrence **267**

– retroperitoneal lymph node
metastases 267, **268**
– seminoma 267, **267**, *268*,
269, *269*
– SUV 269
– teratoma 267, 269
– tumor markers **268**
texture analysis **44**
thallium SPECT 152
theragnostic imaging **334**
therapy response
– cortical bone lesions 148
– Deauville's criteria **148**
– definition of 142
– disease-specific evaluation
criteria **148**
– end of treatment 142
– EORTC criteria 142, *143*
– false negatives 145
– false positives 145
– head and neck **163**
– hepatic, splenic lesions 148
– infection,
inflammation 147, *348*,
348, *349*
– interim PET 142
– lack of baseline PET
study 147
– midtreatment vs.
posttreatment results 144
– non-SUV metrics 142, *145–
146*
– normal response 145
– PERCIST criteria 142, *143*
– principles **142**
– reproducibility 142
– SUV measurement
error 145
– SUV, increases vs.
decreases 145
– variable response 144, *147*
thoracic neoplasms, *see* lung
cancer, small cell lung
cancer
– adenocarcinomas 179, 184
– adrenal hyperplasia *71*, 186
– bronchoalveolar
carcinoma 179, *180*
– carcinoids 179
– dexamethasone
suppression 185
– differential diagnosis *178*,
179, *179*
– dual point imaging 178
– dynamic contrast-enhanced
CT 177
– false negatives 177, 179,
180
– false positives 179, 186
– FDG uptake/SUV 2.5 180
– hamartomas 179
– histology 179
– injected clot *64*, 180
– interpretation 178, *178*
– invasive staging 184
– lack of CT correlate *104*, 180

– large cell carcinomas 179
– lung adenocarcinoma, FDG
avidity 180
– lung base nodules 181
– lung nodules, screening-
detected 181
– lymph node density 185
– lymph nodes, enlarged 184
– mediastinoscopy 183–184
– modality comparison **177**
– nodule size in
evaluation 178
– NSCLC, *see* non-small cell
lung cancer (NSCLC)
– pathologic N2 disease
prediction 184
– pattern of uptake *134–135*,
184
– PET/CT accuracy **177**, **182**,
188
– PET/CT misregistration *104*,
180
– pleural disease, malignant
vs. benign 182, *183*
– pleural dissemination 186
– pulmonary metastasis vs.
benign nodule **181**
– radiation pneumonitis *64*,
188
– round atelectasis 179, *179*
– scan time 178
– small nodule
evaluation 178
– solitary pulmonary
nodules **177**
– squamous cell
carcinomas 179
– staging **181**, *182*
– subsolid nodules 179
– SUV cutoffs 185
– T99 depreotide SPECT 177
– talc pleurodesis 186, *186*
– tuberculosis, PET/CT
accuracy effects 185, *185*
– visual analysis 178, *178*,
185
thoracic veins *104*, *105*
thorax mislocalizations 102
thrombosis 78, *82–83*
thymomas, average SUV 62
thymus
– adults 61, *61–62*
– carcinoma, average SUV 62
– children 61
– hyperplasia *61–62*, 224
– normal variants, benign
findings **61**
– superior mediastinal
activity 62, *62*
– thymic hyperplasia, average
SUV 62
thyroid cancer
– calcitonin levels 174
– CT correlation 170
– differentiated, elevated
serum thyroglobulin/

negative radioiodine
scans *171*, **171**
– diffuse plus focal/multifocal
uptake 171
– diffuse uptake 171
– follicular neoplasms 170
– follicular/papillary 170,
172, *172*
– histology 173
– Hürthle's cell
neoplasms 170
– lymph nodes 170, *171*
– medullary **174**
– modality comparison **172**,
174
– muscle/brown fat
uptake *58*, 173, *174*
– nodule mimics 60, 170
– nodules *169*, **169**
– nodules, incidental 170,
170
– normal variants, benign
findings *59*, *60*
– parathyroid abnormality
60
– PET/CT accuracy **172**, **174**
– prognosis **172**
– pulmonary metastases 173
– recombinant TSH 173
– recurrent *171*, **171**
– staging **171**
– thyroglobulin level 173
thyroiditis *60*
tonsillar carcinoma 55
total lesion glycolysis (TLG)
46
toxoplasmosis **154**
tracer kinetic analysis 43
trastuzumab 47
tuberculosis, PET/CT accuracy
effects 185, *185*
tumor microenvironment
– aerobic glycolysis *23*, 24
– glucose/FDG metabolism
altered pathways 22
– hypoxic environment **23**
tumor-to-background ratio
values 368

U

urinary activity 31, *253*, *265*,
269
urinary tract IV contrast
104
uterus
– endometrial uptake 71, *73*
– IUDs 72
– leiomyomas 70, *72–73*
– normal variants, benign
findings **70**
– post-menstrual 72
– postmenopausal
endometrial uptake 72
– postpartum 72, *74*

V

vascular dementia 356
vascular system
- atherosclerosis 78, *81*
- grafts 78, *84*
- intravenous contrast 104,
  105
- normal variants, benign
  findings **78**
- perivascular tumor
  infiltration 78, *85*
- thrombosis 78, *82–83*
- vasculitis 78, *82*
vasculitis **347**

vertebral body
  hemangioma *76*
vesicular monoamine
  transporter 2 (VMAT2) 364
Vizamyl (18F-
  flutemetamol) **360**, *362*
vocal cord paralysis *58*, 170

W

Warburg effect 22–23